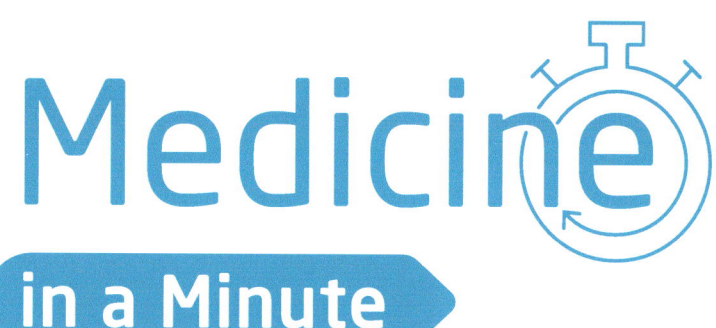

Dedicated to Nick Mills, Chim Lang and Anoop Shah;
for their encouragement in the pursuit of excellence

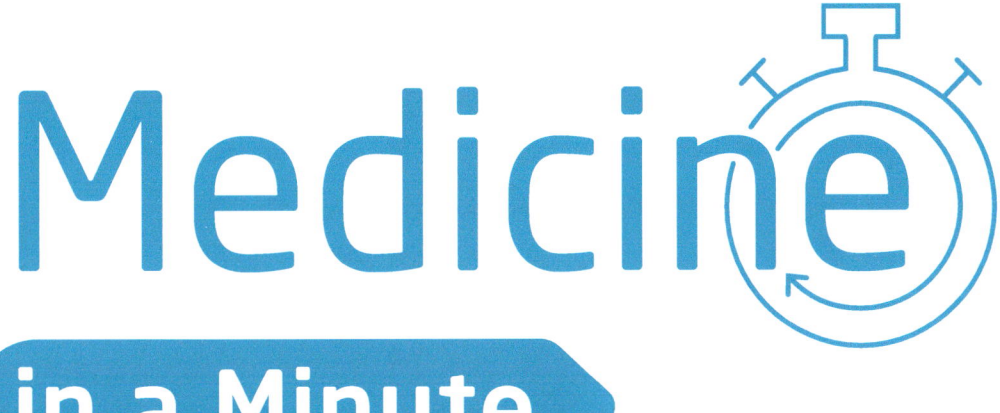

Medicine

in a Minute

Amar Vaswani MBChB
Royal Infirmary of Edinburgh

Hwan Juet Khaw MBChB
Royal Infirmary of Edinburgh

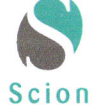

Scion

© **Scion Publishing Limited, 2019**

ISBN 9781907904981

First published 2019

A CIP catalogue record for this book is available from the British Library.

Scion Publishing Limited

The Old Hayloft, Vantage Business Park, Bloxham Road, Banbury OX16 9UX, UK
www.scionpublishing.com

Important Note from the Publisher

The information contained within this book was obtained by Scion Publishing Ltd from sources believed by us to be reliable. However, while every effort has been made to ensure its accuracy, no responsibility for loss or injury whatsoever occasioned to any person acting or refraining from action as a result of information contained herein can be accepted by the authors or publishers.

Although every effort has been made to ensure that all owners of copyright material have been acknowledged in this publication, we would be pleased to acknowledge in subsequent reprints or editions any omissions brought to our attention.

Registered names, trademarks, etc. used in this book, even when not marked as such, are not to be considered unprotected by law.

Cover photos reproduced under licence from stock.adobe.com
Cover design by Andrew Magee Design Ltd
Typeset by Medlar Publishing Solutions Pvt Ltd, India
Printed in the UK
Last digit is the print number: 10 9 8 7

Contents

List of contributors

Adrian Mar MBBS, FACD
Consultant Dermatologist, Monash Health, Melbourne

Amar Vaswani MBChB
Foundation Doctor, Royal Infirmary of Edinburgh

Anastasios Stavrakoglou MBBS, FACD
Consultant Dermatologist, Monash Health, Melbourne

Hwan Juet Khaw MBChB
Foundation Doctor, Royal Infirmary of Edinburgh

Ian Wu MBBS (Aus) MRCP (Edin) MMed
Haematology Registrar, National University Hospital, Singapore

Kelsey Wai Jan Wong MBBS (Hons)
Internal Medicine Core Trainee, Western Health, Melbourne

Kimberly Shuyi Loh MBChB
Foundation Doctor, Southern General Hospital, Glasgow

Li Anne Ong MBBChBAO
Medical Officer, Psychiatry, Singapore General Hospital

Samantha Jingyun Koh MBChB
Foundation Doctor, Royal Infirmary of Edinburgh

Scott D. Dougherty MBChB BMSc MRCP
Cardiology Registrar, Ninewells Hospital, Dundee

Senhong Lee MBBS (Hons)
Clinical Research Fellow, Dermatology, Skin and Cancer Foundation, Melbourne

Tan Chuen Wen MBBS MRCP MMed FRCPath
Consultant Haematologist, Singapore General Hospital

Teo Hooi Khee MBBS MRCP MMed
Cardiology Registrar, National Heart Centre, Singapore

Preface

Many senior clinicians have likened the study and mastery of medicine to drinking out of a fire hydrant. In the course of three short years, students are placed on a merry-go-round of clinical specialties and are expected to take information in by the bucketful.

Most students are able to grasp the relevant concepts quite readily. Why, then, do finals and post-graduate exams induce such fear and trepidation? Apart from the high stakes involved, we believe that the playing field when it comes to medical education has changed in three fundamental ways, and this has greatly impacted the way medicine is taught.

1. Mismatched expectations

There is a great mismatch between what institutions want and what students need. Speaking from experience, many students feel that the materials they are provided with do not suitably prepare them for their exams. Likewise, many doctors feel that their medical school experience has not adequately prepared them for clinical practice.

Studies conducted by the GMC in the last decade echo the problems faced by new foundation doctors, recommending that the curriculum should be structurally overhauled. Our book aims to bridge the gap, as far as possible, providing clarity and empowering students and junior doctors with up-to-date, guideline-based information (which is considered the gold standard), to enable them to progress with confidence.

2. Information overload

This is the era of information overload in medicine, and one amusing anecdote sums up our experience. When we were preparing for our final exams, the official advice was to 'read Up ToDate'.

Up ToDate is a medical reference website, containing a wealth of information, used by practising clinicians across the globe. This advice can be likened to asking a young secondary school student to prepare for their English paper by reading a 30-volume encyclopaedia.

This naturally caused some worry amongst students, as many wondered what the most effective resource was and how best to prepare. (Very few actually used Up ToDate as their sole revision source, though we wouldn't be at all surprised if several students did indeed manage to accomplish this feat.) For the mere mortals among us, we believe our textbook will help reduce the anxiety and stress linked to the information overload that comes when embarking on each new step in your career path.

3. The pursuit of excellence

Ultimately, medicine, more than anything, humbles us all. No amount of study will ever confer complete mastery of the material. Total expertise remains elusive, encouraging each aspirant to strive to do their very best for their patients.

There is a quiet beauty to simplicity – both for ourselves as physicians and for our patients. Mastery develops from this simplicity, as we add layer after layer of bricks and mortar until the foundation is rock solid and well-nigh impregnable. If data are the bricks with which we build, compassion and empathy are most certainly the cement.

Many of our mentors have exemplified these principles in practice, and it would be remiss of us not to share their findings with you. It is our great wish that this foundation will continue to grow stronger, as our readers become more skilled and more compassionate.

Excellence, therefore, is what we must aim for – both in our everyday dealings with patients, and in our commitment to honing our craft. We are indebted to our mentors, who have shown us that the pursuit of excellence can keep us humble, who have encouraged us to hone our craft, and to serve steadfastly.

We hope that this textbook will encourage you to do the same. We wish you the very best in your exams and in your studies, and, for students taking their final exams, we cheer you on in spirit.

Go forth boldly, spurred on by love and support from your family, friends and teachers, and strive to do your best, for it won't be long before it will be your turn to be handed the bleep.

Commit yourself to excellence, and we trust that, in due course, you will find yourself more than ready to take up this calling, like so many who have come before you.

A.V., H.J.K

On behalf of the Medicine in a Minute writing team
September 2018

Acknowledgements

The authors would like to thank the team of contributors for their hard work and dedication in bringing this project to life.

We are also grateful to Dr Calvin Chin, Dr Huang Weiting, Dr Marc Dweck, Dr Santiago Giavedoni, Dr James Tiernan, Dr Ana Volovets, Professor John Plevris, Dr Luke Boyle, Dr Belinda Weller, Dr Peter Johnson, Dr Manish Kaushik, Dr Maciej Piotr Chlebicki, Dr Ross Murphy and Dr Leong Hoo Kwong for supporting us from the very beginning and taking the time to encourage us to keep writing. Writing this type of book is like carrying a pregnancy – fun getting started, nine or so months of agony in between, and pure joy when it's all over.

We would like to thank Dr Jonathan Ray, Mr Simon Watkins and Ms Clare Boomer and the team at Scion Publishing for pointing us in the right direction and reassuring us that the world would not end – and was not indeed flat!

On a more serious note, we are also indebted to the many students who have kindly provided us with valuable feedback over the last year, and this has no doubt tremendously improved the finished product.

Last, but certainly not least, the authors wish to thank their families, friends and long-suffering better halves for their unconditional support and encouragement throughout the writing process.

Abbreviations

25OHD	25-hydroxyvitamin D	AIDS	acquired immunodeficiency syndrome
5-ASA	5-aminosalicylic acid	AIH	autoimmune hepatitis
5-HT	serotonin	AIHA	autoimmune haemolytic anaemia
6-MP	mercaptopurine	AIN	acute interstitial nephritis
A1AT	alpha 1-antitrypsin	AIP	acute intermittent porphyria
A–a gradient	alveolar–arterial gradient	AKI	acute kidney injury
ABG	arterial blood gas	ALD	alcoholic liver disease
ABPA	allergic bronchopulmonary aspergillosis	ALL	acute lymphoblastic leukaemia
ABPM	ambulatory blood pressure monitoring	ALM	acral lentiginous melanoma
		ALP	alkaline phosphatase
ABV	alcohol by volume	ALS	amyotrophic lateral sclerosis
AC	adenocarcinoma	ALT	alanine aminotransferase
ACA	anterior cerebral artery	AMA	anti-mitochondrial antibody
ACD	allergic contact dermatitis	AML	acute myeloid leukaemia
ACE	angiotensin-converting enzyme	AMSAN/AMAN	acute motor/sensory axonal neuropathy
ACh	acetylcholine/acetylcholinergic	ANA	anti-nuclear antibody
AChE	acetylcholinesterase	ANCA	anti-neutrophil cytoplasmic antibody
ACR	albumin:creatinine ratio	ANS	autonomic nervous system
ACS	acute coronary syndrome	APAbs	antiphospholipid antibodies
ACTH	adrenocorticotropic hormone	APCs	antigen-presenting cells
ADH	anti-diuretic hormone	APML	acute promyelocytic leukaemia
ADHD	attention deficit hyperactivity disorder	APS	antiphospholipid syndrome
ADL	activities of daily living	APTT	activated partial thromboplastin time
ADP	adenosine diphosphate	AR	aortic regurgitation
ADPKD	autosomal dominant polycystic kidney disease	ARB	angiotensin receptor blocker
		ARC	AIDS-related complex
AF	atrial fibrillation	ARDS	acute respiratory distress syndrome
AFP	alpha fetoprotein	ARF	acute rheumatic fever
Ag	antigen	ARPKD	autosomal recessive polycystic kidney disease
AHI	apnoea/hypopnoea index		
AIDP	acute immune demyelinating polyneuropathy	ARVC	arrhythmogenic right ventricular cardiomyopathy

ASD	atrial septal defect		CF	cystic fibrosis
ASOT	anti-streptolysin O titre		CHD	congenital heart disease
AST	aspartate aminotransferase		CJD	Creutzfeldt–Jakob disease
AT	angiotensin		CK	creatine kinase
ATG	anti-thymocyte globulin		CKD	chronic kidney disease
ATN	acute tubular necrosis		CK-MB	Creatine kinase, MB isoenzyme
ATP	adenosine triphosphate		CLL	chronic lymphocytic leukaemia
ATRA	all-trans retinoic acid		CML	chronic myeloid leukaemia
AV	atrioventricular		CMT	Charcot–Marie–Tooth
AVM	arteriovenous malformations		CMV	cytomegalovirus
AVNRT	atrioventricular nodal re-entrant tachycardia		CNS	central nervous system
			CO	cardiac output
AVR	aortic valve replacement		COCP	combined oral contraceptive pill
AVRT	atrioventricular re-entrant tachycardia		COHb	carboxyhaemoglobin
			COMT	catechol-O-methyltransferase
AVSD	atrio-ventricular septal defect		COPD	chronic obstructive pulmonary disease
AXR	abdominal X-ray			
BCC	basal cell carcinoma		COX	cyclo-oxygenase
BCS	Budd–Chiari syndrome		CPAP	continuous positive airway pressure
BD	*bis in die*; twice daily		CPP	chronic plaque psoriasis
BE	base excess		CPPD	calcium pyrophosphate deposition
BMD	bone mineral density		CPR	cardiopulmonary resuscitation
BMI	body mass index		CRC	colorectal cancer
BMT	bone marrow transplant		CRH	corticotropin-releasing hormone
BMZ	basement membrane zone		CRP	C-reactive protein
BNP	b-type natriuretic peptide		CRT	cardiac resynchronisation therapy
BPPV	benign paroxysmal positional vertigo		CRT-D	CRT device
Br	bilirubin		CRT-P	CRT pacemaker
BSA	body surface area		CSF	cerebrospinal fluid
C-cells	parafollicular/calcitonin-secreting cells		CST	corticospinal tracts
			CT	computed tomography
CABG	coronary artery bypass grafting		CTD	connective tissue disease
CAD	coronary artery disease		CTZ	chemoreceptor trigger zone
CAG	cysteine-adenosine-guanine		CVA	cerebrovascular accident
CAH	congenital adrenal hyperplasia		CVD	cardiovascular disease
CAP	community-acquired pneumonia		CVI	chronic venous insufficiency
CAPD	continuous ambulatory peritoneal dialysis		CVID	common variable immunodeficiency
			CVP	central venous pressure
CATT	card agglutination test for trypanosomiasis		CVS	cardiovascular system
			Cx	complications
CBD	common bile duct		CXR	chest X-ray
CBT	cognitive behavioural therapy		DAT	direct antigen (Coombs) testing
CCB	calcium channel blocker		DCIS	ductal carcinoma *in situ*
CD	Crohn's disease		DCT	distal convoluted tubule
CEA	carcinoembryonic antigen			

DDAVP	desmopressin
DDx	differential diagnosis
DF	discriminant factor, Maddrey's
DH	dermatitis herpetiformis
DHEA	dehydroepiandrosterone
DI	diabetes insipidus
DIC	disseminated intravascular coagulation
DIF	direct immunofluorescence
DKA	diabetic ketoacidosis
DL_{CO}	diffusion capacity of carbon monoxide
DMARD	disease-modifying anti-rheumatic drugs
DNA	deoxyribonucleic acid
DOT	directly observed therapy
DPP-4	dipeptidyl peptidase-4
DPT	diphtheria pertussis tetanus
DRE	digital rectal examination
DSG	desmoglein
DVT	deep venous thrombosis
DXA scan	dual-energy X-ray absorptiometry scan
EBV	Epstein–Barr virus
ECG	electrocardiogram
EDV	end diastolic volume
EEG	electroencephalogram
EF	ejection fraction
eGFR	estimated glomerular filtration rate
EIA	enzyme immunoassay
ELF	enhanced liver fibrosis
ELISA	enzyme-linked immunosorbent assay
EM	erythema multiforme
EMA	eosin-5-maleimide
EPO	erythropoietin
ERCP	endoscopic retrograde cholangio-pancreatography
ERV	expiratory reserve volume
ESR	erythrocyte sedimentation rate
ESV	end systolic volume
ET	essential thrombocythaemia/thrombocytosis
EUS	endoscopic ultrasound
FAP	familial adenomatous polyposis
FAST	face, arms, speech, time test

FBC	full blood count
FDP	fibrin degradation products
FeNa	fractional excretion of sodium
FeNO	fractional exhaled nitric oxide
FEV_1	forced expiratory volume in 1 second
FFP	fresh frozen plasma
FGFR3	fibroblast growth factor receptor 3
FiO_2	fraction of inspired air
FISH	fluorescent *in situ* hybridisation
FL	follicular lymphoma
FLI	fatty liver index
FNA	fine needle aspiration
FODMAP	fermentable, oligosaccharides, disaccharides, monosaccharides and polyols
FPF	familial pulmonary fibrosis
FRC	functional residual capacity
FSGS	focal segmental glomerulosclerosis
FSH	follicle-stimulating hormone
FTA-abs	fluorescent treponemal antibody absorbed test
FVC	forced vital capacity
FVL	factor V Leiden
G	gauge
G6PD	glucose-6-phosphate dehydrogenase
GABA	gamma-aminobutyric acid
GABHS	group A beta-haemolytic streptococcus
GBM	glioblastoma multiforme
GCA	giant cell arteritis
GCS	Glasgow Coma Scale
GCT	germ cell tumours
GORD	gastro-oesophageal reflux disease
GFR	glomerular filtration rate
GGT	gamma-glutamyl transferase
GH	growth hormone
GHIH	growth hormone inhibiting hormone
GHRH	growth hormone releasing hormone
GI	gastrointestinal
GIST	gastrointestinal stromal tumour
GLP-1	glucagon-like peptide-1
GN	glomerulonephritis
GnRH	gonadotropin-releasing hormone

GPA	granulomatosis with polyangiitis	HRS	hepatorenal syndrome
GSF	Gold Standards Framework	HRT	hormone replacement therapy
GTN	glyceryl trinitrate	HSCT	haematopoietic stem cell transplantation
GVHD	graft-versus-host disease		
H$_2$ antagonist	histamine-2 antagonist	HSE	herpes simplex encephalitis
HAART	highly active anti-retroviral therapy	HSV	herpes simplex virus
HAP	hospital-acquired pneumonia	HTLV	human T-lymphotropic virus
HAV	hepatitis A virus	HTT	huntingtin
Hb	haemoglobin	HUS	haemolytic uraemic syndrome
HbA	haemoglobin a	IAT	indirect antigen testing
HbA1c	glycated haemoglobin	IBD	inflammatory bowel disease
HbA2	haemoglobin A2	IBS	irritable bowel syndrome
HbF	haemoglobin f	ICA	internal carotid artery
HBPM	home blood pressure monitoring	ICC	interstitial cells of Cajal
HbS	sickle cell haemoglobin	ICD	implantable cardiac device
HBV	hepatitis B virus	ICP	intracranial pressure
HCC	hepatocellular carcinoma	ICS	inhaled corticosteroids
hCG	human chorionic gonadotrophin	ICU/ITU	intensive care unit, intensive therapy unit
HCV	hepatitis C virus		
HDL	high-density lipoproteins	IDA	iron-deficiency anaemia
HDU	high dependency unit	IE	infective endocarditis
HER2	human epidermal growth factor receptor 2	IFG	impaired fasting glucose
		IgA	immunoglobulin A
HFpEF	heart failure with preserved ejection fraction	IgE	immunoglobulin E
		IGF-1	insulin-like growth factor 1; somatomedin C
HFrEF	heart failure with reduced ejection fraction		
		IgM	immunoglobulin M
HH3	human herpes virus 3	IGRA	interferon gamma release assay
HHC	hereditary haemochromatosis	IGT	impaired glucose tolerance
HHS/HONK	hyperosmolar hyperglycaemic state/ hyperosmolar non-ketotic coma	IHD	ischaemic heart disease
		ILD	interstitial lung disease
HHT	hereditary haemorrhagic telangiectasia	IM	intramuscular
		INO	internuclear ophthalmoplegia
HHV	human herpes virus	INR	international normalised ratio
Hib	Haemophilus influenzae B	IPF	idiopathic pulmonary fibrosis
HIT	heparin-induced thrombocytopenia	IRV	inspiratory reserve volume
HIV	human immunodeficiency virus	ITP	immune thrombocytopenic purpura
HL	Hodgkin lymphoma	IUCD	intra-uterine contraceptive device
HNPCC	hereditary non-polyposis colon cancer	IV	intravenous
		IVDU	intravenous drug user
HOCM	hypertrophic cardiomyopathy	IVIg	intravenous immunoglobulin
HPAG	hypothalamic–pituitary–adrenal– gonadotropic	JAK2	Janus kinase 2
		JC	John Cunningham (virus)
HPV	human papillomavirus	JVP	jugular venous pressure
HRCT	high-resolution CT		

LA	left atrium		MDRD	modification of diet in renal disease
LABA	long-acting beta agonist		MDS	myelodysplastic syndrome
LACS/LACI	lacunar stroke/infarct		MDT	multi-disciplinary team
LAD	left anterior descending (artery)		MEN	multiple endocrine neoplasia
LADA	latent autoimmune diabetes of adulthood		Men C	meningococcal C
LAMA	long-acting muscarinic antagonist		MERS-CoV	Middle East respiratory syndrome-coronavirus
LBBB	left bundle branch block		MET	metabolic equivalents
LCA	left coronary artery		MF	myelofibrosis
LCX	left circumflex (artery)		MGUS	monoclonal gammopathy of uncertain significance
LDH	lactate dehydrogenase		MI	myocardial infarct
LDL	low-density lipoprotein		MLF	medial longitudinal fasciculus
LFT	liver function test		MM	multiple myeloma
LGN	lateral geniculate nucleus		MMR	measles, mumps, rubella vaccine
LGV	lymphogranuloma venereum		MMSE	mini-mental state examination
LH	luteinising hormone		MND	motor neuron disease
LHRH	luteinising hormone-releasing hormone		MOCA	Montreal cognitive assessment
LIF	left iliac fossa		MODY	maturity onset diabetes of the young
LLSE	left lower sternal edge		MPTP	1-methyl-4-phenyl-1,2,3,6-tetrahydropyridine
LMA	laryngeal mask airway		MR	mitral regurgitation
LMM	lentigo maligna melanoma		MRA	mineralocorticoid receptor antagonists
LMN	lower motor neuron		MRCP	magnetic resonance cholangio-pancreatography
LMWH	low molecular weight heparin		MRI	magnetic resonance imaging
LOS	lower oesophageal sphincter		MRSA	methicillin-resistant *Staphylococcus aureus*
LP	lumbar puncture		MS	multiple sclerosis
LPS	lipopolysaccharide		MSK	musculoskeletal
LSE	Libman–Sacks endocarditis		MSM	men who have sex with men
LTOT	long-term oxygen therapy		MTHF	methyl-tetrahydrofolate
LV	left ventricle (ventricular)		MTP	metatarsophalangeal
LVAD	left ventricular assist device		MVP	mitral valve prolapse
LVEF	left ventricular ejection fraction		MVR	mitral valve replacement
LVF	left ventricular failure		NA	noradrenergic
LVOT	left ventricular outflow tract		NAAT	nucleic acid amplification testing
MAHA	microangiopathic haemolytic anaemia		NAFLD	non-alcoholic fatty liver disease
MALT	mucosa-associated lymphoid tissue lymphoma		NAPQI	*N*-acetyl-*p*-benzoquinone imine
MAO-B	monoamine oxidase B		NASH	non-alcoholic steatohepatitis
MAT	multifocal atrial tachycardia		NBM	nil by mouth
MC&S	microbiology, culture and sensitivity		NBTE	non-bacterial thrombotic endocarditis
MCA	middle cerebral artery		NG	nasogastric
MCP	metacarpophalangeal			
MCV	mean corpuscular volume			

NHL	non-Hodgkin lymphoma		PE	pulmonary embolism
NK	natural killer		PEF	peak expiratory flow
NM	nodular melanoma		PET	positron emission tomography
NMDA	*N*-methyl-D-aspartate		PFO	patent foramen ovale
NMJ	neuromuscular junction		PFT	pulmonary function test
NNRTI	non-nucleoside analogue reverse transcriptase inhibitors		PH	pulmonary hypertension
			Ph	Philadelphia chromosome
NOAC	novel oral anticoagulant		PI	protease inhibitors
NPH	neutral protamine Hagerdorn		PICA	posterior inferior cerebellar artery
NRT	nicotine replacement therapy		PID	pelvic inflammatory disease
NRTI	nucleoside analogue reverse transcriptase inhibitors		PIN	prostate intra-epithelial neoplasia
			PIP	proximal interphalangeal
NSAID	non-steroidal anti-inflammatory drug		PJS	Peutz–Jeghers syndrome
NSCLC	non-small cell lung cancer		PKD/PCKD	polycystic kidney disease
NSTEMI	non-ST elevation myocardial infarction		PML	progressive multifocal leukoencephalopathy
OA	osteoarthritis		PMR	polymyalgia rheumatica
OCD	obsessive–compulsive disorder		PND	paroxysmal nocturnal dyspnoea
OD	once daily		PNH	paroxysmal nocturnal haemoglobinuria
OFT	osmotic fragility test			
OGD	oesophago-gastro-duodenoscopy		PNS	peripheral nervous system
OSA	obstructive sleep apnoea		PO	*per os*; orally
PA	postero–anterior		PO_2	partial pressure of O_2
$PaCO_2$	arterial PCO_2		POCS/POCI	posterior circulation stroke/infarct
PACS/PACI	partial anterior circulation stroke/infarct		PPAR	peroxisome proliferator activated receptor gamma
PAN	polyarteritis nodosa			
PAO_2	alveolar PO_2		PPI	proton pump inhibitor
PaO_2	arterial PO_2		PR	*per rectum*; rectally
PAS	periodic acid–Schiff		PRN	*pro re nata*; as needed
PASI	Psoriasis Area and Severity Index		PSA	prostate-specific antigen
PBC	primary biliary cirrhosis		PSC	primary sclerosing cholangitis
PBG	porphobilinogen		PSGN	post-streptococcal glomerulonephritis
PCA	posterior cerebral artery		PSP	primary spontaneous pneumothorax
PCI; pPCI	(primary) percutaneous coronary intervention			
			PT	prothrombin time
PCO_2	partial pressure of CO_2		PTH	parathyroid hormone
PCOS	polycystic ovarian syndrome		PVT	portal venous thrombosis
PCP/PJP	*Pneumocystis jirovecii (carinii)* pneumonia		QDS	*quarter die sumendus*; four times daily
			QTc	corrected QT interval
PCR	polymerase chain reaction		RA	rheumatoid arthritis
PCT	proximal convoluted tubule		RAAS	renin–angiotensin–aldosterone system
PCWP	pulmonary capillary wedge pressure		RAST	radioallergosorbent
PDA	patent ductus arteriosus		RBBB	right bundle branch block
PDGF	platelet-derived growth factor		RBC	red blood cell

RCA	right coronary artery
REM	rapid eye movement
RF	rheumatoid factor
RFA	radiofrequency ablation
Rh	rhesus
RHD	rheumatic heart disease
RMI	Risk Malignancy Index
RNA	ribonucleic acid
RPGN	rapidly progressive glomerulonephritis
RPR	rapid plasma reagin
RR	respiratory rate
RRT	renal replacement therapy
RTA	renal tubular acidosis
RUQ	right upper quadrant
RV	right ventricle/ventricular
RV	residual volume
SA	sinoatrial (node)
SAAG	serum–ascites albumin gradient
SABA	short-acting beta agonist
SAH	subarachnoid haemorrhage
SALT	speech and language test/assessment
SAM	systolic anterior motion
SAMA	short-acting muscarinic antagonist
SARS	severe acute respiratory syndrome
SAVR	surgical valve replacement
SBP	spontaneous bacterial peritonitis
SC	subcutaneous
SCC	squamous cell carcinoma
SCDC	subacute combined degeneration of the spinal cord
SCID	severe combined immunodeficiency
SCLC	small cell lung cancer
SGLT-2	sodium-glucose co-transporter-2
SIADH	syndrome of inappropriate ADH secretion
SIBO	small intestine bacterial overgrowth
SJS	Stevens–Johnson syndrome
SLE	systemic lupus erythematosus
SLNB	sentinel lymph node biopsy
SMA	anti-smooth muscle antibody
SOB	shortness of breath
SoNS	somatic nervous system

SPECT	single-photon emission computed tomography
SpO_2	peripheral capillary oxygen saturation
SSM	superficial spreading melanoma
SSP	secondary spontaneous pneumothorax
STD	sexually transmitted disease
STEMI	ST elevation myocardial infarction
STK11	serine threonine kinase
SUDEP	sudden unexpected death in epilepsy
SUNCT	short-lasting unilateral neuralgiform headaches with conjunctival injection and tearing
SV	stroke volume
SVCO	superior vena cava obstruction
SVR	systemic vascular resistance
SVT	supraventricular tachycardia
T_3	triiodothyronine
T_4	tetraiodothyronine/thyroxine
TACS/TACI	total anterior circulation stroke/infarct
TAVI	transcatheter aortic valve implantation
TB	tuberculosis
TCC	transitional cell carcinoma
TDS	*ter die sumendum*, three times daily
TEE	transoesophageal echocardiography
TEN	toxic epidermal necrolysis
TF	tissue factor
TFT	thyroid function tests
TGA	transposition of the great arteries
THF	tetrahydrofolate
TI	terminal ileum
TIA	transient ischaemic attack
TIBC	total iron binding capacity
TIPSS	transjugular intrahepatic porto-systemic shunting
TLC	total lung capacity
TNM	tumour/node/metastasis – staging
TOF	tetralogy of Fallot
t-PA	tissue plasminogen activator
TPMT	thiopurine methyltransferase
TRALI	transfusion-related acute lung injury
TRH	thyrotropin-releasing hormone
TRUS	transrectal ultrasound-guided
TSH	thyroid-stimulating hormone

TTE	transthoracic echocardiography		UTI	urinary tract infection
TTP	thrombotic thrombocytopenia purpura		UVB	ultraviolet B
			V/Q	ventilation/perfusion (referring to planar scintigraphy)
TV	tidal volume			
U&Es	urea and electrolytes		VC	vital capacity
UA	unstable angina		VEGF	vascular endothelial growth factor
UC	ulcerative colitis		VF	ventricular fibrillation
UCDA	ursodeoxycholic acid		VSD	ventricular septal defect
UDPGT	uridine-diphosphoglucuronate glucuronosyltransferase		VT	ventricular tachycardia
			VTE	venous thromboembolism
UFH	unfractionated heparin		vWD	von Willebrand disease
UGIE	upper gastrointestinal endoscopy		vWF	von Willebrand factor
ULC	ultralarge complexes		VZV	varicella-zoster virus
UMN	upper motor neuron		WCC	white cell count
URTI	upper respiratory tract infection		WPW	Wolff–Parkinson–White syndrome
US/USS	ultrasonography		ZES	Zollinger–Ellison syndrome

Chapter 1
Cardiology

Amar Vaswani, Teo Hooi Khee and *Scott D. Dougherty*

Basic principles

The cardiovascular system, which consists of the heart and blood vessels, plays a vital role in the maintenance of homeostasis and transport of nutrients, waste compounds and respiratory gases. To achieve this, the heart and blood vessels must work in tandem with the respiratory and haematological systems to achieve adequate tissue and organ perfusion.

Contracting at an average rate of 75 beats per minute (bpm), the human heart is said to contract up to 3 billion times in an average 80-year lifespan.

Bridge to clinical medicine

Anatomy

- The heart is covered by a fibroserous sac called the **pericardium** and is located in the thorax between the lungs, in an area known as the **mediastinum**
- The heart is a four-chambered, muscular structure comprising two atria and two ventricles, which serve to pump deoxygenated (largely venous) blood to the lungs and transport oxygenated (largely arterial) blood to organs and tissues (see *Fig. 1.1*)
- The **right atrium** receives venous drainage from two large systemic veins, the superior vena cava superiorly and the inferior vena cava inferiorly, as well as the coronary sinus (inferiorly) and the anterior cardiac vein anteriorly (draining the anterior heart)
- The right **atrial appendage** or **auricle** is a pouch-like extension of the right atrium
- Blood moves from the right atrium to the right ventricle through the tricuspid valve, which is made up of three leaflets (anterior, posterior and septal)

- The **tricuspid valve** orifice is the largest in the heart and its leaflets are supported by chordae tendineae ('heart strings'), which link the ventricular aspect of the leaflets to the papillary muscles
- The **right ventricle** is composed of the large inlet (sinus) and smaller outlet (conus); the inflow tract is typified by trabeculae carneae (irregular ridges), whereas the outlet tract has smooth walls
- The **infundibulum** is a funnel-shaped muscular structure that forms the right ventricular outflow tract and supports the pulmonary valve, through which deoxygenated blood flows to the lungs via the **pulmonary trunk**
- The true interatrial septum is limited to a shallow depression known as the **fossa ovalis**, which is a remnant of the now closed **foramen ovale**
- The **left atrium** receives oxygenated blood from the four pulmonary veins
- The **left atrial appendage** is a long, hooked and tubular structure that forms part of the left atrium and is important clinically because it is the major site of thrombus formation in atrial fibrillation

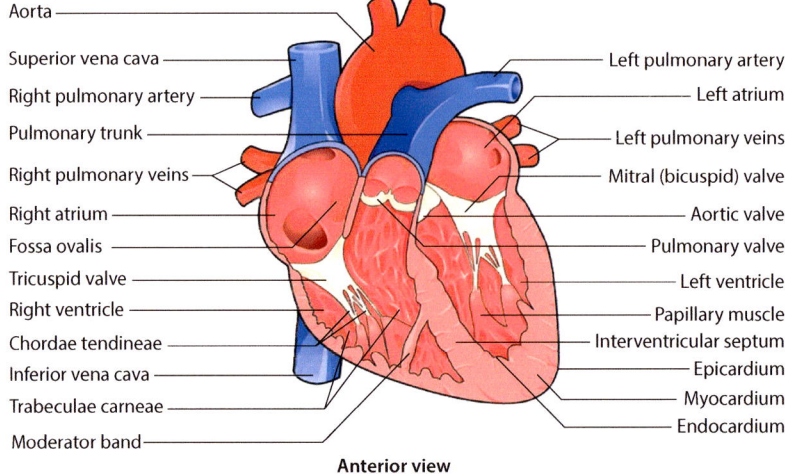

Aorta
Superior vena cava
Right pulmonary artery
Pulmonary trunk
Right pulmonary veins
Right atrium
Fossa ovalis
Tricuspid valve
Right ventricle
Chordae tendineae
Inferior vena cava
Trabeculae carneae
Moderator band

Left pulmonary artery
Left atrium
Left pulmonary veins
Mitral (bicuspid) valve
Aortic valve
Pulmonary valve
Left ventricle
Papillary muscle
Interventricular septum
Epicardium
Myocardium
Endocardium

Anterior view

Fig. 1.1 *Gross anatomy of the heart.*

- As blood moves from the left atrium to the left ventricle, it flows through the **mitral valve**, which has anterior and posterior mitral valve leaflets

> (P) ≫ The mitral valve is so named because of its resemblance to a bishop's mitre (ceremonial head-dress).

- The majority of the blood flow from the left atrium to the left ventricle is passive, with only 30% of flow resulting from left atrial contraction
- Like the right ventricle, the left ventricle consists of a trabeculated inlet and a smooth outlet
- The left ventricle is thicker and larger than the right ventricle because it must generate enough force to push blood around the entire body
- The left ventricle pumps oxygenated blood to the entire body, first through the **aortic valve** and then through the **aorta**
- The aortic and pulmonary valves, which are similar in structure, are each composed of three cusps, and are also known as **semilunar** valves

Coronary circulation

- The heart consumes more oxygen per tissue mass than any other organ in the body: myocardial blood supply occurs via the **right and left coronary arteries**, which arise as the first branches of the aorta at the right and left sinuses of Valsalva, respectively
- The heart is drained mainly by the great, middle and small cardiac veins, and to a lesser extent by other cardiac veins into the **coronary sinus**, which empties into the right atrium

- The **right coronary artery (RCA)** has three major branches (see *Fig. 1.2*):
  - The **sinoatrial (SA) nodal branch**, which supplies the sinoatrial node, the dominant pacemaker of the heart
  - The **atrioventricular (AV) nodal branch**, which supplies the atrioventricular node
  - The **posterior descending artery**
- The **left coronary artery (LCA)**, which supplies a large surface area of the heart, is subdivided into (see *Fig. 1.2*):
  - The **left main stem**
  - The **left anterior descending (LAD) artery**, also known as the 'widowmaker', because occlusion of this vessel can lead to rapid death
  - The **left circumflex (LCX)** artery

> (P) ≫ One might appreciate the beauty of individuality within each heart, perhaps anatomically reflected in the variation observed in arterial supply:
> 1. 90% of the population have a **right dominant** heart, in which the posterior descending artery originates from the terminal branch of the RCA; whereas the LCX normally supplies the posterior descending artery in a **left dominant** heart
> 2. The SA nodal artery is supplied by the RCA in two-thirds of the population, and by the LCX in one-third
> 3. The AV node, on the other hand, is supplied by the RCA in 90% of the population and by the LCX in the remaining 10%.

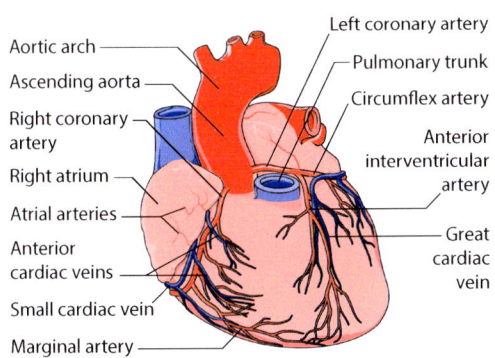

Anterior view

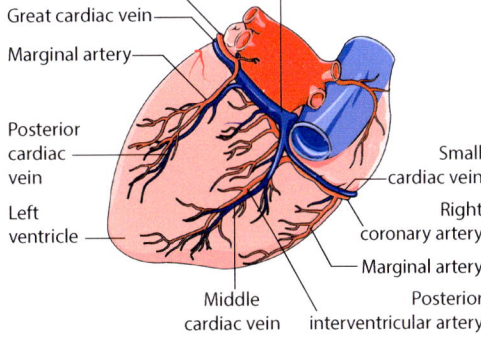

Posterior view

Fig. 1.2 *The coronary circulation.*

Cardiac cycle

The cardiac cycle can be divided into two distinct phases: systole (contraction) and diastole (relaxation).

> **W** »» Coronary blood flow mainly occurs during diastole. When the heart is contracting, the intramuscular blood vessels are compressed and blood flow is at its lowest. During diastole, the myocardium relaxes, allowing blood flow to resume. Any increase in the heart rate reduces diastolic time more than systolic time, thus reducing coronary artery perfusion time. In patients with pre-existing disease (such as coronary artery disease or aortic stenosis), tachycardia may lead to reduced myocardial perfusion.

The cardiac cycle takes place over four major phases (see *Fig. 1.3*):

Conducting system of the heart

- The intrinsic pacemaker of the heart is usually the sinoatrial node (SA node) because it has the fastest rate of automaticity of all cardiac fibres (*see Fig. 1.4*)
- However, other fibres also generate automatic rhythmical impulses (such as the AV node), albeit at slower rates, and these may act as the cardiac pacemaker if there is a problem with the SA node

- The action potential from the SA node is propagated through the atrial myocytes, which have intercalated discs at a structural level, allowing for the action potential to move freely across both atria
- The impulse then travels to the AV node, which lies in the interatrial septum
- Conduction is delayed at the AV node for 0.1 seconds before continuing on towards the bundle of His; this time delay allows for ventricular filling to take place
- Depolarisation then continues through the bundle of His (which subdivides into left and right bundle branches) and then through Purkinje fibres to the ventricular muscle, which provokes contraction

> **P** »» The heart derives its autonomic nervous supply mostly from the parasympathetic vagus nerve (cardio-inhibitor) and the C1–T5 sympathetic ganglia (cardio-accelerator) via superficial and deep cardiac nervous plexuses. The autonomic nervous system plays an important role in controlling the rate of SA node impulse formation and conduction and the strength of muscle contraction. For instance, in the denervated heart (e.g. in heart transplant patients), the resting heart rate is higher (90–110bpm) and the heart rate response is reduced during exercise (chronotropic incompetence).

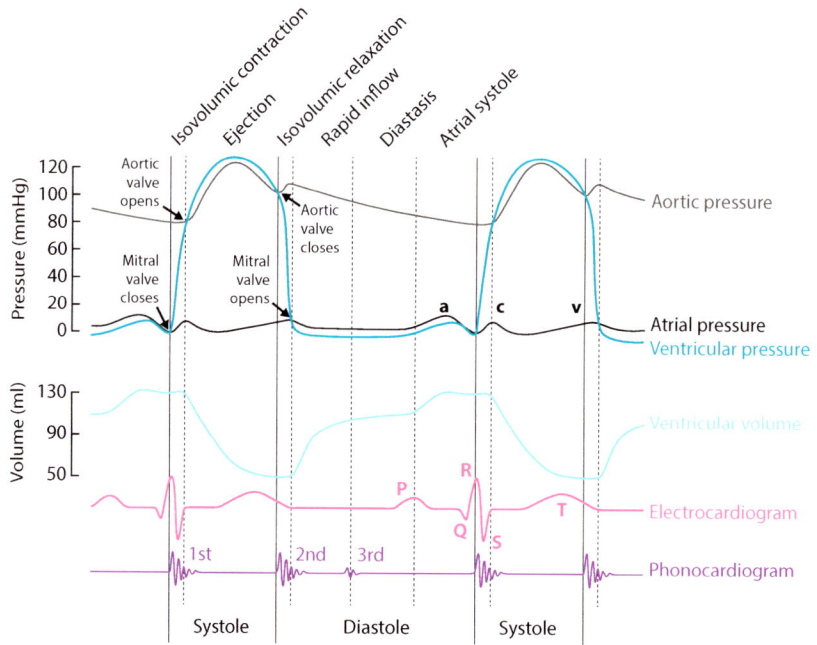

Fig. 1.3 *The cardiac cycle.*

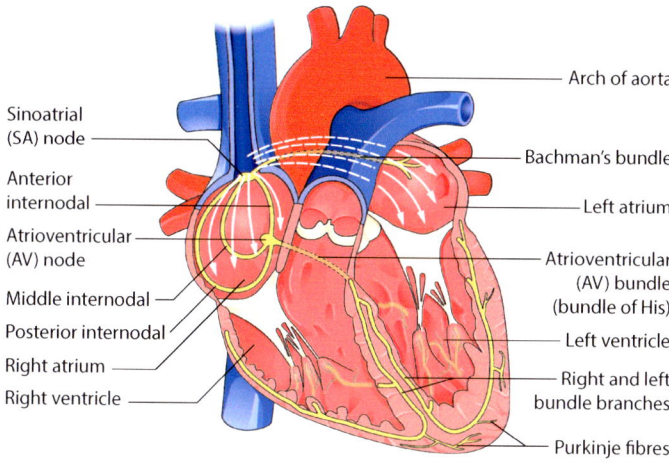

Fig. 1.4 *The conduction system of the heart.*

W ≫ Cardiac pain is not found exclusively in the chest, but often radiates down the medial side of the left arm and up to the neck and jaw. This is because radiation occurs to areas that send sensory impulses to the same level of the spinal cord that receives cardiac sensation. The sensory fibres from the heart then travel up to T1–T4, and radiation occurs in the medial left arm via dermatomes T1–T4.

Cardiac muscle contraction and relaxation

Cardiac myocytes, which differ in cellular structure from skeletal and smooth muscle myocytes, contract at a cellular level by means of a phenomenon known as **calcium-induced calcium release**.

- Depolarisation causes calcium ions to enter the myocyte via L-type voltage-gated calcium channels
- This in turn activates calcium-sensitive calcium release channels (also known as **ryanodine** receptors) in the sarcoplasmic reticulum, which causes sufficient flooding of calcium ions to initiate contraction
- Calcium ions bind to **troponin** C, exposing the actin-binding site
- Myosin then binds to actin, and contraction occurs via actin–myosin interactions secondary to hydrolysis of adenosine triphosphate (ATP)
- As relaxation of the myocyte occurs, calcium ions disengage from troponin C binding sites and are actively transported out of the cytosol via an ATP-dependent cellular pump

Cardiac output

Ensuring an adequate cardiac output is vital for organ perfusion. Regulation of CO occurs via modification of heart rate or stroke volume.

- Cardiac output (CO) = heart rate (HR) × stroke volume (SV)
- Stroke volume (SV) = end diastolic volume (EDV) – end systolic volume (ESV)

Definitions

Table 1.1 *Cardiac physiology terminology*

End diastolic volume (EDV)	Ventricular volume at the end of filling in diastole (approximately 120ml)
End systolic volume (ESV)	Ventricular volume at the end of contraction in systole (approximately 40ml)
Stroke volume (SV)	Volume of blood pumped by each ventricle per beat
Cardiac output (CO)	Volume of blood ejected by each ventricle per minute
Ejection fraction (EF)	Percentage of blood pumped out by each filled ventricle per beat (80/120ml = 66%)

Heart rate

- The normal heart rate is between 60 and 100bpm

Stroke volume

- Affected by **preload**, **afterload** and **contractility**
- Preload
  - Refers to the degree of stretch applied to a resting muscle at the end of diastole; this

1

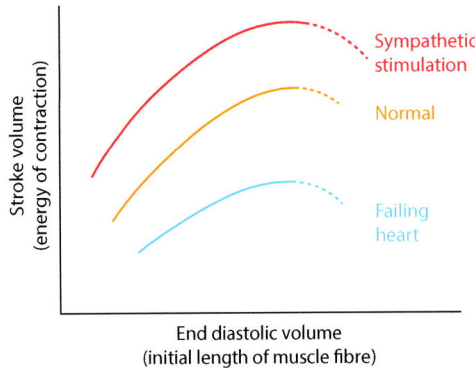

Fig. 1.5 *Frank–Starling curve.*

increased resting muscle length augments the strength of the subsequent muscle contraction
- The Frank–Starling law (see *Fig. 1.5*) illustrates how the initial length of the muscle fibre is proportional to the cardiac contraction
- The greater the stretch of the ventricle during diastole, the greater the force of contraction, and therefore the greater the stroke volume
- Afterload
  - Refers to the load exerted on a muscle after the onset of contraction (e.g. systolic pressure), which must be overcome before the muscle begins to shorten
  - Afterload represents the resistance to ventricular ejection because the afterload force opposes muscle contraction
  - Afterload is inversely proportional to stroke volume
- Contractility refers to the force of myocardial contractility, measured by EF

Blood pressure regulation

- Blood pressure refers to the pressure exerted by circulating blood against the vessel walls
- $BP = CO \times SVR$ (systemic vascular resistance)

Blood pressure is sensed by baroreceptors (mechanoreceptor sensory neurons) at the carotid sinus and aortic arch, which detect changes (e.g. low BP) based on the degree of stretch. Afferent information is then transmitted to the brain, which leads to reflexive vasoconstriction, an increased heart rate and contractility, increasing SV, CO and BP in turn.

Another mechanism that modifies BP is the renin–angiotensin–aldosterone system (RAAS; see *Fig. 1.6*). When the arterial pressure falls, renin is released from the juxtaglomerular cells of the kidney. Renin converts angiotensinogen (released from the liver) into angiotensin I.

Angiotensin-converting enzyme (ACE) then converts angiotensin I into angiotensin II, which mediates its effects, primarily by vasoconstriction and increased water retention.

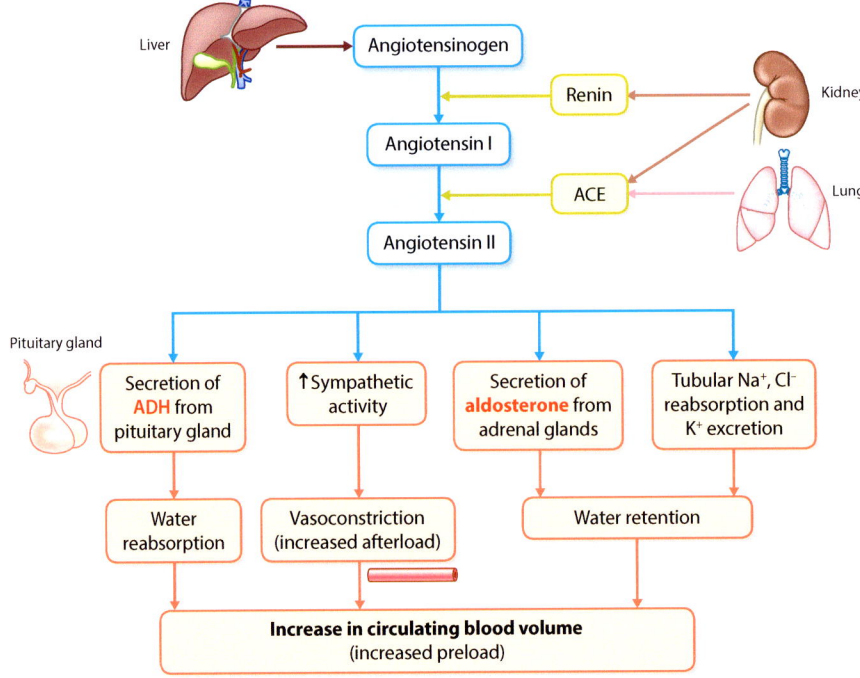

Fig. 1.6 *The renin–angiotensin–aldosterone system (RAAS).*

The jugular venous pressure (JVP)

The JVP is an indirect measure of central venous pressure and can be examined at the bedside.

It has a distinctive double waveform pulsation. Two waves are visible on examination (see *Fig. 1.7*):

- A wave, signifying atrial contraction
- V wave, reflecting atrial venous filling

P ≫ The C wave reflects the tricuspid valve closure, which is not visible on examination. Two descents are present, an X descent (reflecting atrial relaxation) and a Y descent (reflecting ventricular filling).

Table 1.2 *Common JVP waveform abnormalities*

Absent A waves	Atrial fibrillation
Giant A waves	Tricuspid stenosis
'Cannon' A waves	Complete heart block
Giant V waves	Tricuspid regurgitation
Prominent X descent	Cardiac tamponade

E ≫ Six cardinal symptoms should always be asked about during history-taking:

- Chest pain, using the mnemonic '**SOCRATES**' (**S**ite, **O**nset, **C**haracter, **R**adiation, **A**ssociated factors, **T**iming, **E**xacerbating/relieving factors, **S**everity)
- Shortness of breath (including orthopnoea and paroxysmal nocturnal dyspnoea)
- Ankle swelling
- Palpitations
- Syncope or pre-syncope
- Claudication

It is also important to ask about relevant risk factors and family history.

Cardiovascular investigations

Investigations are an essential part of the clinician's arsenal, but must be used judiciously.

a. Blood tests
   - Cardiac biomarkers
     ○ **Troponin** is a component of skeletal and cardiac muscle which facilitates muscle contraction

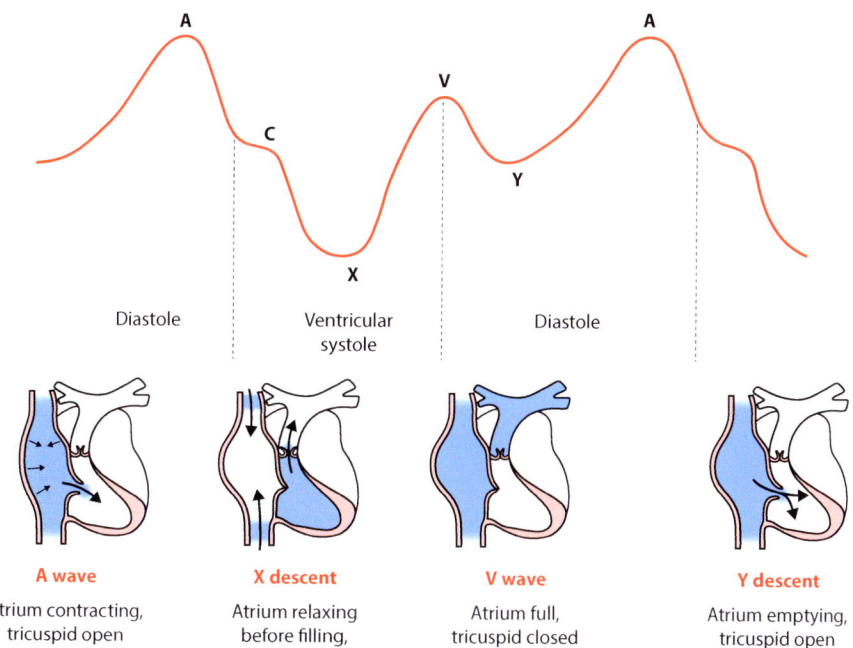

Fig. 1.7 *JVP waveform.*

- Protein complex made up of three subunits troponin T (TnT), troponin I (TnI) and troponin C (TnC)
- TnT and TnI are highly sensitive and specific markers of myocardial injury
  - **Creatine kinase (CK)**
    - CK-MB isozyme is relatively cardiospecific, but the use of CK has largely been superseded by troponin
    - Rises and falls quickly (after 36 hours), and so may have a role in detecting reinfarction
- Lipid panel (a fasting sample is not required)
- Natriuretic peptides

b. Cardiac catheterisation
  - Involves passing catheters into the heart under radiographic guidance
  - May be diagnostic or therapeutic
  - Site of entry is identified, followed by administration of local anaesthetic; a guide wire is used to ensure correct placement of the catheter
  - Classically, the right **radial** (increasingly preferred) or right **femoral** arteries are used for arterial access in **angiography**
  - Haemodynamics may be measured during the process
  - Relatively safe procedure, with a mortality rate <0.1%
  - Complications
    - Contrast reaction, contrast induced nephropathy
    - Arrhythmias
    - Stroke
    - False aneurysm
    - Haemorrhage
    - Coronary artery dissection (which may require emergency coronary artery bypass grafting)

c. Cardiac magnetic resonance imaging (MRI)
  - Non-invasive imaging technique obtained by using controlled magnetic fields to alter hydrogen nuclei alignment
  - No radiation exposure, but expensive
  - Superior to echocardiography in visualising structure and function; not limited by body habitus (physique)
  - Valuable in assessing coronary artery disease, heart failure, cardiomyopathy and congenital heart disease
  - Contraindicated in patients with permanent pacemakers (unless MR-safe), implantable cardioverter defibrillators, jewellery and implants

d. Myocardial perfusion scanning
  - Form of nuclear stress testing

- Observes passage of gadolinium contrast through the heart via T1-weighted sequencing
- Contrast absorbed by myocardium; low signal indicates hypoperfusion
- Assesses for the presence of coronary artery disease
- Agents such as adenosine, dipyridamole and regadenoson are used as vasodilators in myocardial perfusion imaging stress tests

e. Echocardiography
  - Ultrasound allows the physician to visualise the heart and assess its function; may be in two or three dimensions
  - Transthoracic echocardiography (TTE) images the heart through the chest wall, but may yield poorer images in patients with a larger body habitus or with airway disease
  - Transoesophageal echocardiography (TOE) is an alternative, invasive method requiring sedation, which captures images via a probe placed down the oesophagus; TOE has a higher sensitivity and produces higher-quality images, while being particularly effective at imaging the posterior heart
  - Utilising echocardiography
    - Two-dimensional (2D) echocardiography
    - Three-dimensional (3D) echocardiography can be used to answer questions raised by 2D imaging (e.g. viewing valves from multiple angles)
    - Doppler echo
      - Allows for assessment of flow and severity of valvular heart disease
    - Stress echo
      - Echocardiography performed before and after exercise (or with dobutamine if exercise is not possible) to assess the myocardium
    - Myocardial wall motion is used as a surrogate marker for perfusion, because ultrasound cannot visualise blood flow in the arteries

> **W** » Dobutamine, a positive inotrope and chronotrope, is used because it actively simulates exercise, but should not be used in patients with pacemakers or with left bundle branch block.

f. Electrocardiogram (ECG) – see *Table 1.3*.

g. Stress ECG
  - An ECG is recorded at rest and while the patient is exercising on a treadmill

Table 1.3 *Approach to interpreting an ECG*

1. Check calibration	Check length of vertical column at the start of an ECG strip (10mm should equal 1mV)
2. Check patient details	Ensure correct patient name and date of birth; check date and time ECG was taken
3. Calculate the heart rate	300 divided by number of large squares between the R–R interval
4. Assess rhythm	Ensure each P wave is followed by a QRS complex and a T wave
5. Assess cardiac axis	Positive QRS in leads I and II = normal axis Positive QRS lead I, negative QRS lead II = left axis deviation Negative QRS lead I, positive QRS lead II = right axis deviation
6. Review individual waveform morphology	Assess P waves for: a. P pulmonale – right atrial enlargement b. P mitrale – left atrial enlargement c. Absent P waves – atrial fibrillation Assess PR interval (0.12–0.2s) Assess QRS complex
7. Localise lesion	See *Fig. 1.8* and lead location below

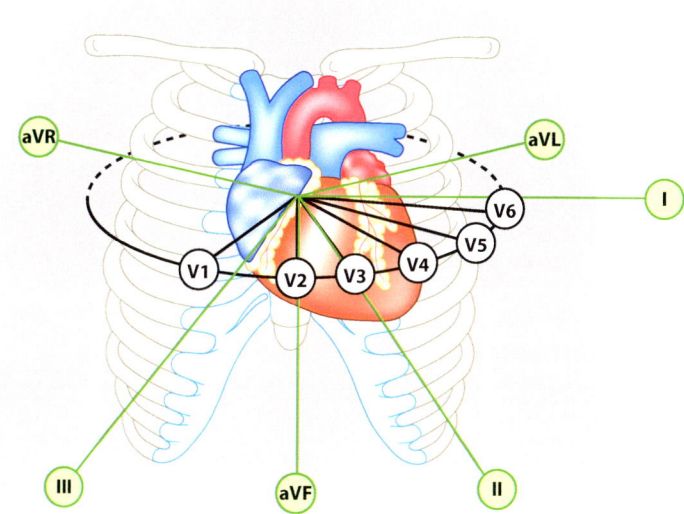

Fig. 1.8 *Views of the heart and their corresponding leads.*

Leads	Location
V1–V2	Anterior wall of right ventricle; posterior wall (reciprocal change)
V3–V4	Anteroseptal wall, anterior wall of left ventricle
V5–V6, I, aVL	Lateral wall
II, III, aVF	Inferior wall

1

- The **Bruce protocol** is the most widely used protocol, and increases myocardial workload in stages
- Traces are recorded up to 15 minutes after exercise has taken place
- ST–T changes may indicate coronary artery disease, but the most reliable of these is horizontal or >1mm downsloping or ST segment depression
- BP is also monitored during the test; a sustained decrease in BP may also suggest coronary artery disease
- Sensitivity and specificity figures vary, but are estimated to be 78% and 70% respectively
- NICE does not recommend the use of stress ECG testing, because of the relatively higher false positive and negative rate – but note that other guidelines (e.g. ESC) do still recommend it as a viable alternative

> **E** ≫ Stress testing is contraindicated if patients have had a recent MI, have severe valvular disease or arrhythmias. The test should be stopped immediately if the patient experiences cardiac symptoms, light-headedness, arrhythmias, >1mm ST elevation or a >10mmHg fall in BP.

When considering stress testing, a general rule of thumb should be to consider exercise treadmill tests if the patient has few comorbidities, and pharmacological testing if the patient has underlying ECG abnormalities or is unable to exercise. Vasodilator agents (such as dipyridamole and adenosine) **should be used with caution** in patients with a history of bronchospasm or carotid stenosis and dobutamine **should not** be used in patients with a history of ventricular arrhythmia.

Cardiac pharmacology

- **ACE inhibitors** are used in the treatment of hypertension and heart failure; the most notable side effects are a dry cough and angioedema, which may be avoided by switching or stopping the medication. ACE inhibitors should be prescribed with caution in patients with hyponatraemia, hyperkalaemia or renal dysfunction, and are contraindicated in pregnancy.
- **Angiotensin receptor blockers (ARBs)** mimic the effects of ACE inhibitors and antagonise the ATII receptor. Likewise, similar considerations and contraindications should be considered when prescribing ARBs. These are good alternatives in

patients who develop ACE inhibitor associated cough.
- **Beta blockers** exert their effect by antagonising the action of epinephrine and norepinephrine at beta adrenergic receptors. They are prescribed to treat heart failure, arrhythmias and coronary artery disease, and should be used with caution in asthmatics.
- **Calcium channel blockers (CCBs)** are generally divided into two main classes – non-rate-limiting (dihydropyridines, e.g. amlodipine, nifedipine) and rate-limiting (non-dihydropyridines, e.g. verapamil, diltiazem).
- **Antiplatelet agents** prevent thrombus formation and are indicated in the prevention and treatment of cardiovascular events. Aspirin inhibits cyclo-oxygenase (COX) to prevent the production of thromboxane A2. P2Y-12 inhibitors (such as clopidogrel, prasugrel and ticagrelor) antagonise the ADP receptor and prevent platelet aggregation.
- **Anticoagulants** interfere with prothrombotic mediators in the coagulation cascade. Warfarin inhibits the synthesis of Vitamin K dependent clotting factors (II, VII, IX and X). Novel oral anticoagulants (NOACs), such as apixaban, dabigatran and rivaroxaban, are used increasingly as they do not require therapeutic monitoring. However, these medications have no direct antidote, except for dabigatran. The FDA approved idarucizumab as an antidote in 2015.
- **Nitrates** are vasodilators that are used in the treatment of angina. Common (usually short-lived) side effects include headaches and flushing. Tolerance is a common complication of nitrate administration.
- **Diuretics** are used to treat oedema and heart failure by increasing urinary sodium excretion and urine output. Hypotension and hyponatraemia are potential side effects in all classes. Thiazide diuretics (e.g. bendroflumethiazide) and loop diuretics (e.g. furosemide) can also cause hypokalaemia, hyperuricaemia and gout. Ototoxicity is specific to loop diuretics. Potassium-sparing diuretics (e.g. spironolactone) can cause hyperkalaemia.
- **Lipid-lowering agents** are exemplified by the statins, which work by inhibiting HMG CoA reductase, thereby reducing synthesis of cholesterol in the liver. (This occurs mostly at night, which is why most statins should be taken at night.) Well-known side effects include myositis and abnormal liver enzyme profiles. Note that deranged LFTs are far more common than myopathy. Rhabdomyolysis is a very rare complication. Other lipid-lowering agents include ezetimibe (which inhibits intestinal absorption of

cholesterol), fibrates (which may increase the risk of developing rhabdomyolysis if co-prescribed with a statin) and bile acid sequestrants. However, it should be borne in mind that, unlike statins, these medications do not lower mortality.

- **Digoxin** inhibits the sodium-potassium pump and is a negative chronotrope and positive inotrope. Patients on digoxin should be monitored for complications (see *Section 1.14.1*).

Atherosclerosis

Atherosclerotic cardiovascular disease is the number one worldwide cause of death and disability. It is a complex process, affecting principally medium- to large-sized arteries. It normally results in luminal stenosis which may be progressive over time. Pathologically, there is focal accumulation within the intimal layer of the arterial wall of cells, lipids, fibrous tissue and complex proteoglycans, eventually leading to the formation of an atherosclerotic plaque. As they advance, these plaques also accumulate calcium, giving rise to the colloquial term 'hardening of the arteries'.

(P) ≫ Smoking is by far the greatest cause of preventable mortality and has been implicated as a risk factor in the development of numerous disease processes. NICE encourages practitioners to discuss smoking cessation with patients when appropriate, advising practitioners as follows:

- Attempt to offer therapy when patients feel ready to quit
- Options include nicotine replacement therapy (NRT), varenicline or bupropion, but none of these should be prescribed together (apart from various subtypes of NRT)
- Bupropion is contraindicated in patients with seizures or eating disorders
- Varenicline is contraindicated in patients with mood disorders (a helpful way to remember this is the phrase 'Varenicline makes your mood decline').
- For most patients, establishing a **target stop date** is key to smoking cessation.

1.1 Stable angina

(E) ≫ Ischaemic heart disease refers to a group of conditions that result from an imbalance between myocardial oxygen supply and demand, leading to tissue hypoxia. This discrepancy is most commonly caused by atherosclerotic disease, although possible non-atherosclerotic causes, such as coronary artery anomalies (younger individuals) and systemic vasculitides (older individuals), should also be kept in mind. Ischaemic heart disease can be categorised as either stable angina or acute coronary syndrome.

(W) ≫ The term 'angina' is a commonly used form of 'angina pectoris', which is derived from the Latin words *angere* and *pectus* which, taken together, mean 'to strangle the chest'. As one might imagine, angina is typically described by patients as 'pressure' or a 'crushing sensation' retrosternally. If the pain is 'stabbing', positional or sharp, the underlying pathological process is less likely to be ischaemic in nature.

Definition: stable angina generally occurs due to a fixed narrowing of the coronary arteries, resulting in symptoms typically associated with exertion, emotion, eating and cold weather. The onset of symptoms is predictable and resolves once the stimulus is removed (e.g. resting after exertion).

Epidemiology:
- Men affected almost twice as much as women; South Asians more likely to be affected
- Modifiable risk factors include diabetes mellitus, hypertension, hyperlipidaemia, smoking and obesity

Aetiology/pathophysiology:
- Coronary artery narrowing by an atherosclerotic plaque reduces blood flow and oxygen delivery to the myocardium
- The atheroma also causes endothelial dysfunction, reducing vasodilator release (e.g. nitric oxide and prostacyclin)
- The demand for increased myocardial oxygen supply (e.g. by walking uphill) is unable to be met due to the stenotic lesion, resulting in myocardial ischaemia
- Ischaemia causes acidosis, decreased ATP production and release of lactate and other chemokines, which stimulate nerve cells in myocytes, producing the sensation of pain

Clinical features

NICE guideline: Chest pain of recent onset
(NICE 2010, CG95)

Key features:

- **Central chest pain** (in reality, stable angina is rarely described as frank 'pain'; rather, the nature of the discomfort may be heaviness, pressure or squeezing)
- Precipitated by **exertion**
- Relieved by **rest** or **nitrates**, usually within 5 minutes

NICE considers a patient with all three features to have **typical angina**, a patient with two features to have **atypical angina**, and a patient with one or none of these features to have **non-anginal pain**.

Investigations

Investigations should be undertaken in the following order.

> **Stepwise plan:**
>
> **1   Obtain an electrocardiogram (ECG)**
>
> **2   Arrange blood tests**
> - FBC, U&Es, LFTs (required for statin therapy), glucose, cholesterol, HDL, LDL and triglycerides
>
> **3   Stratify patients according to clinical risk**

Determining probability (NICE 2010, CG95)

When a person has stable angina, NICE recommends stratifying the probability of coronary artery disease (CAD). Gender (being male), increasing age, typicality of chest pain and associated risk factors (diabetes, smoking, hyperlipidaemia) point to a higher likelihood of CAD.

Likelihood of CAD: shown in *Table 1.4* below.

(E) » Cardiovascular disease refers to a collection of diseases, which include:
- Coronary heart disease (e.g. angina pectoris/myocardial infarction)
- Cerebrovascular disease (e.g. TIA/stroke)
- Peripheral artery disease (e.g. intermittent claudication)

Risk calculators, such as QRISK3 or Framingham, are useful for doctors to predict a patient's risk of developing a CVD within a 10-year period. However, these risk assessment tools are not recommended for use with patients who are type 1 diabetics or those with pre-existing cardiovascular disease.

(P) » Exercise stress testing is no longer recommended by NICE because it is only moderately specific. However, this does not mean that there is little place for stress testing in general. It is still used in many centres, and the European Society of Cardiology (ESC) guidelines still support its use. Stress ECG testing represents a cost-effective alternative to various imaging modalities, and is suitable for evaluating the majority of patients. Stress myocardial perfusion or stress echocardiography (using agents such as dobutamine, which mimic cardiac stress) are more specific investigations than the stress ECG and can be used in patients with contraindications to stress ECG testing, or where ECGs may not be viable (e.g. if the patient has a pacemaker or bundle branch block). Exercise capacity in itself is measured in metabolic equivalents, or METs, which is a strong indicator of prospective mortality. An increase of 1 MET (defined as $3.5ml\ O_2/kg/min$) is said to confer a greater than 10% increase in survival.

Table 1.4 *Approach to CAD investigations*

<10%	**Consider alternative diagnosis**
10–29%	Offer CT calcium scoring: • If calcium score = 0, consider alternative diagnosis • If calcium score 1–400, offer CT coronary angiography • If calcium score >400, consider invasive angiography
30–60%	Offer non-invasive functional testing, e.g. myocardial perfusion scanning
61–90%	Offer coronary angiography if revascularisation is considered, or non-invasive functional testing if not considered
>90%	Treat as per CAD

Management

Stepwise management of stable angina (NICE 2011, CG126)

Ensure that the patient has up-to-date information about their condition. **Aspirin** and **statins** should be prescribed for patients with angina.

1 Optimise diet and lifestyle, prescribe aspirin and a statin

2 Institute pharmacological therapy
- Glyceryl trinitrate (GTN) should be used as and when necessary, repeating a second time after 5 minutes if the pain persists; call an ambulance if the pain persists 5 minutes after a second dose
- First line: beta blocker **or** calcium channel blocker (rate-limiting, e.g. verapamil)
- Increase the dose of monotherapy if still symptomatic
- Second line: beta blocker **and** calcium channel blocker combination therapy (use a non-rate-limiting agent, e.g. nifedipine)
- Third line: if either drug is contraindicated, alternative agents may be tried (ivabradine, nicorandil or ranolazine – of these, ranolazine has the best, albeit limited, evidence); the side effects of ivabradine include visual disturbances, particularly bright spots and luminous phenomena

3 Instituting lipid modification therapy (NICE 2014, CG181)
- Measure a full lipid profile, including total cholesterol, HDL, LDL, triglycerides and liver function tests
- Ratio of total cholesterol to HDL cholesterol is the best predictor of CVD risk, while LDL cholesterol helps guide goals of lipid therapy
- Offer atorvastatin 20mg for primary prevention if estimated 10-year cardiovascular risk using QRISK3 is >10% (note that this is still controversial in some centres)
- Offer atorvastatin 80mg for secondary prevention in patients with pre-existing CVD
- LFTs should be measured within 3 months of starting treatment and at 12 months; statins are safe to start as long as liver transaminase results are less than 3 times the upper limit of normal

E ≫ Coronary artery bypass grafting is recommended in:
- Significant left main disease
- Three vessel disease
- Two vessel disease in diabetics

P ≫ Metabolic syndrome is characterised by having three of any of the following five criteria:
- Hyperinsulinaemia (elevated fasting plasma glucose)
- **Decreased HDL** (as opposed to LDL levels, which are not required in making the diagnosis)
- Central obesity
- Hypertriglyceridaemia
- Hypertension (>130/85)
- This syndrome confers a threefold increase in the risk of cardioembolic events.

Adult Treatment Panel (ATP III) Guidelines

The ATP III Guidelines are also a useful accessory when evaluating lipid-lowering therapy in ischaemic heart disease. Patients are stratified according to their 10-year risk, with >20% risk being a coronary heart disease equivalent; ≤20% conferring moderate risk; and patients with 0–1 risk factor (or a lower than 10% 10-year risk score by default) being regarded as low risk. Target LDL levels are thus recommended, using a fasting lipid panel:
- CHD equivalent (>20%) – target LDL <100mg/dl (<70 in very high-risk patients)
- Moderate risk (≤20%) – target LDL <130mg/dl
- Zero to one risk factors (low risk) – target LDL <160mg/dl

1

1.2 Acute coronary syndrome

Definition: the term acute coronary syndrome (ACS) refers to a group of conditions that result from a sudden and unpredictable disruption in coronary blood flow. ACS exists on a continuum, from myocardial ischaemia (unstable angina) to the development of myocardial infarction and necrosis (NSTEMI or STEMI; see *Fig. 1.9*). Clinically, these conditions are classified according to changes in the electrocardiogram and biochemical markers of myocardial necrosis.

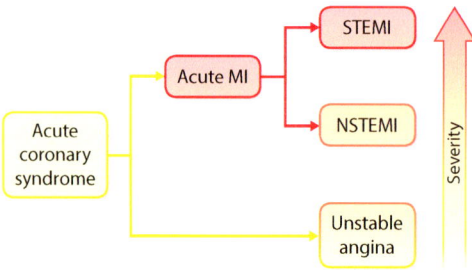

Fig. 1.9 *Acute coronary syndrome.*

Epidemiology:
- ACS accounts for approximately 30% of all deaths worldwide
- While there is a male preponderance, the condition may be underdiagnosed in women
- The GRACE registry suggests that up to 30% of patients with ACS present with STEMI

Aetiology/pathophysiology:
- Atherosclerosis is the most common cause
- Risk factors (see *Table 1.5*)
- ACS usually results from atherosclerotic plaque rupture, promoting thrombus formation which imposes varying degrees of luminal impingement, precipitating an acute coronary event
- If the resultant thrombus occludes the vessel **completely**, myocardial infarction (characterised by ST elevation on ECG) will most often develop
- In the absence of total thrombotic occlusion, an NSTEMI or unstable angina may commonly develop, and ECG changes (such as ST segment depression and/or T wave inversion) may occur

Clinical features:
- Chest pain in ACS is classically acute, central, crushing and retrosternal in nature, with or without radiation to the jaw, neck or arm
- Other symptoms include shortness of breath, sweating, nausea and vomiting

Table 1.5 *Risk factors for ACS*

Modifiable	Non-modifiable
Diabetes mellitus	Age
Obesity and sedentary lifestyle	Male sex
Smoking	South Asian ethnicity
Hypertension	Family history of cardiovascular disease (<55 in men, <65 in women) in a first-degree relative
Dyslipidaemia	Previous myocardial infarction

P ≫ Variant (or Prinzmetal) angina may present similarly to acute coronary syndrome, but the underlying pathophysiological process is usually attributed to **coronary artery vasospasm**. The gold standard for diagnosis is coronary angiography with a provocative agent, such as ergonovine, to induce an attack. The condition is treated with **calcium channel blockers** or **nitrates. Note that the use of aspirin or beta blockers may worsen vasospasm.**

E ≫ ACS may present atypically in some patients, particularly those with autonomic dysfunction (diabetics and the elderly). They may have a silent MI (with no chest pain) or they may present with delirium, hypotension or epigastric pain.

Immediate investigations (see *Fig. 1.10*)

1 Obtain ECGs
- Should be recorded 15–30 minutes apart, looking for dynamic changes, and compared with older ECGs if possible

2 Arrange chest X-ray
- Assess cardiomediastinal contours (e.g. the presence of cardiomegaly, mediastinal widening in aortic dissection), lung fields (e.g. signs of heart failure) and exclude non-cardiac causes of chest pain (e.g. pneumothorax, pneumonia)

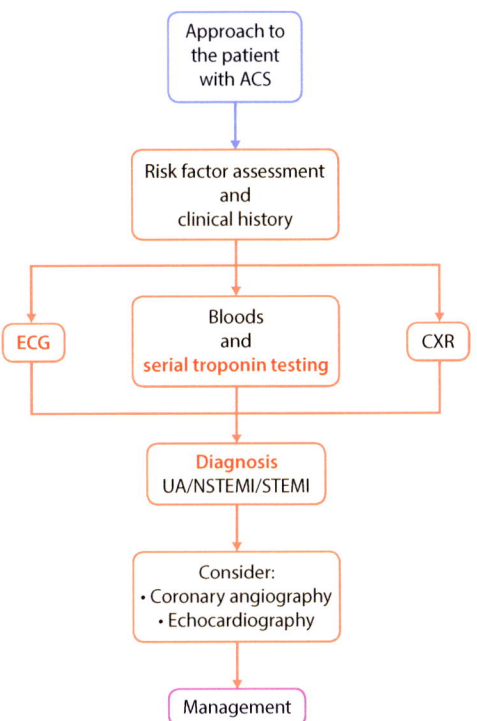

Fig. 1.10 *Approach to ACS.*

3 Arrange blood tests
- Troponin T or I (serial, 6h apart, looking for a peak in the measured values), FBC, U&Es, LFTs

> **W** ≫ With the advent of high-sensitivity troponin assays, very low levels of troponin can be detected. While these newer assays improve diagnostic sensitivity, they are likely to affect clinical specificity. This is primarily because troponin can be elevated in several other conditions: acute heart failure, myocarditis, pericarditis, pulmonary embolism, renal failure and sepsis.

> **P** ≫ Posterior STEMIs are usually characterised by horizontal ST depression, tall R waves and upright T waves (all changes in leads V1–3). The left circumflex or right coronary artery is often implicated. Posterior STEMI is confirmed by placing leads V7–9 (V7 posterior axillary line, V8 at tip of left scapula and V9 left paraspinal region – all leads at same horizontal plane as V6).

Guidelines: Third Universal Definition of Myocardial Infarction (2012)

The joint ESC/ACCF/AHA/WHF task force published the following recommendations for the diagnosis of acute MI in 2012.

A rise and/or fall of cardiac biomarkers (troponin) with at least one value above the 99th percentile of the upper reference limit (URL) in conjunction with evidence of myocardial ischaemia, with at least one of the following:
- Symptoms of ischaemia
- ECG changes indicative of new ischaemia (ST–T changes or new LBBB)
- Development of pathological Q waves in the ECG
- Imaging evidence of new loss of viable myocardium or regional wall motion abnormality
- Identification of an intracoronary thrombus by angiography

Classification of myocardial infarction

Table 1.6 *Types of MI*

Type 1	Spontaneous myocardial infarction related to ischaemia due to a primary event such as plaque erosion and/or rupture, fissuring or dissection
Type 2	Myocardial infarction secondary to ischaemia due to either increased oxygen demand or decreased oxygen supply, e.g. coronary artery spasm, coronary embolism, anaemia, arrhythmias, hypertension or hypotension
Type 3	Myocardial infarction resulting in death when biomarker values are unavailable
Type 4A	Myocardial infarction associated with PCI
Type 4B	Myocardial infarction associated with stent thrombosis detected by angiography or at autopsy
Type 5	Myocardial infarction related to CABG

Stepwise management of acute coronary syndrome

The aim of management is to instigate antiplatelet therapy expeditiously, to re-perfuse the myocardium in STEMI, and to prevent the progression of unstable angina and NSTEMI. The approach to management can be divided into three steps: initial management, advanced management and post-acute management.

1

1 Initial management for ALL patients (MONAC)

- Continuous cardiac monitoring
  - Ideally move to a controlled environment (e.g. Coronary Care Unit)
- Administer (or check) **aspirin** 300mg, plus another antiplatelet agent (e.g. clopidogrel, prasugrel, ticagrelor); antiplatelet agents **lower mortality**
- **Oxygen**: indicated only if SpO_2 <94%; the evidence indicates that oxygen may have a vasoconstrictive effect on the coronary arteries and should be avoided if the patient is not hypoxic
- **GTN**: may be given via the sublingual or buccal route – if minimal to no response, an IV infusion may be considered; **note that GTN should be avoided if systolic BP <90mmHg**
- **IV morphine** for pain: (e.g. 2.5mg boluses, 5 minutes apart), with up-titration if clinically indicated; may also be used for pulmonary oedema, shortness of breath or anxiety
- **IV metoclopramide**: ischaemia and morphine are both emetogenic
- **Tight glucose control**: glucose should be monitored regularly

2 Advanced management

After immediate management, further therapy depends on the type of ACS, STEMI or NSTEMI/UA and the clinical condition of the patient.

a. **STEMI**
  1. Establish diagnosis of STEMI
  2. Primary percutaneous coronary intervention (PPCI)
     - This is the gold standard reperfusion strategy in STEMI

> **E** ≫ Features of STEMI on ECG:
> - ST elevation of ≥1mm in at least 2 adjacent limb leads or ≥2mm in 2 contiguous precordial leads **OR**
> - New onset of LBBB (this is less specific for STEMI)

  - Indicated if symptom onset occurs within 12 hours
  - Procedure should be performed within 90–120 minutes of diagnosis
  - **Bivalirudin** (direct thrombin inhibitor), in combination with aspirin and clopidogrel, is recommended for patients with STEMI undergoing PPCI (although practice may vary between centres)

  - LMWH or unfractionated heparin are the anticoagulants of choice in patients undergoing PPCI who have been treated with prasugrel or ticagrelor
  - NICE recommends against the routine use of glycoprotein IIb/IIIa inhibitors before planned PPCI
  3. Thrombolysis in STEMI
     - Should only be performed if patients are unable to receive PPCI within 90–120 minutes of diagnosis, or where PPCI is contraindicated
     - ECG should be performed 90 minutes after thrombolysis
       - Look for 50% reduction in ST elevation
       - If inadequate response, consider rescue PCI within 6 hours of thrombolysis

b. **NSTEMI/UA**
  1. Establish the diagnosis
     - NSTEMI: positive troponin ± ischaemic changes on ECG (e.g. ST depression, T wave inversion)
     - UA: negative troponin ± ischaemic changes on ECG
  2. Assess risk of future adverse cardiovascular events:
     - NICE recommends the **GRACE score** to predict 6-month mortality
     - If low risk (predicted 6-month mortality <3%):
       - Offer patients anticoagulation (**fondaparinux 2.5mg SC** is recommended for 8 days or until discharge) without early angiography and proceed to post-acute management
     - If intermediate (3–6%) or high risk (>6%):
       - Consider IV glycoprotein IIb/IIIa inhibitors and anticoagulation (bivalirudin or unfractionated heparin recommended)
       - Arrange coronary angiography within 96 hours of admission and consider PCI

3 Post-acute management

- **Antiplatelet agents**
  - **Aspirin** 75mg lifelong following ACS
  - **P2-Y12 inhibitors:** (clopidogrel, ticagrelor, prasugrel) for **12 months**
- **Statin therapy** lowers mortality; NICE recommends atorvastatin 80mg
- **Beta blockers** lower mortality and provide symptomatic relief

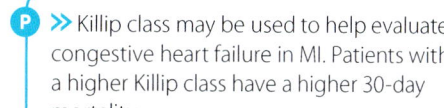

- **Nitrates**, regular (if required), and PRN (for all patients)
- **ACE inhibitors** lower mortality, and prevent ventricular remodelling and subsequent heart failure
- **Structured cardiac rehabilitation and lifestyle modification**
  - Driving limitations:
    - If angioplasty – 1 week
    - No angioplasty – 4 weeks
  - Sexual intercourse:
    - Generally best avoided for at least 1 week after an uncomplicated MI
    - Patients who are able to carry out physical activity may be advised to resume sexual activity on a case-by-case basis
  - Air travel:
    - Avoid for 2 months

> **(E)** >> **Complications of acute coronary syndrome**
> This can be memorised using the popular mnemonic 'Sudden Death on PRAED Street'.
> Sudden Death
> **P**ump failure or **P**ericarditis
> **R**upture (e.g. of LV free wall, septum or papillary muscle)
> **A**neurysm or Arrhythmia
> **E**mbolism
> **D**ressler syndrome

Complications of myocardial infarction

Careful monitoring of patients post MI is essential because of the risk of complications. These include:
- **Recurrent MI or re-occlusion**
- Should be suspected with recurrent or new chest pain post MI; may have new ECG changes
  - CK-MB may be useful in detecting re-infarction, as troponin levels take 14 days to normalise
  - Rare complication, requires angiography and potential revascularisation to treat
  - In-stent thrombosis incidence is reduced by appropriate adherence to antiplatelet therapy
- **Acute pulmonary oedema** (see *Chapter 12*)
  - Common complication
- **Cardiogenic shock**
- **Arrhythmia:**
  - Ventricular tachycardia and ventricular fibrillation may result in sudden death in up to one-fifth of patients

> **(P)** >> Killip class may be used to help evaluate congestive heart failure in MI. Patients with a higher Killip class have a higher 30-day mortality.
> Class I: no clinical signs of heart failure
> Class II: presence of crackles, elevated JVP or third heart sound
> Class III: acute pulmonary oedema
> Class IV: cardiogenic shock

- Bradycardia and heart block are more commonly associated with an inferior wall MI; heart block associated with inferior MIs is usually self-limiting but should be monitored closely
- Bradycardia and heart block in the setting of an **anterior** wall MI are associated with a poorer prognosis, and pacing should be considered
- **Ventricular septal rupture:**
  - Uncommon, often occurs within a week of MI
  - Associated with anterior MI
  - Septal rupture may be associated with the **sudden onset** of shock and pulmonary oedema
  - Development of a new systolic murmur best heard at the lower left sternal border
  - Echocardiography is first line (transoesophageal is superior to transthoracic, but this depends on the stability of the patient); alternatively, catheterisation demonstrates characteristic **stepping up** in oxygen saturation in right ventricle
  - Requires **surgical closure**
- **Ventricular free wall rupture:**
  - Leads to pericardial tamponade and imminent death if left untreated
  - Urgent pericardiocentesis and surgery are essential

> **(E)** >> LV aneurysm typically develops after 4–5 weeks, presenting with LV failure, VT and systemic emboli. ECG shows persistent ST elevation. Treat with anticoagulation and/or excision.

- **Papillary muscle rupture:**
  - Associated with acute mitral regurgitation and inferior infarctions in particular; life-threatening complication
  - Holding treatments include reducing afterload (e.g. treating with sodium nitroprusside), inotropes, diuretics, ventilation, followed by urgent surgical repair/replacement

1

- **Right ventricular failure:**
  - Associated with inferior wall MI
  - Suspect if clear lung fields, elevated JVP and systemic hypotension
  - Fluid boluses that augment RV preload are required (e.g. 250ml 0.9% NaCl over 10 minutes)
  - **Avoid** prescribing nitrates and diuretics

> ≫ Nitrates and diuretics reduce preload, which will worsen the condition of right ventricular failure, as filling of the right side of the heart is already impaired.

- **Mural thrombus**
- **Cholesterol embolus**
  - May affect various organs, e.g. renal failure if kidneys are affected
  - Classically presents with gangrene of the extremities, particularly the toes, if emboli lodge in the lower limbs
  - Suspect if the patient develops distal ischaemia, renal failure or hypertension

- **Pericarditis**
  - Common complication, particularly in the first few days, following transmural infarcts
  - May be clinically silent or the patient may experience pleuritic chest pain that classically improves on sitting up
  - There may be a pericardial rub and evidence of a pericardial effusion on chest X-ray or echocardiography

> ≫ Late pericardial inflammation is termed Dressler syndrome. This is an autoimmune condition that presents 2–6 weeks post MI with recurrent pericarditis, fever and effusions. Often associated with large pericardial and pleural effusions, the former predisposing to cardiac tamponade. Treatment is with aspirin, colchicine or steroids. NSAIDs may also be used, but the evidence, while not particularly clear, does suggest that they may in some way interfere with myocardial healing.

1.3 Heart failure

Definition: heart failure refers to the inability of the heart to produce a cardiac output sufficient to meet the body's metabolic demands.

Epidemiology:
- Incidence and prevalence increase with age
- Affects 1–2% of the population in the western world

Aetiology:
- The most common causes of heart failure are ischaemic heart disease, valvular heart disease, cardiomyopathy and hypertension
- Other causes include infiltrative disease, toxins, infections (e.g. Chagas disease) and drugs

Pathophysiology: the pathophysiological process that takes place in heart failure involves a complex interplay of many factors. As cardiac output begins to decline, compensatory mechanisms (both mechanical and neurohumoral in nature) are activated in an attempt to sustain adequate tissue perfusion. These may initially be beneficial, but will lead to worsening heart failure over time as their ability to compensate declines.
- Mechanical compensatory mechanisms include Frank–Starling forces (stretch on myocardial fibres increases subsequent stroke volume)
- Neurohumoral compensatory mechanisms include increased sympathetic nervous system stimulation and activation of the renin–angiotensin–aldosterone system

Classification of heart failure

Heart failure can be classified as follows:

1. Anatomical

Left heart failure (LHF)

- The left side of the heart is usually affected first
- Poor ventricular contraction causes blood to 'back up' into the lungs
- This increases the pulmonary vein hydrostatic pressure, resulting in extravasation of fluid into the interstitium. This phenomenon is known as pulmonary oedema

Right heart failure (RHF)

- The most common cause of right heart failure is **left heart failure**
- An increase in the pressure of the pulmonary vasculature causes the right side of the heart to pump against increased resistance
- The right heart compensates with ventricular hypertrophy, but this leads to progressive dilatation and eventual failure
- Less commonly, isolated RHF may occur secondary to lung disease such as pulmonary hypertension or pulmonary emboli. When this happens, it is termed **cor pulmonale**
- Rarer causes are related to pulmonary and tricuspid valve pathology

2. Functional

Systolic heart failure

- Also known as heart failure with reduced ejection fraction (HFrEF)
- Impaired left ventricular systolic function is a key feature
- Poor ventricular contraction leads to reduced ejection fraction (<40%)
- Commonly seen as a result of ischaemic heart disease (IHD) or myocardial infarction (MI)

Diastolic heart failure

- Also known as heart failure with preserved ejection fraction (HFpEF)
- These patients have preserved LV systolic function
- Ventricles are unable to relax due to stiffness, resulting in inadequate filling of the heart during diastole (EF >50%)
- Seen in restrictive cardiomyopathy and constrictive pericarditis

Low-output heart failure

- Compensatory mechanisms eventually fail, resulting in reduced cardiac output
- Caused by failure of the pump (heart), increased preload or increased afterload
- Low-output states are seen in IHD and aortic stenosis
- Characterised by cool peripheries and weak pulses

High-output heart failure

- Inability of the heart to meet increased metabolic demands of body tissues despite normal or increased cardiac output
- This is rare and is seen in thyrotoxicosis, AV fistula, beriberi (thiamine deficiency), pregnancy and severe anaemia
- Conversely, this form is characterised by warm peripheries and normal pulses

3. Temporal

Acute heart failure

- Acute heart failure is a medical emergency
- This may occur in the context of an episode of decompensation of chronic heart failure, which is termed 'acute-on-chronic' heart failure
- Decompensation in a previously stable patient with heart failure is triggered by factors such as poor compliance with medication, infection, arrhythmias and fluid overload
- Acute heart failure can also occur *de novo* in a patient with no prior chronic heart failure (i.e. in ACS and malignant hypertension)

Chronic heart failure

- The term 'heart failure', when used in clinical practice, is often synonymous with patients who present with the chronic form of this condition

1

New York Heart Association (NYHA) classification of the extent of heart failure

Table 1.7 *NYHA classification of heart failure*

NYHA class	Physical activity limitation	Symptoms with ordinary physical activity
I	Physical activity not limited	No symptoms
II	Slight limitation	Mild symptoms with ordinary activity
III	Marked limitation	Symptomatic with less than ordinary activity such as walking short distances (20–50 metres)
IV	Symptoms present at rest (mostly bed-bound patients)	Symptoms present at rest

Clinical features

- Dyspnoea
- Orthopnoea and paroxysmal nocturnal dyspnoea
- Other symptoms include a nocturnal cough, chest discomfort, peripheral oedema and fatigue
- Note that individual symptoms may differ based on the aetiological cause of the heart failure and the duration of onset
- The presence of two major, or one major and two minor, criteria in the Framingham criteria may also be used to help suggest the diagnosis of heart failure

E ≫ **Examination findings:**
- Signs of right heart failure: elevated JVP, hepatomegaly, ascites, significant peripheral oedema
- Signs of left heart failure: displaced apex beat, S3, pulmonary congestion
- Note that in clinical practice both types of heart failure often occur simultaneously, which is termed congestive cardiac failure.

Investigations

Investigations should be undertaken in the following order.

Stepwise plan:

1 **Arrange blood tests**
- FBC, U&Es, LFTs, TFTs, lipid levels and glucose

2 **Assess B-type natriuretic peptide (BNP)**
- This is released in response to myocardial stretch:
  - If levels of BNP ≥100pg/ml, investigate further and arrange for specialist referral within 6 weeks
  - If levels of BNP ≥400pg/ml, refer for specialist referral and echocardiography within 2 weeks

3 **Obtain chest X-ray**
- Characteristic 'ABCDE' features (see *Fig. 1.11*)

4 **Arrange for echocardiogram**
- Key investigation in suspected heart failure

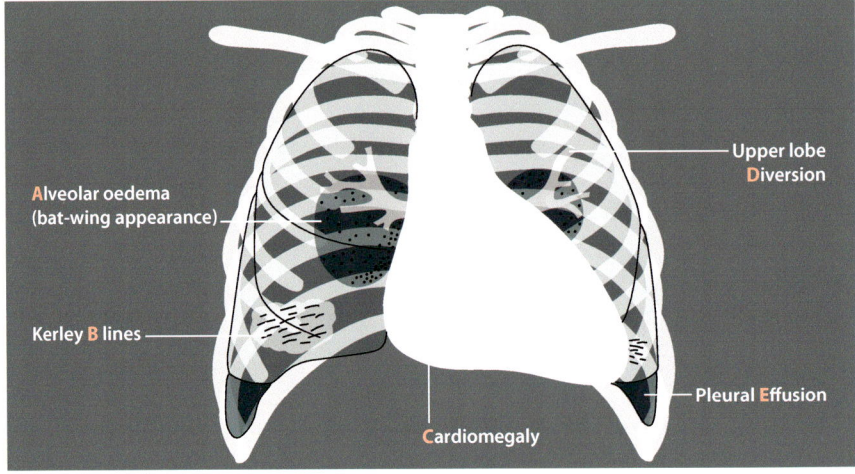

Fig. 1.11 *Classic 'ABCDE' findings on a CXR in a patient with heart failure.*

- Enables assessment of ventricular function, wall motion abnormalities and valvular or structural abnormalities

5 Obtain ECG
- Useful in evaluating potential causes

6 Arrange other investigations
- May include angiography, CT scanning and cardiac MRI

P ≫ BNP levels above 400pg/ml are associated with a poor prognosis. BNP levels decrease once treatment is initiated. A higher BNP level correlates with higher mortality, and a BNP level below 100pg/ml has a very high (approximately 95%) negative predictive value in excluding heart failure. **NICE, SIGN and the ESC guidelines all recommend the use of BNP in the assessment of heart failure.**

Management of heart failure (NICE CKS, 2015)

General principles: the aim of management is to ensure treatment of all underlying pathology, encourage lifestyle changes (including treating sleep apnoea, which has been linked to poorer outcomes), manage symptoms and prevent episodes of acute decompensation as far as possible. Weighing the patient daily may also help provide an assessment of fluid status.

Stepwise management of heart failure

1 Lifestyle modification
- Smoking cessation
- Adequate fluid and salt restriction (<3g salt/day)
- Restrict alcohol, optimise diet and exercise

2 Diuretics
- Loop diuretics prescribed first line (e.g. furosemide)
- Symptomatic relief of fluid overload
- Does **not** reduce mortality
- **Introduce one drug at a time;** once the person is stable on the first drug, add the second drug

3 ACE inhibitors
- **Improve morbidity and mortality**
- Improve ventricular function
- Switch to an angiotensin receptor blocker (ARB) if cough (common side effect) not tolerated

4 Beta blockers
- **Improve morbidity and mortality**

- Bisoprolol, carvedilol and nebivolol are recommended in the treatment of heart failure
- Titrate dose **slowly** and incrementally, preferably every 2 weeks if dosage requires adjustment

P ≫ NICE recommends using clinical judgment when deciding which drug to start first.

For example, the preferred initial treatment might be:
- a beta blocker, if the person has angina
- an ACE inhibitor, if the person has diabetes
- a diuretic and ACE inhibitor, if the person still has signs of fluid overload.

E ≫ Note that beta blockers are still the first-line choice for rate control when managing heart failure with accompanying atrial fibrillation. Digoxin is used as an alternative.

5 Mineralocorticoid receptor antagonists (MRAs)
- **Improve mortality**
- MRA therapy is used early in post-STEMI patients who have evidence of heart failure
- Added to treatment regimen if still symptomatic despite use of ACE inhibitors, beta blockers and loop diuretics
- Eplerenone is more expensive, but has fewer endocrine side effects compared to spironolactone

6 Ivabradine
- Note that ivabradine is not recommended for use if AF is present
- Indicated if patient's symptoms fail to improve on triple therapy with beta blockers, ACE inhibitors and aldosterone antagonists, or if beta blockers are contraindicated in the first instance

7 Hydralazine plus nitrate
- **Improves mortality**
- Recommended for patients whose symptoms are still not controlled, and this treatment is particularly recommended for Afro-Caribbean patients

8 Device therapy and surgical management
- **Cardiac resynchronisation therapy pacemaker (CRT-P)**
  - **Improves mortality**
  - Indicated in severe heart failure with LVEF <35% and **broad QRS** complexes on ECG

1

- **Implantable cardioverter defibrillator**
  - Indications include previous ventricular fibrillation/ventricular tachycardia and a reduced ejection fraction
  - Can be integrated with CRT devices (CRT-D)
- **Left ventricular assist device (LVAD)**
  - Used as a bridge to transplantation or recovery
- **Cardiac transplantation**
  - Rarely undertaken, utilised in particular for young patients with refractory end-stage disease

P » One of the newest agents to emerge in the past few years is the combination tablet valsartan/sacubitril. Two major trials, PARADIGM-HF and PARAMOUNT, were instrumental in establishing that combination therapy with valsartan/sacubitril improves mortality and is far more effective in reducing frequency of admissions than enalapril therapy alone. This was seen in both HFrEF and HFpEF. Sacubitril, the newer agent, is an angiotensin receptor neprilysin inhibitor (ARNI), which exerts its effects by causing increased peptide degradation and promoting natriuresis.

1.4 Hypertension

Definition: blood pressure is a continuous variable, with a skewed normal distribution (bell-shaped curve) that varies with race, sex and age. The definition of hypertension is therefore arbitrary, although the higher the diastolic and/or systolic blood pressure, the greater the risk of cardiovascular disease, stroke and renal disease. Evidence shows that this increased risk begins with any blood pressure over 120mmHg systolic. Hypertension is therefore usually defined as a BP that increases the risk of cardiovascular morbidity and mortality, the treatment of which results in more benefit than harm.

Epidemiology:
- Affects around one-third of patients aged 45–54
- Affects approximately 70% of patients aged 75 and over

Aetiology/pathophysiology:
- 95% of cases are classified as **essential** – i.e. having no underlying discernible cause
- The remaining 5% are classified as **secondary** and may be due to:
  - Renal disease (e.g. diabetic nephropathy, glomerulonephritis, polycystic kidneys, renovascular disease)
  - Endocrine disease (e.g. Conn syndrome, phaeochromocytoma)
  - Others: pre-eclampsia, coarctation of the aorta

Clinical features:
- Hypertension is usually **asymptomatic**
- Symptoms observed may be related to an underlying secondary cause (e.g. headaches, palpitations and sweating in phaeochromocytoma)

W » Essential hypertension is a multifactorial environmental and genetic condition. There is a greater prevalence of hypertension in first-degree relatives with hypertension, and a high concordance in identical twins. The exact pathophysiology, however, remains undefined.

Guidelines: Defining hypertension (NICE 2011, CG127)

Stage 1 hypertension
- Clinic blood pressure (CBP) = 140/90mmHg or higher **and**
- Ambulatory blood pressure monitoring (ABPM) average or home blood pressure monitoring (HBPM) average = 135/85mmHg or higher

Stage 2 hypertension
- Clinic blood pressure = 160/100mmHg or higher **and**
- ABPM/HBPM average = 150/95mmHg or higher

Severe hypertension
- Clinic **systolic BP** ≥180mmHg **OR**
- Clinic **diastolic BP** ≥110mmHg

Investigations (NICE 2011, CG127)
Investigations should be undertaken in the following order.

Stepwise plan:

1 **Take blood pressure at clinic**
- Measure ABPM or HBPM if clinic reading is ≥140/90

2   Arrange for ABPM or HBPM readings
- ABPM: at least 2 readings per hour every waking hour, with an average of 14 readings required for diagnosis
- HPBM: BP measured twice a day, with each entry being the average of 2 readings taken at least 1 minute apart with the patient sitting down

3   Additional investigations
- U&Es, creatinine, eGFR and assessment of renal function
- Renal ultrasound
- Echocardiogram
- ECG
- Fasting blood glucose and lipid profile
- Additional investigations if a secondary cause is suspected

Complications of hypertension
Hypertension predisposes patients to:
- Acute coronary syndrome
- Stroke (ischaemic or haemorrhagic)
- Chronic kidney disease (note that chronic kidney disease may itself cause hypertension)
- Hypertensive retinopathy
- Aortic dissection/aneurysm

Management
General principles: treatment should be initiated for patients with stage 1 hypertension, under the age of 80, with end organ damage, cardiovascular or renal disease or diabetes. **All** patients with stage 2 hypertension should be offered treatment. Encourage patients to modify specific lifestyle factors, such as preventing obesity, stopping smoking, and adopting a low salt diet.

E ≫ Treatment targets
Under 80 years: CBP <140/90mmHg
Over 80 years: CBP <150/90mmHg
Diabetics: CBP <130/80mmHg

Stepwise management of hypertension (see *Fig. 1.12*)

1   ACE inhibitors or calcium channel blockers
- Below 55 years of age, offer ACE inhibitor or ARB if intolerant
- If above 55 years of age, or of Afro-Caribbean origin, offer calcium channel blocker

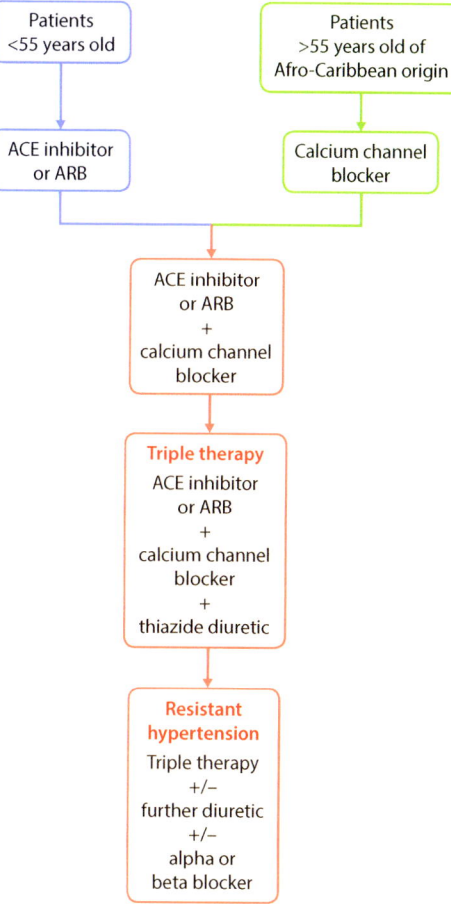

Fig. 1.12 *Stepwise management of hypertension.*

P ≫ Newer agents, such as direct renin inhibitors (e.g. aliskiren) block the conversion of angiotensinogen to angiotensin I. At present, they are recommended if patients are unable to take other anti-hypertensive agents.

Some patients may present with a hypertensive emergency (accelerated or malignant hypertension) or hypertensive urgency, all of which encompass a severely elevated BP (usually systolic BP >220mmHg or diastolic BP >120mmHg) but are differentiated by the degree of end organ damage.

With hypertensive urgency, there is no end organ damage. Accelerated hypertension presents with evidence of hypertensive retinopathy, no worse than grade 3 (e.g. flame haemorrhages, soft exudates) and without papilloedema. The definition of malignant hypertension requires papilloedema.

1

End organ damage is not necessarily limited to hypertensive retinopathy. Encephalopathy (headache, visual disturbances, altered consciousness, seizures), myocardial ischaemia (angina, LV failure) or renal failure are also common presentations in a hypertensive emergency.

Hypertensive emergencies may present as part of another condition too, including aortic dissection, catecholamine excess (pheochromocytoma, recreational drug overdose), or pregnancy (eclampsia/pre-eclampsia).

Deterioration can be acute and rapid, and requires urgent treatment, for which there are various approaches. One option is to commence oral therapy as soon as possible (e.g. atenolol or amlodipine). This helps facilitate weaning from IV treatment (e.g. labetalol, nitroprusside), which forms the mainstay of initial management.

One regimen for BP reduction is to lower SBP by 10% in the first hour, followed by 15% in the following few hours. (This helps reduce the risk of organ hypoperfusion.) However, there are some exceptions to this, most notably with aortic dissection, where a more rapid reduction in BP is mandated (if tolerated), with a target SBP <120mmHg.

2 Combination therapy
- Add second drug
- Offer ACE inhibitor with calcium channel blocker
- Offer thiazide diuretic (e.g. chlorthalidone or indapamide) at this stage if intolerant of CCBs

W ≫ One of the common side effects of ACE inhibitors is a dry cough. ACE inhibitors prevent the breakdown of bradykinin, substance P and prostaglandins, which contribute to the presence of a cough.

3 Triple therapy
- Combination of ACE inhibitor, CCB and thiazide diuretic

E ≫ First-line therapy in all diabetics is an ACE inhibitor, regardless of age.

4 Additional therapies
- Increase dose of thiazide diuretic, if potassium >4.5mmol/L
- Offer aldosterone antagonists (e.g. spironolactone/eplerenone), if potassium <4.5mmol/L
- If further diuretic therapy is not tolerated, offer an alpha blocker or a beta blocker

1.5 Pericarditis

Definition: pericarditis refers to inflammation of the pericardium, the membranous sac enclosing the heart.

Epidemiology:
- Accounts for up to 5% of non-MI chest pain in the emergency department
- Approximately 1% of emergency cases with ST elevation

Aetiology/pathophysiology:
- Up to 90% of cases are idiopathic or viral in origin
  - The most common viruses implicated are Coxsackie, echovirus and EBV
- May also occur as sequelae of autoimmune disease (e.g. SLE, sarcoidosis) or as part of an acute MI or Dressler syndrome (see *Section 1.2*)
- Drugs: hydralazine, isoniazid, procainamide, penicillin
- Uraemia

W ≫ The pericardium is an avascular sac and contains serous fluid that reduces friction as the heart contracts. It is, however, well innervated, which accounts for the sensation of pain when inflammatory changes occur. In pericarditis, the inflamed visceral and parietal pericardial layers rub against one another, resulting in pain. The friction between these two layers can sometimes be heard as an audible rub on the stethoscope.

Clinical features:
- **Sharp** retrosternal or left-sided chest pain occurs in up to 95% of patients
- Pain is classically described as worse on leaning back, and better on sitting forward

- Viral prodrome of low-grade pyrexia, tachycardia and malaise may also be seen

> **E** ≫ Muffled heart sounds, hypotension and a raised JVP (Beck's triad) suggest cardiac tamponade (see *Chapter 12*).

Investigations

Investigations should be undertaken in the following order.

> **Stepwise plan:**

1   Obtain ECG
- First-line investigation
- Classically depicts widespread ST elevation
- **PR segment depression** is the most specific finding

2   Arrange for blood tests
- Elevated white cell count, acute phase reactants like CRP
- Troponin may be elevated in pericarditis

3   Carry out chest X-ray and echocardiogram (see *Fig. 1.13*)
- May reveal a pericardial effusion (cardiomegaly on CXR)

> **Stepwise management of pericarditis (ESC 2015)**

1   NSAIDs or aspirin
- Given until symptoms resolution or CRP normalisation, usually within 2 weeks of treatment

2   Colchicine
- May be used as monotherapy but generally used as adjunct to **prevent recurrence**
- Patients should be warned about possible gastrointestinal upset (e.g. diarrhoea), as this is a common side effect with the use of colchicine

> **P** ≫ Post-MI pericarditis should be managed with aspirin and colchicine, as the administration of NSAIDs may interfere with the healing of the myocardium.

3   Corticosteroids
- Should only be given in connective tissue disease, uraemic or immune-mediated pericarditis, or if NSAID and colchicine therapy are contraindicated or ineffective

1.5.1 Constrictive pericarditis

Constrictive pericarditis refers to the progressive thickening, fibrosis and calcification of the pericardium, limiting cardiac chamber filling. Around 9% of patients with acute pericarditis may develop constrictive pericarditis. It is usually caused by tuberculosis, but other possible causes include mediastinal irradiation, cardiac surgery (resulting in pericardial trauma) and tissue disease. Patients typically present with features of right heart failure (e.g. oedema, ascites) due to a low cardiac output, resulting in dyspnoea on exertion and fatigue.

> **P** ≫ **K**onstrictive pericarditis may have a pericardial **K**nock and **K**ussmaul sign (paradoxical rise in JVP during inspiration).

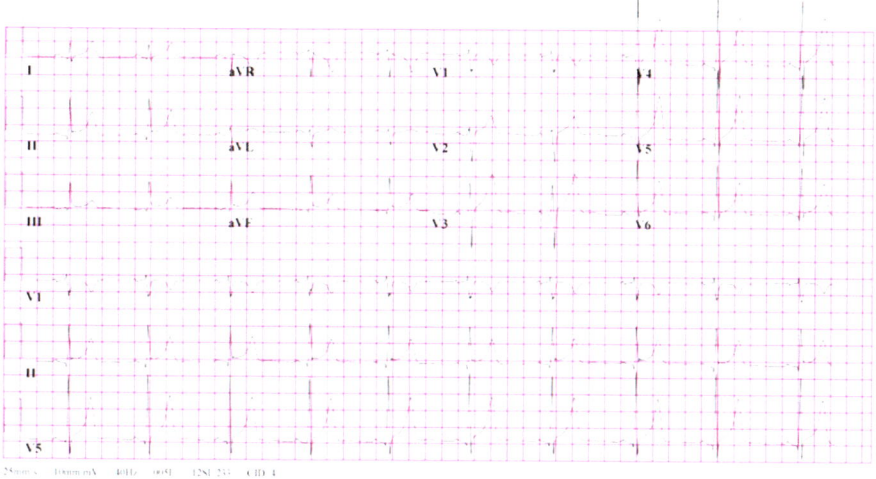

Fig. 1.13 *An ECG showing widespread concave ST elevation and PR depression, characteristic of pericarditis.*

1

Echocardiography may demonstrate a restrictive mitral filling pattern and pericardial thickening.

A chest X-ray may show **pericardial calcification**, which is pathognomonic in the presence of heart failure and elevated JVP. Pericardectomy is the only definite treatment. Medical therapy may involve a trial of diuretics and NSAIDs, steroids or colchicine.

1.6 Rheumatic fever

Definition: acute rheumatic fever (ARF) is a neglected disease that remains endemic in the developing world. It is a multisystem disorder that occurs as a result of an autoimmune mediated reaction to Group A streptococcal pharyngitis or skin infection. Its only long-term sequela is rheumatic heart disease (RHD), which progresses after repeated episodes of ARF. The pathognomonic lesion in RHD is mitral stenosis but mitral and aortic regurgitation are also commonly seen.

Epidemiology:
- Rare in developed countries
- Most commonly seen in children aged 5–14 in developing countries, where there is poor access to healthcare (Australian Aboriginals have the highest rates of ARF in the world)

Aetiology/pathophysiology:
- Immune mediated reaction to rheumatogenic strains of Group A streptococcus in susceptible individuals

> W ≫ During an infection, monoclonal antibodies are formed against Group A streptococcal antigens. Due to molecular mimicry between antigens and human host tissue, these antibodies can cross-react with cardiac proteins (carditis) as well as proteins in synovial (arthritis), neuronal (chorea), subcutaneous (subcutaneous nodules) and dermal tissues (erythema marginatum), producing inflammation that gives rise to the clinical features of rheumatic fever. Although molecular mimicry is thought to play a central role, we still do not fully understand the exact pathogenesis.

- Poor sanitation and overcrowded housing are largely implicated in the transmission of Group A streptococci
- Genetic susceptibility in 3–6% of individuals

Clinical features:
- In most of the world, the 2015 Jones criteria provide the gold standard for ARF diagnosis

- Two major (or one major and two minor) criteria, **plus** evidence of a preceding streptococcal infection, are required for the diagnosis of initial ARF
- The Jones criteria are now divided into low-risk criteria (for high-resource populations) and moderate to high risk criteria (for low-resource populations) because ARF is more common in the latter

> E ≫ The mnemonics '**ACES$_2$**' and '**FRAPP**' can be used to help remember the major and minor Jones criteria (the following criteria are for low-risk populations)
>
> **Major:**
> **A**rthritis (polyarthritis only)
> **C**arditis (e.g. murmur)
> **E**rythema marginatum
> **S**ubcutaneous nodules
> **S**ydenham chorea
>
> **Minor:**
> **F**irst-degree AV block
> **R**aised acute phase reactants
> **A**rthralgia (polyarthralgia)
> **P**yrexia >38.5°C
> **P**revious rheumatic fever

Investigations
Investigations should be undertaken in the following order.

Stepwise plan:

1 **Demonstrate evidence of streptococcal infection**
- Antistreptolysin O or anti-DNAse B antibodies
- Throat swab is often negative

2 **Arrange blood tests**
- Elevated white cell count, acute phase reactants (Jones criteria: ESR ≥60mm/h and/or CRP ≥3.0mg/dl
- Blood cultures to exclude infective endocarditis

3 Obtain ECG and echocardiogram
- ECG may demonstrate AV block or features of pericarditis
- Accelerated junctional rhythm is specific for ARF
- Echocardiogram is mandatory in suspected/confirmed ARF to look for carditis and assess LV size and function

Stepwise management of rheumatic fever

1 General
- Bed/chair rest reduces pain and cardiac workload
- Only patients with severe carditis should gradually be re-commenced on ambulation, especially during the first four weeks
- Patients with less severe carditis can mobilise as soon as their arthritis or other symptoms sufficiently subside

2 Eradication of Group A streptococci
- Single dose benzathine penicillin G IM (first line) or oral penicillin V (500mg TID PO) for 10 days

3 Arthritis
- The arthritis in rheumatic fever almost always responds to aspirin within 72 hours, and should be continued until all joint symptoms have resolved

4 Carditis
- Treatment is mainly aimed at the management of heart failure, with fluid restriction, diuretics and ACE inhibitors
- Corticosteroids are sometimes recommended in patients with acute severe carditis with heart failure

5 Chorea
- Is usually self-limiting (weeks to months)

P ≫ Long-term secondary prophylaxis is recommended to prevent recurrence of acute rheumatic fever and development/progression of rheumatic heart disease. The WHO and AHA advise IM benzathine penicillin G every 3 to 4 weeks as the most effective therapy. Duration:
- If severe and debilitating chorea is present, carbamazepine or valproic acid are effective
- No carditis or valvular disease: 5 years or until age 18
- With carditis but no valvular disease: 10 years or until age 21
- With carditis and valvular heart disease: 10 years or until 40 years; some patients may require lifelong prophylaxis
- After valvular surgery: lifelong

1.7 Infective endocarditis

Definition: infective endocarditis (IE) refers to the infection of the endocardium and all its related structures, including cardiac valves and chordae tendineae. It may be acute, subacute or chronic.

Epidemiology:
- Males are predominantly affected
- May arise as a complication of rheumatic heart disease
- Most commonly occurs in older patients, and incidence argued to be increasing because of increased prevalence of medical intervention, prosthetic valves and intravenous drug users (IVDUs)

Aetiology/pathophysiology:
- Majority of cases occur secondary to infection
  - *Staph. aureus* is most common cause overall
  - *Strep. viridans* is the most common cause of subacute IE, and native valve endocarditis
  - Rare aetiological agents include the HACEK group: *Haemophilus, Actinobacillus, Cardiobacterium, Eikenella, Kingella*
- Non-infective causes include:
  - Systemic lupus erythematosus (SLE)
  - Autoimmune disorders, malignancy
- **Risk factors** for the development of IE include advancing age, being male, **dental procedures**, intravenous drug use, structural heart disease, prosthetic heart valves and immunodeficiency.

P ≫ Libman–Sacks endocarditis (LSE) is a type of non-bacterial thrombotic endocarditis (NBTE) characterised by valvular vegetations that might be seen in patients with SLE. A helpful way to remember this is that SLE causes LSE.

Clinical features:
- The presentation of IE is highly variable and depends on the microorganism involved. Some features are:
  - Fever (most common symptom), rigors, night sweats
  - Embolic phenomena (e.g. to the lung, brain or spleen)
  - New or changing heart murmur

W ≫ Normally, the valvular endothelium is resistant to bacterial colonisation. IE is usually preceded by endocardial injury and bacteraemia with a suitably pathogenic organism, which then 'buries' into a protective matrix of platelets and fibrin, forming vegetation, usually on valvular surfaces.

- – 'Textbook' stigmata of IE are rare – these include Roth spots, splinter haemorrhages (see *Fig. 1.14*), Osler nodes (see *Fig. 1.15*) and Janeway lesions (see *Fig. 1.16*)
- The **modified Duke Criteria** is the gold standard diagnostic tool and is both sensitive (92%) and specific (99%) for IE

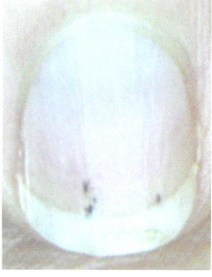

Fig. 1.14 *Splinter haemorrhages.*

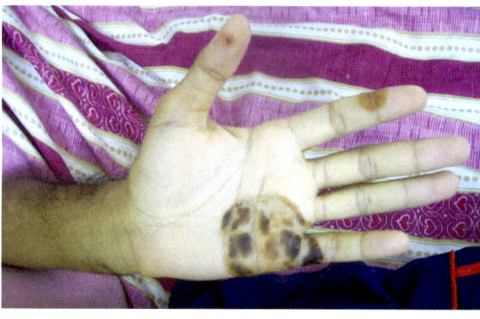

Fig. 1.15 *Osler node.*

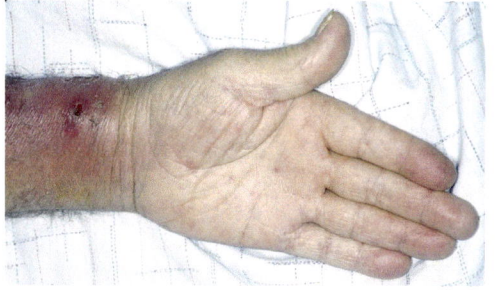

Fig. 1.16 *Janeway lesions.*

Investigations (ESC 2009)

Investigations should be undertaken in the following order.

Stepwise plan:

1 Obtain blood cultures
- First-line investigation and most important lab test
- **Three** sets of blood cultures, taken at least 12 hours apart

2 Arrange echocardiography
- Key investigation
- Transthoracic echocardiography (TTE) is the best initial choice, but transoesophageal echocardiography should be performed if clinical suspicion remains
- Hallmark finding is an oscillating irregular mass/vegetation (see *Fig. 1.17*)

3 Arrange other investigations
- Blood tests (FBC, U&Es, ESR/CRP, LFTs)
- Urinalysis (looking for haematuria and proteinuria)
- CXR and ECG
- Dental evaluation

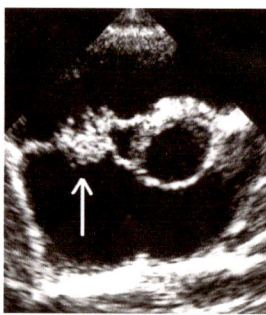

Fig. 1.17 *Vegetation on the tricuspid valve seen on a transoesophageal echocardiogram.*

E ≫ The modified Duke criteria can be remembered using the mnemonic '**BE PVP FIT**'. The diagnosis of definite IE can be made if there are: 2 major criteria **or** 1 major and 3 minor criteria **or** 5 minor criteria.

Major criteria:
Blood cultures
- Two or more separate blood cultures demonstrating typical organisms, e.g. *Strep. viridans*, *Staph. aureus*
- Two positive cultures >12 hours apart **or** three positive cultures **or** a majority of ≥4 positive blood cultures ≥1 hour apart

1

- Serology: single positive blood culture for *C. burnetii* **or** an antiphase 1 IgG antibody titre of ≥1/800

Echocardiography
- Positive echo demonstrating oscillating mass, abscess or dehiscence of prosthetic valve
- New valvular regurgitation

Minor criteria:
Positive blood culture or echo findings not met in major criteria
Vascular phenomena (e.g. arterial emboli)
Predisposing heart disease
Fever >38°C
Immunological phenomena (e.g. glomerulonephritis, Osler nodes, RF)
Tests (e.g. PCR)

Stepwise management of infective endocarditis (ESC 2009)

1   IV antibiotics
- Empirical treatment of **native** valves: e.g. vancomycin (or flucloxacillin) with gentamicin; duration of 4–6 weeks

- Empirical treatment of **prosthetic** valves: vancomycin with gentamicin with rifampicin; duration at least 6 weeks
- **Fungal** endocarditis should be treated using flucytosine IV with fluconazole orally; amphotericin B may be needed in some cases

2   Surgical management
- Consider in:
  - Acute MR or AR with heart failure
  - Persistent bacteraemia or valve dysfunction
  - Fungal endocarditis
  - Prosthetic valve endocarditis
  - Recurrent emboli
  - Annular abscess

E ≫ The efficacy of antimicrobial prophylaxis against IE is unknown and remains a highly controversial area. Since 2008, NICE has advised against antibiotic prophylaxis for any dental, gastrointestinal, genitourinary or respiratory tract procedure.

P ≫ Patients with a culture positive for *Strep. gallolyticus* (previously known as *Strep. bovis*) should also be investigated with colonoscopy, as this organism is associated with concomitant colorectal tumours.

1.8 Arrhythmias

Approach to arrhythmias

Arrhythmia is the term given to any disorder of heart rhythm. The following algorithm is a helpful systematic approach for any arrhythmia:

1. Check rhythm: regular or irregular? (Map P–P and R–R intervals)
2. Look at the **heart rate** – is there a **tachycardia** (>100bpm) or **bradycardia** (<60bpm)?
3. If it is a **bradycardia** and
   - symptomatic, suspect an **AV** block
   - asymptomatic, consider sinus bradycardia, but AV block should still be ruled out
4. If it is a **tachycardia**, examine whether it is **narrow complex** (QRS <0.12s) or **broad complex** (QRS >0.12s)
   - Narrow complex tachycardias are **generally** supraventricular in origin
5. P wave: always present? One per QRS complex?
6. PR interval (0.12s–0.2s)

7. QRS complex: duration (<0.12s), voltage, Q waves
8. ST segment: isoelectric, elevated or depressed
9. QT interval (QTc <0.44s)
   - As a very general rule of thumb, all broad complex tachycardias should be considered ventricular in origin, as these patients are commonly haemodynamically unstable
10. Check for missing or extra beats

1.8.1 Bradycardias

Definition: bradycardia is defined as a heart rate that is less than 60 beats per minute in adults, though some dispute this and define it as a heart rate less than 50 beats per minute. It occurs in the setting of a normal sinus rhythm.

Aetiology/pathophysiology:
- Bradycardia may be **physiological** in athletes and young people, and is common during sleep

- Medications such as beta blockers, calcium channel blockers, anti-arrhythmics and digoxin may cause bradycardia
- Infiltrative disease, infection (e.g. myocarditis), sick sinus syndrome (see later section) and metabolic abnormalities (hypothyroidism, hypothermia) may also cause bradycardia

> **P** ≫ The pathophysiology leading to bradycardia may be multifactorial: **intrinsic** disease occurs as a result of ageing or ischaemic disease, while **extrinsic** factors such as drugs and metabolic imbalances suppress SA node activity by reducing automaticity via vagal stimulation.

> **W** ≫ The SA nodal artery is a branch of the right coronary artery (RCA) in 90% of the population. Thus, an inferior myocardial infarction, for example, may lead to ischaemia of the SA node and sinus bradycardia.

1.8.1.1 Sinus bradycardia

Clinical features:
- Physiological causes of sinus bradycardia are asymptomatic
- Pathological causes may result in dizziness, fatigue and syncope

Investigations
Investigations should be undertaken in the following order.

> **Stepwise plan:**
>
> **1 Obtain an ECG (see *Fig. 1.18*)**
> - First-line investigation
> - If symptoms are potentially intermittent, consider **ambulatory** monitoring
>
> **2 Arrange electrolytes, thyroid function tests and toxicology**
> - To exclude any other underlying causes

> **Stepwise management of bradycardia**
>
> **1 Symptoms and heart rate**
> - Management depends on clinical assessment of the patient and the risk of asystole
> - Clinical assessment, level of consciousness, dizziness, BP (<90mmHg) HR (<40bpm), any ventricular arrhythmias, signs of heart failure
> - Risk of asystole: recent asystole, Mobitz II heart block, complete heart block with wide QRS, ventricular pause >3s
> - If there are any adverse signs on clinical assessment or there is a risk of asystole, first-line management is to give atropine
>
> **2 Atropine**
> - 0.5mg IV may be used in symptomatic patients, repeated up to a maximum of 3mg

> **P** ≫ Beta blocker overdose or toxicity may produce hypotension and bradycardia if symptomatic. High-dose glucagon (for which no upper limit has been defined; watch for symptomatic improvement) is first line. Calcium channel blocker toxicity is treated with calcium and adrenaline.

> **3 Other therapies**
> If patients do not respond to atropine, consider:
> - Isoprenaline or adrenaline infusion
> - Temporary pacing (emergency: temporary transcutaneous followed by transvenous pacing – although both rarely required)

1.8.1.2 Sick sinus syndrome

Definition: sick sinus syndrome refers to a syndrome of SA node dysfunction that encompasses, either singularly or in combination, sinus bradycardia, sinoatrial block (see *Fig. 1.19*) or sinus pause (see *Fig. 1.20*).

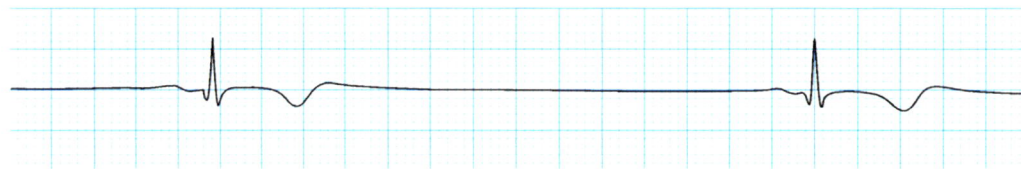

Fig. 1.18 *Sinus bradycardia.*

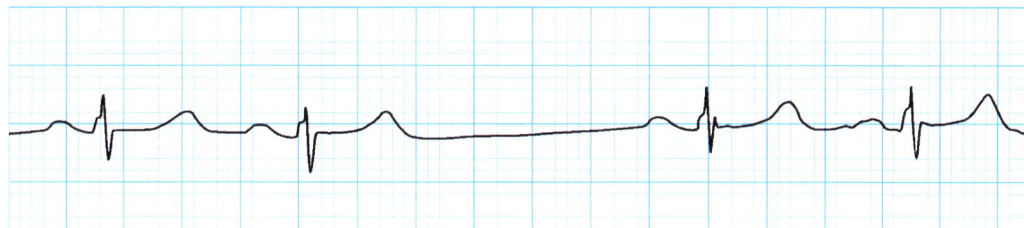

Fig. 1.19 *Sinus node exit block. There is a missing P wave. The sinus node has 'fired' but the impulse has failed to propagate into the atrium.*

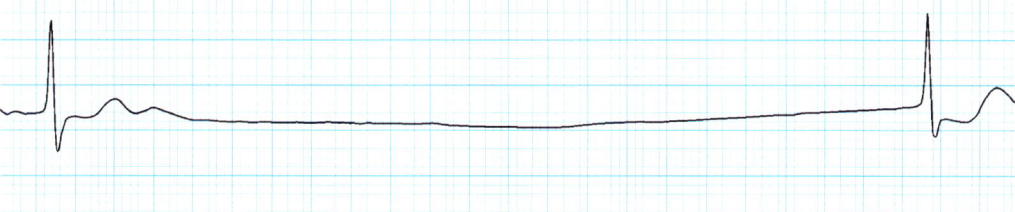

Fig. 1.20 *A long sinus pause (>3s) is seen as a result of SA node failure; the subsequent beat is a junctional escape.*

Aetiology/pathophysiology:

- The most common cause is idiopathic fibrosis of the SA node
- It may also be caused by infiltrative, metabolic and ischaemic conditions as well as drugs

Clinical features:

- This condition may present with associated paroxysmal atrial arrhythmias (e.g. atrial tachycardia, AF, or flutter), giving rise to tachy-brady syndrome
- Tachy-brady syndrome may present with dizziness, palpitations, syncope or chest pain

Management

- Management involves treating the underlying cause, where possible
- IV atropine and temporary pacing may be useful in patients with severe symptoms

> **P** >> Holter monitoring can be used to detect paroxysmal arrhythmias. It is an outpatient ECG recorder, small enough to be carried around by the patient, and is usually attached for 24, 48 or 72 hours. Data is usually produced for leads V1, V3 and V5. Patients are advised to keep the electrodes dry (e.g. avoiding showers during the test period).

Guidelines (NICE 2014, TA324)

NICE recommends dual-chamber pacemaker implantation for all patients with symptomatic bradycardia due to sick sinus syndrome, with or without the presence of AV conduction block.

1.8.1.3 Atrioventricular conduction blocks

First-degree heart block: first-degree heart block is characterised by delayed atrioventricular conduction, resulting in a **prolonged** PR interval (see *Fig. 1.21*). This may be due to idiopathic degeneration of the conduction system, ischaemia or drug related, but it can be physiological in athletes or during sleep. The condition is usually asymptomatic, and treatment is not usually required.

Second-degree heart block: second-degree heart block involves intermittent failure of atrioventricular conduction, resulting in dropped beats.

Mobitz type I (Wenckebach block): this involves successive prolongation of the PR interval until a beat is dropped (see *Fig. 1.22*). Treatment is generally not indicated unless symptoms are severe.

Mobitz type II: this involves an AV conduction deficit that results in intermittent dropped beats without changes in the PR interval (see *Fig. 1.23*), and may have a fixed ratio block (e.g. 2:1, 3:1). Patients with Mobitz type II second-degree heart block may present with dizziness, syncope or sudden cardiac death.

Haemodynamic compromise should be treated with IV atropine initially, failing which adrenaline or isoprenaline may be used IV. In emergency situations, temporary pacing (transcutaneous, then transvenous) may be attempted.

> **E** ≫ A permanent pacemaker is indicated for this condition in all patients, even those who are asymptomatic.

Third-degree (complete) heart block:
third-degree (or complete) heart block refers to complete failure of AV conduction, causing the atria and ventricles to beat asynchronously (see *Fig. 1.24*). Common causes include idiopathic degeneration of the conduction system or anterior/inferior MIs.

Clinical features: patients may present with symptoms of low cardiac output (a result of low ventricular rate) – dizziness, syncope, breathlessness or Stokes-Adams attacks.

> **P** ≫ Stokes–Adams attacks involve transient episodes of syncope, characterised by a sudden unexpected collapse, up to several minutes of unconsciousness, and then rapid recovery, and are caused by paroxysmal arrhythmias.

Palpitations or intermittent **cannon A waves** on JVP may be observed on examination. These waves occur

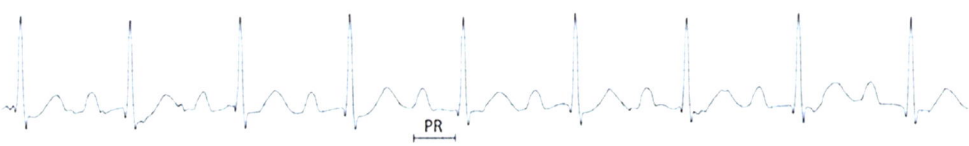

Fig. 1.21 *First-degree heart block.*

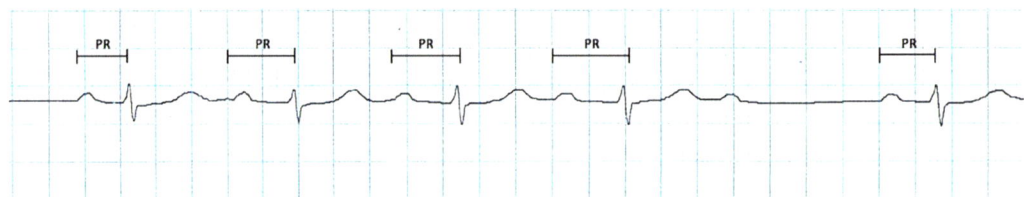

Fig. 1.22 *Wenckebach block.*

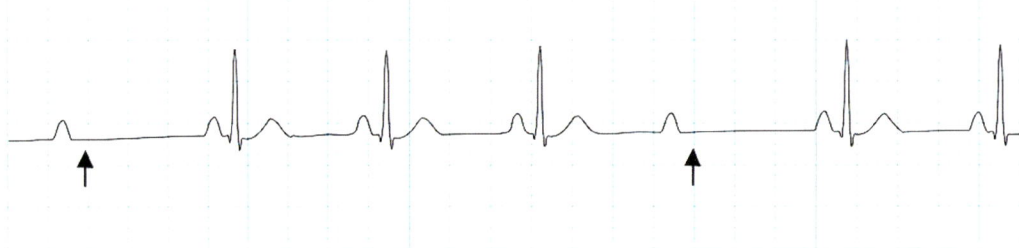

Fig. 1.23 *Mobitz type II; arrows point to P waves with blocked AV conduction.*

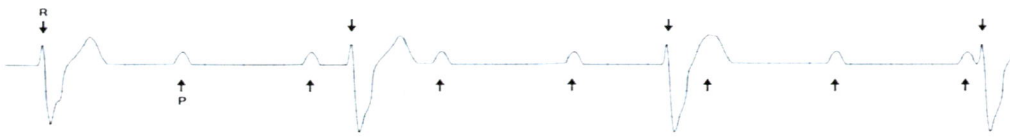

Fig. 1.24 *Complete heart block; note that the P wave (atrial) and ORS complexes (ventricular) are independent of each other.*

as a result of contraction of the right atrium against a closed tricuspid valve.

Management: all patients should have a permanent pacemaker implanted if no reversible causes are identified. Management of symptomatic and emergency bradycardia remains the same.

1.8.1.4 Bundle branch blocks

Definition: the bundle of His splits into the left and right bundle branches, and these subsequently divide into Purkinje fibres, which transmit electrical impulses to ventricular myocytes, resulting in depolarisation and then contraction.

> ⓦ ≫ Left or right bundle branch block is the result of a delay or block in one of these bundles, delaying depolarisation of the ipsilateral ventricle, which must then be depolarised indirectly via the other bundle branch. This delayed ventricular depolarisation results in widening of the QRS complex and asynchronous ventricular contraction, reducing cardiac output.

Right bundle branch block (RBBB)

RBBB causes a delay in right ventricular depolarisation. While it may be a normal variant, it is commonly associated with RVH, right heart strain and pulmonary stenosis or emboli.

A simple diagnostic approach for LBBB or RBBB is to remember the name William Morrow. For LBBB, the QRS looks like a 'W' in V1 and an 'M' in V6 (WiLLiaM; see *Fig. 1.25*). In RBBB, the QRS looks like an 'M' in lead V1 and a 'W' in lead V6 (MoRRoW; see *Fig. 1.26*).

Left bundle branch block (LBBB)

LBBB invariably indicates underlying pathology, such as IHD, cardiomyopathy or LV hypertrophy.

> ⓦ ≫ Left bundle branch blocks may be divided into left anterior fascicular blocks (LAFB) and left posterior fascicular blocks (LPFB) (also known as hemiblock).
> Bifascicular block: RBBB + LAFB/LPFB
> Trifascicular block: bifascicular block + prolongation of PR interval

Clinical features: a new LBBB on ECG, particularly if associated with chest pain, warrants clinical suspicion of an acute myocardial infarction.

Investigations

Investigations for a newly discovered LBBB include echocardiography and a coronary angiogram.

Management: management of trifascicular block requires a permanent pacemaker, and sometimes for bifascicular block.

1.8.2 Tachycardias

Definition: the majority of tachycardias seen in clinical practice are narrow complex in nature, and generally supraventricular in origin (i.e. they originate from the atria, SA or AV node).

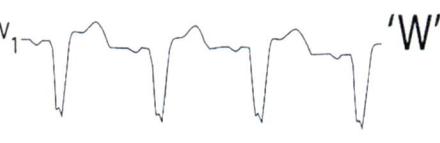
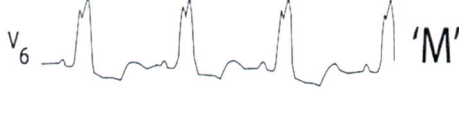

Fig. 1.25 *Dominant broad S wave in V₁ and rSR' pattern in V₆ (WiLLiaM).*

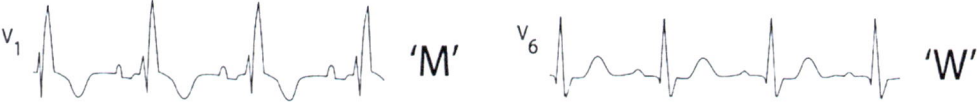

Fig. 1.26 *Typical rSR' in V₁ and wide slurred S wave in V₆ (MoRRoW).*

1

Narrow complex tachycardia

1.8.2.1 Sinus tachycardia

Definition: sinus tachycardia is an increase of the heart rate to more than 100bpm with normal sinus rhythm (see *Fig. 1.27*). Sinus tachycardia may be physiological and occur during exercise, but it may occur as a result of a myriad of pathological processes. These include (but are not limited to) pulmonary embolism, ischaemic heart disease, hyperthyroidism, infection, substance abuse and other conditions. Patients may complain of palpitations, shortness of breath or dizziness.

Management: management involves treating the underlying cause. Beta blockers may be used in chronic cases. Radiofrequency ablation is performed if the patient is refractory to medical therapy, but this is rarely required.

1.8.2.2 Atrial fibrillation (AF)

Definition: AF is characterised by very rapid and uncoordinated atrial activity that results in an irregularly irregular rhythm. While the rhythm is in and of itself benign, its sequelae are not, and can have important electromechanical consequences.

Epidemiology:
- Commonest cardiac rhythm disorder with an estimated worldwide prevalence of 2.8%
- Ageing is the most consistent independent risk factor for AF; >70% of patients are >65 years old
- Can affect 3–6% of those admitted to hospital

 E >> Classifying AF (see *Fig. 1.28*):
- Acute: <48 hours
- Paroxysmal: <7 days, self-limiting episode, may recur
- Persistent: >7 days, not self-limiting, may become permanent
- Permanent: more than 1 year, resistant to treatment

Aetiology/pathophysiology:

 P >> **Causes of atrial fibrillation**
Remember the mnemonic '**ATRIALE-PIBI**':
Alcohol and caffeine
Thyrotoxicosis
Rheumatic fever and mitral valve pathology
Ischaemic heart disease
Atrial myxoma
Lungs (pulmonary hypertension)
Electrolyte disturbances
Pharmacological
Iatrogenic
Blood pressure
Infections

Binge drinking may also prompt an episode of AF, which is usually self-limiting. This is known as **holiday heart syndrome.**

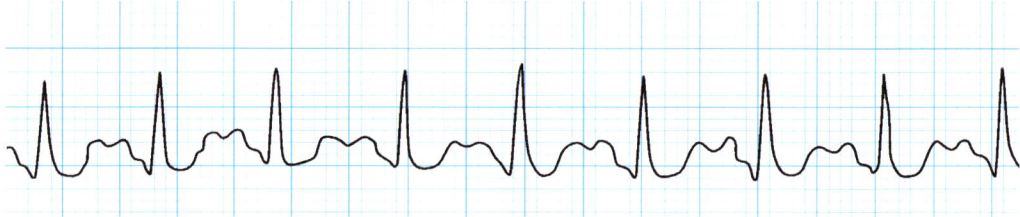

Fig. 1.27 *Sinus tachycardia. Note the 'camel hump' appearance, as a result of the fusion of preceding T waves onto the next P waves.*

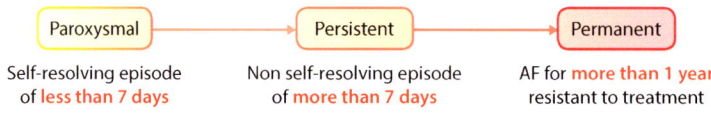

Fig. 1.28 *Types of AF (temporal classification).*

Clinical features:

- Patients may be **asymptomatic**
- NICE recommends performing manual pulse palpation to assess for the presence of an irregularly irregular pulse that may indicate AF in patients presenting with any of the following: (NICE 2014, CG180)
  - Breathlessness/dyspnoea
  - Palpitations
  - Syncope/dizziness
  - Chest discomfort
  - Stroke/TIA (2006)

Investigations (NICE 2014, CG180)

Investigations should be undertaken in the following order.

Stepwise plan:

1 **Obtain an ECG (see *Fig.1.29*)**
- First-line investigation
- Perform whether or not patient is symptomatic, particularly if irregularly irregular pulse has been detected
- Holter monitor may be used for patients with suspected paroxysmal AF

W ≫ AF is often 'triggered' by an **ectopic focal firing** which usually arises from the pulmonary veins. Maintenance of AF occurs by one of three mechanisms:
- One or more rapidly discharging atrial foci
- One or a small number of **primary re-entry circuits** (called rotors)
- Multiple functional re-entry circuits

This electrical activity is disorganised, and the atria fibrillate rather than contract, leading to pooling of blood (particularly in the left atrial appendage) and a **predisposition to thrombus formation or emboli**. AF also reduces cardiac output by up to 20%.

2 **Arrange blood tests**
- To identify underlying cause
- FBC (leucocytosis for infection, anaemia), U&Es (hypokalaemia, hypomagnesaemia), LFTs
- **TFTs**

3 **Obtain echocardiography**
- This allows assessment of LV systolic function, mitral valve, LA size (a dilated LA provides the substrate for persistent AF) and the presence of an intracardiac thrombus
- Arrange transthoracic echo if:
  - Consideration of rhythm control including cardioversion
  - High suspicion of structural heart disease
  - Additional information needed for anticoagulation risk stratification
- Arrange a transoesophageal echo if TTE is difficult or inadequate or demonstrates an abnormality that requires further imaging

4 **Arrange assessment of need for/risks of anticoagulation**

Management of atrial fibrillation (NICE 2014, CG180): general principles:

treatment goals include **treating any underlying cause** (including addressing **heart failure**), **controlling the arrhythmia** and providing **adequate thromboprophylaxis**.

P ≫ Do not offer aspirin monotherapy to patients with AF solely for stroke prevention.

E ≫ Synchronised DC cardioversion refers to the process of administering an electrical shock that synchronises with the QRS complex (because shocking during repolarisation (R wave) may precipitate VF), in order to restore sinus rhythm. Defibrillation refers to administration of a shock that isn't in synchrony with the QRS in order to return the heart to sinus rhythm (e.g. pulseless VT or VF).

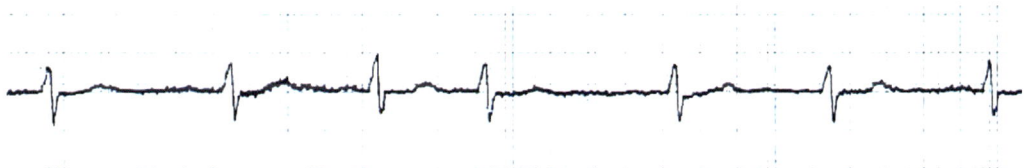

Fig. 1.29 *Atrial fibrillation – irregularly irregular rhythm and missing P waves.*

Table 1.8 CHA$_2$DS$_2$Vasc and HAS-BLED scores

CHA$_2$DS$_2$Vasc to assess risk of stroke	HAS-BLED to assess risk of bleeding if on therapy
C – History of congestive heart failure (1)	H – Hypertension (SBP >160mmHg) (1)
H – Hypertension (1)	A – Abnormal liver/renal function (1 point each)
A – Age (65–74 = 1, ≥75 = 2)	S – Stroke history (1)
D – Diabetes	B – Bleeding history/predisposition (1)
S – Stroke, venous thromboembolism (2)	L – Labile INR (1)
S – Sex (Female = 1)	E – Elderly (>65)
Vasc – Vascular disease (1)	D – Drugs (NSAIDs, antiplatelets) or alcohol (1)
• *Score of 0 in men or 1 in women, recommend no anticoagulation* • *Score of ≥1 in men, consider anticoagulation* • *If score of ≥2, offer anticoagulation*	• *Score ≥3 does not preclude anticoagulation, but caution is warranted, with regular review*

Treating acute atrial fibrillation

 ≫ Carry out immediate synchronised DC cardioversion in patients presenting with new onset AF and haemodynamic instability, with no need for anticoagulation.

Patients with AF for <48h

Haemodynamically stable individuals with atrial fibrillation for less than 48 hours should be anticoagulated with heparin, and may be cardioverted electrically or pharmacologically (using flecainide in the absence of structural heart disease, and amiodarone if it is present).

 ≫ If AF is present for >48 hours, it carries with it an increased (up to 5%) risk of embolism after cardioversion – hence the rationale for anticoagulation. At this point, options also include transoesophageal echocardiography (to look for an intracardiac thrombus). If no thrombus is present on echocardiography, the patient may be heparinised and cardioverted within the next 24 hours. Note that anticoagulation should **continue** after cardioversion for 3–4 weeks. After this time, and if the patient remains in sinus rhythm, the anticoagulation may be stopped.

Patients with AF for >48h

In patients with atrial fibrillation that has been present for longer than 48 hours (or an uncertain time period)

and if the patient is considered a good candidate for long-term rhythm control, delay cardioversion until they have been maintained on therapeutic anticoagulation for a minimum of 3 weeks. During this period, offer rate control as appropriate. NICE also recommends using electrical, rather than pharmacological, cardioversion for AF that has persisted for longer than 48 hours.

In addition, in high-risk individuals, consider amiodarone or dronedarone therapy for up to 4 weeks before cardioversion and up to 12 months after. A broad flowchart may help summarise the management of AF (based on CG180) – see *Appendix 1*.

Stepwise management of chronic atrial fibrillation

There are, very broadly speaking, two treatment modalities in the approach to atrial fibrillation – rate and rhythm control.

1 Rate or rhythm control?
- NICE recommends offering **rate control** as a **first-line strategy, UNLESS**:
  - There is a reversible cause
  - New onset AF
  - Heart failure is present
  - Rhythm control is more suitable, based on clinical judgment
  a. Rate control
    - Offer a **beta blocker** (except sotalol) or a rate-limiting calcium channel blocker as monotherapy first line, considering symptoms and comorbidities

1

- If monotherapy does not control symptoms, offer combination therapy with any two of:
  - Beta blocker
  - Diltiazem
  - Digoxin

b. Rhythm control
- This is generally preferred if patients have concomitant heart failure or in younger patients (<65 years of age), but AF frequently recurs after restoration of sinus rhythm
- Offer a beta blocker for long-term rhythm control

P ≫ Note that beta blockers are used as both rate and rhythm control strategies in atrial fibrillation. Digoxin is recommended as an alternative first-line monotherapy if there is concomitant heart failure or if the patient is very sedentary (this may vary between centres).

2   Anticoagulation
- Anticoagulation should be offered after consideration of stroke and bleeding risk (see scores in preceding section)
- Warfarin or novel oral anticoagulants (NOACs), e.g. dabigatran, apixaban or rivaroxaban
- INR targets for patients are 2–3, with targets set higher (2.5–3.5) if patients have had recurrent thromboembolic events on anticoagulation, or if a metallic mitral valve is present
- The use of NOACs has not been validated in 'valvular AF', i.e. patients with mechanical heart valves, those with RHD or mitral stenosis, and in those with moderate/severe heart failure who are likely to require a valve replacement in the future; until further evidence emerges, warfarin should be used in these patients

- Bleeding risks with NOACs are largely confined to the GI tract (particularly dabigatran in the elderly), whereas bleeds with warfarin tend to be intracranial

3   Electrophysiological therapy
- Radiofrequency ablation may be offered in intractable cases of atrial fibrillation that do not respond to medical therapy

W ≫ One of the most important properties of the AV node is decremental conduction. This property refers to the innate ability of the AV node to conduct impulses to the ventricles far slower as it receives increasingly faster signals from the atria. This is also why atrial fibrillation does not, in the vast majority of cases and in the absence of an accessory pathway, lead to ventricular fibrillation.

1.8.2.3 Atrial flutter

Definition: atrial flutter is an atrial tachyarrhythmia characterised by a regular, rapid atrial rate. It has many similarities with AF, but is less common. Flutter may be caused by ischaemic heart disease, right atrial dilatation (e.g. pulmonary embolus, valvular heart disease or heart failure) or certain medications. Atrial flutter may have no discernible cardiac cause in up to one-third of patients.

Clinical features:
- Atrial flutter occurs secondary to a macro re-entrant circuit, most commonly revolving around the tricuspid annulus in an anti-clockwise fashion
- This results in a rapid atrial rate of approximately 300bpm, producing characteristic 'saw tooth' waves on ECG (F waves, see *Fig. 1.30*)
- As with AF, the filtering ability of the AV node determines the ventricular rate, with conduction usually 2:1 (i.e. HR 150bpm or 4:1 (75bpm) and rarely 1:1 (300bpm)
- It should always be suspected in tachycardias with a **fixed** conduction ratio (2:1)

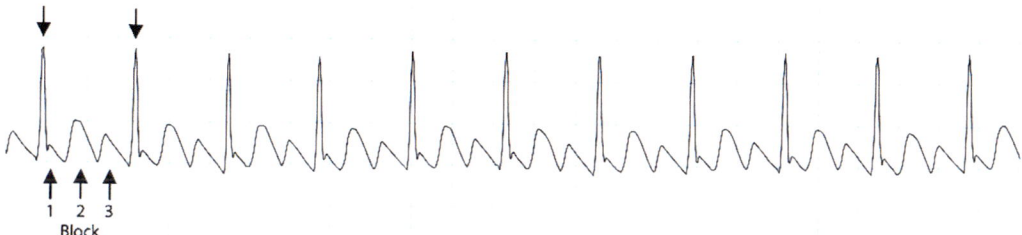

1 2 3
Block

Fig. 1.30 Atrial flutter.

1

Investigations

- Investigation and management of atrial flutter is similar to that of atrial fibrillation (including anticoagulation for stroke prevention), but it should be noted that achieving rate control in flutter is more difficult
- 60% of patients with flutter present acutely, and cardioversion is recommended in this group
- Radiofrequency ablation is highly recommended in patients with chronic atrial flutter, as therapy can induce high rates of remission (90%)

1.8.2.4 Supraventricular tachycardia (SVT)

Definition: the term supraventricular tachycardia (SVT), broadly speaking, typically refers to paroxysmal episodes of tachycardia that are not ventricular in origin. These include atrioventricular nodal re-entrant tachycardia (AVNRT), atrioventricular re-entrant tachycardia (AVRT), atrial and junctional tachycardia.

Aetiology/pathophysiology:

- SVT is primarily caused by **re-entry mechanisms**, or **impulse initiation disorders**, producing automatic tachycardias
- Re-entrant tachycardias:
  - **AVNRT** – caused by a **non-anatomical pathway** involving dual pathways with **fast and slow conduction velocities**; typically, conduction via the slow pathway is anterograde, and the fast pathway is retrograde
  - **AVRT** – caused by an anatomically defined re-entrant circuit involving one or more accessory pathways (e.g. **Wolff–Parkinson–White syndrome**)

> **E** ≫ AVNRT is the most common type of SVT, accounting for up to 60%.

- Automatic tachycardias:
  - **Junctional tachycardia** – secondary to abnormal impulses from the junctional region, usually from the AV node or bundle of His
  - **Atrial tachycardia** – a tachycardia that is initiated and maintained irrespective of the SA node, AV junction, accessory pathways or ventricular tissue

> **P** ≫ Multifocal atrial tachycardia (MAT) is an arrhythmia caused by three or more ectopic regions of atrial tissue. It presents with variable P waves and P–R intervals and is commonly associated with **lung disease, classically COPD**. Verapamil or metoprolol are commonly used first line.

Clinical features:

- A range of symptoms may be observed, from palpitations and dizziness to breathlessness and chest discomfort
- Haemodynamic compromise (e.g. low BP, altered consciousness) and syncope may occasionally occur

Investigations

Investigations should be undertaken in the following order.

> **Stepwise plan:**
>
> 1 **Obtain an ECG (see *Fig. 1.31*)**
> - First-line investigation
> - If symptoms are intermittent, consider **ambulatory** monitoring
>
> 2 **Arrange for electrolytes, thyroid function tests and toxicology**
> - To exclude any other underlying causes
> - Digoxin levels – digoxin may predispose to SVT

> **Stepwise management of supraventricular tachycardia (SVT)**
>
> 1 **Assess haemodynamic status**
> - If the patient is haemodynamically **unstable**, arrange for **sedation and urgent DC cardioversion**
> - If the patient is haemodynamically **stable**, proceed **to Step 2**
>
> 2 **Vagal manoeuvres**
> - Carotid sinus massage, Valsalva or facial immersion in cold water are recommended

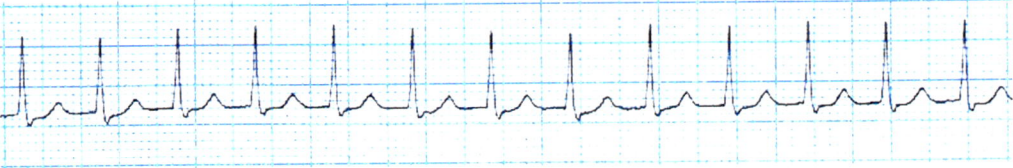

Fig. 1.31 *Supraventricular tachycardia. Note the rate of 150bpm and non-visible (buried) P waves.*

first line to attempt to terminate the arrhythmia

(E) ≫ Carotid sinus massage should be attempted with care in older individuals, particularly if they have an audible carotid bruit, because of the risk of precipitating an artery to artery embolic stroke.

3 Adenosine

If vagal manoeuvres are unsuccessful, prescribe IV adenosine (given rapidly via a large-bore cannula in the antecubital fossa, followed by a saline flush):
- Initially, 6mg bolus IV, 12mg if unsuccessful, then a further 12mg
- Offer IV verapamil as an alternative if adenosine is contraindicated (e.g. asthma)
- If administration of adenosine is unsuccessful, consider the use of digoxin, beta blocker or amiodarone; if medical therapy remains unsuccessful, attempt synchronised DC cardioversion

(W) ≫ Administration of adenosine may prove to be unpleasant for some patients, as it is associated with chest tightness, an 'impending sense of doom', breathlessness and discomfort. It is helpful to warn the patient about these side effects before administering the drug.

4 Radiofrequency ablation
- May be used as a curative therapy
- Generally reserved for patients who are refractory to anti-arrhythmic therapy or for whom drug therapy is contraindicated

1.8.2.5 Wolff–Parkinson–White syndrome

Definition: Wolff–Parkinson–White syndrome (WPW), results from an accessory pathway (i.e. a conducting pathway between the atrium and ventricle) known as the bundle of Kent. This pathway can conduct in both an antegrade (i.e. atrium to ventricle) and retrograde fashion.

(E) ≫ Classic ECG features of WPW (but may not be present, see *Fig. 1.32*):
- Short PR interval (<0.2s)
- Broad QRS (>0.12s)
- Delta wave – slurring of the QRS upstroke

Clinical features:
- There are two types of WPW – Type A and Type B
- As a general rule, Type A typically presents with upright delta waves and a QRS complex in V1
- Type B generally presents with a negative delta wave and QRS complex in V1

(W) ≫ Accessory pathway conduction is faster than AV nodal conduction (because the AV node briefly delays depolarisation). Thus, ventricular depolarisation usually happens early via the pathway (pre-excitation), and is then followed by normal AV nodal depolarisation. Patients with accessory pathways are more likely to develop AF. If antegrade conduction occurs via the accessory pathway (and not the AV node), this will lead to pre-excited AF, which is very dangerous because pre-excited AF may degenerate into VF.

Management: catheter ablation of the accessory pathway usually provides definitive treatment. Note that drugs that block AV conduction (e.g. digoxin and calcium channel blockers) are contraindicated in WPW syndrome, because they promote conduction through the accessory pathway.

Broad complex tachycardias

Broad complex tachycardias combine, by definition, tachycardia (HR>100) with wide QRS complexes (>0.12s). They are often ventricular in origin, but may also be supraventricular with an aberrant conduction. They may be regular (monomorphic ventricular

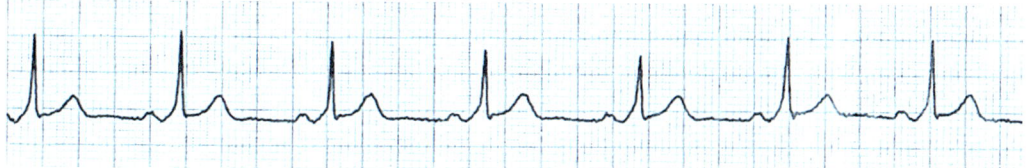

Fig. 1.32 *Upslurring 'delta' wave characteristic of Wolff–Parkinson–White syndrome.*

1

tachycardia) or irregular (torsades de pointes, polymorphic ventricular tachycardia) in nature.

1.8.2.6 Ventricular tachycardia (VT)

Definition: ventricular tachycardia (VT) is a tachyarrhythmia that originates from the ventricles, producing three or more successive broad QRS complexes at a rate of more than 100 beats per minute (see *Fig. 1.33*).

Epidemiology:
- VT and ventricular fibrillation (VF) are the most common causes of sudden cardiac death

Aetiology/pathophysiology: common causes include:
- Ischaemic heart disease
- Structural heart disease (e.g. cardiomyopathy)

> **P** ≫ Torsades de pointes, a form of polymorphic VT associated with a prolonged corrected QT interval, is French for 'twisting of the points' (see *Fig. 1.34*). Primary causes include congenital or acquired long QT syndrome, or electrolyte abnormalities or medications.

- Electrolyte abnormalities (e.g. potassium, magnesium)
- Medications (e.g. digoxin toxicity)
- The mechanisms underlying VT include:
  - Re-entrant circuit (most common) – usually due to myocardial scarring post MI

> **P** ≫ Unlike sustained monomorphic VT, which may be well tolerated, sustained polymorphic VT is not, and haemodynamic collapse is inevitable, necessitating urgent DC cardioversion. For patients with non-sustained polymorphic VT, management involves treating the underlying cause, e.g. by stopping a causative drug or correcting electrolyte abnormalities. Treatment also involves administration of IV magnesium or IV lidocaine, or pacing if the patient is resistant to drug therapy.

Clinical features:
- Haemodynamically stable patients may present with:
  - No symptoms
  - Palpitations
  - Dizziness
- Haemodynamically unstable patients may present severely hypotensive and tachycardic, and may have severe dyspnoea and dizziness or syncope, which may lead to cardiac arrest

> **Stepwise management of monomorphic ventricular tachycardia (VT)**
>
> **1 If the patient is haemodynamically unstable:**
> - Immediate resuscitation
> - Emergency synchronised DC cardioversion plus an IV amiodarone infusion (150–300mg)
> - ICD implantation should be considered once stable

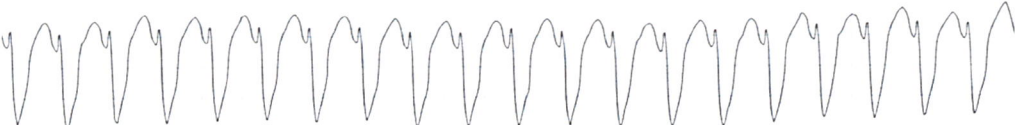

Fig. 1.33 *Monomorphic ventricular tachycardia.*

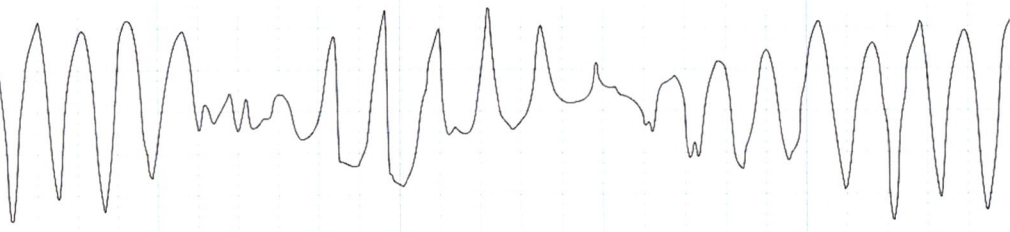

Fig. 1.34 *Torsades de pointes.*

2 If the patient is haemodynamically stable, the management depends on the underlying cause:

- IV amiodarone or IV lidocaine
- Overdrive pacing (transvenous pacing using a pacing wire in the RV and set at 15–20bpm faster than the VT) will terminate the rhythm in 80–90% of cases
- Synchronised DC cardioversion may be indicated if resistant to medical therapy

1.8.2.7 Brugada syndrome

Definition: Brugada syndrome is an autosomal sodium channelopathy associated with sudden cardiac death.

Epidemiology:
- It is **most prevalent in Asia**
- Has a high male predominance (8:1)

Clinical features:
- Defective sodium channels impair influx of sodium ions, resulting in shorter action potentials; ECG features are shown in *Figure 1.35*
- Brugada syndrome classically presents with **syncope** and **sudden cardiac arrest** (most likely secondary to VF) in a third of otherwise asymptomatic patients

Management: ICD implantation is the only definitive treatment.

1.8.2.8 Long QT syndrome

Definition: long QT syndrome refers to a group of inherited or acquired conditions characterised by prolongation of the corrected QT interval (QTc), which is calculated using Bazett's formula.

Aetiology/pathophysiology:
There are a vast number of causes of long QT syndrome, some of which include:
- Inherited mutations (LQT1 to LQT13; all variants of specific mutations)
  - Of these, LQT1 and LQT2 are the most common
- Electrolyte abnormalities, e.g.
  - Hypocalcaemia, hypokalaemia, hypomagnesaemia
- Medications, e.g.
  - Erythromycin, tricyclics, **methadone** and amiodarone
- Hypothermia

> **P** ≫ Jervell and Lange-Nielsen syndrome is an autosomal recessive variant of long QT syndrome associated with deafness. Romano–Ward syndrome is an autosomal dominant variant **not** associated with deafness.

Clinical features:
- Patients may present with syncope, sudden death or seizures
- Also at increased risk of developing **polymorphic ventricular tachycardia** (torsades de pointes)

Management: treatment involves avoidance of drugs that prolong the QT interval, and prevention of sudden cardiac death with ICDs if necessary.

1.8.2.9 Ventricular fibrillation (VF)

Definition: ventricular fibrillation (VF) refers to a rapid and uncoordinated life-threatening ventricular arrhythmia that results in haemodynamic collapse. If left untreated, it is a lethal arrhythmia and the

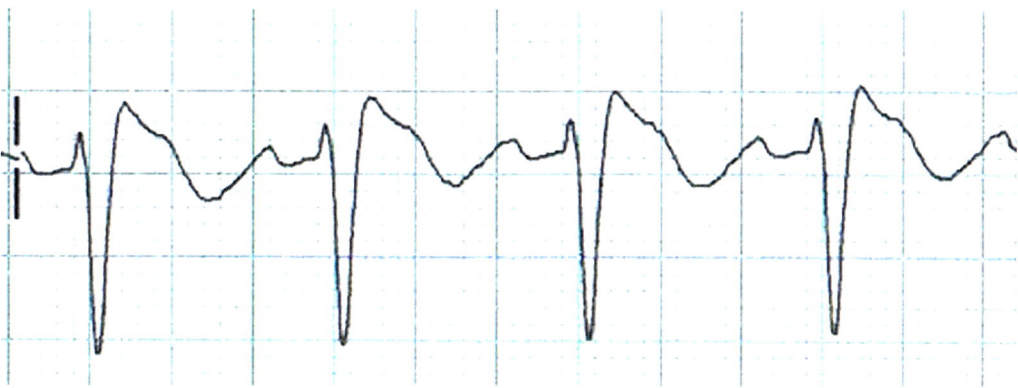

Fig. 1.35 *An ECG of Brugada syndrome showing 'Brugada' sign (downsloping coved ST elevation followed by an inverted T wave); note that this is only present in leads V1 and V2.*

1

patient will lose consciousness within 10–15 seconds of onset.

Epidemiology:

- 1–8% occur outside hospital and are usually fatal
- 90% of the deaths from acute MI are due to VF

Aetiology/pathophysiology:

- Common causes include:
  - Ischaemic heart disease (relatively common following an MI)
  - Electrolyte abnormalities (particularly hyperkalaemia)
  - Structural heart disease
- The pathogenesis of VF involves continuous micro re-entrant circuits forming within the ventricles and very rapid irregular electrical activity (see *Fig. 1.36*), resulting in unsynchronised, ineffective ventricular contractions and no cardiac output

Management:

- Immediate management:
  - Advanced cardiac life support (see *Chapter 12*)

> **P** ≫ Community survival rate is 5–33% depending on factors such as prompt, high-quality bystander CPR and duration of CPR to defibrillation time.

1.8.2.10 Extra beats

Definition: **premature atrial ectopics** are beats that originate from an ectopic focus within the atria, and are more common in patients with conditions that cause elevated atrial pressures (e.g. mitral valve disease, heart failure). These are usually benign, and represent a normal electrophysiological phenomenon (see *Fig. 1.37*). Patients who experience symptoms (dizziness, palpitations) may be offered beta blockers or calcium channel blockers.

Premature ventricular ectopics refer to beats originating from an ectopic focus within the ventricles. The incidence increases with age, and they are more common in patients with concomitant ischaemic heart disease. These are usually **benign** as well. However, as with premature atrial ectopics, they may present with palpitations in symptomatic individuals.

Investigations: patients with **recurrent** premature ventricular ectopics (not sustained episodes) should be evaluated for underlying heart disease, as this may increase the risk of arrhythmias and sudden death.

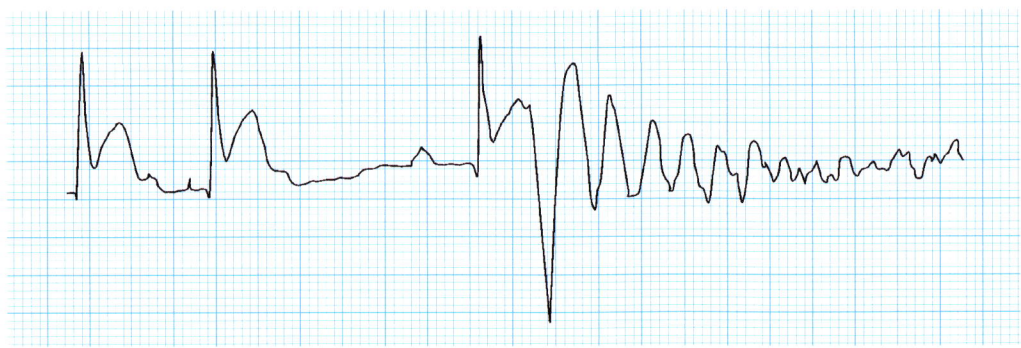

Fig. 1.36 *Ventricular fibrillation.*

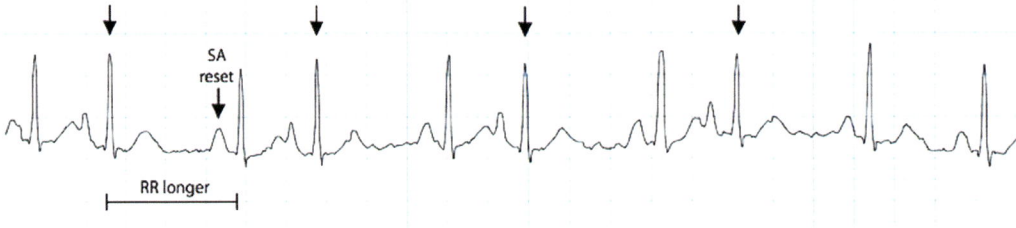

Fig. 1.37 *This rhythm strip shows premature atrial ectopics (arrows), followed by compensatory pauses.*

1.9 Cardiomyopathy

The cardiomyopathies are a diverse group of disorders that affect the heart muscle. The diseases often manifest as mechanical and/or electrical dysfunction, are often progressive, and the underlying cause is frequently genetic.

Although it is common practice, strictly speaking, the term **cardiomyopathy** should not be associated with other cardiovascular disorders (e.g. ischaemic cardiomyopathy or hypertensive cardiomyopathy) and should be restricted to conditions primarily involving the myocardium.

1.9.1 Dilated cardiomyopathy

Definition: dilated cardiomyopathy is characterised by dilatation and systolic dysfunction of the left and/or right ventricles (see *Fig. 1.38*). The left ventricle is frequently affected in isolation, and the ventricular walls may be abnormally thin.

Aetiology/pathophysiology: around 50% of cases are idiopathic, but several important associations exist:
- Chronic alcohol consumption
- Genetic (at least 20% are familial)
- Viral infections
- Hypothyroidism
- Peripartum cardiomyopathy
- Chemotherapy (e.g. doxorubicin, trastuzumab/Herceptin)

Clinical features:
- Patients may present with symptoms of heart failure, dyspnoea and thromboembolism
- Or patients may be asymptomatic

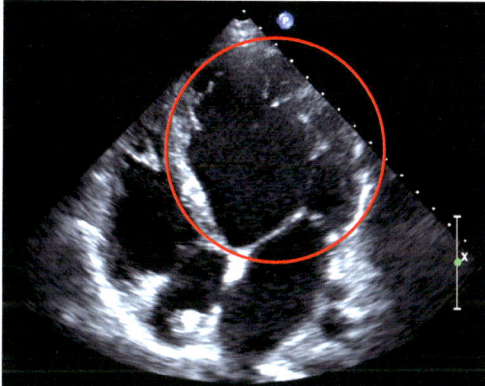

Fig. 1.38 *Echocardiogram showing significant left ventricular dilatation.*

E ≫ It is important to rule out alcohol as an aetiological factor because dilated cardiomyopathy that is secondary to chronic alcohol consumption is potentially reversible.

Management: echocardiography is the gold standard investigation, and patients may require management of heart failure symptoms and anticoagulation. Some patients may need an ICD or CRT.

1.9.2 Hypertrophic cardiomyopathy

Definition: hypertrophic cardiomyopathy (HCM) is the most common genetic cardiac disorder and is inherited in an **autosomal dominant** fashion (although around 50% of cases are sporadic). It is characterised by asymmetrical left ventricular hypertrophy and **diastolic** dysfunction.

W ≫ HCM involves narrowing of the left ventricular outflow tract due to a thickened interventricular septum. The anterior mitral valve is sucked towards the hypertrophied septum, which may lead to obstruction. This is known as systolic anterior motion (SAM) of the mitral valve. These patients are prone to mitral regurgitation, but this is not a major feature of this condition.

Aetiology/pathophysiology:
- Increased prevalence in **males** and **Afro-Caribbean/Asian patients**
- Obstructive form i.e. hypertrophic obstructive cardiomyopathy (HOCM) is seen in 25% of cases; other cases are non-obstructive
- Most common cause of sudden death in patients under 35 years old
- Genetic

Clinical features:
- Most people with hypertrophic cardiomyopathy are **asymptomatic**
- May present with angina, dyspnoea or syncope if left ventricular outflow tract (LVOT) obstruction occurs
- Sudden death is usually caused by arrhythmias or severe LVOT obstruction

1

P ≫ The majority of mutations are mis-sense mutations, related to genes encoding for myocardial contractile proteins, particularly cardiac troponins T and I, as well as myosin regulatory light chains. Troponin T mutations, in particular, result in a high risk of sudden death (and may not be associated with regional wall thickening). Beta myosin heavy chain defects are the most common type of defect.

E ≫ Valsalva manoeuvre (forced expiration against a closed glottis) reduces venous return to the heart and will increase the murmur intensity by bringing the hypertrophied septum closer to the mitral valve and increasing obstruction to blood flow. In contrast, the murmur of aortic stenosis will decrease in intensity as flow is reduced.

Investigations:
- Echocardiography is gold standard – dilatation is not seen; most patients have a thickened interventricular septum (see *Fig. 1.39*)
- Increased septal wall thickness is associated with a poorer prognosis

Stepwise management of hypertrophic cardiomyopathy

  1   Manage the LVOT and SAM:
- Avoid volume depletion as this worsens LVOT obstruction
- Administer beta blockers or rate-limiting calcium channel blockers first line

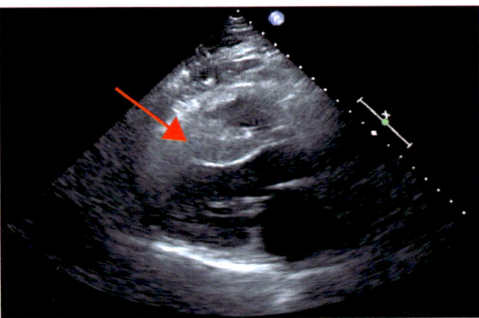

Fig. 1.39 Long-axis view on echocardiogram showing a thicker-walled left ventricle.

- Surgical myectomy is recommended for patients who are unresponsive to best medical therapy
- Alcohol septal ablation is another treatment option (alcohol injected directly into the coronary artery, causing a small iatrogenic MI to reduce septal thickness)
- Worsening heart failure can be managed with cautious use of diuretics
- Heart transplantation may be required in severe cases

  2   Prevent sudden cardiac death:
- ICD implantation

  3   Offer screening:
- First-degree relatives should be offered ECG and echocardiography

1.9.3 Restrictive cardiomyopathy

Definition: restrictive cardiomyopathy involves contraction of atria against stiff, non-dilated ventricles with near normal systolic function.

Aetiology/pathophysiology:
- Almost always due to fibrosis or accumulation of substances in the myocardium
- Remains the least common cardiomyopathy
- More commonly seen in developing countries
- In developed countries, the most common cause is **amyloidosis**, but systemic diseases (such as sarcoidosis, haemochromatosis and malignancy) may also predispose to its development
- Stiff ventricles lead to impaired diastolic filling, congestive heart failure and reduced cardiac output

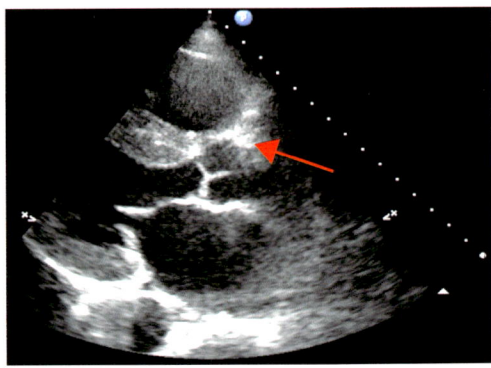

Fig. 1.40 Amyloid infiltration into the interventricular septum, seen as white speckles on echocardiography.

Management: echocardiography is **first line** (see *Fig. 1.40*), with endomyocardial biopsy being the gold standard. CT, MRI and diagnostic angiography are also helpful in distinguishing restrictive cardiomyopathy from constrictive pericarditis, as the latter may be correctable with surgery. Management involves treating the underlying cause, anticoagulation and treatment of heart failure.

> **E** ≫ Remembering the different types of dysfunction:
> - **D**ilated cardiomyopathies have a **D**ad bod – they can't lift weights (systolic dysfunction)
> - **H**ypertrophic cardiomyopathies are **H**ulked-out bodybuilders – they're always flexed and can't relax (diastolic dysfunction)
> - **R**estrictive cardiomyopathies are so **stiff** they can't **R**elax (diastolic dysfunction)

1.9.4 Arrhythmogenic right ventricular cardiomyopathy

Definition: arrhythmogenic right ventricular cardiomyopathy (ARVC) is a form of cardiomyopathy that can present with arrhythmia or sudden death.

Genetic mutations in the desmosomes of the cardiac myocyte lead to eventual **fibro-fatty infiltration of the myocardium**, leading to impaired RV function.

Management: diagnosis is challenging and requires a combination of ECG changes, echocardiography (see *Fig. 1.41*) and cardiac MRI. Patients are described as having 'notching' of the QRS complex, known as an **epsilon wave** and T wave inversion on ECG. Patients should be treated symptomatically and be offered ICDs for the prevention of sudden cardiac death.

1.9.5 Takotsubo cardiomyopathy

Definition: takotsubo cardiomyopathy, also known as broken heart syndrome, is thought to be a catecholamine-mediated response to severe stress events (e.g. death of a family member).

Clinical features: signs and symptoms may mimic MI but patients have **non-obstructive coronary arteries** on angiography (see *Fig. 1.42*). **Apical ballooning** of the left ventricle is pathognomonic on ventriculography. The condition is usually self-limiting, but there is a risk of death due to arrhythmia or ventricular free wall rupture.

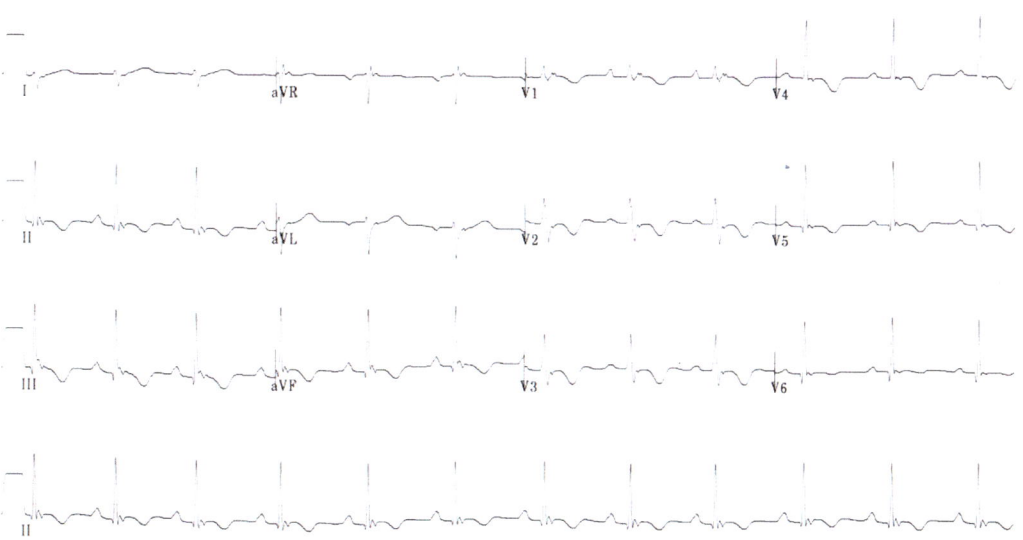

Fig. 1.41 *An ECG showing widespread T wave inversion and the characteristic epsilon wave in V1, seen in 30% of patients with ARVC.*

1

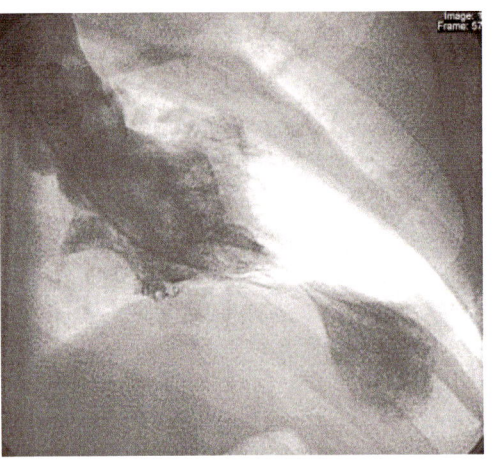

Fig. 1.42 *Apical ballooning on left ventriculogram seen in takotsubo cardiomyopathy.*

Management: most physicians recommend monitoring in the early stages of treatment with beta blockers and ACE inhibitors.

1.10 Myocarditis

Myocarditis refers to acute inflammation of the myocardium due to infection, toxins or autoimmune disease. Viral infections are the most common cause (specifically **Coxsackie** and **influenza A and B)**. Other specific causes include Lyme disease, cocaine, drug allergy or lead toxicity. The condition is generally self-limiting and carries a good prognosis. In a small number of patients, myocarditis may progress to dilated cardiomyopathy or predispose to life-threatening arrhythmias. **Note that myocarditis is also associated with a rise in troponin.**

1.11 Cardiac tumours

Primary heart tumours are extremely rare and are usually benign. The most common type are atrial myxomas, which are usually surgically excised. A small number are malignant, and these tumours are usually detected incidentally on echocardiography (see *Fig. 1.43*).

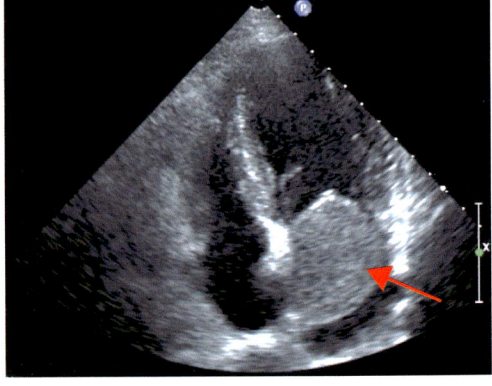

Fig. 1.43 *A large atrial myxoma seen on echocardiography.*

1.12 Valvular heart disease

Broadly speaking, heart valves can be affected in two ways – having their openings narrowed (**stenosis**) or having blood flow back through them (**regurgitation**). A stenosed valve may cause its preceding chamber to experience **pressure overload, which may lead to chamber hypertrophy**. Regurgitation, on the other hand, tends towards **volume overload, which may lead to chamber dilatation and failure. Mixed valve disease** occurs when both stenosis and regurgitation affect the same valve.

> **E** ≫ A murmur is defined as a pathological heart sound, produced over a region of turbulent blood flow. Murmurs can be graded from I to VI, using the **Levine scale**, as follows:
> Grade I – very faint, almost inaudible
> Grade II – quiet, audible
> Grade III – clearly audible
> Grade IV – loud with associated thrill
> Grade V – very loud, with thrill, audible with rim of stethoscope
> Grade VI – audible without stethoscope placed on chest

1.12.1 Mitral stenosis

Definition: mitral stenosis refers to the narrowing of the mitral valve orifice and most commonly occurs as a result of fusion of the leaflet commissures.

Epidemiology:
- Peak incidence age 40–50
- Rare in developed countries
- Women are three times more likely to develop mitral stenosis from rheumatic fever than men

> **W** ≫ The carditis of rheumatic fever causes post-inflammatory changes to the mitral valve, leading to commissural fusion, but this can take many years to manifest. This causes valve narrowing and stenosis, leading to increased pressure on the left atrium and left atrial dilatation over time, which can also predispose to thromboembolism.

Aetiology/pathophysiology:
- **Acute rheumatic fever** is the **most common** cause (up to 95%)

- Mitral stenosis secondary to ARF is called rheumatic heart disease
- Other causes include age-related degenerative calcification, a congenital valve deformity, rheumatological disorders or amyloidosis

Clinical features:
- Symptoms tend to mimic those of heart failure
  - Dyspnoea (pulmonary congestion and interstitial oedema)
  - Fatigue
- Strong association with **atrial fibrillation** (47%)
- Examination findings may include
  - Tapping apex beat
  - Loud S1
  - Opening snap
  - Rumbling mid-diastolic murmur
  - Malar flush and longer duration of the murmur are associated with more severe disease

> **P** ≫ Hoarseness and dysphagia can result from a large left atrium compressing the recurrent laryngeal nerve and oesophagus. This phenomenon is known as Ortner syndrome.

> **W** ≫ A loud first heart sound is due to an increase in the difference in pressure between the left atrium and left ventricle. This is often accompanied by an opening snap, which is thought to occur because of the tension of the chordae tendineae and the stenotic valve leaflets.

Investigations: investigations should be undertaken in the following order.

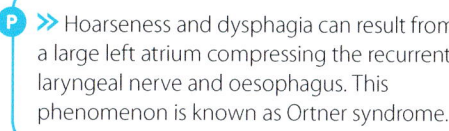

> **Stepwise plan:**

1 Obtain an echocardiogram
- First-line investigation, diagnostic (see *Fig. 1.44*)
- Recommended in all patients
- Transoesophageal echo may provide a more complete assessment of the valve

2 Obtain an ECG
- Left atrial dilatation and AF are common

3 Arrange a chest X-ray
- Left atrial enlargement may be seen

1

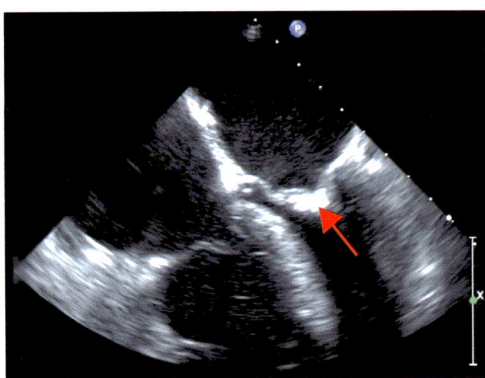

Fig. 1.44 *Four-chamber view on echocardiography showing significant calcification of the mitral valve.*

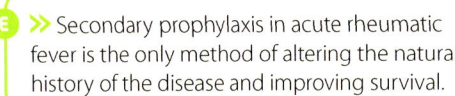
Stepwise management of mitral stenosis

General principles: symptomatic management and prevention of embolic events

1   Anticoagulation
- Warfarin should be given if AF is present
- Treat AF

2   Symptomatic relief

The onset of symptoms necessitates intervention. If this is not viable, then consider medical therapy:
- Diuretics
- Beta blockers

E ≫ Secondary prophylaxis in acute rheumatic fever is the only method of altering the natural history of the disease and improving survival.

3   Valve intervention
- **Percutaneous mitral balloon commissurotomy is first line** (if commissures are not heavily calcified)
- The philosophy for mitral valve intervention (particularly in the young) should always be repair rather than replace

1.12.2 Mitral regurgitation

Definition: mitral regurgitation refers to the backflow of blood from the left ventricle into the left atrium as a result of an incompetent (leaky) mitral valve.

Aetiology/pathophysiology:
- Any aberration to the mitral valve apparatus
- Acute mitral regurgitation
  - Papillary muscle infarction
  - Ruptured chordae tendineae

  - Infective endocarditis
  - Trauma
- Chronic mitral regurgitation
  - **Mitral valve prolapse** (most common cause in developed countries)
  - **Ischaemic mitral regurgitation** (widening of the mitral valve annulus secondary to ventricular dilatation)
  - **Rheumatic heart disease** (most common cause in developing nations)
  - Mitral valve calcification
  - Connective tissue disease
  - Coronary artery disease

P ≫ Mitral regurgitation reduces the forward cardiac output. It also results in volume overload of the left atrium and left ventricle. If severe, these chambers will both dilate. Over time, these changes also result in reduced systolic function of the left ventricle.

Clinical features:
- Acute mitral regurgitation
  - Presents as an emergency
  - Sudden onset severe dyspnoea and rapidly progressive pulmonary oedema
  - Hypotension and cardiogenic shock
- Chronic mitral regurgitation
  - Asymptomatic if mild or moderate
  - Symptoms occur when left heart failure develops in severe mitral regurgitation
  - At risk for AF (due to LA dilatation)
- Examination findings may include:
  - Displaced apex beat
  - Blowing apical pansystolic murmur radiating to the axilla

W ≫ The murmur of mitral regurgitation is usually pansystolic (i.e. it occurs throughout systole) because the murmur starts as soon as the valve closes. Blood flow through the valve may continue even after the second heart sound, as the pressure difference between the left atrium and the left ventricle has not yet equalised. There is often radiation to the axilla, marking the usual direction of flow of the regurgitant jet, although eccentric jets may radiate in a different direction.

Investigations: investigations should be undertaken in the following order.

Stepwise plan:

1 Obtain an echocardiogram
- First line, diagnostic (see *Fig. 1.45*)
- Can help assess ventricular size and function and severity of regurgitation

2 Obtain an ECG
- Detection of AF, P mitrale, acute/old MI

3 Arrange a chest X-ray
- Look for cardiomegaly, signs of heart failure or pulmonary oedema (particularly in the acute setting)

4 Arrange cardiac catheterisation
- Useful **second-line** investigation to assess coronary arteries or if echo is inconclusive

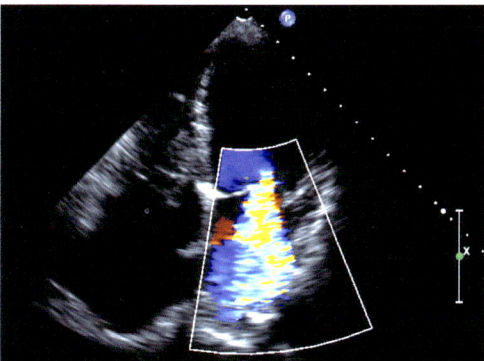

Fig. 1.45 *Doppler echocardiography showing the back flow of blood (blue – signifying flow away from the probe) from the left ventricle into the left atrium.*

Stepwise management of chronic mitral regurgitation

1 Anticoagulation
- If AF or severe LA dilatation present

2 Medical management
- Diuretics, beta blockers and ACE inhibitors for symptomatic relief

3 Surgical intervention
- Indicated in severe symptomatic mitral regurgitation
- Indicated in severe asymptomatic mitral regurgitation with pulmonary hypertension or new onset AF or LV dysfunction
- Surgical options include valve repair or replacement
- Patients require careful follow-up

1.12.3 Mitral valve prolapse

Definition: mitral valve prolapse (MVP), also known as Barlow syndrome, refers to one or both of the mitral valve leaflets prolapsing and projecting into the left atrium.

Aetiology/pathophysiology:
- Commonly caused by mxyomatous degeneration (accumulation of proteoglycans by an unknown mechanism), connective tissue disorders or cardiomyopathy

E » MVP is the most common valvular heart disease (prevalence approximately 3%).

Clinical features:
- Most patients have mild to trivial MR
- The condition is usually asymptomatic, but patients may complain of atypical chest pain or palpitations
- A mid-systolic click is often described on examination

Management: echocardiography is diagnostic. Reassurance should be provided for asymptomatic patients, with appropriate lifestyle advice (e.g. reducing caffeine intake) and beta blockers for patients with chest pain or palpitations.

1.12.4 Aortic stenosis

Definition: aortic stenosis refers to narrowing of the aortic valve orifice. **Aortic sclerosis**, the preclinical phase to aortic stenosis, refers to calcification and thickening of the aortic valve but without significant blood flow obstruction.

Epidemiology:
- Third most common cardiovascular disease after coronary artery disease and hypertension in developed countries
- Prevalence increases with age, affecting 25% of those >65 years and almost 50% of those >85 years

Aetiology/pathophysiology:
- **Calcific aortic stenosis (age-related)** – overwhelmingly the most prevalent form of AS worldwide
- Congenital bicuspid aortic valve
- Rheumatic heart disease – mostly in the developing world

1

P ›› Aortic stenosis is often erroneously labelled a 'degenerative' disease, but evidence suggests that it is an active process involving, for example, lipoprotein deposition, chronic inflammation and osteoblast-mediated calcification of the aortic valve. The narrowed orifice results in increased afterload, leading to adaptive LV hypertrophy. Over time, this increased pressure load leads to LV failure.

Clinical features:

- Classic triad of 'SAD' symptoms on exertion
  - **S**yncope (e.g. hypotension, transient arrhythmia)
  - **A**ngina
  - **D**yspnoea (most common symptom)

Symptomatic aortic stenosis indicates a poorer prognosis and a reduced life expectancy if left untreated. 10% risk of sudden death.

- Examination findings include:
  - Slow rising and delayed pulse (*pulsus parvus et tardus*)
  - Narrow pulse pressure
  - Crescendo-decrescendo ejection systolic murmur

Investigations: investigations should be undertaken in the following order.

Stepwise plan:

1. **Obtain an echocardiogram**
- First line, narrow valve area is diagnostic (see *Fig. 1.46*)
- Severe AS (EAE/ASE 2009)
  - Peak gradient ≥4m/s
  - Mean transvalvular gradient >40mmHg
  - AV area ≤1cm

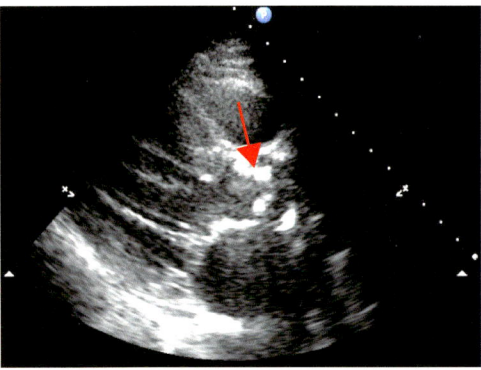

Fig. 1.46 Long-axis view showing calcified aortic valve leaflets.

2. **Obtain an ECG**
- Detection of LV hypertrophy, bundle branch block

3. **Second line**
- Cardiac MRI
- Cardiac catheterisation (particularly if there is co-existing angina)

Stepwise management of aortic stenosis

1. **Symptomatic or asymptomatic?**
- As a general rule of thumb, patients who are asymptomatic should be routinely followed up
- Coronary artery disease is common in patients with aortic stenosis, and risk factors should be optimised

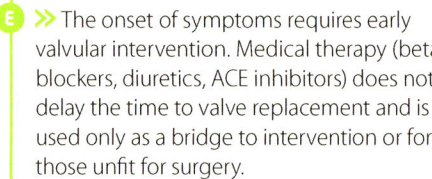

E ›› The onset of symptoms requires early valvular intervention. Medical therapy (beta blockers, diuretics, ACE inhibitors) does not delay the time to valve replacement and is used only as a bridge to intervention or for those unfit for surgery.

2. **Surgical or percutaneous intervention**
- **Aortic valve replacement (AVR) or transcatheter aortic valve implantation (TAVI)**
- Improves survival and quality of life

Guidelines: Surgical Management of Aortic Stenosis (AHA/ACC 2014)

The American Heart Association and American College of Cardiology taskforce published guidelines on the surgical management of aortic stenosis in 2014. Indications for surgery include:
- Symptomatic severe AS
- Asymptomatic AS and LVEF <50%
- Patients with severe AS undergoing cardiac surgery for other indications
- Reasonable in asymptomatic, very severe AS
- Reasonable in asymptomatic, severe AS with decreased exercise tolerance

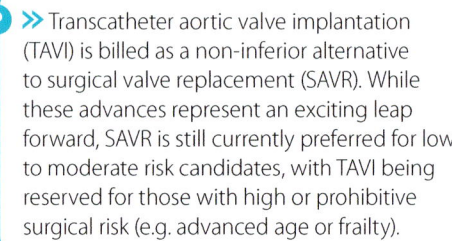

P ›› Transcatheter aortic valve implantation (TAVI) is billed as a non-inferior alternative to surgical valve replacement (SAVR). While these advances represent an exciting leap forward, SAVR is still currently preferred for low to moderate risk candidates, with TAVI being reserved for those with high or prohibitive surgical risk (e.g. advanced age or frailty).

E ≫ Mechanical valves are typically used in younger patients, but be aware that their use necessitates anticoagulation. Bioprosthetic valves are used more often in older patient populations but they do not last as long and do not require anticoagulation if the patient is not in AF. A biological AVR will usually last longer than a biological MVR.

E ≫ As you raise the patient's arm, gravity promotes arterial blood flow back towards the heart. An aortic valve with defect will have blood regurgitating from the aorta back into the ventricles. The flowing of blood back to the heart will result in a palpable 'collapsing' pulse.

1.12.5 Aortic regurgitation

Definition: aortic regurgitation (AR) results from incomplete closure of the AV leaflets.

Aetiology/pathophysiology:
- Acute
  - Infective endocarditis (valve destruction and leaflet perforation)
  - Aortic dissection or chest trauma
  - Acute AR is a **surgical emergency**
- Chronic
  - Rheumatic heart disease
  - Congenital anomalies (including bicuspid aortic valve)
  - Connective tissue disorders (e.g. Marfan syndrome, Ehlers–Danlos syndrome)
  - SLE
  - Rheumatoid arthritis
  - End-stage syphilis (very rare)

W ≫ Blood flows back into the left ventricle from the aorta, meaning that the left ventricle has to overcome the increased volume in its subsequent contraction. A sharp increase in end diastolic volume with a relatively non-compliant left ventricle causes an increase in heart rate and contractility to counteract the increasing preload.

Clinical features:
- Acute AR typically presents with severe dyspnoea and features of pulmonary oedema, hypotension
- Chronic AR is usually asymptomatic for many years, before presenting with symptoms of heart failure
- Examination findings include:
  - Pulsus bisferiens
  - Wide pulse pressure
  - High-pitched early diastolic murmur, best heard on expiration at LLSE
  - Collapsing (waterhammer) pulse

P ≫ The following eponymous signs are associated with **severe**, **rip-roaring** AR:
- Corrigan sign: carotid pulsation
- De Musset sign: head nodding with each heartbeat
- Quincke sign: capillary pulsation in nail beds
- Duroziez sign: diastolic femoral murmur
- Traube sign: 'pistol shot' sound auscultated over femoral arteries

Investigations: investigations should be undertaken in the following order.

Stepwise plan:

1 **Obtain an echocardiogram**
- Regurgitant jet is diagnostic, LV dilatation also seen (see *Fig. 1.47*)

2 **Obtain an ECG and CXR**
- LV hypertrophy on ECG; cardiomegaly, pulmonary oedema on CXR

3 **Second line**
- Cardiac catheterisation

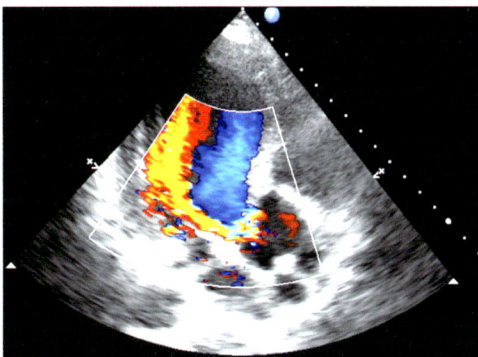

Fig. 1.47 *Doppler echocardiography showing the back flow of blood (red – signifying blood flow towards the probe) from the aortic root into the left ventricle.*

1

Stepwise management of aortic regurgitation

1 Medical therapy
- Treatment of hypertension is recommended in all
- Symptomatic patients require surgery; medical therapy is not a substitute
- Medical therapy includes beta blockers and ACE inhibitors

2 Surgical intervention
- Definitive treatment is **aortic valve replacement**
- Indications:
  - Symptomatic severe AR
  - Asymptomatic severe AR with decreased LVEF (<50%), or if normal LVEF but increased end-systolic dimension (>50mm)
  - Patients with AR undergoing cardiac surgery for other indications

1.12.6 Right-sided valvular heart disease

Valvular heart disease affecting the right side of the heart is relatively uncommon. However, these conditions are important differentials to consider when confronted with a murmur.

Tricuspid stenosis
- Rheumatic heart disease is **most common cause**; other causes include infective endocarditis/congenital (rare)
- Tends to present with fatigue, ascites and peripheral oedema; early diastolic murmur
- Echo is diagnostic, manage with diuretics and surgery

Tricuspid regurgitation
- Causes: physiological (70% of adults), left heart failure, rheumatic fever, endocarditis, congenital
- Fatigue, right upper quadrant pain, oedema, dyspnoea
- **Giant V waves** in the JVP, pansystolic murmur
- Treat underlying cause, manage with diuretics and ACE inhibitors and surgery

Pulmonary stenosis
- Most commonly congenital (Turner syndrome, tetralogy of Fallot)
- Presents with dyspnoea, fatigue, oedema and ejection systolic murmur
- Balloon valvuloplasty is the treatment of choice

Pulmonary regurgitation
- Generally caused by pulmonary hypertension
- Decrescendo murmur is early diastolic (at LLSE)
- This murmur is called a Graham Steell murmur if secondary to mitral stenosis and pulmonary hypertension

1.13 Congenital heart disease

Congenital heart disease may range from haemodynamically insignificant lesions to complex, severe disease, and is very common, affecting up to 1% of all births.
- People of East Asian descent are more likely to be affected
- Ventricular septal defects (VSD) are the most common form of congenital heart disease

There is no known aetiology for CHD, but there are important associations to be aware of:
- Down syndrome
- Maternal alcoholism and smoking

Other risk factors:
- Preterm infants
- Familial: a family history of congenital heart disease in first-degree relatives increases the risk from 1% to 4%
- Maternal factors: pregnant mothers with poorly controlled diabetes, hypertension, rubella infection or systemic lupus erythematosus (SLE) have a higher risk of having a baby with CHD
- Marfan syndrome, DiGeorge syndrome
- Teratogenic drugs: e.g. lithium (specifically Ebstein anomaly, a CHD with displacement of the tricuspid valve and atrialisation of the right ventricle), certain anticonvulsants and ACE inhibitors; warfarin may predispose to an atrial septal defect or a patent ductus arteriosus.

Shunt reversal – Eisenmenger syndrome

Increased pulmonary blood flow that occurs as a result of a left-to-right shunt (e.g. caused by a septal defect) can progressively lead to increased pulmonary artery pressures due to the increased resistance of blood flow in the lungs, resulting in pulmonary hypertension. The pulmonary artery pressure and its corresponding right ventricular muscle mass may then eventually become greater than the left-sided

P ≫ **Down syndrome**: occurs as a result of trisomy 21. Features include learning difficulties, epicanthic folds and a single palmar crease. Around 50% of children with Down syndrome will have a CHD, half of which are atrio-ventricular septal defects (AVSD).

DiGeorge syndrome: occurs as a result of 22q11 deletion. Features include learning difficulties, cleft palate, hypoparathyroidism, bone and muscle deformities. Children with DiGeorge syndrome suffer from a wide range of CHDs, including tetralogy of Fallot and persistent truncus arteriosus.

Marfan syndrome: autosomal dominant condition resulting from a mutation in a gene coding for fibrillin, a structural protein. Features include arachnodactyly, tall stature and lens dislocation. Aortic root dilatation, resulting in aortic regurgitation, is commonly seen.

Noonan syndrome: an autosomal dominant condition involving a mutation in the *ras* family of genes. Features include short stature, learning difficulties, webbed neck and coagulopathy. Pulmonary stenosis, ASD and hypertrophic cardiomyopathy are commonly seen.

Edwards syndrome: occurs as a result of trisomy 18. Features include organ malformation, omphalocoele, cranio-facial abnormalities and severe learning difficulties. A ventricular septal defect, atrial septal defect and a patent ductus arteriosus are commonly seen.

Turner syndrome: occurs as a result of missing part or all of an X chromosome (i.e. 45XO). Features include short stature, infertility (primary amenorrhoea), webbed neck and learning difficulties. A bicuspid aortic valve and coarctation of the aorta occur in 25% of children.

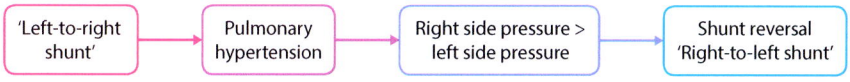

Fig. 1.48 *Progression of Eisenmenger syndrome.*

pressure, causing a reversal of the shunt from right to left. The onset of Eisenmenger syndrome marks the point at which the pulmonary hypertension is irreversible, and can develop from as young as 12 months old. *Fig. 1.48* shows the natural progression of Eisenmenger syndrome.

1.13.1 Patent ductus arteriosus

Definition: a patent ductus arteriosus (PDA) refers to a congenital heart defect caused by a failure of closure of the ductus arteriosus soon after birth. This condition accounts for 10% of all congenital heart diseases and is more common in premature infants.

W ≫ The ductus arteriosus is provoked to close after birth by a rise in blood oxygen tension and reduced prostaglandins.

Clinical features:
- The condition is usually asymptomatic if small, and is characterised by a **continuous machinery-like murmur** on examination
- A larger shunt may produce a bounding pulse and symptoms of heart failure (poor feeding and faltering growth in children)

Management: echocardiography is the investigation of choice (see *Fig. 1.49*).

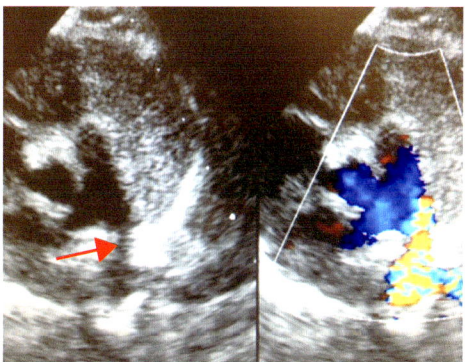

Fig. 1.49 *PDA on echocardiography.*

Premature neonates (<37 weeks) may have their PDA closed using an NSAID such as indomethacin or ibuprofen. This is not recommended in term neonates. Term neonates should receive transcatheter closure of the PDA, or surgical repair if the defect is too large.

1.13.2 Coarctation of the aorta

Definition: coarctation of the aorta refers to a narrowing of the aorta that is almost always congenital, but may in very rare instances, be acquired due to trauma, Takayasu arteritis, or rarely, atherosclerosis.

Aetiology/pathophysiology:
- Accounts for 6–8% of all congenital heart disease
- Most commonly occurs after the aortic isthmus (termed post-ductal coarctation), as opposed to pre-ductal coarctation (if occurring before the aortic isthmus), which is very rare

> **E** » Key associations:
> - Bicuspid aortic valve
> - Cerebral 'berry' aneurysms
> - Turner syndrome

Clinical features:
- Patients may present with symptoms of heart failure
- May have radio-femoral or radio-radial pulse delays or an absent femoral pulse in children
- Differences in BP and oxygen saturation may also be seen

Management: echocardiography is first line (see *Fig. 1.50*).

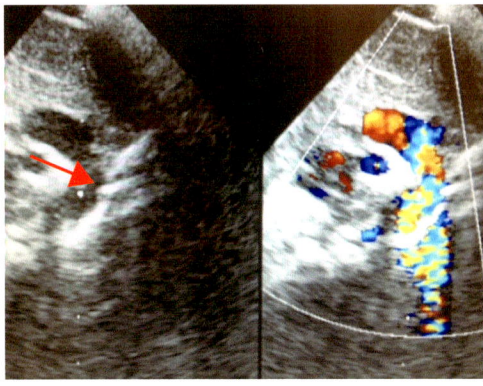

Fig. 1.50 *Coarctation of the aorta seen on echocardiography.*

There are severe complications if a coarctation is not repaired, such as aortic dissection and left ventricular failure. Surgical repair should be attempted early on in childhood, as late repair may lead to persistent or recurrent hypertension. The choice of balloon angioplasty and stenting versus surgery depends on the presentation of the disease, in the context of symptoms and the size of the defect.

1.13.3 Atrial septal defect

Definition: an atrial septal defect refers to a communication between the left and the right atria.

Aetiology/pathophysiology:
- Accounts for up to 10% of all congenital heart defects
- Most commonly arises as a result of the foramen ovale failing to close
- Ostium secundum defects are the most prevalent

Clinical features:
- ASDs are usually asymptomatic (recall that this is a left-to-right shunt)
- A systolic murmur may be heard at the upper left sternal edge, with characteristic **fixed splitting of the second heart sound** as a result of pulmonary valve delay closure
- Atrial fibrillation may occur later on in life, as might heart failure secondary to progressive right heart dilatation

Management: echocardiography is the gold standard investigation (see *Fig. 1.51*). Transcatheter closure may be used for most defects, but very large ASDs and primum ASDs require surgical closure.

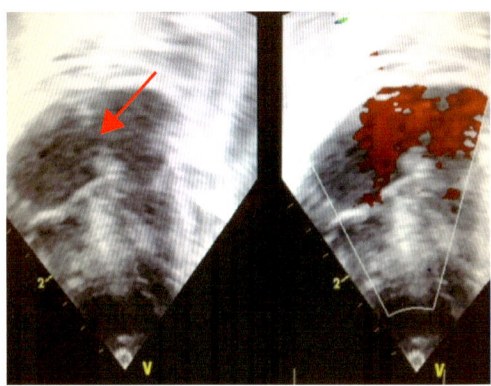

Fig. 1.51 *Atrial septal defect.*

1

1.13.4 Patent foramen ovale

The foramen ovale (FO) is a normal communication between the atria *in utero*. In some patients, this fails to close as it normally would after birth. Patients with PFO are **generally asymptomatic** but the most important clinical association is **cryptogenic stroke**. Diagnosis is based on echocardiography. PFOs may be closed percutaneously or surgically.

> **P** ≫ The term cryptogenic stroke is used when the aetiology is not due to cardioembolism, artery–artery embolism (e.g. secondary to carotid artery atherosclerosis), or small artery disease. Potential causes of cryptogenic stroke include a PFO or thrombophilia.
>
> The mechanism of stroke in the setting of a PFO results from a paradoxical embolism, where a venous thrombus enters the systemic circulation (via the PFO) and occludes and end-artery, causing a stroke or limb ischaemia, for example.

1.13.5 Ventricular septal defect

Definition: a ventricular septal defect (VSD) refers to a communication between the left and right ventricles.

Aetiology/pathophysiology:
- Most common congenital heart defect, accounting for 30% of all defects at birth
- Only accounts for 10% of CHD in adults, because many close spontaneously

Clinical features:
- A small VSD is asymptomatic
- Symptoms such as dyspnoea, faltering growth and poor feeding in children may occur in larger VSDs due to the effects of a large shunt
- A pansystolic murmur is best heard at the LLSE
- A small VSD will produce a louder murmur than a large VSD

Management: echocardiography is key in clinching the diagnosis (see *Fig. 1.52*). Management depends on the extent of the defect, and involves a choice between percutaneous closure or surgical repair.

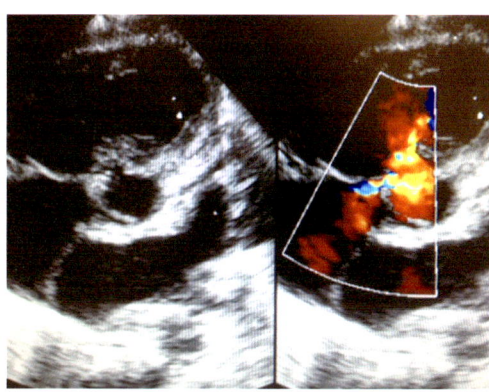

Fig. 1.52 *Ventricular septal defect on echocardiogram.*

1.13.6 Tetralogy of Fallot

Tetralogy of Fallot is a combination of the following four defects (which can be remembered using the mnemonic 'PROVe'):
- **P**ulmonary stenosis
- **R**ight ventricular hypertrophy
- **O**verriding aorta
- **Ve**ntricular septal defect

Tetralogy of Fallot is an early cyanotic disease, the severity of which depends on the degree of pulmonary stenosis. Cyanosis around the time of birth warrants close examination, as this is more likely to be transposition as opposed to tetralogy.

> **P** ≫ Hypercyanotic spells sometimes occur because RV outflow obstruction is exacerbated by adrenergic stimulation. There are two hypercyanotic phenomena:
> - Tet spells (previously known as Fallot spells), where an infant presents increasingly cyanotic, typically after crying. This is life-threatening and requires immediate intervention.
> - Older children may display the Fallot sign, describing a child squatting down during a hypercyanotic spell, increasing systemic vascular resistance and easing the effect of the shunt.

Echocardiography demonstrates the anomaly and allows for pre-operative evaluation (see *Fig. 1.53*). Complete surgical repair is indicated, preferably before the child turns five years old.

1

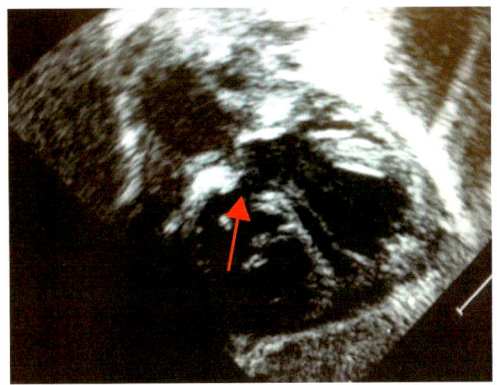

Fig. 1.53 *An echocardiogram showing a VSD with overriding aorta.*

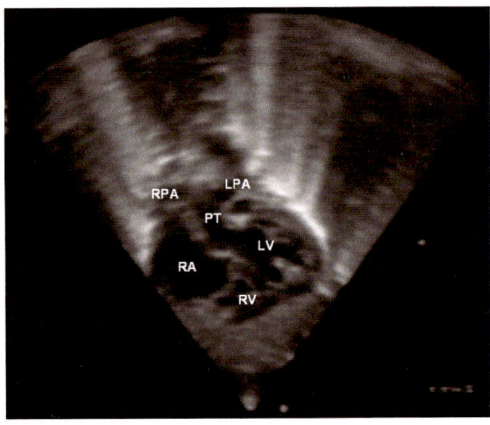

Fig. 1.54 *An echocardiogram showing the pulmonary trunk (PT) originating from the left ventricle (LV).*

1.13.7 Transposition of the great arteries

Transposition of the great arteries (TGA) refers to the phenomenon in which the great arteries (aorta and pulmonary trunk) are transposed and originate from the opposite ventricular outflow tract.

It presents with early, profound cyanosis. Echocardiography demonstrates the defect (see *Fig. 1.54*), and prompt surgical repair should be carried out, ideally within the first few weeks of life.

> W ≫ This is also one instance in which a PDA is favourable, as it promotes mixing of the circulation. Recall that indomethacin, a prostaglandin inhibitor, is used to close a PDA. In this case, we are aiming for the opposite effect, and prostaglandin E2 infusion should be used to keep the ductus patent (as a stop-gap measure) before surgical repair is carried out.

1.14 Miscellaneous cardiac conditions

1.14.1 Digitalis toxicity

Definition: therapeutic toxicity from digoxin is relatively common because of the narrow therapeutic window.

Aetiology/pathophysiology:
- Typically associated with **hypokalaemia**, but can also occur in the setting of renal insufficiency, hypercalcaemia and hypomagnesaemia
- Drugs such as amiodarone, rate-limiting CCBs and spironolactone can also precipitate toxicity by increasing serum digoxin levels

Clinical features:
- Symptoms include lethargy, nausea, vomiting, delirium and xanthopsia (yellow flashes/discoloration of vision)
- ECG may show bradycardia, prolonged QT interval, AV block, ventricular ectopics VT, or downsloping ST depression (see *Fig. 1.55*)

Management: treatment depends on presentation and may involve correcting electrolyte abnormalities, treating arrhythmias and administering digoxin antibodies (Digibind) for severe poisoning. Digibind rapidly corrects arrhythmias and hyperkalaemia, although is rarely used.

1.14.2 Postural hypotension

Definition: defined as a drop in systolic BP of >20mmHg or >10mmHg diastolic BP; or, if standing, causes symptoms within 3 minutes of standing up from a lying or sitting position.

Aetiology/pathophysiology:
- Patients who are older
- Patients being treated with anti-hypertensive medications (e.g. ACE inhibitors)
- Or patients who are dehydrated

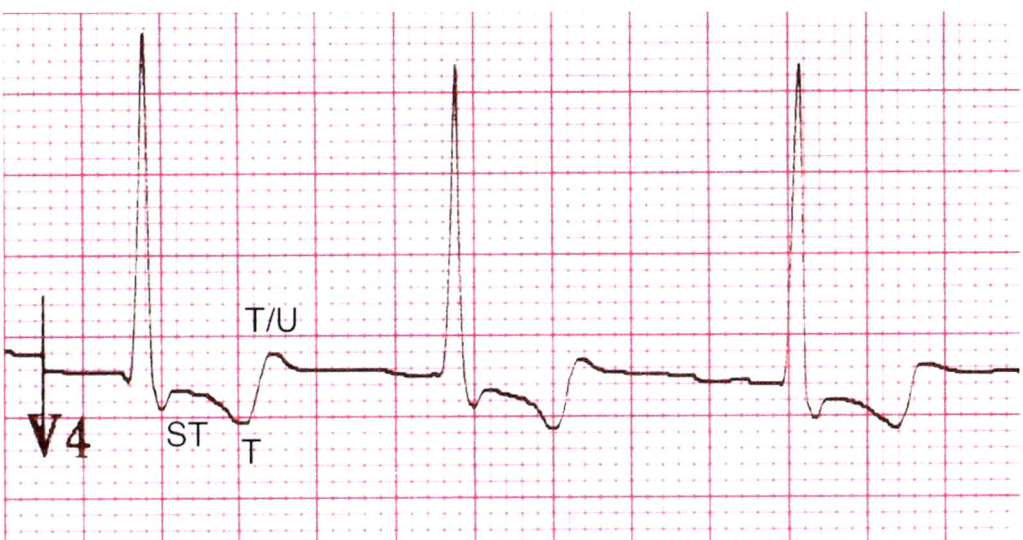

Fig. 1.55 *'Reverse tick' sign (downsloping ST depression) seen as a result of digoxin use. Note that this may be a normal ECG finding.*

Clinical features:
- Patients are typically older and experience dizziness, nausea, headache or syncope
- Blood is generally pooled in the lower extremities
- Reflex mediated vasoconstriction protects from a decrease in BP

Management: diagnosis is made based on lying/standing BP or a tilt table test in uncertain cases. Management involves stopping or reducing culprit drugs (e.g. such as anti-hypertensives), increasing salt and fluid intake, or mineralocorticoid therapy if the condition does not remit.

1.14.3 Cardiac syndrome X and Prinzmetal angina

Cardiac syndrome X: cardiac syndrome X refers to anginal chest pain on exertion, ST depression on treadmill testing, and **normal coronary** arteries on angiography. There is no known aetiology, but the postulated pathogenesis may involve coronary microvascular dysfunction and increased sensitivity to cardiac pain. It is a diagnosis of exclusion. Management involves reassurance and nitrates. The condition is unlikely to promote MI or increase the risk of other cardiovascular sequelae.

Prinzmetal angina: Prinzmetal (or vasospastic) angina is characterised by nitrate-responsive chest pain, transient ECG changes, and angiographic evidence of coronary artery spasm. There is usually focal or diffuse spasm of a major coronary artery. CCBs (e.g. nifedipine) are first line, with nitrates added if response is inadequate. Avoid non-selective beta blockers and high-dose aspirin, as they can worsen the vasospasm.

Chapter 2
Respiratory medicine

Amar Vaswani

Basic principles

The primary role of the respiratory system (see *Fig. 2.1*) is to facilitate gas exchange, oxygenate the blood and remove waste gases, particularly carbon dioxide. Alveolar and capillary walls, with their simple squamous epithelium, allow for rapid gas exchange to take place, also involving interaction between the cardiovascular and haematological (circulatory) systems. The lungs are thus exposed to a plethora of infective and environmental agents. Defence (both structural and immunological) is therefore another important key function of the system.

Bridge to clinical medicine

Anatomy and physiology

- Air is warmed and humidified after inhalation, travelling from either nose or mouth to the trachea, then the left and right main bronchi (which divide segmentally into secondary and tertiary bronchi), followed by terminal bronchioles; no gas exchange takes place throughout the tract up to this point – this makes up the **anatomical dead space** (estimated at 150ml)
- Terminal bronchioles give rise to respiratory bronchioles, which is where the alveoli are situated

> **E** ≫ The right main bronchus is shorter, wider and more vertical than the left, and aspirated material is therefore more likely to lodge in the right main bronchus.

- The bronchi are lined by pseudostratified ciliated columnar epithelium; the cilia 'beat' unwanted substances and pathogens towards the larynx – and this defence mechanism is known as the mucociliary escalator

- The **alveoli** are lined by type I pneumocytes, which have pores of Kohn, allowing for gas exchange across adjacent alveoli
- Type I pneumocytes are derived from type II pneumocytes; type II pneumocytes produce surfactant, a lipoprotein complex – the main component, dipalmitoylphosphatidylcholine, reduces the surface tension of the alveoli and increases lung compliance
- The lung is divided into two lobes (superior and inferior) with a cardiac notch on the left, and three lobes (superior, middle and inferior) on the right
- A **bronchopulmonary segment** is a division of a lobe; a lobe may contain many segments, and in some cases, when disease takes place, a particular segment can be removed surgically without affecting adjacent segments
- Deoxygenated blood is carried by the pulmonary artery to the alveoli, where gas exchange takes place, exiting via pulmonary veins, which now carry oxygenated blood
- The diaphragm is a major organ of respiration

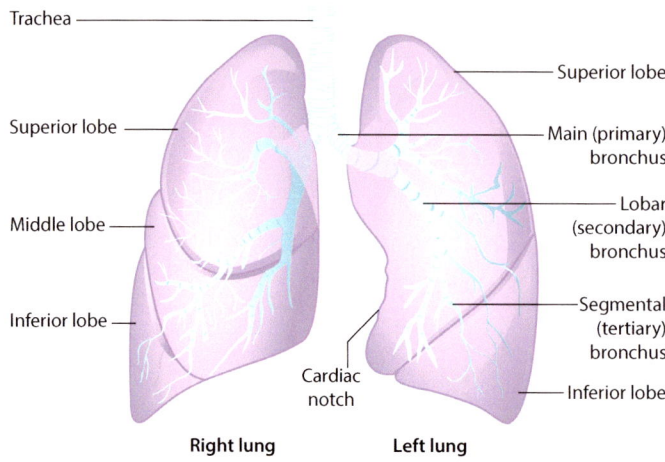

Trachea

Superior lobe

Superior lobe

Main (primary) bronchus

Middle lobe

Lobar (secondary) bronchus

Inferior lobe

Segmental (tertiary) bronchus

Cardiac notch

Inferior lobe

Right lung   **Left lung**

Fig. 2.1 *Gross anatomy of the respiratory system.*

W ≫ Hiccups occur as a result of involuntary contraction of the inspiratory muscles and the diaphragm. The distinctive sound produced is caused by an abrupt inhalation of air, which causes the glottis to close spontaneously. These are often self-limiting, but intractable cases can be treated with haloperidol or chlorpromazine. Alternatively, some patients may benefit from baclofen or domperidone.

- The lungs are lined by visceral pleura, and parietal pleura lines the thoracic wall; pleural fluid secreted within this space reduces friction as the lungs expand and relax
- Control of respiration is achieved by poorly localised neurons in the pons and medulla, with arterial pH and $PaCO_2$ driving respiration, with chemoreceptor feedback

Respiration, ventilation and perfusion

- Pulse oximeters are a cheap and effective way to measure oxygen saturation

P ≫ The oximeter emits red and infrared light across the nailbed and finger. Oxygenated blood absorbs red light more readily, while deoxygenated blood absorbs infrared light more readily. The combination of light absorption is determined and processed by the device, providing a saturation level. This also explains why the presence of nail varnish, carbon monoxide poisoning and excessive movement may result in an inaccurate reading.

- Respiration involves inspiration (active) and expiration (normally passive, but active during exercise); the accessory muscles of respiration include the sternocleidomastoid muscles and the scalenes
- **Ventilation (V)** refers to the movement of gas between the external environment and the alveoli
- **Perfusion (Q)** refers to the amount of blood delivered to the alveolar capillaries for gas exchange to occur
- A V/Q ratio therefore refers to the ratio of the air reaching the alveoli to the amount of blood available; an ideal V/Q ratio is 1, but because of differences in ventilation and perfusion across the lung apex and base and gravitational forces, the average 'normal' V/Q is estimated at 0.8
- A **V/Q mismatch** (exemplified by a low V/Q ratio) is seen in conditions such as asthma, while a high

V/Q ratio (seen in conditions such as pulmonary embolism) is secondary to over-ventilation of the alveoli with gas, as the embolus interferes with oxygenation of the blood

Pulmonary function tests and spirometry

Pulmonary function tests are a reliable method of categorising various respiratory diseases and assessing their severity, including function after treatment. Bear in mind that spirometry must be carried out with the proper technique, or results may appear variable.

- FEV_1: forced volume of expiration at 1 second from the point of maximal inspiration
- FVC: forced vital capacity – volume of air that can be expelled, from the point of maximal inspiration to the point of maximal expiration
- The FEV_1/FVC ratio is a key determining factor in evaluating obstructive versus restrictive disease
- DL_{CO}: diffusing capacity of carbon monoxide; CO has a high affinity for erythrocytes, and is used to evaluate gas transfer

E ≫ A low DL_{CO} is observed in conditions involving impaired alveolar surface area, such as fibrosis. A high DL_{CO}, on the other hand, is observed with increased pulmonary blood volume and alveolar haemorrhage.

Lung volumes and pulmonary function

Lung volumes represent the volume of air in the lungs at various stages of inspiration and expiration. Capacities are calculated based on these volumes (see *Fig. 2.2*).

- TV: tidal volume – the volume of air inspired or expired during a single breath
- RV: residual volume – the volume of air remaining in the lungs after **maximal expiration**
- IRV/ERV: inspiratory/expiratory reserve volume – the additional volume of air inspired/expired after a normal inspiration/expiration
- FRC: functional residual capacity – volume of air remaining in the lungs after **normal expiration** (FRC = ERV + RV)
- VC: vital capacity – maximum amount of air that can be expelled after maximal inspiration (VC = IRV + TV + ERV)
- TLC: total lung capacity (TLC = IRV + TV + ERV + RV)

Alveolar-arterial gradient (A–a gradient)

A rudimentary formula for the A–a gradient is P_AO_2 (alveolar PO_2) – P_aO_2 (arterial PO_2). An elevated A–a

2

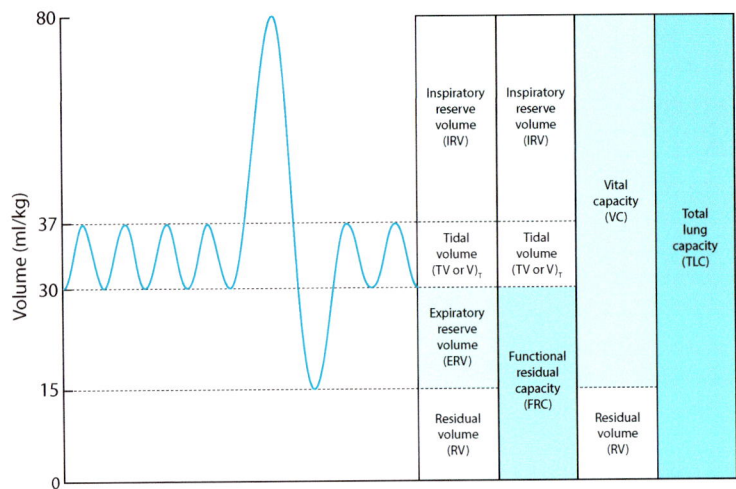

Fig. 2.2 *Spirometry – pulmonary function tests.*

gradient reflects a defect in gas exchange. This may be helpful in evaluating hypoxaemia, particularly when determining whether it is intra- or extra-pulmonary. An **increased** A–a gradient reflects hypoxaemia, except at high altitudes and in hypoventilation. A normal A–a gradient in healthy individuals is 5–15mmHg.

Minute ventilation

Respiratory minute volume (amount of air inhaled or exhaled per minute) is an important parameter because it is inversely proportional to blood carbon dioxide levels. For instance, a high minute volume will reflect lower blood levels of carbon dioxide. Minute volume is calculated thus:

- Minute volume = tidal volume x respiratory rate (RR)

> **E** ≫ Cardinal respiratory symptoms include:
> - Cough
> - Sputum
> - Haemoptysis
> - Dyspnoea (including orthopnoea and PND)
> - Wheeze
> - Chest pain
>
> Remember to ask about these symptoms when evaluating a patient's respiratory symptoms or during a systems review.
>
> An additional tool to help assess the effect of respiratory dysfunction is the 6-minute walk test, which can be carried out at intervals to assess a patient's level of impairment in chronic lung disease.

Arterial blood gas analysis

Arterial blood gas (ABG) analysis is useful when evaluating clinically unwell patients in order to assess severity, oxygenation and acid–base balance. ABGs are usually performed on the radial artery, but samples may also be obtained from the brachial or femoral artery if necessary.

A modified Allen test should ideally be performed before attempting an ABG, in order to assess collateral circulation before puncturing the radial artery. Guidelines recommend the use of local anaesthetic before obtaining a sample, but this is not usually reflected in clinical practice.

Normal ABG values
- **pH: 7.35–7.45**
- **PaO_2: 10.5–13.5 kPa**
- **$PaCO_2$: 4.7–6.0 kPa**
- **HCO_3^-: 21–26**
- **H^+: 35–47**
- **Base excess (BE) typically reflects the degree of metabolic disturbance observed. Normal range: −2 to +2**

> **W** ≫ Lactate is a useful tool when evaluating unwell patients. Recall that lactate (and lactic acidosis, by extension) is built up as a result of anaerobic respiration through the glycolytic pathway. Conditions such as sepsis and volume depletion may adversely affect cellular metabolism, increasing lactate levels, which may help in assessing the severity of the presentation, particularly early on.

Consider ABG as a whole, but emphasis should be given to pH, PCO_2 and HCO_3^-.

1 **Determine if the patient is acidotic or alkalotic (pH)**

2 **Identify if the acidosis or alkalosis is respiratory, metabolic or mixed in origin**
- Begin by observing **PaCO$_2$**, and then look at the pH. As a rule of thumb, an elevated PaCO$_2$ with acidosis implies a respiratory cause; and if the bicarbonate is low, it implies a metabolic cause

3 **Calculate the anion gap, identify possible compensation and consider if it is a mixed picture**

The anion gap

Anion gap = $[Na^+] - ([Cl^-] + [HCO_3^-])$

The anion gap refers to the difference in specifically measured cations and anions in serum, plasma or urine, and is helpful when trying to identify a potential cause of metabolic acidosis.

> **E** ≫ **Causes of a high anion gap metabolic acidosis**
> These can be easily remembered using the mnemonic **'MUDPILES'**.
> **M**ethanol
> **U**raemia
> **D**KA
> **P**araldehyde
> **I**soniazid
> **L**actic acidosis
> **E**thylene glycol
> **S**alicylates

2.1 Obstructive lung disease

2.1.1 Asthma

Definition: asthma is characterised by recurrent episodes of breathlessness, wheezing and bronchoconstriction secondary to **reversible** obstruction and hyper-reactivity of the airways.

Epidemiology:
- Globally, affects 300 million people
- Affects 30 million people in Europe alone
- Adult-onset asthma is more severe
- Boys with asthma are less likely to suffer relapses after puberty

Aetiology:
- Involves an interplay of genetic (atopic) and environmental factors
- Often a hypersensitivity response to allergens such as the house dust mite, fungi, pollen **(may be occupational)**
- The hygiene hypothesis suggests that exposure to a variety of microbes may be protective, but management strategies are, as yet, undefined
- May be associated with cold weather, exercise, gastro-oesophageal reflux disease (GORD) or emotion

> **P** ≫ Asthma may also occur as part of a clinical syndrome. Around 90% of patients with Churg–Strauss disease have had a history of asthma or atopy. Aspirin-exacerbated respiratory disease, or aspirin-induced asthma, is also known as Samter syndrome, and presents with a triad of nasal polyps, aspirin intolerance and asthma.

Pathophysiology:
- Airway inflammation occurs due to a complex interaction of inflammatory mediators and cytokines
- Primarily mast cell degranulation and histamine release as a result of allergen exposure in the acute phase, causing mucus plugging and airway bronchoconstriction

> **E** ≫ Diseases such as asthma, chronic bronchitis, emphysema and bronchiectasis are obstructive respiratory diseases. As a result, conditions with FEV$_1$/FVC ratios <0.7 are considered obstructive, while ratios that are near normal or possibly increased are likely to be considered restrictive in nature (e.g. pulmonary fibrosis, sarcoidosis, neuromuscular disorders). The severity of the condition can be assessed by observing the FEV$_1$ in obstructive disease, and the TLC in restrictive disease.

Approach to asthma

According to SIGN and BTS guidelines (2016), the diagnosis of asthma is largely clinical. The objective is to ascertain the probability of asthma – high, intermediate, or low, based on a patient's clinical presentation.

2

Determining probability (BTS/SIGN 2016)

A structural clinical assessment should be performed to evaluate the initial probability of asthma. Risk factors include:

- Episodic symptoms of wheeze, chest tightness and cough exacerbated by allergens, or exposure to cold or medications (e.g. NSAIDs, beta blockers)
- Evidence of diurnal variability – i.e. symptoms that are worse at night/early morning
- Observation of wheeze by a healthcare professional
- Past medical or family history of atopy (i.e. eczema, allergic rhinitis)
- Absence of symptoms suggestive of other diagnoses (e.g. extensive smoking history, coryzal symptoms, peripheral tingling and light-headedness)

Patients presenting with these clinical features are considered to have a high clinical probability of asthma. Patients who have some, but not all, of these features have intermediate probability; and those who do not have any of these features have a low probability. *Figure 2.3* illustrates the line of investigation used, based on a patient's diagnostic probability.

Stepwise management of asthma in adults (BTS/SIGN 2014)

Encourage good inhaler technique, avoidance of potential allergens, regular monitoring of response to treatment and regular peak flow measurements. The BTS guidelines recommend pharmacological management in a stepwise fashion. However, it is important to start treatment at a level that is appropriate for the initial severity of the asthma.

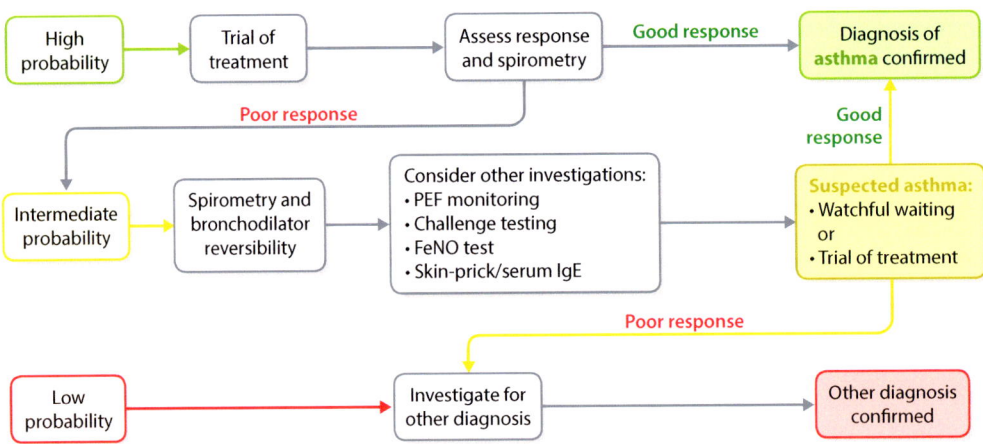

Fig. 2.3 *Diagnostic algorithm of asthma (adapted from BTS/SIGN 2016 Asthma guidelines).*

Table 2.1 *Investigation used in a patient with suspected asthma*

Investigation	Explanation
Spirometry	Preferred first-line test; an obstructive picture (FEV_1/FVC <0.7) and reversibility with bronchodilators increases the likelihood of asthma diagnosis
Peak expiratory flow (PEF)	Usually normal between attacks; reduced PEF during symptomatic episodes is suggestive of an obstructive lung disease
Challenge testing	Involves using either a histamine or methacholine in a safe environment, to provoke symptoms which may help confirm the diagnosis
Fractional exhaled nitric oxide (FeNO)	Indirect marker of airway inflammation; increased levels are seen in patients with asthma; it may also be used to predict responsiveness to treatment and monitor adherence
Skin-prick and serum IgE	Investigation of atopy; normal levels reduce the probability of asthma

1   **Inhaled short-acting B2 agonist as required**

2   **Add inhaled corticosteroid 200–800 micrograms (mcg) per day**
- **400mcg is an appropriate starting dose**

3   **Add a long-acting beta agonist (LABA) and assess response, consider a leukotriene receptor antagonist**
- If good control, continue LABA
- If there is benefit from LABA, but condition is still not controlled, continue LABA and increase inhaled corticosteroid dose to 800mcg per day
- If no response to LABA, stop LABA, and increase inhaled corticosteroid dose to 800mcg per day; if control still inadequate, consider leukotriene receptor antagonist

4   **Consider increasing inhaled corticosteroid dose to 2000mcg per day, or adding another drug, such as a leukotriene receptor antagonist**

5   **If control is still persistently poor, offer a daily steroid tablet, while maintaining inhaled corticosteroid at 2000mcg per day**
- Consider other treatments to minimise use of the steroid tablet, and refer the patient for specialist care; such treatment modalities include omalizumab, a monoclonal antibody against IgE, preventing mast cell degranulation (note that this is only used in very specific cases, with consideration of IgE levels); or bronchial thermoplasty, in which smooth muscle is singed off using heat, but the use of this therapy is not widespread

2.1.2 Chronic obstructive pulmonary disease

Definition: COPD is a preventable, treatable condition in which there is airflow limitation, secondary to abnormal inflammation caused by poisonous substances or stimuli, that is not fully reversible. This condition encompasses emphysema and chronic bronchitis.

Epidemiology:
- Fifth leading cause of death and disability worldwide
- Rates of COPD are often associated with level of social deprivation

Aetiology:
- Tobacco smoking is by far the most common aetiological factor

- Air pollution and exposure to toxic substances may also be implicated

W ≫ A genetic cause (i.e. alpha-1 antitrypsin deficiency) should be suspected in younger patients with emphysematous symptoms, particularly if they also have liver disease. Alpha-1 antitrypsin prevents the breakdown of elastin by neutrophil elastase. Breakdown subsequently causes destruction of alveolar walls, leading to emphysema. Congestion of the liver with the enzyme alpha-1 antitrypsin (which is produced there in an attempt to compensate) eventually causes destruction of hepatocytes, leading to liver disease. Not all patients with the deficiency will present with liver disease.

P ≫ The type of emphysema seen in smokers differs from that seen in patients with alpha-1 antitrypsin deficiency. Smokers tend to develop **centrilobular** emphysema which typically affects proximal acini and the upper lung, whereas patients with alpha-1 antitrypsin deficiency tend to develop **panlobular** emphysema, broadly affecting the lower lung. The allele classification includes PiMM (normal), PiSS (alpha-1-antitrypsin levels at 50% of normal) and PisZ (alpha-1-antitrypsin levels at 10% of normal, which indicates severe deficiency).

E ≫ The most common organism implicated in infective exacerbations is *Haemophilus influenzae*.

Clinical features:
- The diagnosis of COPD is suspected based on risk factors (particularly smoking), symptoms and signs, and is supported by spirometry (NICE 2010)
- Symptoms include exertional breathlessness, wheeze
- Regular sputum production and bronchitis in the winter
- Ask also about haemoptysis, weight loss and occupational hazard

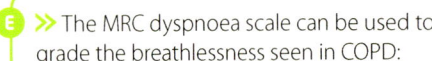

2

E >> The MRC dyspnoea scale can be used to grade the breathlessness seen in COPD:
- Grade 1: not troubled by breathlessness except on exertion
- Grade 2: shortness of breath (SOB) on walking or hurrying up a hill
- Grade 3: walks slower than contemporaries on level ground, or has to stop for breath at own pace
- Grade 4: stops for breath after 100m or after a few minutes
- Grade 5: too breathless to leave house, or upon dressing

Pathophysiology:
- Airway remodelling occurs secondary to chronic inflammation of lung structures, parenchyma and vasculature as a response to inhaled stimuli (e.g. tobacco smoke)
- COPD may be divided into two subtypes: emphysema, in which there is alveolar wall destruction due to inflammatory changes; and chronic bronchitis, in which there is goblet cell hyperplasia and increased mucus secretion, leading to chronic cough

Investigations
A combination of assessment of risk factors and observation of symptoms can help practitioners diagnose and investigate COPD. Investigations should be undertaken in the following order.

Stepwise plan:

1 **Arrange spirometry**
- Spirometry is the best initial test for COPD, and may help diagnose and classify it

2 **Grade breathlessness with MRC dyspnoea scale**
- Obtain SpO_2, BMI

3 **Obtain CXR to exclude any other pathology**
- Lung field hyperinflation may be seen (see *Fig. 2.4*)

4 **A sputum culture may be helpful in identifying organisms**

5 **The BODE index (B – BMI; O – obstruction of airway; D – dyspnoea; and E – exercise capacity) may be helpful in assessing prognosis**

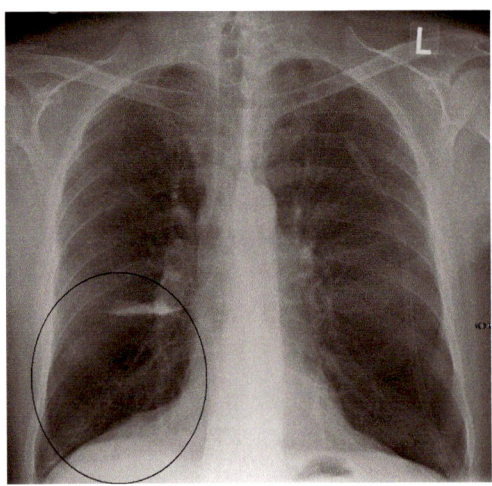

Fig. 2.4 *CXR showing a hyper-inflated chest and a large bulla (circle).*

Grading of severity of airflow obstruction (NICE 2010, CG101)
Note that the FEV_1/FVC ratio is <0.7 in the following grading scale:
- Stage 1 (Mild): FEV_1 >80% predicted
- Stage 2 (Moderate): FEV_1 = 50–79% predicted
- Stage 3 (Severe): FEV_1 = 30–49% predicted
- Stage 4 (Very severe): FEV_1 <30% predicted

Management
General principles: encourage good inhaler technique, obtain an up-to-date smoking history and offer smoking cessation help (nicotine replacement therapy, varenicline or bupropion, as appropriate). Annual influenza vaccination is also linked to fewer exacerbations. A single pneumococcal vaccination should also be offered.

Physiotherapy (and by extension, pulmonary rehabilitation) is also a useful adjunct in the management of COPD.

E >> Varenicline is contraindicated in mental illness and bupropion is contraindicated in epilepsy. (Varenicline leads to a lower mood.)

Stepwise management of stable COPD (NICE 2010, CG101)

Smoking cessation is the single most effective intervention and confers the greatest mortality benefit in patients who continue to smoke.

1 **Short-acting beta-2 agonists (SABAs) OR short-acting muscarinic antagonists (SAMAs) as first-line treatment**
- If control is inadequate using SAMA QID, offer LAMA OD

2 **Use FEV$_1$ levels to guide further treatment**
- If FEV$_1$ >50%, offer **LABA** (e.g. salmeterol) **or LAMA** (e.g. tiotropium), and discontinue SAMA
- If FEV$_1$ <50%, offer **LABA + ICS** (inhaled corticosteroid) combination therapy **or LAMA**

3 **Additional therapies**
- **Theophylline** and **mucolytics** may be considered
- There is insufficient evidence to recommend prophylactic antibiotics
- Routine use of corticosteroids is **not** recommended

4 **Long-term oxygen therapy (LTOT)**
- Indicated if PaO$_2$ <7.3kPa when stable or PaO$_2$ <7.3–8kPa with secondary polycythaemia, nocturnal hypoxaemia, or pulmonary hypertension; note that these values should be taken twice, three weeks apart
- LTOT improves mortality, and patients should be using LTOT for at least 15 hours per day; greater benefit is seen at up to 20 hours per day

5 **Surgical therapy (after CT)**
- Lung volume reduction therapy, **bullectomy** or **lung transplant** is the final step in management

Bear in mind that the GOLD guidelines are also recommended for treatment of COPD. These guidelines take into account severity, frequency of exacerbations and associated risk in classification.

2.1.3 Bronchiectasis

Definition: bronchiectasis is characterised by recurrent episodes of infection, chronic cough with purulent sputum and bacterial infection secondary to irreversible dilatation of the airways.

Epidemiology:
- Globally, burden of disease is unknown
- Prevalence increases with age and has been increasing as a whole

Aetiology:
- Immunodeficiency – seen in hypogamma-globulinaemia
- Seen in some other conditions such as rheumatoid arthritis and inflammatory bowel disease

- Genetic: Kartagener syndrome (a triad of primary ciliary dyskinesia, situs inversus in which body organs lie on the other side of the body habitus or dextrocardia, and bronchiectasis) or Young syndrome (bronchiectasis associated with normal sperm production but obstructive azoospermia)

> W >> A motor protein in cilia, dynein, is dysfunctional in patients with Kartagener syndrome, leading to impaired clearance of airway secretions by defective cilia. This protein also affects flagella, accounting for commonly presenting male infertility. Situs inversus is believed to occur as a result of defective rotation during the embryological phase of development, in which normal ciliary movement is thought to be necessary.

- Cystic fibrosis
- Yellow nail syndrome – extremely rare, presents with yellow nails, oedema, pleural effusion and bronchiectasis
- Post-infectious states, e.g. childhood infections or pneumonia (most common implicated cause)

Clinical features:
- Wheeze, breathlessness and cough, particularly with copious amounts of purulent sputum produced
- Coarse inspiratory crepitations and finger clubbing may be present in some cases

Pathophysiology
- The irreversible airway dilatation seen in bronchiectasis occurs as a result of chronic inflammation caused by immune response to infection
- The dilatation creates a vicious cycle in which the airway is more susceptible to repeat colonisation, causing recurrent episodes

Investigations
If a diagnosis of bronchiectasis is suspected, proceed stepwise.

Stepwise plan:

1 **Arrange CXR in primary care**
- May show tram-tracks/fluid levels (see *Fig. 2.5*)

2 **Arrange a high-resolution CT scan (HRCT) in secondary care (see *Fig. 2.6*)**
- This is the **gold standard investigation**, which helps diagnose the condition and assess severity

3 **Arrange spirometry**

4 **Obtain a sputum sample for culture and microscopy**

5 **Arrange additional tests**
- FBC, U/E, serum immunoglobulins, *Aspergillus* antigen test
- Assessment of genetic disease e.g. cystic fibrosis, Kartagener syndrome, Young syndrome should be carried out if symptoms suggest them
- Bronchoscopy may be indicated in certain cases, largely in investigating obstruction

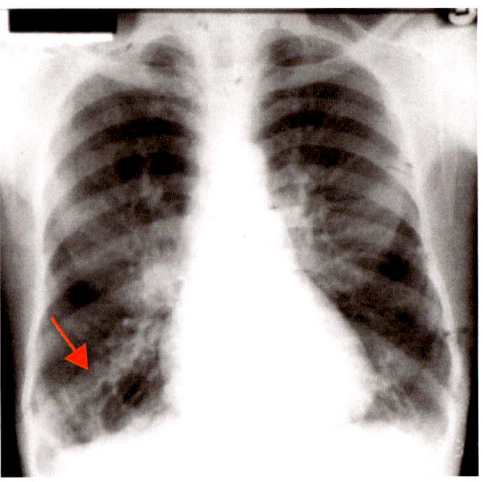

Fig. 2.5 *CXR showing tram-tracking characteristic of bronchiectasis.*

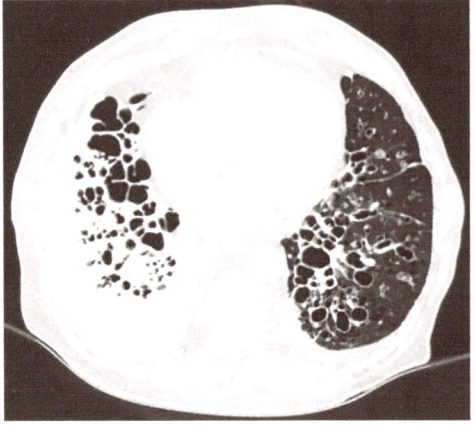

Fig. 2.6 *HRCT showing extensive 'signet ring' pattern and tree bud appearance characteristic of bronchiectasis.*

Management of non-cystic fibrosis bronchiectasis (BTS 2010)

General principles: airway clearance is paramount, with regular chest physiotherapy and mucolytic

therapy. Antibiotic and bronchodilator therapy are the mainstays of therapy, with surgical management playing a supporting role. The goal of therapy is to reduce exacerbations, maintain or improve pulmonary function and to achieve normal growth and development in children. These patients should be managed as part of a multidisciplinary team.

> **Stepwise management of non-CF bronchiectasis (BTS 2010)**

1 **Airway clearance**
- All patients with a chronic cough and evidence of mucus plugging on HRCT should be taught airway clearance by an experienced chest physiotherapist
- Pulmonary rehabilitation should be offered to individuals who are having difficulty with ADL (activities of daily living)

2 **Assess response to beta-2 agonists and anticholinergic bronchodilator therapy**
- **Oxygen therapy** should be considered

> **E** ≫ Note that the evidence does not support the use of inhaled or oral corticosteroids in bronchiectasis.

3 **Start empirical antibiotic therapy (local guidelines may differ), which specifically includes inhaled antibiotics while awaiting sputum microbiology**
- Initial therapy – **amoxicillin** or **clarithromycin**; high-dose amoxicillin for *H. influenzae* colonisation
- Early pseudomonas eradication is also encouraged

4 **If poor response, consider lung surgery**
- Lung resection surgery or lung transplant surgery may be considered in patients with poor response to medical therapy

2.1.4 Cystic fibrosis

Definition: cystic fibrosis (CF) is an autosomal recessive disease that affects multiple organs as the result of a defect in the CFTR gene on chromosome 7.

Epidemiology:
- Approximate burden at 70,000 worldwide
- More commonly affects people with European ancestry

Clinical features:
- Respiratory: wheeze, breathlessness and cough with purulent sputum and finger clubbing

 >> The exact cause of finger clubbing is unknown, but growth factor secretion, such as PDGF, and prostaglandin overexpression have been implicated in its development.

- Paediatrics: in neonates, this condition is exemplified by features such as jaundice, failure to thrive and intestinal obstruction secondary to meconium ileus
- Reproductive: male infertility with absence of the ductus deferens bilaterally; female subfertility
- Gastrointestinal/endocrine: diabetes mellitus, pancreatic insufficiency, steatorrhoea, liver disease and gallstones, osteoporosis

Pathophysiology
- CFTR gene mutation typically affects chloride ion transport, causing secretions that are unusually viscous
- In the pancreas, build-up of these secretions causes blockage of ducts and damages the pancreatic cells
- Gastrointestinally, viscous secretions may affect intestinal transport and lead to blockage of the bile ducts
- Secretions also build up in the lungs, which pre-disposes the individual to chronic infection and colonisation by infective agents

Investigations
The age at which symptomatic CF presents may vary.

Stepwise plan:

1 Arrange a sweat test
- If clinically suspected, the best initial test is a **sweat test**
- Pilocarpine is applied topically to stimulate sweating, and the sample is collected
- A chloride ion concentration >60mmol/L on two different occasions is diagnostic
- Genetic testing may aid the diagnosis

2 CXR, HRCT and spirometry to assess respiratory function

3 Sputum microscopy and culture
- *Aspergillus* serology should also be tested

4 Arrange relevant blood tests
- FBC, U&Es, LFTs (including vitamin A, D, E and K levels)

P >> Colonisation with *Burkholderia cepacia* is indicative of a poor prognosis.

Management of cystic fibrosis
General principles: the management of cystic fibrosis is complex, and requires a multi-disciplinary team with specialist input. While the treatments classified here are arranged by system, in clinical practice the patient is usually treated concurrently, and acute exacerbations of bronchiectasis are managed as and when they occur.

Stepwise management of cystic fibrosis

1 Respiratory
- Most common cause of morbidity and mortality, exemplified by chronic infection and bronchiectasis
- Regular chest physiotherapy is essential
- SABA PRN
- Mucolytics: dornase alfa (recombinant human DNAse)
  - Note that dornase alfa should only be used in CF bronchiectasis; for non-CF bronchiectasis, alternative agents such as acetylcysteine may be used
- Nebulised tobramycin, if patient is >6 years of age and affected by *P. aeruginosa*
- Oral antibiotics are used in mild exacerbations; IV in severe exacerbations
- Prophylactic azithromycin is recommended in patients with *P. aeruginosa*
- Corticosteroid use is recommended for acute exacerbations or superimposed *Aspergillus* infections

2 Gastrointestinal/endocrine
- Pancreatic enzyme (Creon) and fat-soluble vitamin supplementation with high-calorie meals and optimised nutrition
- Ursodeoxycholic acid in hepatobiliary disease
- Stool softeners, laxatives and adequate hydration to assist intestinal motility

3 Other
- Ensure that the patient is coping with the disease psychologically, screen for depression
- Assess for presence of diabetes
- Assessment of fertility and genetic counselling
- Increased risk of osteoporosis: offer calcium supplementation, bisphosphonates and DXA scans
- Life expectancy is estimated at 40–50 years

2

2

2.1.5 Bronchiolitis obliterans

Definition: bronchiolitis obliterans refers to an inflammatory fibrotic process that occurs in patients, leading to scarring of the bronchioles. Progressive narrowing of the airways occurs, leading to irreversible changes and airflow obstruction.

Epidemiology:
- Patients typically at risk of this condition include those who present with autoimmune disease, **transplant rejection** and those exposed to various industrial chemicals
- Chemicals classically linked to bronchiolitis obliterans include **diacetyl** (a chemical used to provide artificial butter flavouring in snacks, and also found in e-cigarettes), amine dyes and chlorine

Investigations:
- The diagnosis is difficult to arrive at, with a combination of history, physical examination, transfer factor, spirometry and HRCT being required for accurate diagnosis
- The condition is also frequently misdiagnosed as COPD or asthma

Management of bronchiolitis obliterans
Therapy involves lung transplantation, but – being transplant recipients themselves – patients are again at risk of the condition recurring.

2.2 Interstitial lung disease

Definition: interstitial lung disease (ILD) is a broad term that encompasses a variety of conditions (estimated at over 200!). It is related to lung disease associated with the interstitium, or tissue around the alveoli.

Aetiology:
- The most common presentation is idiopathic pulmonary fibrosis
- ILD can also occur as a result of medication use, autoimmune disease such as systemic sclerosis or lupus, or occupational exposure to inhaled substances

2.2.1 Idiopathic pulmonary fibrosis

Definition: pulmonary fibrosis encompasses a spectrum of diseases with multiple aetiologies causing interstitial lung disease. Idiopathic pulmonary fibrosis (IPF), formerly known as cryptogenic fibrosing alveolitis (CFA), is characterised by progressive scarring and fibrosis of the lung interstitium. Note that while there are many causes of pulmonary fibrosis (drugs, etc.), IPF is a term used when there is no discernible underlying cause.

> **P** >> Drugs such as methotrexate, amiodarone and bleomycin are commonly associated with fibrosis of the lung as a side effect.

Epidemiology:
- Most common interstitial lung disease
- Two-thirds of people who present with IPF are over 60 years old

- No ethnic or regional factors have been implicated, but a familial variant (FPF) exists

Aetiology:
- Unknown, although tobacco smoking has been implicated in its development

Pathophysiology:
- While the exact aetiological mechanism is unknown, characteristic fibrosis and inflammation takes place secondary to cytokine activation and mediation
- The normal tissue repair process is adversely affected
- Fibroblastic foci are formed in the interstitium, leading to disruption of the normal lung parenchyma and a subsequent decrease in function

Clinical features:
- Patients generally present at an older age
- Persistent, progressive dyspnoea that is worse on exertion
- Cough
- Finger clubbing may be present
- Bilateral inspiratory crackles on auscultations
- PFTs demonstrate a restrictive type pattern in IPF

Investigations (NICE 2013, CG136)
According to NICE, the following steps should be followed.

> **Stepwise plan:**

1 **Conduct an adequate history and physical examination**
- Be familiar with the clinical features of IPF (detailed above)

2 Perform blood tests
- Blood tests will help you exclude alternative diagnoses and consider history of environmental and occupational exposure

3 Perform PFTs and gas transfer (reduced DL_{CO} in IPF)
- Spirometry shows a restrictive pattern (FEV_1 normal/decreased, with FEV_1/FVC increased)

4 Review CXRs
- CXRs will show bilateral lower zone reticulo-nodular shadows

5 Perform high-resolution CT of the thorax
- This **gold standard** investigation may demonstrate a 'ground-glass appearance' (see *Fig. 2.7*)

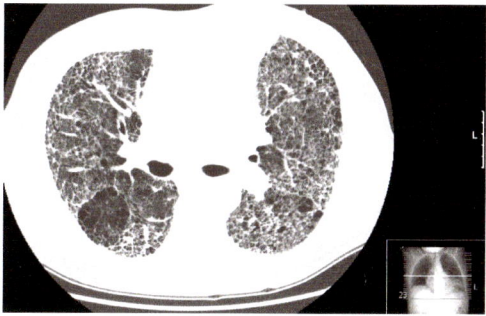

Fig. 2.7 *HRCT showing ground-glass appearance characteristic of pulmonary fibrosis.*

Management of idiopathic pulmonary fibrosis (NICE 2013, CG136)

General principles: pulmonary rehabilitation and supportive care have been the mainstay of treatment in IPF. Medical therapy has been proven to have little benefit, though the guidelines do recommend the use of tyrosine kinase inhibitors or pirfenidone (antifibrotic medication), neither of which confers a mortality benefit. Corticosteroids are also not recommended. Selected patients may be offered lung transplant. Do note that the prognosis is unfortunately poor, with the average life expectancy ranging from 3 to 5 years from the time of diagnosis.

2.2.2 Sarcoidosis

Definition: sarcoidosis refers to a chronic granulomatous disorder of unknown cause affecting multiple organ systems and is characterised histologically by **non-caseating** granulomas.

Epidemiology:
- Worldwide prevalence of 6 per 100,000
- Higher incidence in Afro-Caribbean and Scandinavian populations
- Traditionally affects people in their second to fourth decade

Clinical features:
- Affects multiple systems
- Generally presents with a flu-like illness, in which the patient may be pyrexial
- Pulmonary features are the most common symptoms
- Patients may present with a dry cough and dyspnoea
- Cutaneous changes, such as maculopapular rash and erythema nodosum (see *Fig. 2.8*), may be seen on the legs

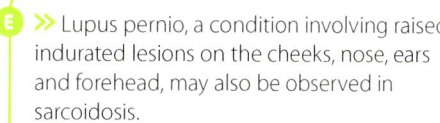 E ≫ Lupus pernio, a condition involving raised indurated lesions on the cheeks, nose, ears and forehead, may also be observed in sarcoidosis.

- Associated with Lyme disease
- Dry eyes and anterior uveitis (see *Fig. 2.9*) may also be present

P ≫ Löfgren syndrome is characterised by fever, erythema nodosum, bilateral hilar lymphadenopathy and polyarthralgia. This is an acute presentation of sarcoidosis and has a good prognosis. Treat with bed rest and NSAIDs.

- Bell palsy, polyarthritis and hypercalcaemia (caused by a disturbance in vitamin D metabolism secondary to granulomatous change in the disease) are also features, with features of hypercalcaemia developing as well

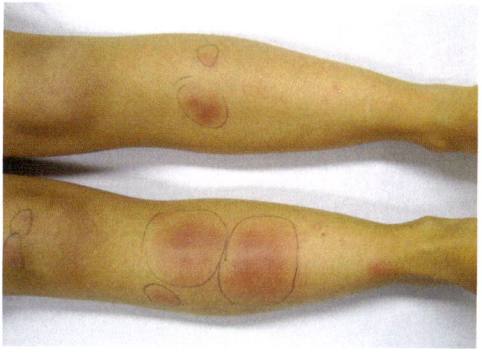

Fig. 2.8 *Erythema nodosum.*

2

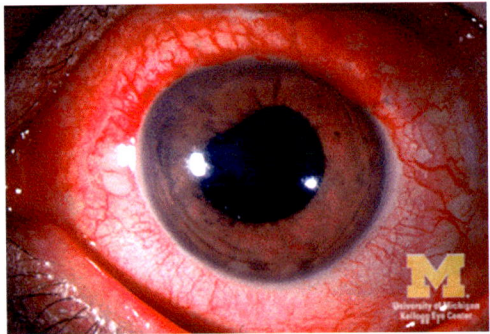

Fig. 2.9 *Anterior uveitis.*

Pathophysiology:

- Characterised by the development of non-caseating granulomas in response to the disease state
- Aetiology is unknown

Investigations

There is a wide differential diagnosis for sarcoidosis, and judicious investigation may be carried out depending on the presenting symptoms.

Stepwise plan:

1 **Arrange a CXR**
- Staging of sarcoidosis can be carried out based on CXR findings (see *Figs 2.10–2.13*)

2 **Arrange blood tests**
- Levels of calcium, ESR and serum ACE (limited diagnostic role) may be elevated; LFTs may also be deranged

3 **Arrange spirometry**

4 **Perform a tuberculin skin test**
- These tests will be negative in patients with sarcoidosis

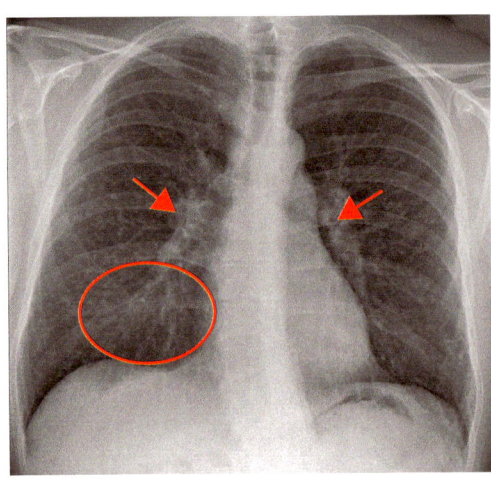

Fig. 2.11 *Stage 2 – bilateral hilar lymphadenopathy and infiltrates (note nodularities predominantly in the bases).*

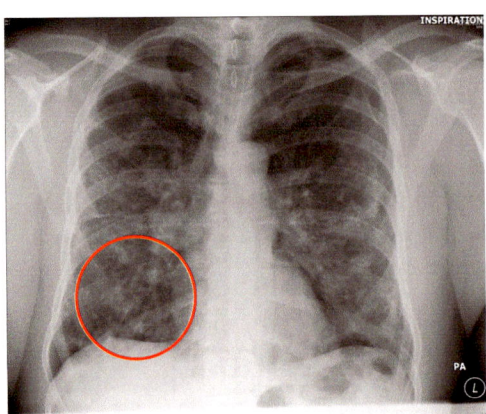

Fig. 2.12 *Stage 3 – infiltrates only.*

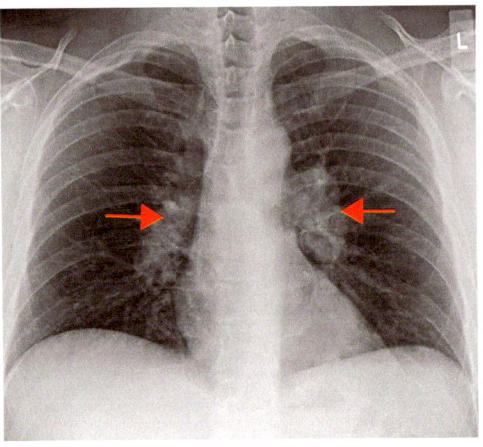

Fig. 2.10 *Stage 1 – bilateral hilar lymphadenopathy only.*

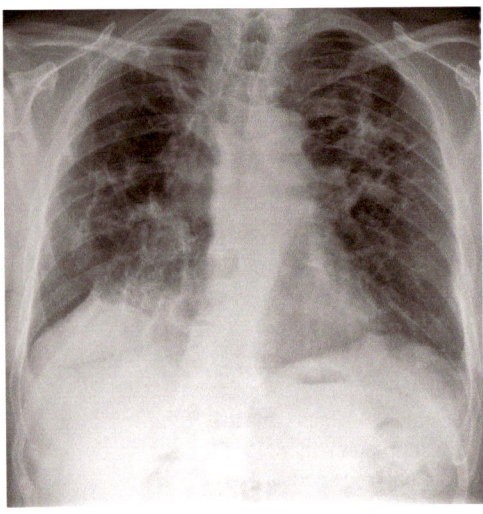

Fig. 2.13 *Stage 4 – fibrosis.*

Management of sarcoidosis

In practice, the management of sarcoidosis is fairly complex and requires a specialist referral.

Stepwise management of sarcoidosis

1 If asymptomatic with bilateral hilar lymphadenopathy, observe

2 If symptomatic Stage 2, 3 or 4, offer oral or inhaled corticosteroids first line
- Treat with cytotoxics (such as methotrexate or hydroxychloroquine) if severe or unresponsive

3 Consider treatment with topical corticosteroids
- Corticosteroids are helpful in dealing with cutaneous and ocular manifestations of sarcoidosis

2.2.3 Acute respiratory distress syndrome

Definition: acute (or adult) respiratory distress syndrome (ARDS) refers to non-cardiogenic pulmonary oedema and lung inflammation that leads to severe respiratory difficulty.

Aetiology:
- ARDS can develop as a result of many different pathologies
- Sepsis, particularly lung-related sepsis, is a common cause
- Other causes include aspiration, pancreatitis, pneumonia and disseminated intravascular coagulation (DIC)

> **P** >> Diagnostic criteria (Berlin Criteria)
> 1. Dyspnoea and ARDS is of acute onset (less than one week)
> 2. Bilateral infiltrates on CXR (see *Fig. 2.14*)
> 3. Classification of ARDS into mild, moderate and severe using $PaO_2:FiO_2$ (inspired air) 201–300 (mild), 200–100 (moderate), <100 (severe)
> 4. Non-cardiogenic pulmonary oedema

Pathophysiology
- Lung injury that occurs secondary to ARDS is not fully understood, but is thought to be a result of leakage of protein-rich fluid into the alveolar air space
- The mechanism by which this occurs (along with accompanying endothelial injury) is not always clear, but it invariably leads to inflammation, hypoxia and subsequent respiratory distress

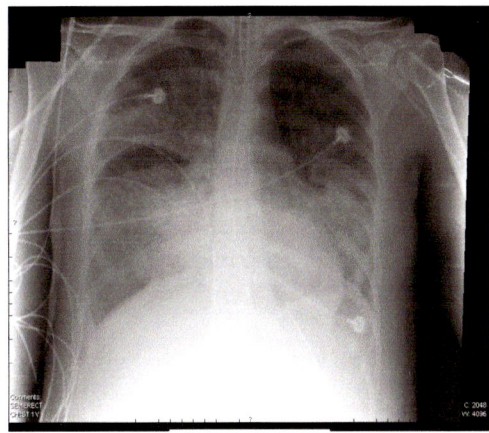

Fig. 2.14 *Bilateral infiltrates suggestive of pulmonary oedema.*

Investigations
Investigations should be undertaken in the following order.

Stepwise plan:

1 Arrange a CXR
- Use CXR to look for bilateral infiltrates (see *Fig. 2.14*)

2 Arrange relevant blood tests
- FBC, U&Es and an ABG

3 Obtain blood, sputum or urine cultures if an underlying infection is suspected

4 Arrange an echocardiogram
- An echocardiogram may be useful, and will be normal in ARDS

> **W** >> Utilising pulmonary capillary wedge pressures as a diagnostic tool is extremely helpful. An elevated PCWP suggests cardiogenic pulmonary oedema, while a lower PCWP may help indicate ARDS.

Management

Stepwise management of ARDS

The aims of ARDS treatment are to provide supportive care, optimise oxygenation and prevent complications.

1 Optimise oxygenation
- Low tidal volume ventilation has been shown to reduce mortality (4–6ml/kg of ideal body weight)

- Sedation may be required to improve ventilation by reducing patient/ventilator dyssynchrony, especially in patients with refractory hypoxia (low sats despite high FiO_2)
- Putting patients in the prone position is helpful with homogenous ventilation, as this is said to alter chest wall mechanics, and has been shown to improve outcomes in patients already on a low lung volume strategy

2 Adjunct care and treat underlying sepsis
- Strict fluid balance and DVT prophylaxis are important
- Commence appropriate antibiotic therapy for underlying sepsis

2.3 Occupational lung disease

Occupational lung disease (OLD), according to the American Thoracic Society, refers to a group of diagnoses caused by the inhalation of dusts, chemicals or proteins.

> **E** ≫ Note that asthma can be occupational in nature. This is typified by a patient with a history of asthma during the week, with relative improvement over the weekend. This is a clue that the asthma may be related to the workplace.
>
> Common causes include isocyanates (spray paints), resin, platinum salts, flour.
>
> If occupational asthma is suspected:
> - Carry out serial peak flow measurements at work and at home (this will vary)
> - Confirm diagnosis with IgE assay, skin prick test, specific inhalation testing
>
> If the asthma is sensitiser-induced, there is a latent period between exposure and symptoms.
>
> If the asthma is irritant-induced, symptoms start within hours of exposure.

2.3.1 Extrinsic allergic alveolitis (hypersensitivity pneumonitis)

Definition: extrinsic allergic alveolitis (EAA), also known as hypersensitivity pneumonitis, refers to the process in which granulomatous inflammation occurs in the lung due to inhaling organic or chemical antigens or proteins.

Aetiology:
There are several types of EAA, with different causes.
- Farmer's lung, linked to the inhalation of material in mouldy hay; chief antigen involved – *Saccharopolyspora rectivirgula*

- Bird fancier's lung, linked to inhalation of organic proteins in bird droppings
- Malt worker's lung, linked to inhalation of *Aspergillus clavatus* when working with mouldy malt
- Mushroom worker's lung

Clinical features:
- Symptoms, such as an expectorant cough, shortness of breath and a flu-like illness, may present up to 8 hours after exposure
- In many instances, patients recover within a week

Management
Acute forms can be managed supportively, as these generally resolve within the next few days.

Chronic forms of the disease occur with gradually decreasing exercise tolerance, weight loss, recurrent symptoms and crackles on lung examination. They are also managed with supportive therapy and removal of the offending antigen, which may warrant a change of occupation. Progressive or severe disease may require the use of corticosteroids.

2.3.2 Coal worker's pneumoconiosis and silicosis

Definition: pneumoconiosis, often associated with coal workers and their exposure to harmful dusts and particles (including silica), is exemplified by fibrosis that occurs secondary to repeated inflammation caused by these particles.

Aetiology:
- Silica exposure also occurs in coal mines, but does not exclusively present in coal miners
- Patients with silicosis often have histories involving occupations in bricklaying, tunnelling and the pottery and ceramic industry
- Silicosis similarly causes fibrosis and is clinically indistinguishable from pneumoconiosis on CXR

> **P** ≫ Coal worker's pneumoconiosis with associated rheumatoid arthritis is known as Caplan syndrome.

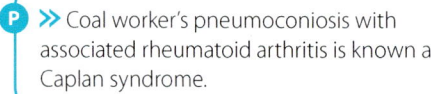

2

Management

In patients with occupational lung disease, it is important to obtain a thorough occupational history and also to consider the social side of their management, as patients may be eligible for financial compensation. Both social and emotional support should be given to these patients. Coal worker's pneumoconiosis is a **notifiable** disease. Silicosis and pneumoconiosis unfortunately have no specific therapy, but symptomatic management should be offered.

2.3.3 Asbestos-related lung disease

Definition: exposure to asbestos fibres, considered high risk in individuals who work at shipyards, train lines and in the plumbing industries for instance, can lead to asbestos-related lung disease.

Aetiology:

- Broadly classified, asbestos exposure can lead to benign pleural plaques and interstitial lung disease (asbestosis)
- It can also predispose an individual to the development of lung cancer, particularly cancer of the pleura, known as mesothelioma

Management

Patients who develop asbestos-related disease may be eligible for financial compensation, and it may be helpful to discuss this with them.

Benign pleural plaques

These plaques **are not premalignant**, and are generally asymptomatic. They may be visualised on CXR (see *Fig. 2.15*), but CT scans are a lot more precise. This is the most common form of asbestos-related lung disease.

Asbestosis

This refers to interstitial lung disease caused by asbestos exposure, and it is directly proportional to the amount and duration of the exposure. There is no specific therapy available. Treatment should focus on minimising further exposure to asbestos, as well as smoking cessation and managing any other co-morbid lung disease.

> E >> Asbestos exposure is an independent risk factor in the development of lung cancer.

Mesothelioma

Chronic exposure to asbestos can predispose to the development of lung cancer, particularly cancer of the pleura, known as mesothelioma. Chest pain, shortness of breath and weight loss may be presenting symptoms in these patients. Breathlessness may also be caused by a pleural effusion. This condition has a very poor prognosis.

- Investigations include a CXR (see *Fig. 2.16*), CT scan and pleural biopsy
- Treatment is supportive, with pleural surgery being indicated for palliative symptomatic relief

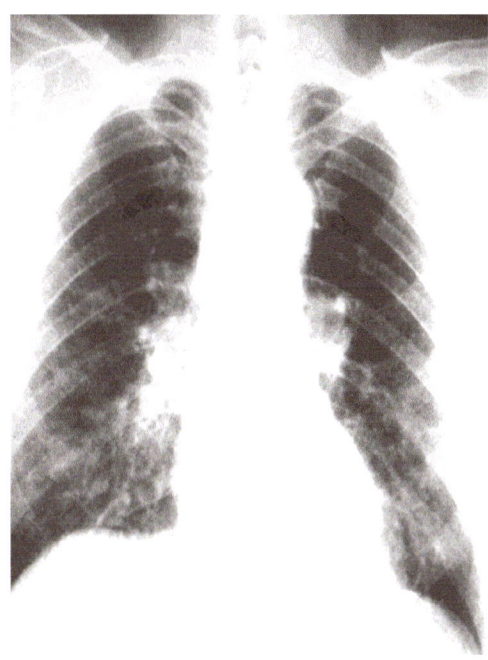

Fig. 2.15 *Asbestosis on a CXR. Note the haziness at the outer borders of the lungs.*

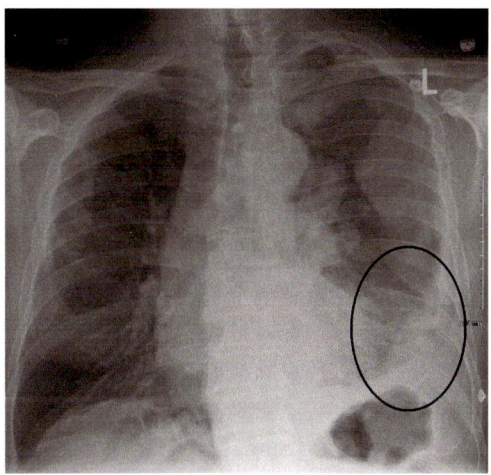

Fig. 2.16 *Left-sided mesothelioma. There is also blunting of the costophrenic angles, suggestive of a paramalignant effusion.*

2.4 Infections of the respiratory system

2.4.1 Pneumonia

Definition: pneumonia, often colloquially referred to as a 'chest infection', refers to lung inflammation associated with consolidation or infiltrates secondary to infection.

Aetiology:

There are several types of pneumonia, with different causes.

- Community-acquired pneumonia (CAP) refers to patients with a pulmonary parenchymal infection who present with symptoms of an acute infection from the community
- Hospital-acquired pneumonia (HAP) presents after at least 48 hours in a hospital setting
- Healthcare-associated pneumonia (HCAP) refers to pneumonia that develops in patients who reside in nursing homes, long-term care facilities or haemodialysis centres or who have had recent chemotherapy. This term is increasingly being phased out, with patients with this type of pneumonia falling into the HAP bracket
- Aspiration pneumonia is caused by inhalation of contents (e.g. vomitus) in patients with altered mental status/stroke, causing lung injury and subsequent infection; treatment is with **intravenous antibiotics** and supportive care
- Ventilator-assisted pneumonia is likely to occur 48–72 hours after endotracheal intubation
- *Pneumocystis jirovecii* pneumonia (previously known as *Pneumocystis carinii* pneumonia or PCP) is caused by an opportunistic infection in HIV patients; diagnosis is made by identifying the organism in sputum; treatment is with **co-trimoxazole**
- Atypical pneumonia (e.g. mycoplasma)

Clinical features:

- Fever
- Cough with purulent sputum which may be blood-stained
- Shortness of breath
- Malaise, loss of appetite and myalgia

Pathophysiology

- A chest infection may occur for several reasons, and these factors are usually intertwined – e.g. the type and amount of pathogen present, the host's immune status, risk factors and current lung function, as well as stroke or altered mental status
- The lungs are constantly exposed to particulate matter and microbes, which are present in the upper respiratory tract
- The lower respiratory tract typically remains sterile because of pulmonary defence mechanisms, but can be overwhelmed for the reasons stated above, which contribute to the development of an infection

Investigations

Investigations should be undertaken in the following order.

> **Stepwise plan:**
>
> 1 **Arrange CXR (see *Fig. 2.17*)**
>
> 2 **Arrange blood tests**
> - FBC, U&Es, LFTs, CRP and blood cultures
>
> 3 **Obtain sputum for microscopy and culture**
>
> 4 **Test for urinary antigen for *Legionella***
>
> 5 **Arrange additional special tests (if necessary)**
> - e.g. serology for mycoplasma

P >> Various organisms that cause pneumonia are typically associated with a collection of symptoms in the histories seen in clinical practice:

- *Strep. pneumoniae* is the most common cause of CAP, and typically affects the elderly and immunocompromised
- *Staph. aureus* pneumonia is more likely to occur following an influenza infection
- *Klebsiella pneumoniae* is typically associated with alcoholics and diabetics

- *Legionella* infections are associated with air conditioning or a recent history of travel to a foreign country; **hyponatraemia** and **deranged LFTs** are also features
- Mycoplasma infections present with a flu-like illness and may be associated with erythema multiforme and cold autoimmune haemolytic anaemia; treatment is with **erythromycin.**

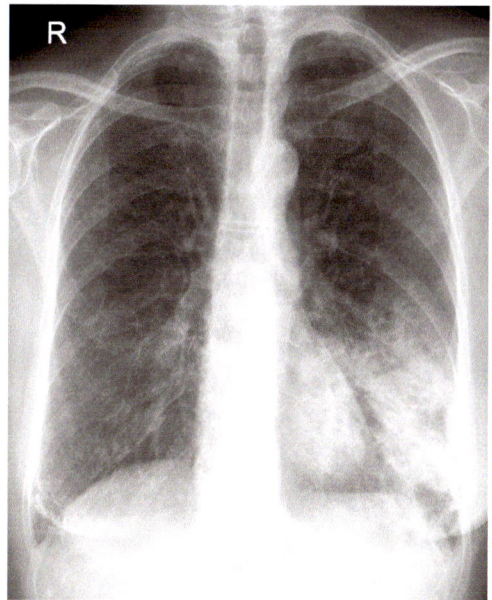

Fig. 2.17 *Left lower lobe consolidation on CXR.*

E ➤ CURB-65 is an excellent tool in predicting 30-day mortality in community-acquired pneumonia. The BTS recommends the use of a CURB score to assess severity of CAP and help guide treatment. The maximum number of points obtainable for a CURB-65 score is 5.
- **C**onfusion (abbreviated mental test score <8)
- **U**rea >7
- **R**espiratory rate >30
- **B**P <90 **OR** DBP <60 (either one scores one point; if both are present, the score remains one point for both)
- **65** – Age ≥65

Management
General principles: assess severity using CURB-65. Provide appropriate smoking cessation advice and vaccination (pneumococcal and influenza). Note that antibiotic regimens differ from location to location, and the following choices represent a sample regimen.

Stepwise management of community-acquired pneumonia (NICE 2014, CG191)

1   **If CURB-65 score 0–1, outpatient treatment (mild)**
- Amoxicillin 500mg TDS **OR** clarithromycin 500mg BD for **5 days** (oral)

2   **If CURB-65 score 2, inpatient treatment (moderate)**
- Amoxicillin 500mg tds **AND** clarithromycin 500mg bd for **7 days** (**oral or IV**)

3   **If CURB-65 score ≥3, consider ITU admission (severe)**
- Co-amoxiclav 1.2g TDS IV **AND** clarithromycin 500mg BD **IV** for **7 days**
- Consider ICU involvement

Stepwise management of hospital-acquired pneumonia

1   **Offer antibiotic therapy as soon as possible, and certainly within 4 hours of diagnosis**

2   **Consider a course of antibiotics for 5–10 days in accordance with local hospital protocol for HAP**

2.4.2 Lung abscess

Definition: a lung abscess refers to the development of necrotic lung tissue and cavity formation secondary to infection. Patients with a history of alcohol excess, diabetes, cystic fibrosis and risk factors for aspiration are at much greater risk of developing an abscess. The condition may occur as primary or secondary disease.
- Primary disease:
  - Existing pneumonia or lung disease
  - Untreated pneumonia can cause abscess formation
- Secondary disease:
  - Aspiration
  - Alcoholics
  - Septic emboli from right-sided infective endocarditis

Clinical features:
- Swinging fevers
- Night sweats
- Productive cough with purulent sputum

Management
Diagnosis is made on CXR, CT and sputum culture. Bronchoscopic aspirates can be assessed for organisms, and may also provide symptomatic relief. Treat with IV broad-spectrum antibiotics; the majority of cases will resolve. If refractory to medical therapy, surgical resection may be considered.

2

2.4.3 Tuberculosis

Definition: tuberculosis (TB) is a granulomatous disease caused by mycobacteria, the most common of which is *M. tuberculosis*. It presents with primarily pulmonary symptoms, but may have extra-pulmonary manifestations as well.

> **E** ≫ Tuberculosis is a notifiable disease.

Epidemiology:
- More than 50% of cases are in southeast Asia and the western Pacific
- TB is particularly devastating in immuno-compromised individuals
- More than 90% of TB deaths occur in countries with low to middle incomes

Clinical features:
- Pulmonary TB presents with an expectorant cough, fever, haemoptysis, malaise and weight loss
- May have extra-pulmonary manifestations, such as arthritis, meningitis, Pott spine, erythema nodosum and finger clubbing
- Risk factors include patients from endemic regions, alcoholics, homeless patients, the immunocompromised and close contacts of patients with existing tuberculosis; clinical suspicion should be raised when assessing patients with relevant risk factors

Pathophysiology:
- Tuberculous infection occurs via droplet transmission when mycobacteria are engulfed and replicate within alveolar macrophages
- Mycolic acid, a substance associated with mycobacteria, prevents degradation of the mycobacterium; as a result, **caseating** granuloma formation occurs, attempting to prevent further spread in a healthy individual. The individual is then said to have latent TB, and TB infections typically occur as a reactivation of dormant disease (active TB)
- Disseminated disease in the immunocompromised individual results in widespread TB (miliary TB), named after its 'millet seed' appearance on CXR (see *Fig. 2.18*)

> **W** ≫ TB typically affects the apical and upper zones of the lungs. The reason for this is not completely understood, but it is thought to occur here because these parts of the lungs have better air flow and reduced lymphatic drainage.

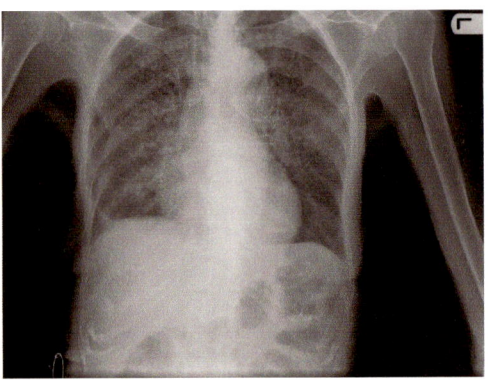

Fig. 2.18 *Miliary TB on CXR. Note the widespread 'seed' appearance.*

Investigations

Investigations should be undertaken in the following order.

A clear history and assessment of risk factors should be considered alongside appropriate investigation.

> **Stepwise plan (NICE 2016, NG33):**

1 **ISOLATE patient appropriately**

2 **Arrange CXR**
- This may show central apical changes or pleural effusions

3 **Obtain sputum samples**
- **At least three samples** (with one early-morning sample) are required to make a diagnosis
- A Ziehl–Neelsen stain should be used, looking for acid-fast bacilli
- Culture using the Löwenstein–Jensen medium takes 4–8 weeks, and is therefore not expedient
- Nucleic acid amplification testing (NAAT) should be used on at least one sample to isolate the organism

4 **Arrange blood tests**
- FBC, U&Es, LFTs (baseline, particularly because anti-TB medications tend to be hepatotoxic)

> **P** ≫ In patients without symptoms of active TB, a tuberculin (Mantoux) skin test or interferon gamma release assays (IGRAs) may be used to investigate latent TB.

> **E** ≫ Treatment should be started without waiting for culture results if there is strong clinical suspicion of TB.

2

1   APPROPRIATELY ISOLATE patient and seek SPECIALIST INPUT
- Assess HIV status and risk assessment for TB drug resistance, and screen for concomitant diabetes mellitus

2   Drug therapy – 6 months total
- **2 months of isoniazid, rifampicin, pyrazinamide and ethambutol**
- Further **4 months of isoniazid and rifampicin only**
- Daily dosing should be administered in patients with active TB
- Alternatively, thrice-weekly dosing regimen should be considered for patients receiving **directly observed therapy (DOT)**

3   Carry out appropriate CONTACT TRACING

Treatment for extra-pulmonary TB requires specialist input and is not covered in this section. However, extra-pulmonary TB generally requires longer duration of therapy. Various strains of mycobacteria have emerged in recent times. Multi-drug resistant strains of TB (MDR-TB) may require use of secondary agents. There are also some extensively-drug resistant strains of TB (XDR-TB), for which – in some cases – there is no cure.

E ≫ TB drug side effects, with 'pronunciation' mnemonics:
- Ethambutol (**Eye-thambutol**) – optic neuritis, renal impairment
- Rifampicin (**Red-famipicin**) – reddish orange secretions, hepatitis
- Isoniazid (**Iso-neuro-zid**) – peripheral neuropathy (supplement with Vit B6 to prevent), agranulocytosis, hepatitis
- Pyrazinamide (**Pyr-ouch-zinamide**) – hyperuricaemia causing gout, myalgia and hepatitis

2.4.4 *Aspergillus*-related lung disease

Aspergillus spp. are a group of fungal moulds that may precipitate lung disease. Inhalation of spores causes various types of respiratory ailment, but cutaneous manifestations may occur.

E ≫ Cutaneous manifestations of aspergillosis usually occur secondary to existing disease, but may occur as a primary form of the condition in a small number of patients or in the immunocompromised. Aspergillosis typically affects the nails, and may in some cases (particularly in secondary cases), present as a localised cellulitis or ulcer with a necrotic centre. Diagnosis may be made on biopsy, and treatment involves systemic antifungal therapy (e.g. voriconazole), with or without surgical excision.

The most common implicated organism is *Aspergillus fumigatus*. Forms of *Aspergillus*-related disease include:

- **Aspergilloma**
  - An aspergilloma, also known as a mycetoma, is essentially a fungal 'ball' that is located in a lung cavity, usually secondary to another disease process such as TB
  - May present with haemoptysis, producing large amounts of blood
  - CXR demonstrates a rim of air around an opacification (see *Fig. 2.19*)
  - CT scan is more sensitive
  - Treatment is **surgical removal** of the aspergilloma, with long-term itraconazole

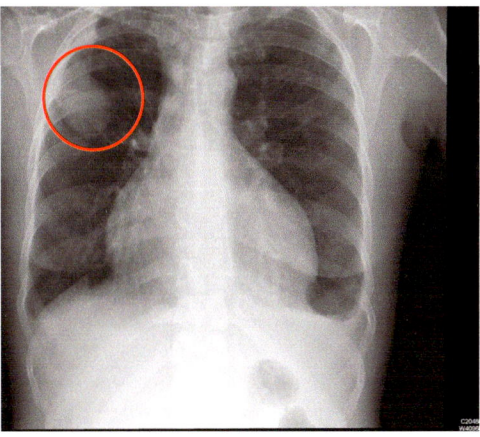

Fig. 2.19 *CXR showing an aspergilloma (mycetoma) in the right upper lobe.*

- **Allergic bronchopulmonary aspergillosis (ABPA)**
- **Invasive aspergillosis**
  - Typically affects immunocompromised individuals

2

– Usually a disseminated fungal infection; **aflatoxin** (antigen produced by *A. flavus*) exposure may also result in hepatocellular carcinoma
– Patients may be systemically unwell, with cough, pyrexia and haemoptysis being key features
– Treatment should be initiated without waiting for results of culture; treat with **voriconazole**

2.4.5 Allergic bronchopulmonary aspergillosis (ABPA)

Definition: allergic bronchopulmonary aspergillosis (ABPA) is characterised by respiratory difficulty caused by a hypersensitivity reaction to *Aspergillus* spp., often seen in patients with a history of atopy.

Epidemiology:
- More common in patients with **asthma** or **cystic fibrosis**
- Seen in 22% of patients with a history of atopy, versus 2% of patients without reported atopy

Clinical features:
- Patients largely present with cough and haemoptysis, and are generally systemically unwell
- Fungal sinusitis may also be a presenting feature

Investigations
Investigations should be undertaken in the following order.

> **Stepwise plan:**

> 1 **Obtain CXR and CT scan demonstrating disease**

2 **Arrange blood tests**
- Elevated IgE, eosinophilia and *Aspergillus* serum precipitins

3 **Check for *Aspergillus* in sputum or on skin tests (*Fig. 2.20*)**

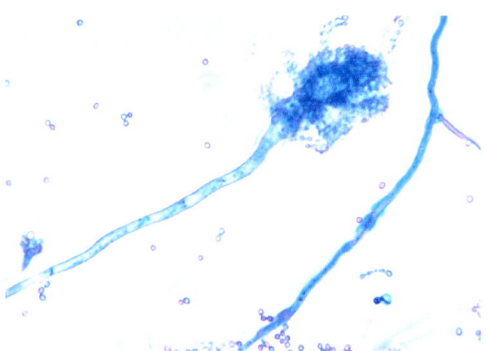

Fig. 2.20 Aspergillus fumigatus *on microscopy.*

> **Stepwise management of allergic bronchopulmonary aspergillosis**

> 1 **Treat with oral CORTICOSTEROIDS and ITRACONAZOLE**

> 2 **Steroid therapy may be required for up to 6 months**

> 3 **Prescribe bronchodilator treatment for asthma and manage cystic fibrosis as per recommendations**

2.5 Diseases of the pleura

2.5.1 Pleural effusion

Definition: a pleural effusion results when a greater than normal amount of fluid collects within the pleural space.

Aetiology/pathophysiology:
- May occur as a result of myriad processes
- Effusions can be helpfully classified into **transudates** and **exudates**, but be aware that blood and chyle can also build up in the pleural space

- Exudates generally occur due to increased capillary permeability, while transudates generally occur as a result of increased capillary hydrostatic pressure or decreased oncotic pressure
- Causes of a transudate may include heart failure, liver failure, hypoalbuminaemia, **Meig syndrome** (a triad of right-sided pleural effusion, ascites and a benign ovarian tumour) and pulmonary embolism
- Causes of an exudate can include inflammatory, neoplastic or infective conditions such as pneumonia, TB and lung cancer

Clinical features:
- May be asymptomatic or may present with
  dyspnoea or pleuritic chest pain
- Signs on examination may include tracheal
  deviation (for large effusions), dullness (classically
  stony dull) on percussion, reduced air entry and
  chest expansion

**Stepwise management of a pleural effusion
(BTS 2010)**

1 Perform a PA (postero-anterior) CXR
- Perform a PA CXR in cases of suspected pleural
  effusion (see *Fig. 2.21*)

2 Check whether effusion is a transudate
- Check the history and clinical picture to
  ascertain whether the effusion is a transudate
  (e.g. LVF, dialysis, hypoalbuminaemia)
- If so, and **particularly if pleural effusion is
  bilateral**, do not perform aspiration of pleural
  fluid

**3 Arrange pleural aspiration if an exudate
   is suspected**
- BTS guidelines recommend the use of
  ultrasound
- Ultrasound guidance significantly increases
  the likelihood of successful pleural fluid
  aspiration and reduces the risk of organ
  puncture
- A diagnostic pleural fluid sample should be
  aspirated with a fine-bore (21G) needle and a
  50ml syringe

4 Arrange for pleural fluid testing
- Pleural fluid should always be sent for protein,
  LDH, Gram stain, cytology and microbiological
  culture
- Record appearance of pleural fluid and any
  associated odour

- All patients with an effusion with a
  superimposed infective condition (e.g.
  pneumonia) require pleural fluid sampling

5 Apply the Light criteria as necessary
- This makes it possible to distinguish between
  a transudate and an exudate

6 Treat the underlying cause
- Tapping pleural fluid may relieve symptoms,
  and chest drains may be utilised as well
- Chest drains are indicated, particularly in cases
  of pleural infection

7 Utilise pleurodesis if necessary
- Pleurodesis (adhering parietal and visceral
  pleura with substances such as talc) may
  also be utilised in refractory cases, such as
  malignant, recurrent effusions

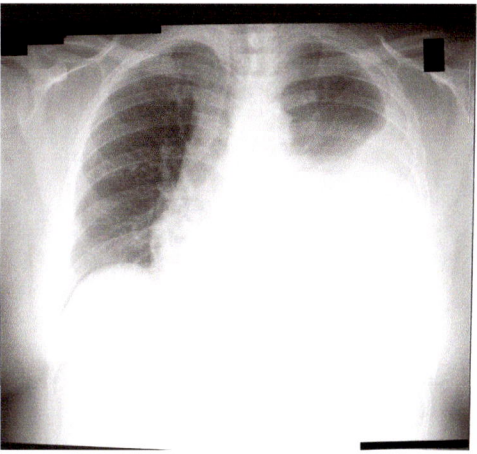

Fig. 2.21 *A large left-sided pleural effusion on CXR.*

P >> A pleural fluid pH <7.2 should prompt
suspicion of **empyema** or a para-pneumonic
effusion (non-infected pleural effusion with
a background of pneumonia). Note that
these require both antibiotics and chest tube
drainage to treat.

E >> The safe triangle is a virtual triangle
bordered by:
- Mid-axillary line
- Imaginary horizontal line at the nipple
- Lateral border of the pectoris major

The drain is usually sited at the fourth, fifth or
sixth intercostal space.

2

2.5.2 Pneumothorax

Definition: a pneumothorax refers to the process by which an abnormal amount of air accumulates within the pleural space.

Epidemiology:

- Pneumothoraces are more likely to occur in smokers, particularly men, and the likelihood of developing a pneumothorax is directly related to the amount of smoking
- Almost 50% of patients with chest trauma develop a pneumothorax

Aetiology:

- May be open (communicating with the exterior), closed (chest wall is intact, with accumulation of air in the pleural space), or tension (air enters the pleural cavity via a one-way valve and compresses surrounding structures)
- Non-tension spontaneous pneumothoraces can be classified into primary and secondary spontaneous pneumothoraces
- **Primary spontaneous pneumothorax (PSP)** occurs in healthy individuals, with no underlying lung disease; classically associated with young, tall, thin men and smokers
- **Secondary spontaneous pneumothorax (SSP)** usually occurs in individuals with underlying lung disease, such as COPD, infection, TB, etc.
- Pneumothorax can also be traumatic or iatrogenic in nature (e.g. occur as a procedural complication, as with insertion of CVP line)

P ≫ A catamenial pneumothorax refers to a pneumothorax that occurs at the time of menstruation (linked to endometriosis involving the pleura).

Clinical features:

- Patient presents with sudden-onset dyspnoea or pleuritic chest pain
- Signs on examination include decreased chest expansion, reduced breath sounds and hyper-resonance on percussion

E ≫ Tension pneumothorax is a medical emergency: the diagnosis here is essentially clinical, and a CXR should not be performed. Treatment of a tension pneumothorax involves insertion of

W ≫ Subcutaneous emphysema refers to the phenomenon in which there is trapped air in the subcutaneous tissue. This can usually be felt as crepitus on the face, chest and neck. It (usually) occurs as a result of air travelling from the respiratory system or GI tract, and may be caused by pneumothoraces, gunshot wounds or infections (e.g. gas gangrene/*Clostridium perfringens*). It may also occur iatrogenically or secondary to a surgical procedure, in which case it is termed surgical emphysema. Palpating the skin causes crackling, which is virtually pathognomonic of the condition.

Pathophysiology

The pressure in the alveoli is generally lower than in the intra-pleural space. Gas accumulates in the pleural space because there is a pressure gradient between the alveoli and the pleural space, and gas flow continues in this direction until sealed.

Management

Management algorithm as per BTS 2010.

Stepwise management of a spontaneous pneumothorax (BTS 2010)

1 **Perform a PA CXR in suspected pneumothorax (see *Figs 2.22* and *2.23*)**

2 **Ascertain the degree of breathlessness from the history and clinical examination**
- The degree of breathlessness influences management (see *Fig. 2.24*)

3 **Distinguish between a primary and secondary spontaneous pneumothorax**
- As a rule of thumb, SSPs involve underlying lung disease and are less well tolerated than PSPs

a large-bore cannula into the second intercostal space at the mid-clavicular line, with subsequent chest drain insertion after the emergent case has been dealt with.

2

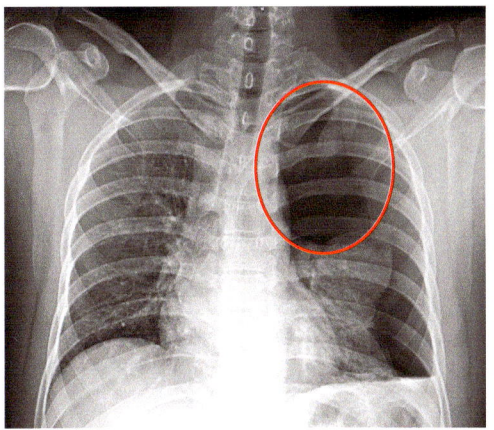

Fig. 2.22 *A large right-sided pneumothorax. Note no lung markings over left lung field.*

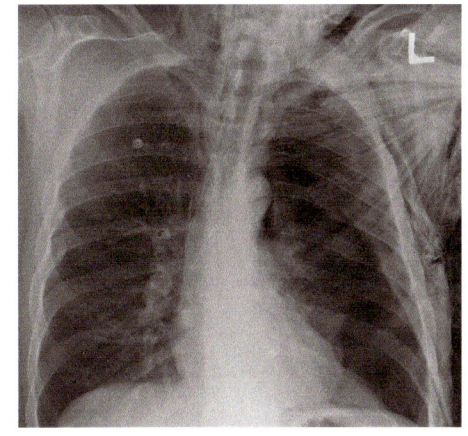

Fig. 2.23 *Tension pneumothorax of the left lung. Note that this CXR should not be done clinically.*

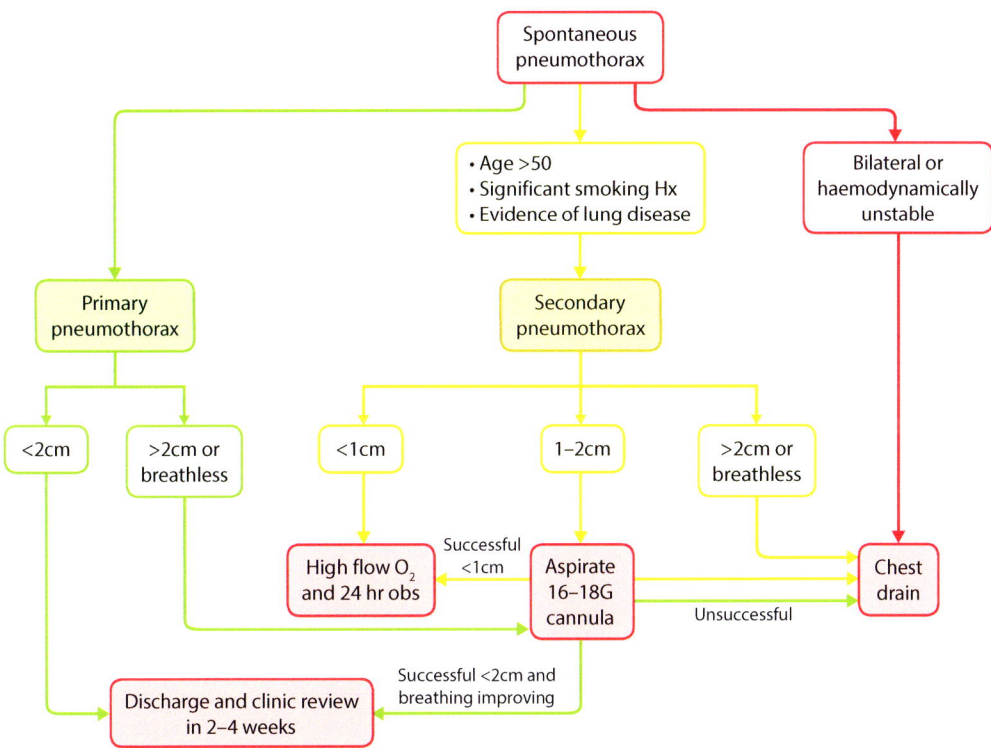

Fig. 2.24 *Management of pneumothorax.*

2

2.6 Lung cancer

Definition: lung cancer is characterised by primary neoplastic change in cells in the bronchi or lung, or the invasion of the lung secondarily by metastatic lesions from elsewhere in the body.

Epidemiology:

- 90% of lung cancer is linked to cigarette smoking
- 58% of lung cancer is found to occur in less developed countries
- Lung cancer is implicated in 1.59 million deaths annually worldwide

Aetiology/pathophysiology:

- The vast majority of primary lung tumours are bronchial in origin; histological classification of the type of lung cancer can help influence management and help ascertain prognosis
- Primary lung tumours are traditionally classified into two groups: small-cell lung cancer (20% SCLC); and non-small cell lung cancer (80% NSCLC)
- SCLC is characterised by rapid proliferation and has often metastasised by the time it is diagnosed
- Neoplastic change originates from endocrine APUD cells. These cancers are usually centrally located, near the bronchi. This type of lung cancer may also be associated with Cushing syndrome, as a result of **ectopic ACTH secretion**. While SCLC is extremely sensitive to chemotherapy, prognosis remains poor due to extensive metastasis
- **Lambert–Eaton myasthenic syndrome** is also most commonly associated with SCLC
- Of the NSCLCs, several important subtypes include:
  1. Adenocarcinoma – this is the most common sub-type in **non-smokers** and people with exposure to asbestos. These tumours arise from mucous cells, and generally metastasise outside the lung, primarily to bone, and can present with metastasis at diagnosis. These tumours are peripherally located.
  2. Squamous cell carcinoma – these tumours are **centrally located**, and locally invasive. As they metastasise late, patients with this type of lung cancer are good surgical candidates, provided there is good cardiorespiratory function and no extensive spread. These are also associated with **ectopic PTH secretion**, and may present with an elevated serum calcium.
  3. Large cell carcinoma – poorly differentiated tumours histologically, which also metastasise early and are associated with a poor prognosis. They are peripherally located.
  4. Carcinoid tumours – rare neuroendocrine tumours that arise from the enterochromaffin cells. Usually clinically silent, but may present with weight loss or localised pain.

 E ≫ **S**mall and **S**quamous are **S**-entrally located tumours.

Clinical features:

- Patients with lung cancer may present with a variety of symptoms; typically, these include shortness of breath, weight loss, chest pain and haemoptysis
- A long-standing history of tobacco smoking is usually present
- Hoarseness may indicate laryngeal nerve involvement, typified by a 'bovine cough'

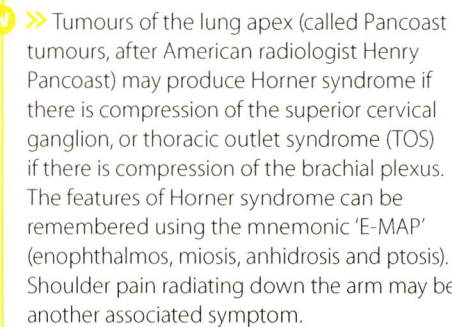 **W** ≫ Tumours of the lung apex (called Pancoast tumours, after American radiologist Henry Pancoast) may produce Horner syndrome if there is compression of the superior cervical ganglion, or thoracic outlet syndrome (TOS) if there is compression of the brachial plexus. The features of Horner syndrome can be remembered using the mnemonic 'E-MAP' (enophthalmos, miosis, anhidrosis and ptosis). Shoulder pain radiating down the arm may be another associated symptom.

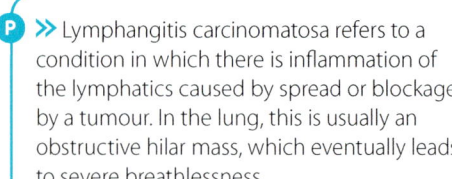 **P** ≫ Lymphangitis carcinomatosa refers to a condition in which there is inflammation of the lymphatics caused by spread or blockage by a tumour. In the lung, this is usually an obstructive hilar mass, which eventually leads to severe breathlessness.

E ≫ Superior vena cava obstruction (SVCO) is another important complication of lung cancer, and lung cancer is described as its most common cause. Patients with SVCO present with acute-onset dyspnoea, neck and face plethora and swelling, and dilated superficial veins. They may also experience syncope. SVCO is also associated with a positive Pemberton sign, in which raising both hands above the patient's head produces facial congestion, cyanosis and transient respiratory distress.

Investigations

Investigations should be undertaken in the following order.

If a diagnosis of lung cancer is clinically suspected, proceed stepwise:

1 **Perform a (PA) CXR**
- The CXR may show a 'coin lesion', suggestive of neoplasia, hilar enlargement or pleural effusion (see *Fig. 2.25*)
- If clinical suspicion is high, despite a normal CXR, further investigation is warranted (NICE 2017, NG12); offer an urgent CXR within 2 weeks if patient is ≥40, smokes and has 1 of the following unexplained symptoms (or is a non-smoker with 2 of the following unexplained symptoms): cough, fatigue, SOB, weight loss, appetite loss or chest pain

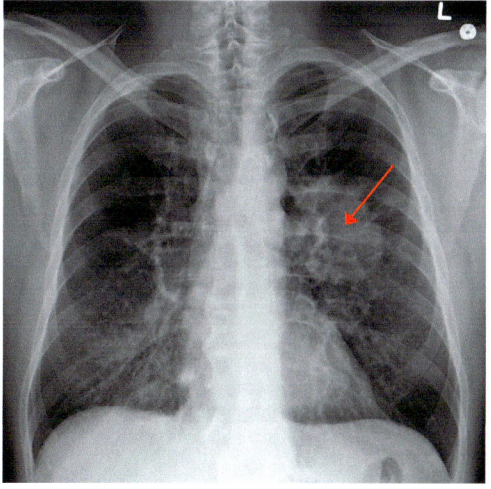

Fig. 2.25 *Solitary 'coin lesion' in the left upper lobe suspicious of lung cancer.*

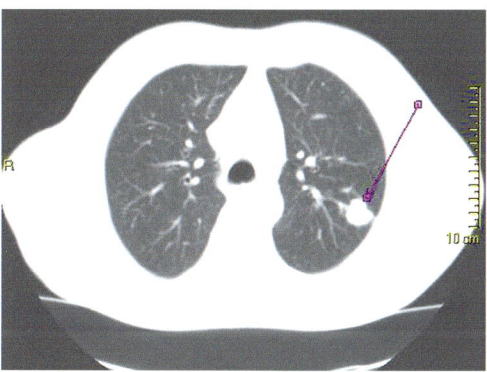

Fig. 2.26 *CT chest showing a peripheral left upper lobe lesion.*

2 **If the CXR suggests lung cancer, involvement of a multi-disciplinary team is recommended**

3 **If lung cancer is known or suspected, offer a contrast-enhanced CT scan**
- Patients with known or suspected lung cancer should be offered a contrast-enhanced CT scan (see *Fig. 2.26*) to further diagnose and stage (TNM – tumour/node/metastasis) the disease
- Note that all patients potentially suitable for curative therapy should be offered a PET-CT before treatment

4 **Arrange further investigations if necessary**
- Offer fibre-optic bronchoscopy to patients with central lesions, and CT or ultrasound-guided needle biopsy to patients with peripheral lung lesions
- Lymph nodes can also be appropriately sampled if necessary

General principles: encourage coordinated campaigning to increase awareness of lung cancer and highlight the importance of early diagnosis. Find out how much the patient knows and ensure that there is good communication. A specialist lung cancer nurse should be involved if possible. Smoking cessation should also be encouraged. Patients who may benefit from palliative care should be referred to a specialist without delay.

For NSCLC:

1 **Use a risk score (Thorascore)**
- Use a risk score (Thorascore) to evaluate risk if surgery is being considered
- Optimise cardiorespiratory function

2 **Consider surgical therapy**
- Surgical therapy is the treatment of choice in patients with Stage I or II disease if there is curative intent

3 **Consider radical radiotherapy**
- Radical radiotherapy is indicated in patients with Stage I, II or III NSCLC if there is curative intent
- Note that all patients should undergo PFTs first

4 Consider chemotherapy
- Consider chemotherapy for patients with Stage III or IV NSCLC to improve survival and quality of life

5 Consider multi-modality therapy
- Multi-modality therapy (surgery, radiotherapy and chemotherapy) should be discussed with an oncologist and thoracic surgeon and an MDT

For SCLC:

1 Offer chemotherapy
- Offer patients with limited-stage disease SCLC four to six cycles of cisplatin-based combination chemotherapy first line
- A multi-drug regimen should be used

2 Offer concurrent radiotherapy

P >> Guidelines recommend consideration of surgical therapy in SCLC if limited disease is present, i.e. no lymph node involvement or metastasis. However, it is important to keep in mind that disease is generally disseminated in various types of lung cancer at presentation, and this is particularly the case in SCLC.

E >> Surgery contraindications
- Disseminated disease or malignant pleural effusion
- FEV_1 <1.5L
- Vocal cord paralysis or local infiltration
- SVCO

2.7 Pulmonary vascular disease

2.7.1 Pulmonary embolism

Definition: a pulmonary embolus (PE) arises as a consequence of a thrombus forming in the deep veins of the lower limbs. This spectrum of thromboembolic disease, encompassing risk, deep vein thrombosis (DVT) and subsequent embolus, is collectively termed venous thromboembolism (VTE).

Epidemiology:
- PE is considered a medical emergency
- No exact epidemiology, but estimated to affect 65 per 100,000 in the general population
- Mortality rates are higher in men

Aetiology:
- Note that a pulmonary embolus can also occur as a result of a fat embolus from a long bone fracture or an air embolus secondary to trauma as well.

E >> Predisposition to thrombosis is exemplified by the Virchow triad: hypercoagulability of blood, venous stasis and endothelial damage.

P >> **PE risk factors**
Risk factors can be memorised using the mnemonic '**SPAM HD**':
Surgery
Pregnancy
Age
Malignancy
Hormones (COCP/HRT)
DVT

Clinical features:
- Symptoms pertaining to PE may be non-specific, but are generally acute; these include chest pain, dyspnoea, haemoptysis and syncope in severe cases
- The most common signs observed are tachypnoea and tachycardia; a lowered SpO_2 may also be present
- The traditional 'S1Q3T3' pattern traditionally described in PE is far less common in clinical practice (see *Fig. 2.27*)

E >> Patients with a massive pulmonary embolus who present with haemodynamic instability, acute breathlessness and features of shock should be treated with thrombolysis. This should be performed in a high-dependency setting.

Pathophysiology
- Emboli in the lung are inextricably linked to thrombus formation in the deep veins of the lower limbs
- It is uncommon for a thrombus to develop in the pulmonary vasculature
- Evidence suggests that a PE is more likely when the lower (rather than upper) limbs are involved

Investigations
The approach to a pulmonary embolism begins, according to NICE guidelines, with an assessment of the patient using a focused history and examination, followed by a CXR to exclude other pathology. Investigations should be undertaken in the following order.

2

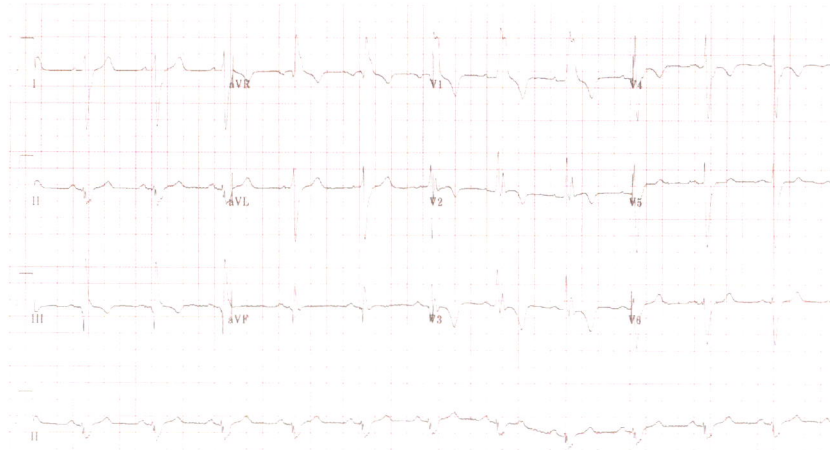

Fig. 2.27 *ECG showing sinus tachycardia, RBBB, T-wave inversion in V1-V3 and the S1Q3T3 pattern, suggestive of a pulmonary embolism.*

Stepwise plan (NICE 2012, CG144):

1   Use a two-level PE Wells score
- Use a two-level PE Wells score to estimate the clinical probability of PE (see *Table 2.2*)

2   Check whether score is more or less than 4
- A PE is likely if the score is more than 4, and unlikely if the score tallies at 4 points or less

3   Check whether PE is clinically likely or unlikely
- (A) If a PE is clinically likely, proceed with an immediate computed tomography pulmonary angiogram (CTPA, see *Fig. 2.28*); if a CTPA cannot be carried out immediately, arrange intermediate anticoagulant therapy
- (B) If a patient has an allergy to contrast media, renal failure or is unsuitable to receive radiation, consider a V/Q SPECT scan (see *Fig. 2.29*). If a PE is unlikely based on the score, arrange a D-dimer test. If D-dimer is negative, consider an alternative diagnosis. If D-dimer is positive, arrange a CTPA for a definitive diagnosis

Table 2.2 *Wells score*

	Score
Signs and symptoms of DVT	3
Alternative Dx less likely than PE	3
Tachycardia (>100 bpm)	1.5
Immobility >3 days or surgery in last 4 weeks	1.5
Previous DVT/PE	1.5
Haemoptysis	1
Malignancy	1

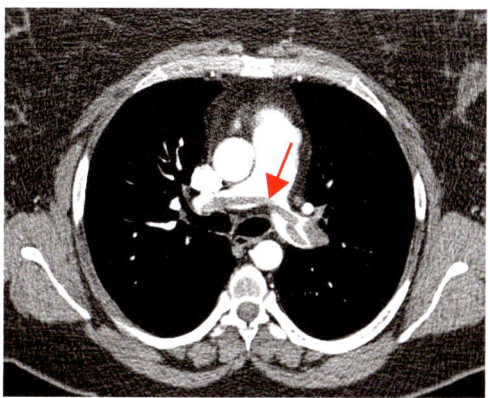

Fig. 2.28 *CTPA showing a saddle embolus sitting across the pulmonary arteries.*

Stepwise management of pulmonary embolism (NICE 2012, CG144)

General principles: in an acute case, ensure the patient is given oxygen and is sitting up. Note that **thrombolysis** is considered first-line treatment for a massive pulmonary embolus in which there is circulatory failure.

1   Administer pharmacological therapy
- Offer LMWH or fondaparinux first line as soon as PE is diagnosed
- Use unfractionated heparin (UFH) if the patient has renal failure or is at particularly high risk of bleeding
- Continue LMWH/fondaparinux for five days or until the international normalised ratio (INR) is ≥2 for more than 24 hours

2

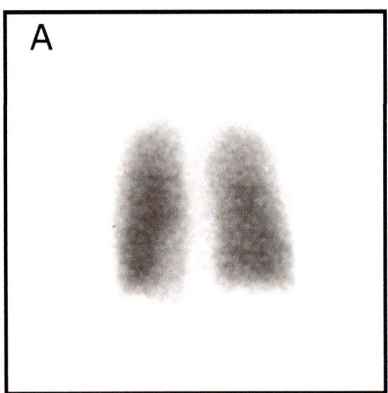
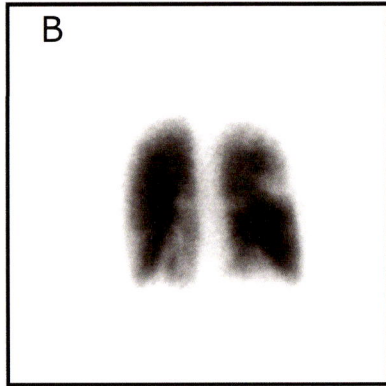

Fig. 2.29 *Ventilation (A)/Perfusion (B) SPECT scan revealing deficits in both the right and left lungs as a result of a PE.*

2   **If the patient has active cancer, offer LMWH for six months and reassess**

3   **Use warfarin for a patient with a provoked (meaning that an attributable cause can be discerned) DVT/PE for three months and reassess**

4   **If the patient had an unprovoked DVT/ PE, consider extending warfarin therapy beyond three months**

5   **Consider a vena cava filter in patients with recurrent emboli despite anticoagulation**

6   **Consider rivaroxaban**
   - According to the latest guidelines, rivaroxaban (novel anticoagulant) is a suitable alternative to warfarin but do bear in mind the cost of the drug

2.7.2 Pulmonary hypertension

Definition: pulmonary hypertension (PH) is defined by the ESC as an increase in mean pulmonary arterial pressure ≥25mmHg at rest or ≥35mmHg with exercise.

It can be classified as follows:
- **Group I: idiopathic pulmonary hypertension**
  - Rare
  - Elevated pulmonary artery pressure, normal PCWP
  - Presents with SOB on exertion, fatigue
- **Group II: PH secondary to left heart disease (most common variant)**
  - Systolic, diastolic or valvular heart disease
- **Group III: PH secondary to lung disease and hypoxia**
  - e.g. COPD, ILD, high altitudes
- **Group IV: chronic thromboembolic pulmonary hypertension (CTEPH)**

Patients typically present with SOB on exertion, fatigue, oedema and may also present with angina type pain.

- **Group V**: pulmonary hypertension due to miscellaneous causes, e.g. sarcoidosis, histiocytosis X

Management
Right heart catheterisation is confirmatory, but other tests should be carried out, such as blood tests, autoimmune screening (especially for **scleroderma**), ECG, spirometry and echocardiography.

Stepwise plan:

Management involves treating the underlying cause.

1   **Carry out acute vasodilator testing**
   a.   If positive, offer oral calcium channel blockers
   b.   If negative, offer:
      i.   Prostacyclin analogues
      ii.   Endothelin receptor antagonists, e.g. bosentan
      iii. Phosphodiesterase inhibitors e.g. sildenafil

2   **Provide oxygen, diuretics and anticoagulation with warfarin**

2.7.3 Cor pulmonale

Definition: cor pulmonale refers to an alteration of structure and function of the right ventricle secondary to lung disease, most commonly COPD and pulmonary hypertension.

Clinical features:
- Worsening shortness of breath (particularly on exertion)
- Fatigue
- Oedema
- Haemoptysis

Management

Diagnosis is made based on echocardiography and right heart catheterisation. ECG demonstrates right ventricular hypertrophy and peaked P waves.

Treatment of cor pulmonale involves treating the underlying cause (e.g. COPD in chronic disease, or VTE in acute cor pulmonale). Patients should be advised to stop smoking.

Further management recommendations:
- Long-term oxygen therapy (LTOT) improves survival and reduces pulmonary artery resistance
- Diuretics
- Long-acting calcium channel blockers, e.g. nifedipine
- Transplantation, in severe, intractable disease

2.8 Other conditions

2.8.1 Allergic rhinitis

Definition: allergic rhinitis refers to inflammation of the nasal mucosa secondary to an IgE-mediated response to an allergen.

Epidemiology:
- Peak incidence in children and young adults; boys are affected more than girls
- Highest prevalence in UK, Australia, New Zealand and Ireland
- Prevalence is increasing in younger age groups

W » The hygiene hypothesis, which refers to the idea that infective agents help strengthen host immunity and prevent the development of immune-mediated disease, has been put forward as an explanation of the increasing prevalence of allergic rhinitis. As the rates of infection decrease in more developed countries, the rates of autoimmune disease have seemingly increased.

Aetiology:
- A history of atopy or a family history of atopy is implicated in the development of this disease
- The development of allergic rhinitis is said to be multifactorial, with both genetic susceptibility and particulate environmental allergens playing a role
- Common allergens include pollen/grass (hay fever) and the house dust mite

Clinical features:
- Sneezing, nasal congestion and post-nasal drip
- Watery eyes, redness, swelling or itching, particularly in the nose and palate

Pathophysiology
Individuals with a genetic susceptibility to particular environmental antigens experience an IgE-mediated reaction upon exposure to the allergen. This leads to mast cell degranulation and histamine release, which in turn leads to gland stimulation, producing symptoms of nasal congestion and rhinorrhoea.

Investigations

Stepwise plan:

Generally, allergic rhinitis may be diagnosed by identifying characteristic features and excluding infectious and irritant causes. Investigations should be undertaken in the following order.

1 Identify whether cause is infective, irritant or allergic
- An infective cause is more likely when there are acute symptoms of an upper respiratory tract infection, pyrexia or lymphadenopathy
- An irritant cause is more likely if there is known physical or chemical exposure

2 Perform an allergy test
- A skin prick test is the first-line investigation
- This is followed by radioallergosorbent (RAST) or enzyme-linked immunosorbent assay (ELISA) second line, if symptoms persist, or the aetiology (infective, irritant or allergic) is unclear

3 Proceed with second-line allergen testing if patient is on antihistamine or corticosteroid
- Note that the results of a skin prick test may be affected by antihistamine or corticosteroid use; if the patient is on these medications, proceed with second-line allergen testing

Stepwise management of allergic rhinitis

1 Advise the patient to avoid the offending allergen

2 Offer oral or nasal antihistamines as required first line

2

3   **Offer intranasal corticosteroids if symptoms persist, particularly if nasal blocking and polyps are predominant**

4   **Nasal douching with normal saline can be used as an adjunct**

2.8.2 Sinusitis

Definition: sinusitis refers to the inflammation of one or more of the paranasal sinuses (frontal, maxillary, sphenoidal and ethmoid).

Epidemiology:
- 25 per 100,000 person-years in the general practice setting in UK
- Most common chronic illness in the USA

Aetiology/pathophysiology:
- Aetiology is thought to be multifactorial in origin, predisposing to inflammation of the sinuses
- Sinusitis occurs when mucus drainage is obstructed
- Structural abnormalities (such as a deviated nasal septum), infective agents (such as *Strep. pneumoniae* or *H. influenzae*) and environmental agents (such as smoking) may further increase the chance of developing sinusitis

Clinical features:
- Facial pain, typically over the affected sinus (note that all but the sphenoidal sinus can be palpated to elicit tenderness)
- Rhinorrhoea or post-nasal drip with or without hyposmia

Investigations
Investigations should be undertaken in the following order.

> **Stepwise plan:**

Generally, sinusitis is diagnosed based on history and examination findings. NICE recommends diagnosing sinusitis when the following are present:

1   **Check for nasal blockage, discoloured discharge, headache and/or impaired sense of smell**
- Check for nasal blockage (obstruction/congestion) or discoloured nasal discharge (anterior/posterior nasal drip) with facial pain/pressure or headache and/or reduction in loss of sense of smell

2   **Distinguish between acute and chronic sinusitis**
- Acute sinusitis generally refers to these symptoms lasting under 12 weeks, whereas

chronic sinusitis refers to symptoms persisting for more than 12 weeks

3   **Consider further investigations if diagnosis is still uncertain**
- Imaging (X-rays, CT and MRI) and sinus puncture may be considered in uncertain cases, but are generally not recommended

> **Stepwise management of acute sinusitis**

1   **Ascertain whether there is orbital involvement**
- Examples include conditions such as peri-orbital oedema or cellulitis, or **intracranial involvement** (symptoms of meningitis or focal neurology)
- If these are present, arrange urgent admission

2   **Provide analgesia**
- Paracetamol or ibuprofen to reduce pain and swelling

3   **Irrigate nose and apply face packs**
- Irrigation of nose with saline may reduce congestion
- Application of warm face packs may provide localised relief

4   **Consider prescribing antibiotic if necessary**
- Only prescribe an antibiotic for patients when acute bacterial sinusitis is present or if they have relevant underlying comorbidities

5   **Consider prescribing intranasal corticosteroids**
- Corticosteroids should only be prescribed for patients with prolonged or severe symptoms

6   **Consider referring patient to ENT**
- ENT referral is only appropriate for patients who have frequent, recurrent episodes of sinusitis (more than three episodes requiring antibiotics a year)

E ≫ Treatments that are **not** recommended include **steam inhalation, oral corticosteroids** or complementary therapies.

2.8.3 Obstructive sleep apnoea

Definition: obstructive sleep apnoea (OSA) refers to intermittent complete or partial blockage of the airway during sleep, resulting in unrefreshing sleep at night and excessive daytime sleepiness.

Epidemiology:
- Common condition, affecting more men than women
- More common in Hispanics and Asians
- Associated with an increased risk of road traffic accidents

Aetiology:
- Particularly associated with obesity, diabetes, insulin resistance, polycystic ovary syndrome (PCOS) and metabolic syndrome
- Obesity is cited as the greatest risk factor
- Other risk factors include a deviated nasal septum, smoking, and sedative drug and alcohol use
- Anatomy of the jaw and pharynx may play a role in the development of OSA

Clinical features:
- Patients commonly present with daytime sleepiness
- Partners may report snoring, restlessness, apnoeic periods and waking at night
- A high index of suspicion should be reserved if patients complaining of these symptoms are obese
- Observe for a large neck circumference and ascertain if there are any jaw abnormalities present
- Dry mouth and gingivitis may be additional associated symptoms, particularly if mouth-breathing

P >> In contrast, central sleep apnoea occurs with lowered respiratory effort secondary to impaired neurological control of breathing or respiratory muscle weakness. Treatment is more difficult and involves treating the underlying cause, although CPAP (see 'Management' below) is a viable treatment modality.

Investigations
Investigations should be undertaken in the following order.

Stepwise plan:

1 **Ascertain sleep/wake cycles from patient's partner**
- Ask about mood and work performance

2 **Assess jaw anatomy, body habitus and neck circumference**
- Neck circumference greater than 40cm confers an increased risk

3 **Assess daytime sleepiness using the Epworth Sleepiness Scale**

4 **Polysomnography (sleep studies) are the gold standard investigation**
- Diagnosis is made based on the apnoea/hypopnoea index (AHI), i.e. the number of apnoea or hypopnoea episodes, divided by the number of hours during the study
- Moderate AHI = 15–30 per hr
- Severe AHI >30 per hr

Stepwise management of obstructive sleep apnoea

1 **Lifestyle modification, including weight loss and optimising risk factors, is first line**

2 **The use of mandibular splints may help moderate sleep apnoea**

3 **CPAP (continuous positive airway pressure) is gold standard therapy**
- But bear in mind that patients may find the use of CPAP uncomfortable or disruptive, and may not adhere to treatment

W >> Diagnosing and treating obstructive sleep apnoea is important, as these patients may go on to develop hypertension, AF and other cardio-metabolic sequelae. This process is thought to occur because arousal from sleep provokes catecholamine release. The frequency with which this occurs over time leads to an increased associated risk of these conditions.

Chapter 3
Gastroenterology and hepatobiliary medicine

Hwan Juet Khaw and *Samantha Jingyun Koh*

Basic principles

The digestive system is one of the largest systems in the human body. Its main function is to transport and break down the foods that we eat, absorb their nutrients and eliminate unwanted by-products. This intricate system also regulates the synthesis of both exocrine and endocrine hormones, allowing it to function synergistically with other body systems. As the alimentary tract is constantly being exposed to foreign antigens, it is protected by both innate and acquired immunological mechanisms.

Bridge to clinical medicine

The alimentary tract is a continuous one-way tube measuring approximately 7m, starting at the mouth and terminating at the anus. Initial digestion occurs in the mouth, as salivary enzymes are released to facilitate the breakdown of complex carbohydrates.

Oesophagus

- A 25cm muscular tube, connecting the pharynx to the stomach

E ≫ Histologically, the upper two-thirds of the oesophagus is lined by stratified squamous epithelium, which transitions distally into squamo-columnar epithelium.

- There are two natural narrowing points along the oesophagus, namely the upper oesophageal sphincter and the lower oesophageal sphincter

- Dysfunction of these sphincters (particularly the lower sphincter) will result in gastro-oesophageal reflux disease (GORD)

Stomach

- The stomach is lined with a specialised columnar epithelium, adapted with gastric pits that contain **chief** cells and **parietal** cells (see *Fig. 3.1*)
- Chief cells are responsible for producing pepsin, and parietal cells secrete hydrochloric acid and release intrinsic factor

E ≫ Intrinsic factor binds to vitamin B12, which essentially primes it to be absorbed in the terminal ileum.

- Because of the stomach's low pH environment, it is protected by surface cells that secrete mucus and bicarbonate
- It connects to the duodenum via the pyloric sphincter

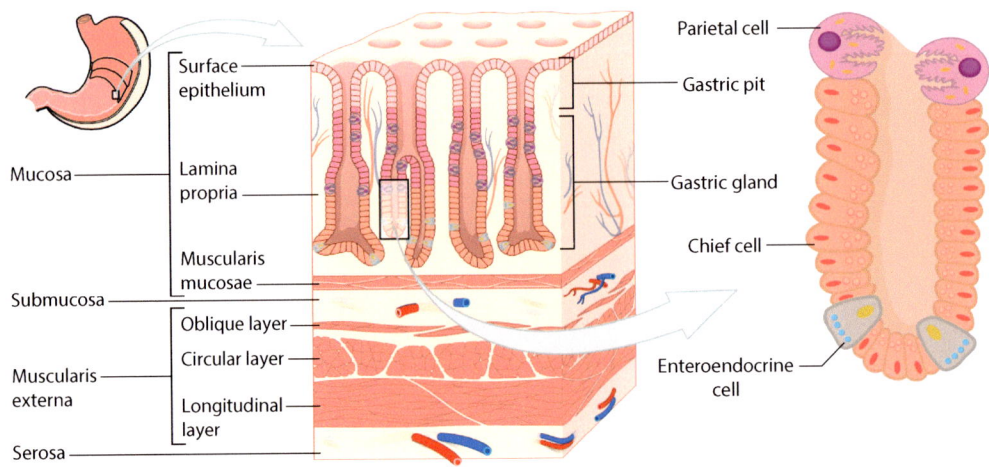

Fig. 3.1 Histology of the stomach.

Small intestine

- At 2–3m long, this is the longest segment of the alimentary tract
- It is divided into three sections: the duodenum (around 25cm), jejunum (0.9m) and ileum (1.8m)
- The duodenum is an important structure, as it is the site where the biliary and pancreatic systems communicate with the intestinal tract via the **ampulla of Vater**

> **P** » The ampulla of Vater is situated at the midpoint of the second part of the duodenum, which is also the embryological landmark at which the foregut becomes the midgut.

- The epithelium of the small intestine is uniquely adapted for its function of nutrient absorption
- Villi and microvilli, finger-like projections formed by the unique arrangement of enterocytes, provide a large absorptive surface area
- Specialised Paneth cells, located at the crypts of the intestinal glands, produce an alkaline mixture of mucus and enzymes

Large intestine

- Terminal segment of the alimentary tract, which can be subdivided into the caecum, colon (see *Fig. 3.2*), rectum and anus
- Primarily responsible for water and electrolyte reabsorption

- Communicates with the terminal ileum via the ileocaecal valve, which functions to regulate flow into the colon
- Food residue then travels up the ascending colon, through the transverse colon, down into the descending colon and inferiorly through the sigmoid colon
- The rectum receives the food residue and acts as a storage site before the anal canal
- Faecal continence is maintained by both the external (voluntary) and internal (involuntary) anal sphincter muscle tone

Pancreas

- An oblong, retroperitoneal structure (see *Fig. 3.3*), located posterior to the stomach, which has both endocrine (2%) and exocrine functions (98%) – the endocrine pancreas will be discussed in *Chapter 4*
- The exocrine cells of the pancreas, known as **acinar cells**, secrete enzyme-rich pancreatic juice into the terminal ends of pancreatic ducts

> **P** » To prevent auto-digestion, only pre-activated forms of protein-digesting enzymes (i.e. trypsinogen and chymotrypsinogen) are produced by the pancreas.

- The pancreas also produces amylase and lipase – for carbohydrate and lipid digestion, respectively
- The pancreatic duct eventually merges with the common bile duct, which empties into the duodenum via the ampulla of Vater

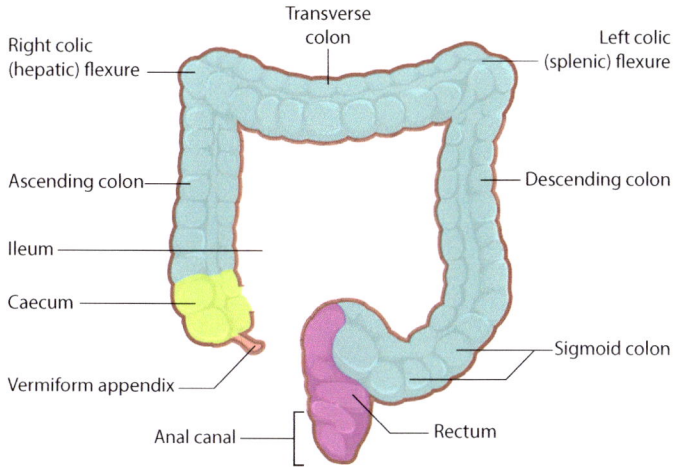

Right colic (hepatic) flexure

Transverse colon

Left colic (splenic) flexure

Ascending colon

Descending colon

Ileum

Caecum

Vermiform appendix

Sigmoid colon

Anal canal

Rectum

Fig. 3.2 *Anatomy of the colon.*

3

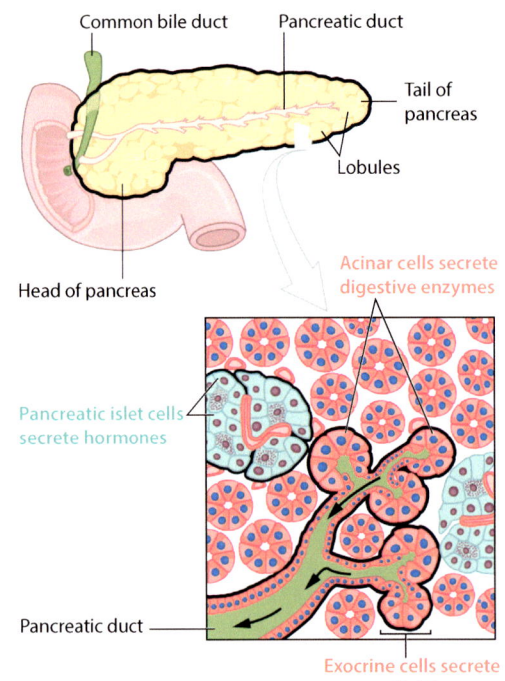

Fig. 3.3 *Anatomy and histology of the pancreas.*

Liver and the biliary system

- The largest internal organ of the body, weighing 1.2–1.5kg
- Can be divided into right and left lobes, with further subdivision into eight segments
- It has a dual blood supply – 25% via the hepatic artery and the other 75% from the portal venous system

> **W** ›› This means that all blood from the alimentary tract flows through the liver. As a result, the liver is a common site for cancer metastasis.

- Role of the liver:
  - **Carbohydrate metabolism** – conversion of glucose to glycogen for storage after a meal, as well as gluconeogenesis during fasting
  - **Lipid metabolism** – the liver is primarily involved in the synthesis of LDL and HDL

> **E** ›› Statins, HMG-CoA enzyme inhibitors, target this metabolic pathway to reduce cholesterol production.

  - **Synthesis of albumin** – albumin is a vital plasma protein that plays a central role in transporting hormones and electrolytes (e.g. Ca) as well as regulating vascular oncotic pressure
  - **Synthesis of clotting factors** – coagulation factors (II, VII, IX, X) are produced in the liver via vitamin K-dependent metabolic pathways
  - **Immunological function** – specialised liver macrophages (known as Kupffer cells) reside in the hepatocyte environment and are responsible for triggering both local and systemic inflammatory responses
  - **Bilirubin metabolism** and **bile production** (see *Fig. 3.4*)
  - **Drug and toxin metabolism**
- Haem from red blood cells is broken down into biliverdin, which is subsequently converted into bilirubin (see *Fig. 3.4*)
- This bilirubin is then transported (albumin-bound) to the liver, to be conjugated by the UDP-glucuronyl enzyme
- Conjugated bilirubin is excreted in the bile and into the gastrointestinal (GI) tract, where it is oxidised into stercobilinogen by colonic bacteria and subsequently stercobilin. Both these products are excreted in stools, giving them their characteristic brown colour
- Some of the stercobilinogen is reabsorbed into the enterohepatic circulation and converted into urobilinogen, which then either re-enters the liver or gets excreted in the urine as urobilin
- Bile produced by the liver is transported to the gall bladder, to be concentrated and stored

> **P** ›› The release of bile from the gall bladder is stimulated by cholecystokinin, which is produced by the duodenum.

- The complex system of ducts that connects the liver to the gall bladder, as well as the pancreas and the rest of the GI tract, is known as the biliary tract (see *Fig. 3.5*)

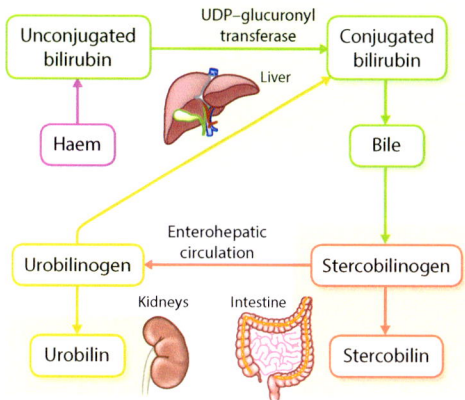

Fig. 3.4 *Bilirubin metabolism.*

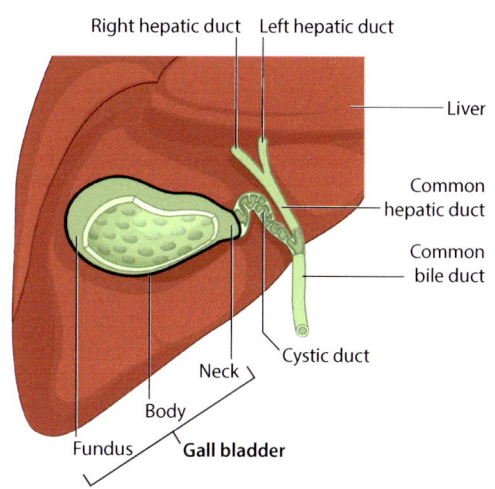

Fig. 3.5 *The biliary tree.*

3.1 Disorders of the mouth

3.1.1 Oral ulcerations

Mouth ulcers are very common, occurring in 5–20% of the population. Most are benign, but some can be serious and potentially even life-threatening. The oral cavity is lined with a thin and fragile, non-keratinised squamous epithelium. It is therefore susceptible to direct trauma as well as systemic inflammatory processes.

Common causes of oral ulceration:
- Recurrent aphthous ulcers (stomatitis)
- Trauma
- Nutritional deficiencies (iron, B12, folate)
- Viral and fungal infections (HSV, Coxsackie, HIV, candidiasis)
- Leukoplakia **(pre-malignant)**
- Inflammatory bowel disease (Crohn's disease)

> **P** ≫ Kaposi sarcoma (reddish-blue oral macule) and oral hairy leukoplakia (white patches) on the lateral borders of the tongue, secondary to Epstein–Barr virus (EBV), are early signs of HIV infection due to immunosuppression.

> **W** ≫ Variations in the tongue mucosa may exist – **geographic tongue** (inflammation of the mucosa causing loss of papillae, a **burning sensation** and a map-like appearance, from where it gets its name) and a **hairy tongue (not the same as oral hairy leukoplakia!)** (abnormal proliferation of keratin). Both conditions are benign.

Other causes/manifestations of systemic disease:
- Oral cancer
- Lichen planus
- Behçet's disease
- Dermatological disorders and drug reactions (see *Chapter 11*)
- Rheumatological disorders (systemic lupus erythematosus [SLE], Sjögren syndrome; see *Chapter 10*)

3.2 Disorders of the oesophagus

The most common presentation of oesophageal disorders is dysphagia. Dysphagia can be defined as 'difficulty swallowing'. It is often described as 'food sticking' or 'a lump in the throat' and is occasionally associated with pain (odynophagia).

Approach to dysphagia

The cause of dysphagia can be elicited just by taking a clinical history in 80% of cases. See *Fig. 3.6* for a stepwise approach to evaluating a patient presenting with dysphagia.

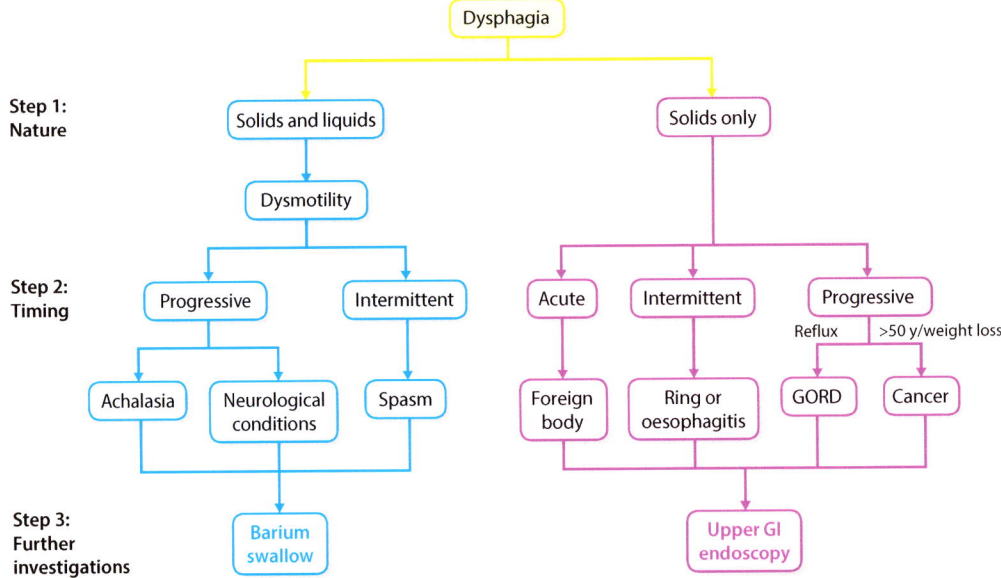

Fig. 3.6 *Evaluation of dysphagia (adapted from the World Gastroenterology Organisation Global Guidelines, Dysphagia 2014).*

3.2.1 Achalasia of the oesophagus

Definition: a motility disorder characterised by aperistalsis of the oesophagus and inadequate relaxation of the lower oesophageal sphincter.

Epidemiology:
- Most commonly presenting in the fifth decade of life
- Annual incidence of 1–2% per 100,000

Pathophysiology:
- The exact aetiology of achalasia is unknown
- Degeneration of the ganglionic cells in the myenteric plexus within the oesophageal wall and lower sphincter has been reported
- As a result, parasympathetic tone is reduced, which leads to inappropriate peristalsis and hypertonia of the lower oesophageal sphincter

Clinical features:
- **Progressive** dysphagia affecting both **solids and liquids**
- Regurgitation is common and often relieves symptoms
- Retrosternal chest pain may also be present
- Small associated risk of developing squamous cell carcinoma (SCC) of the oesophagus

Investigations
If a diagnosis of achalasia is suspected, proceed stepwise.

Stepwise plan:

1 **Arrange a barium swallow examination**
- There may be a classic **'bird's beak'** appearance, as the proximal oesophagus is dilated and very narrow at the lower sphincter (see *Fig. 3.7*)

2 **Obtain a chest X-ray (CXR)**
- CXR may reveal a widened mediastinum as a result of a dilated oesophagus behind the heart

3 **Arrange for manometry to be carried out**
- Manometry is the gold standard investigation
- High resting pressure of the lower oesophageal sphincter is diagnostic

4 **Consider upper GI endoscopy**
- Upper GI endoscopy is often performed to rule out malignancy

> **W** ≫ Oesophageal cancer is a rare and late complication of long-standing achalasia.

Management:
- Surgical myotomy (the Heller procedure) is a more invasive but effective treatment option, and is generally **first line** if the patient is fit
- Endoscopic pneumatic dilatation of the lower sphincter is effective and generally used in older patients with comorbidities

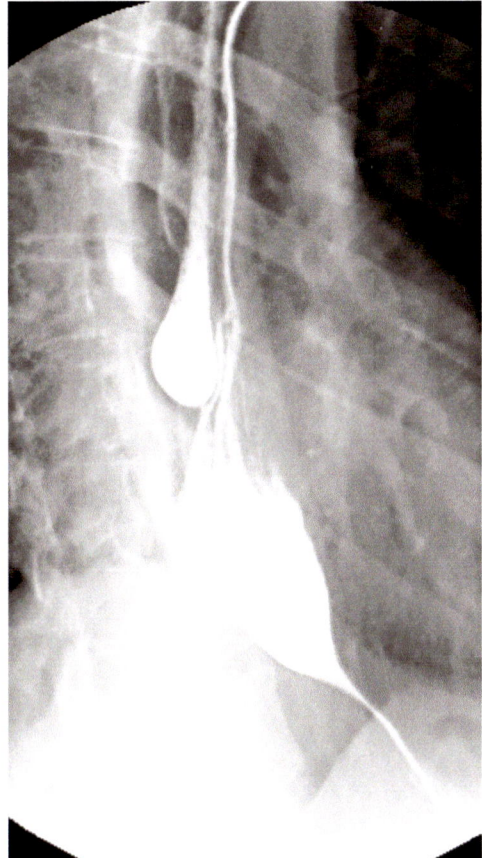

Fig. 3.7 *Barium study showing the characteristic bird's beak appearance of achalasia.*

- Some patients may require botulinum injections directly into the sphincter, but disease frequently recurs. This option may be used in patients who are unfit or unwilling to proceed with invasive treatment
- Calcium channel blockers (CCBs) or nitrates only provide symptomatic relief (poor efficacy)

P ≫ Secondary achalasia can occur in certain situations, e.g. extraluminal compression after a fundoplication.

3.2.2 Diffuse oesophageal spasm

This is an oesophageal motility disorder that typically presents with transient retrosternal chest pain and intermittent dysphagia.
- Barium studies often reveal a **'corkscrew' oesophagus**
- Treatment is initiated with a trial of proton pump inhibitors (PPIs)

- Second-line options are usually nitrates and CCBs
- Pneumatic dilatation and surgical myotomy may be considered as final-line options

Nutcracker oesophagus
This variant of diffuse oesophageal spasm, with similar presentation, is a condition characterised by coordinated high-amplitude contraction peristalsis.

E ≫ Both diffuse oesophageal spasm and nutcracker oesophagus often mimic anginal attacks, and are therefore important differentials of chest pain.

3.2.3 Pharyngeal pouch (Zenker diverticulum)

Definition: this is a rare condition characterised by a posteromedial outpouching of the oesophagus through the Killian dehiscence (weak area of the cricopharyngeus muscle). Food debris accumulates in the pouch, eventually compressing the oesophageal body.

Management
Progressive dysphagia, regurgitation and halitosis are common symptoms. Barium swallow is the investigation of choice (see *Fig. 3.8*). Surgical intervention may be necessary if the patient becomes symptomatic.

E ≫ Endoscopy is strongly discouraged as the initial investigation, as perforation of the pouch may occur as a complication.

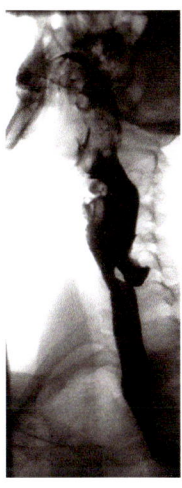

Fig. 3.8 *Barium swallow showing a pharyngeal pouch.*

3

3.2.4 Gastro-oesophageal reflux disease (GORD)

Definition: gastro-oesophageal reflux disease is the condition in which symptoms such as heartburn are produced when reflux of gastric contents into the oesophagus or oral cavity is present.

Epidemiology:
- 2–3 times more common in men
- Affects 10–20% of the western world's population

Aetiology:
- Lower oesophageal sphincter (LOS) dysfunction
  - The LOS is responsible for regulating the passage of food from the oesophagus into the stomach
  - The resting tone of the LOC is important in preventing back-flow of gastric contents into the lower oesophagus
  - In GORD, the resting tone of the LOC is decreased, resulting in acid reflux
- Hiatus hernia
  - Herniation of the upper stomach through the diaphragm into the thoracic cavity eliminates the natural thoraco-abdominal pressure gradient that prevents reflux

> **P** ≫ Hiatus hernias are typically classified as **sliding** (80%), **rolling** or **mixed**. Patients with rolling hiatal hernias should be considered for repair, as there is an increased risk of strangulation with rolling hiatal hernias.

- Lifestyle factors (smoking, alcohol, coffee)
- Increased intra-abdominal pressure (obesity, pregnancy)
- Annual incidence of 1–2% per 100,000

Pathophysiology:
- Reflux of gastric contents into the lower oesophagus exposes the mucosal epithelium to damage
- This triggers an inflammatory response, resulting in reflux oesophagitis

Clinical features:
- Most common symptom is heartburn, a burning sensation originating from the stomach that gets worse after meals and lying down
- Acid brash (a metallic taste as a result of acid regurgitation)
- Dysphagia and atypical chest pain

Investigations

> **Stepwise plan:**

The diagnosis of GORD is a clinical one and rarely requires investigations.

1 Consider proton pump inhibitors (PPIs)
- Young patients and patients with typical symptoms can be treated empirically with a trial of high-dose PPI (course of 4–8 weeks)

2 Consider an upper GI endoscopy (UGIE)
- However, if the diagnosis is uncertain, or the patient presents over the age of 55 years or with 'ALARM' symptoms, a UGIE is recommended

> **E** ≫ **ALARM** symptoms are red flag symptoms associated with dyspepsia that warrant further investigation with UGIE. These symptoms can be easily remembered using the mnemonic 'ALARMS':
> **A**naemia
> **L**oss of weight
> **A**norexia
> **R**ecent onset of progressive symptoms
> **M**elaena, haematemesis
> **S**wallowing difficulty

3 Consider ambulatory intraluminal pH monitoring
- Ambulatory intraluminal pH monitoring may be indicated if surgical intervention is being considered. A pH of less than 4 at more than 4% of the time is diagnostic

> **Stepwise management of GORD (NICE 2014, CG184)**

1 Lifestyle modification
- Smoking cessation, dietary advice, weight reduction and self-treatment (e.g. antacids)
- Patients should elevate the head of the bed, and avoid food likely to provoke GORD (e.g. spicy/fatty food, citrus fruits and chocolate), especially before bed

> **P** ≫ NICE advises against the use of continuous antacids/alginate therapy as it only provides short-term symptomatic relief and does not prevent further episodes.

2 Full-dose PPI therapy for 4–8 weeks
- Patients with a history of oesophageal intervention (i.e. previous dilatation) should remain on lifelong therapy

3 Offer low-dose PPI therapy or switch to a H₂ antagonist, if symptoms persist or recur

4 Consider laparoscopic fundoplication
- This is appropriate for patients who have a confirmed diagnosis of GORD (with pH monitoring) and have responded to PPI therapy but:
  - Do not wish to be on long-term PPI therapy
  - Are unable to tolerate long-term PPI therapy
  - Have severe disease

> **W** ⟩⟩ Patients who undergo a Nissen fundoplication may experience dysphagia, abdominal bloating or recurrence of GORD as complications. The dysphagia, in particular, occurs due to the constrictive effect of wrapping the gastric fundus around the oesophagus too tightly.

Complications of GORD
- Oesophagitis
- Barrett oesophagus
- Oesophageal carcinoma
- Benign oesophageal stricture

> **E** ⟩⟩ Another differential to consider is eosinophilic oesophagitis, which presents with symptoms such as dysphagia and vomiting. This should be suspected in patients with a history of atopy (e.g. asthma, eczema). An endoscopic biopsy is likely to demonstrate oesophageal eosinophilia. The mainstay of treatment is aerosolised glucocorticoids, with oral glucocorticoid therapy in more severe cases.

3.2.5 Barrett oesophagus

Definition: a pre-malignant condition, occurring in 10–20% of patients exposed to chronic acid reflux. Extended exposure to chemical injury causes metaplastic transformation of the normal oesophageal squamous epithelium into columnar gastric epithelium.

Clinical features:
- Most patients are asymptomatic apart from their GORD symptoms

- Diagnosis requires multiple endoscopic biopsies to determine the extent of dysplasia (see *Fig. 3.9*)

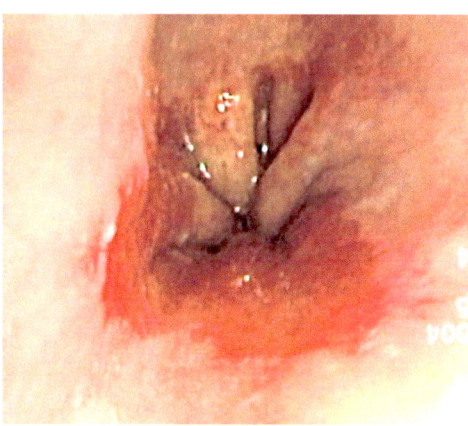

Fig. 3.9 *Barrett disease at the distal oesophagus seen during endoscopy.*

> **Stepwise management of Barrett oesophagus (NICE 2010, CG106)**

1 Regular endoscopic surveillance
- Every 1–3 years to monitor disease progression and dysplasia change

2 Consider continuous surveillance
- Patients with low-grade dysplasia or no dysplasia may be treated conservatively with continuous surveillance

3 Consider surgical oesophagectomy
- In patients with high-grade dysplasia, surgical oesophagectomy is the standard treatment

4 Consider other treatments
- Alternatively, endoscopic radiofrequency ablation, photodynamic therapy and mucosal resection may be considered

3.2.6 Oesophageal cancer

Definition: mucosal neoplasm originating from oesophageal epithelium. There are two histological subtypes, namely squamous cell cancer (SCC) and adenocarcinoma (AC).

> **E** ⟩⟩ Adenocarcinomas tend to originate in the lower oesophagus, as this is the most common site affected by Barrett change. Conversely, the squamous subtype often arises in the middle-third of the oesophagus.

3

Epidemiology:

- Twice as common in men, compared to women
- Annual incidence of 15 per 100,000
- In the western world, AC is the most common subtype, whereas SCC remains more common in Asia and Africa

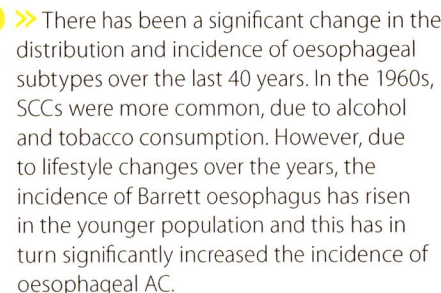 There has been a significant change in the distribution and incidence of oesophageal subtypes over the last 40 years. In the 1960s, SCCs were more common, due to alcohol and tobacco consumption. However, due to lifestyle changes over the years, the incidence of Barrett oesophagus has risen in the younger population and this has in turn significantly increased the incidence of oesophageal AC.

Aetiology/risk factors:

- Smoking and alcohol
- Pre-existing GORD and Barrett oesophagus
- Obesity (risk factor for AC but protective for SCC)
- Paterson–Brown–Kelly syndrome (see below)

Clinical features:

- Often asymptomatic until later stages
- Progressive dysphagia for liquids followed by solids
- Haematemesis or melaena
- Late stages – hoarseness (mediastinal invasion), weight loss
- Annual incidence of 1–2% per 100,000

Pathophysiology:

Exposure to carcinogens (i.e. cigarette smoke) and chronic exposure to acid reflux (as described in Barrett oesophagus) predispose to dysplastic changes within the oesophageal mucosa. This local invasion may then spread to adjacent structures (e.g. trachea, aorta) or metastasise further to local lymph nodes, lungs and liver.

Investigations

Stepwise plan:

This is a stepwise approach to investigating a patient with suspected oesophageal cancer.

1 Arrange blood tests
- Perform baseline **FBCs** (to look for anaemia secondary to occult GI bleed), **U&Es** (to check suitability for staging CT scan), **LFTs** (changes may indicate liver mets)

2 Arrange urgent oesophagogastroduodenoscopy (OGD)
- Urgent **OGD**, with brushings and biopsies to confirm grade

3 Staging imaging
- **Chest and abdominal CT scan**, often performed concurrently with a **PET scan** (CT-PET), to screen for any evidence of metastasis
- TNM staging is performed

Management

As with the treatment of other cancers, the management of oesophageal cancer depends on staging, the patient's nutritional status and other comorbidities, requiring a multidisciplinary approach.

- **Around 70%** of patients present with metastatic disease, meaning that **palliative** therapy is the only option
- Palliative chemo(radio)therapy and oesophageal stenting may provide symptomatic relief of dysphagia
- However, the treatment of choice for patients who are fit, and present with local disease, is **surgical resection**; alternatively, this can be performed endoscopically, if the patient is unsuitable for surgery
- Neoadjuvant **chemoradiotherapy** may also be considered

3.2.7 Oesophageal stricture/web/ring

Narrowing of the oesophagus may be caused by an oesophageal stricture, web or ring. These vary in location and underlying cause. An oesophageal stricture can be either benign (mostly) or malignant. They are primarily caused by long-standing GORD.

An oesophageal web, on the other hand, affects the upper oesophagus in the post-cricoid region and usually occurs as a rare complication of an SCC or associated with Paterson–Brown–Kelly syndrome.

P >> Paterson–Brown–Kelly syndrome (or Plummer–Vinson syndrome) is a condition where iron-deficiency anaemia is associated with post-cricoid webs. The pathogenesis remains controversial, with early reports postulating that a decrease in iron-dependent enzymes results in myasthenic changes in muscles within the oesophageal body. This subsequently causes mucosa atrophy and predisposes to web formation.

Rings most commonly arise in the lower oesophagus, and they are known as Schatzki rings when they affect the gastric-oesophageal junction. They are due to submucosal fibrosis, often with muscle involvement.

Patients usually present with dysphagia and usually require endoscopic dilatation or surgery to relieve symptoms.

3.2.8 Oesophageal varices

Oesophageal varices will be discussed in *Section 3.6.3.2*. The management of an acute oesophageal variceal bleed is discussed below, in *Section 3.2.9*.

3.2.9 Acute upper gastrointestinal bleeding

Acute upper gastrointestinal bleeding is a common medical emergency associated with 10% mortality. Haematemesis is defined as bloody vomit originating from a site proximal to the distal duodenum. Haematemesis can either be frank (pre-stomach) or coffee-ground (post-stomach).

The causes of upper GI bleeding are shown in *Table 3.1*.

> **W** >> The coffee-ground appearance of vomitus is caused by exposure of haem molecules in blood to gastric acid, resulting in iron oxidation.

Table 3.1 *Causes of UGI bleed*

Origin	Causes
Oesophagus	Varices (secondary to portal hypertension) Oesophagitis Mallory–Weiss tear Oesophageal cancer
Gastric	Peptic/duodenal ulcer (secondary to *H. pylori* or NSAID use) Gastritis (secondary to NSAID or alcohol use) Angiodysplasia Gastric cancer

> **Stepwise plan:**

Initial assessment:

1   **Obtain a quick history**
- AMPLE (previous bleeds, liver status, known ulcers)

2   **Assess for signs of hypovolaemic shock**
- Tachycardia, hypotension, low urine output (catheterise), cool peripheries

3   **Identify cause of bleed**
- The two most common causes of UGI bleed are ulcer bleeds and variceal bleeds

Initial resuscitation:

1   **Ensure oxygen supply**
- Ensure patient is maintaining airway, and supplement with high-flow O_2 if patient is desaturating

2   **Obtain IV access**
- Preferably with a wide-bore cannula in each arm

3   **Send off urgent bloods**
- FBCs (to check extent of anaemia and platelets), LFTs (to check for pre-existing liver disease), U&Es (to check co-existing AKI, **urea rise**), clotting/ coagulation screen and **cross-match blood**

> **W** >> A significantly high urea with normal creatinine is suggestive of a UGI bleed. Urea is the end metabolic product of protein hydrolysis. When blood that is rich in haem and other plasma proteins is present in the GI tract, it mimics a heavy protein meal, and urea is produced.

- Monitor vital signs, in particular blood pressure and heart rate
- Initiate fluid resuscitation with IV crystalloid fluid challenges
- Blood products should be transfused appropriately
- NICE (2016, CG141) recommends, for a patient who is actively bleeding:
  - If they have a platelet count $<50 \times 10^9$/L, offer platelet transfusion
  - If they have an APTT/PT >1.5 greater than normal, offer FFP

> **Stepwise management of acute upper GI bleeding**

1   **All patients should undergo risk assessment using:**
a. **Blatchford score** at first assessment
b. **Rockall score** after endoscopy

2   **Arrange urgent UGIE within 24 hours of presentation**
- Aimed at haemorrhage source control
- This can be achieved by thermal coagulation, thrombin injection with adrenaline or banding (for oesophageal varices)

3 Consider use of octreotide/terlipressin and prophylactic antibiotic therapy
- For patients with suspected variceal bleed
- Seek specialist input prior to commencing terlipressin

4 In high-risk patients, start 72-hour IV PPI infusion

5 Repeat UGIE is usually required
- This should be considered in high-risk patients, particularly those with variceal bleeding

6 Consider other modalities to stop bleeding, if refractory
- Include a balloon tamponade with a Sengstaken–Blakemore tube, or transjugular intrahepatic porto-systemic shunting

3.3 Diseases of the stomach

Dyspepsia

Dyspepsia primarily refers to bloating and discomfort associated with the upper abdomen (see *Fig. 3.10*). Dyspepsia is a term often used very loosely and NICE has included GORD symptoms in the term. Most patients do not require investigations and can be treated conservatively, using:
- Medication review – steroids, bisphosphonates, NSAIDs, etc.
- Lifestyle modification – alcohol cessation, dietary change
- Trial of antacids or alginates

As with GORD, if the patient presents with an 'ALARM' symptom (see *Exam Essentials* in *Section 3.2.4*), or is above the age of 55, or is younger but remains unresponsive to conservative therapy, further investigations may be necessary. NICE recommends a **'test and treat'** approach.

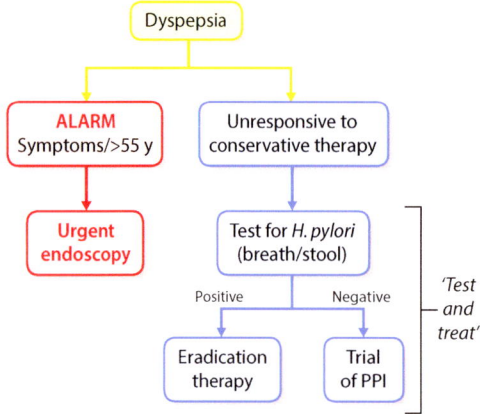

Fig. 3.10 *Evaluation of a patient presenting with dyspepsia (based on NICE CG184).*

3.3.1 Gastritis

Gastritis refers to inflammation of the stomach and is primarily a histological diagnosis. This can be divided into acute and chronic gastritis, each of which is caused by very different pathologies.

Table 3.2 *Causes of acute and chronic gastritis*

Acute gastritis	Chronic gastritis
• *H. pylori* infection • Alcohol • NSAIDs, aspirin • Stress-induced • Bile acid reflux (usually post-gastric surgery)	• Chronic *H. pylori* infection • Crohn's disease • Sarcoidosis • Autoimmune (atrophic)

E ≫ Autoimmune gastritis is a chronic atrophic condition associated with the autoimmune destruction of parietal cells of the stomach. Severe gastric atrophy will result in insufficient **intrinsic factor** production, leading to pernicious anaemia. The development of autoimmune gastritis is strongly associated with other autoimmune disorders such as Addison's, T1DM and autoimmune thyroid disease.

3.3.2 Peptic ulcer disease

Definition: disease of the stomach or duodenal mucosa involving a break in the layer, and loss of surface tissue.

Epidemiology:
- Accounts for 13% of investigated dyspepsia
- Prevalence of less than 1% in the western population

P >> There has been a declining incidence of peptic ulcer disease over the last 50 years, as a result of eradication therapy and declining NSAID use.

Aetiology:

- *Helicobacter pylori* infection
- Drugs – aspirin, NSAIDs
- Rare causes include:
  - Zollinger–Ellison syndrome (see *Section 3.3.3*)
  - Crohn's disease
- Gastric ulcers may occur secondary to:
  - Intracranial neurology (known as a **Cushing** ulcer)
  - Burns or trauma (known as a **Curling** ulcer)

Clinical features:

- Epigastric pain with post-prandial association
- Bloating, abdominal distension
- Nausea
- Annual incidence of 1–2% per 100,000

E >> Peptic ulcers are largely duodenal or gastric in nature (duodenal ulcers are significantly more common). The epigastric pain related to duodenal ulcers is classically improved upon eating, while the pain related to gastric ulcers is typically described as worse on eating.

Pathophysiology:

H. pylori, a Gram-negative, urease-producing bacterium (enabling it to survive in low pH conditions), lives in the stomach and duodenal mucosa. It affects approximately 50% of the population over the age of 50. The pathogen stimulates gastrin production as well as inhibiting somatostatin production, resulting in an increase in acid secretion, which ultimately leads to gastric and duodenal ulceration.

W >> NSAIDs are associated with peptic ulcer disease because they inhibit the cyclo-oxygenase, COX-1 enzyme that functions to protect the gastric mucosa. This is why patients requiring NSAID therapy who have concomitant peptic ulcer disease are also offered (after consideration) COX-2 inhibitors (only celecoxib is currently licensed). Note that COX-2 inhibitors, while useful in managing pain without aggravating the GI tract, are associated with a higher number of cardiovascular complications.

Investigations

H. pylori can be detected in several ways, using:
- Carbon-13 urea breath test

E >> Note that PPI medications should be stopped 2 weeks prior to testing, as they may result in false positive breath tests.

- Stool antigen testing
- Laboratory-based serology testing

Offer an upper GI endoscopy if the patient is above the age of 55 years or presents with any of the 'ALARM' symptoms (see *Exam Essentials* in *Section 3.2.4*).

Stepwise management of peptic ulcer disease (NICE 2014, CG184)

Eradication therapy (*H. pylori* positive disease)

1 **7-day course of triple therapy**
- Regime usually consists of a **7-day course of triple therapy** (a high-dose PPI with 2 twice-daily antibiotics)
  - **Typical regime**: high-dose PPI + amoxicillin + clarithromycin/metronidazole
  - Penicillin allergic: high-dose PPI + clarithromycin + metronidazole

2 **Re-test at 6–8 weeks**
- Perform re-testing at 6–8 weeks with carbon-13 urea breath test to confirm successful eradication

3 **Second-line eradication therapy**
- Offer second-line eradication therapy to patients who remain symptomatic after first-line regime (e.g. bismuth – warn patients that this will result in black stools)

H. pylori negative disease

1 **Stop offending medications and offer drug therapy for 8 weeks**
- Stop any offending medications (NSAIDs, aspirin) and offer full-dose PPI or H2R antagonist (e.g. ranitidine) therapy for 8 weeks

2 **Offer lifestyle medication advice**
- e.g. smoking cessation, dietary changes

Chronic or recurrent disease

1 **Exclude other diagnoses**
- e.g. malignancy, Zollinger–Ellison syndrome, Crohn's disease

3

2 Offer long-term low (maintenance) dose PPI

Complications
- Acute upper GI haemorrhage
- Perforation or bleeding

> **E** ≫ Spilling of gastric or intestinal contents into the abdominal cavity will result in severe peritonitis and is a surgical emergency. Anterior duodenal ulcers are likely to cause perforation, while posterior duodenal ulcers are likely to cause bleeding because of their proximity to the gastroduodenal artery.

- Gastric outlet obstruction – chronic ulceration of the pylorus/duodenum will result in fibrotic stricturing
- Malignant transformation

3.3.3 Zollinger–Ellison syndrome

Definition: a rare condition caused by a gastrin-secreting gastrinoma usually of pancreatic origin (90%). It is thought to have an annual incidence of 1–2 per million. The syndrome is characterised by hypersecretion of gastric acid, resulting in extensive peptic ulceration.

> **P** ≫ Zollinger–Ellison syndrome (ZES) is associated with multiple endocrine neoplasia (MEN) type 1, with as many as 20% of ZES patients having MEN 1. The gastrinoma is likely to be malignant in and of itself.

Clinical features:
- Epigastric pain as a result of ulcerations and GORD
- Diarrhoea

> **W** ≫ High gastric acid secretion inactivates pancreatic enzymes and may induce damage in the proximal small bowel, leading to incomplete digestion, eventually resulting in diarrhoea (steatorrhoea).

Investigations
The diagnosis of ZES requires both biochemical and radiological confirmation of disease.
- Perform FBC (may reveal microcytic anaemia secondary to chronic ulcer bleed)

- Check **fasting serum gastrin levels** (usually >1000pg/ml is diagnostic) and consider measuring basal acid output
- If ZES is suspected, check calcium, PTH and prolactin levels as part of a MEN 1 screen
- **Endoscopic ultrasound** (EUS) is the best radiological modality for tumour localisation. CT imaging may be used but is unable to pick up tumours <1cm in size (40% of gastrinomas). However, CT scans are useful to detect sites of metastasis.

Management
The aims of the treatment of ZES are gastric acid suppression and surgical resection of the tumour.
- First-line option is to offer long-term **high-dose PPI** therapy. This usually alleviates the majority of symptoms
- In a small proportion of patients with localised disease, **surgical resection** may be considered
- **Somatostatin analogues** and **chemotherapy** may be considered in metastatic disease (to inhibit tumour growth)

3.3.4 Gastric cancer

Definition: gastric cancer refers to a neoplasm that arises from the stomach mucosa. It is typically of adenocarcinoma histology. Other gastric tumours (<5%) consist of lymphomas and leiomyosarcoma.

Epidemiology:
- The second most common cause of global cancer-related deaths
- Twice as common in men
- Higher incidence in Asia compared to the western world (more common in Japan, possibly because of high consumption of raw fish)

Aetiology/risk factors:
- *H. pylori* infection
- Alcohol consumption and smoking
- Consumption of salted and smoked foods
- Autoimmune atrophic gastritis
- Familial adenomatous polyposis

> **W** ≫ Nitrate/nitrite-rich foods, such as smoked and pickled processed products, are converted into N-nitroso-compounds by the stomach's commensal bacteria, which predisposes the stomach to neoplastic changes.

Clinical features:
- Usually asymptomatic in early stages
- Non-specific dyspepsia

- Progressive dysphagia, vomiting ± haematemesis
- Weight loss, anorexia
- Iron-deficiency anaemia

P ≫ Linitis plastica ('leather bottle' appearance) is a rare form of **diffuse** gastric cancer that is generally unrelated to *H. pylori* infection.

E ≫ Metastatic spread to distal sites is associated with eponymous signs – supraclavicular nodes (Virchow node), umbilicus (Sister Joseph nodules) and ovaries (Krukenberg tumour).

Investigations

Tests should be carried out in the following order when investigating a patient with suspected gastric cancer.

Stepwise plan:

1 **Check baseline bloods**
- FBC (may reveal microcytic anaemia), LFTs (deranged values may indicate liver metastasis)

2 **Arrange for urgent upper GI endoscopy with tissue biopsies**

3 **Arrange for staging CT chest, abdomen and pelvis**
- To complete the TNM staging

Management

As with the treatment of other cancers, the management of gastric cancer depends on staging, the patient's nutritional status and other comorbidities, requiring a multidisciplinary approach.
- Patients with early-localised disease can usually be treated with **curative surgical resection** with a consideration of neoadjuvant or peri-operative chemoradiotherapy
- However, for patients with advanced inoperable disease, **palliative chemotherapy** and **palliative stenting** may be offered for symptomatic relief
- Capecitabine, in combination with a platinum-based agent, is the regime of choice; **trastuzumab** is recommended in patients with human epidermal receptor 2 positive metastatic disease (NICE 2010, TA208)

3.3.5 Gastrointestinal stromal tumours (GIST)

GISTs are submucosal tumours originating from the interstitial cells of Cajal (ICC). They are rare but their incidence is increasing, with a current annual incidence of 15 per million of population. They occur as a result of an oncogenic KIT receptor tyrosine kinase. The majority of patients are treated by resection. **Imatinib** may be considered as an adjuvant therapy or as part of palliative therapy in metastatic disease.

P ≫ ICC function as native pacemakers of the myenteric system, stimulating smooth muscle cells within the intestinal wall.

3.4 Diseases of the small bowel and colon

Approach to diarrhoea

Diarrhoea can be defined as an increase in stool liquidity and/or increase in stool frequency. Diarrhoea can be further divided, based on duration, into acute (<14 days) and chronic (>4 weeks).

Acute diarrhoea is very common and usually has an infective pathology. Drugs, such as antibiotics, PPIs, NSAIDs and digoxin, may also be responsible. It may also be a first presentation of inflammatory bowel disease.

The most common cause of chronic and relapsing diarrhoea is irritable bowel disease, which often presents with alternating bouts of constipation and diarrhoea. Other aetiologies are shown in *Fig. 3.11*.

Approach to constipation

Constipation is a heterogeneous symptom that has multiple definitions, which vary according to patients' perspectives. It is commonly described as incomplete emptying, excessive straining or reduced stool frequency (<3 times/week). Constipation persisting for longer than 6 weeks is termed chronic constipation. Careful history-taking is important to elicit red flags (necessitating urgent investigation) as well as to identify a possible cause.

3

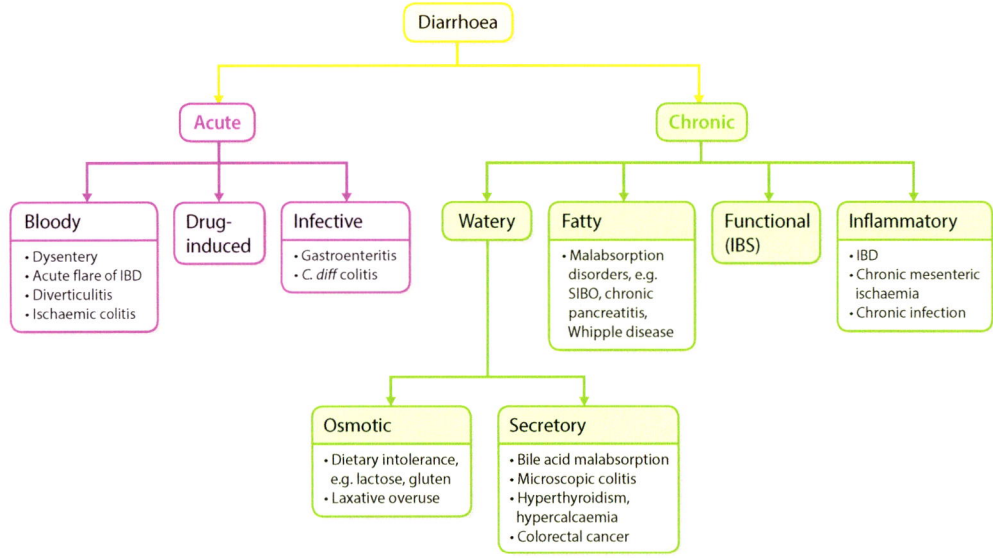

Fig. 3.11 *Causes of acute and chronic diarrhoea.*

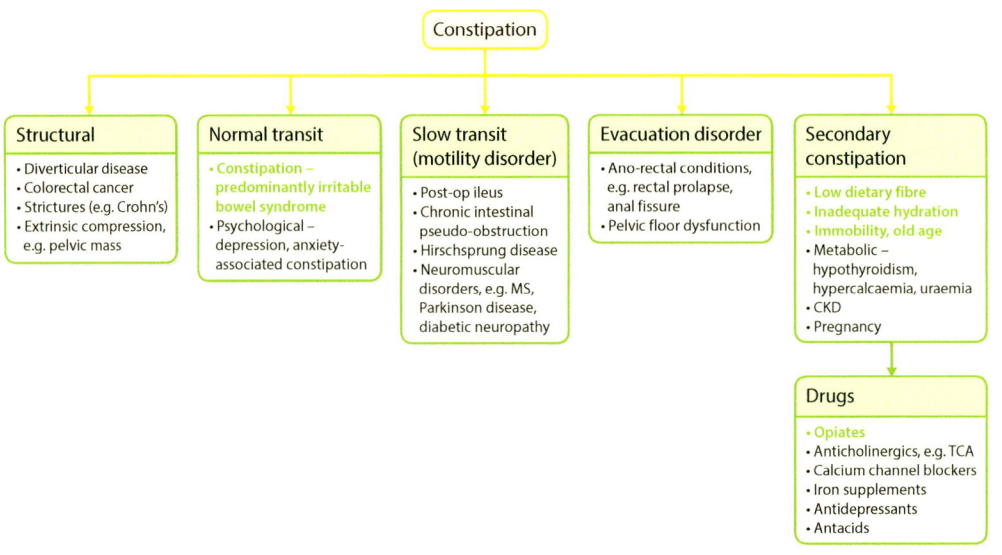

Fig. 3.12 *Causes of constipation (common causes are in **green**).*

E   ≫ Red flag symptoms include – obstructive symptoms, weight loss, PR bleeding, recent-onset constipation, iron-deficiency anaemia and patients over the age of 50 without any previous cancer screening.

Opiate-associated constipation remains the most common type. Some of the aetiologies of constipation are shown in *Fig. 3.12*.

3.4.1 Gastroenteritis

Gastroenteritis is a non-specific term used to characterise symptoms of acute diarrhoea, nausea and vomiting and abdominal pain. It's often used loosely to be synonymous with infective diarrhoea. It is a very common condition, affecting up to 20% of the population each year. Causative agents may include:

- Bacterial, e.g. *Campylobacter*, *E. coli*, *Salmonella*
- Viral (30–40%), e.g. norovirus, rotavirus
- Parasites, e.g. giardiasis, cryptosporidiosis

The causative organism is rarely isolated in the majority of patients, as up to 90% of cases are self-limiting. Some of the more common organisms are listed in *Table 3.3*, along with their source, clinical presentation and management.

3.4.2 *Clostridium difficile-associated disease*

Definition: *Clostridium difficile* (*C. diff*) is a Gram-positive, anaerobic, spore-forming bacterium. It is present in approximately 3–5% of the adult population, remaining dormant in the presence of other normal gut flora. However, this natural balance can be disrupted by the use of antibiotics, resulting in opportunistic infection, causing *C. diff* (pseudomembranous) colitis.

> **E** >> The use of the 'C' antibiotics (i.e. co-amoxiclav, cephalosporins, ciprofloxacin and clindamycin) is hugely associated with *C. diff* colitis. Symptoms typically manifest 5–10 days after antibiotic therapy.

Clinical features:
- Patients usually complain of profuse watery diarrhoea, colicky abdominal pain and fevers and rigors in severe cases
- Severe abdominal pain is an uncommon feature
- Annual incidence of 1–2% per 100,000

Pathophysiology:
C. diff produces enterotoxins A and B. These toxins trigger an inflammatory response within the colonic membrane. This subsequently leads to an increase in vascular permeability and pseudomembrane formation. The accumulation of inflammatory cells, fibrin and necrotic debris contributes to this pseudomembrane (see *Fig. 3.13*).

Investigations
Investigations should be undertaken in the following order.

Stepwise plan:

1 Arrange blood tests
- FBC (↑WCC), ↑CRP, ↓albumin, may show deranged U&Es secondary to dehydration

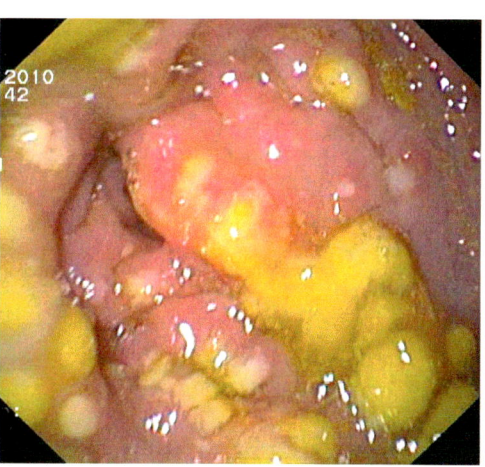

Fig. 3.13 *Pseudomembranous colitis seen on colonoscopy.*

2 Arrange stool testing
- Stool samples should be sent for MC&S including *C. diff* cytotoxin analysis

3 Obtain imaging
- AXR may show colonic dilatation

4 Consider colonoscopy/flexi sig
- Not routinely performed but may be useful if there is diagnostic uncertainty

Stepwise management of *C. diff* colitis

The treatment of *C. diff* colitis involves assessing the severity of disease, infection control, supportive care and antibiotic therapy.

1 Infection control
- Patients should be isolated to a side room with barrier nursing precautions

> **E** >> Alcohol hand gels should be avoided.

2 Medication review
- Stop all causative agents, particularly antibiotics and PPIs

3 Antibiotic therapy
- Offer a 10 to 14-day course of 400mg oral metronidazole in non-severe cases
- Severe disease: IV metronidazole + **ORAL** vancomycin

4 Consider surgery
- Surgery may be indicated in fulminant disease

3

Table 3.3 *Common organisms causing gastroenteritis*

Organism	Source	Clinical features	Management
Campylobacter jejuni (most common bacterial cause)	• Contaminated water • Animal droppings • Unpasteurised milk	• Fever and dysentery (bloody diarrhoea) • Cx: Guillain–Barré syndrome (seen in up to 10% of patients) • Reactive arthritis	• Self-limiting in the first 7 days • More severe forms may respond to erythromycin
Salmonella spp.	• Contaminated water • Eggs, poultry, meat	• Dysentery and vomiting • Abdo pain and low-grade fever • Cx: reactive arthritis	• Usually self-limiting • Ciprofloxacin may be used if there is bacteraemia
Shigella	• Faecal–oral (poor hygiene) • Contaminated food, water	• Dysentery and colicky abdo pain ± fever • Cx: reactive arthritis	• Ciprofloxacin • Improve hand hygiene/ sanitation
Bacillus cereus	• Reheated rice or sauces	• Watery diarrhoea and profuse vomiting	• Self-limiting (recovery usually within 24 to 48 hours)
Listeria monocytogenes	• Unpasteurised milk, cheese • Raw meat (pâtés)	• Watery diarrhoea, colicky abdo pain and vomiting • Cx: pneumonia, meningoencephalitis	• Ampicillin
Clostridium perfringens	• Incompletely cooked contaminated meat	• Watery diarrhoea and colicky abdo pain	• Self-limiting
Clostridium botulinum	• Bottled/canned food (e.g. beans or honey)	• Short period of watery diarrhoea • Symmetrical descending flaccid paralysis • No sensory impairment	• Anti-toxin • Benzylpenicillin and metronidazole
Staph. aureus	• Dairy products, cooked meats	• Profuse vomiting is the initial symptom • Diarrhoea presents later	• Self-limiting (rapid recovery)
Escherichia coli (ETEC)	• Most common causative organism of traveller's diarrhoea	• Watery diarrhoea and vomiting	• Self-limiting (within 3 to 5 days) • Ciprofloxacin may be considered
E. coli (EHEC, O157:H7)	• Contaminated food products, usually occurs as outbreaks	• Dysentery and constant abdo pain • Cx: haemolytic uraemic syndrome (HUS)	• Supportive as antibiotic therapy may worsen symptoms • Haemodialysis if necessary
Yersinia enterocolitica	• Pork, milk	• Abdo pain, watery diarrhoea ± fever • Cx: mesenteric adenitis, reactive arthritis	• Ciprofloxacin
Giardia lamblia	• Contaminated water • Common in the tropics	• Explosive, offensive diarrhoea, vomiting • Abdo pain and distension	• Tinidazole stat and metronidazole for 10 days
Cryptosporidiosis	• Only seen in immunocompromised patients • Contaminated water	• Profuse diarrhoea • Intermittent abdo pain	• Usually self-limiting • If severe, co-trimoxazole for 7 days

Table 3.3 (continued)

Organism	Source	Clinical features	Management
Entamoeba histolytica	• Faecal–oral, contaminated food	• Dysentery with intermittent constipation • Cx: liver abscesses – swinging fever, RUQ pain	• Metronidazole or tinidazole should be given in the acute phase • Paromomycin or diloxanide should be given for up to 10 days to eliminate intra-intestinal cysts
Strongyloides	• Endemic in the tropics and sub-tropics	• Triad of abdo pain, diarrhoea and urticaria • Systemic disease is associated with immune suppression (e.g. HIV, steroid use)	• Ivermectin for 2 days or albenazole for 3 days
Norovirus	• Common in adults	• Profuse watery diarrhoea, projectile vomiting • Colicky abdo pain	• Self-limiting, contact precaution
Rotavirus	• Common in children	• Watery diarrhoea and vomiting	• Self-limiting, contact precaution
Vibrio cholerae	See *Chapter 9 (Infectious disease)*		

3.4.3 Malabsorption disorders

3.4.3.1 Coeliac disease

Definition: an autoimmune disorder triggered by gluten consumption, resulting in small bowel inflammation and subsequent malabsorption.

Epidemiology:
- Affects 1% of the UK population
- Annual incidence of 1–2% per 100,000
- Bimodal age distribution – first peaking in infancy and also in the fourth to fifth decade of life, though it can present at any age
- Twice as common in women

Clinical features
Many patients with coeliac disease are asymptomatic (*silent disease*), and those who **are** symptomatic usually present with vague and non-specific signs and symptoms (see *Table 3.4*).

Pathophysiology:
- The aetiology of coeliac disease involves a complex interplay of genetic and environmental factors
- Coeliac disease is highly associated with the HLA-DQ2 haplotype (seen in up to 90% of patients), present on specific antigen-presenting cells (APC), responsible in the inflammatory cascade

Table 3.4 *Clinical presentation of patients with coeliac disease*

GI	• Malabsorption (steatorrhoea, abdo pain, flatus) • Unexplained weight loss
Metabolic	• Iron deficiency (microcytic anaemia) • B12 and folate deficiency (anaemia, polyneuropathy, epilepsy, neuropsychiatric symptoms) • Hypocalcaemia (tetany, osteomalacia, osteoporosis) • Faltering growth/failure to thrive in infants
Dermatological	• Dermatitis herpetiformis (see *Fig. 3.14*) • Severe aphthous oral ulcers
Associated conditions	• Autoimmune – Type 1 DM, thyroid disease, PBC • Cancer – lymphoma, breast, small bowel

- Gliadin peptides, derived from gluten in wheat and other prolamins in rye and barley, are resistant to naturally occurring digestive enzymes and tend to remain in the lumen or sub-endothelium of the small bowel
- In coeliac disease, there is a loss of intact immune tolerance, mediated by HLA-DQ2-associated APC, resulting in an immune response

W ≫ Dermatitis herpetiformis is an associated cutaneous manifestation of coeliac disease, occurring in up to 20% of patients. It is a pruritic, vesicular rash, mainly affecting the extensor surfaces. Deposition of IgA complexes in the dermis is thought to be responsible for the development of these lesions. They usually respond to a gluten-free diet but may require dapsone in resistant cases.

P ≫ Patients are advised to continue a gluten-rich diet, with at least one gluten-containing meal per day for at least 6 weeks prior to testing. This ensures test accuracy.

2 Obtain duodenal biopsy
- This gold standard investigation allows for a histopathological diagnosis (see *Fig. 3.15*)

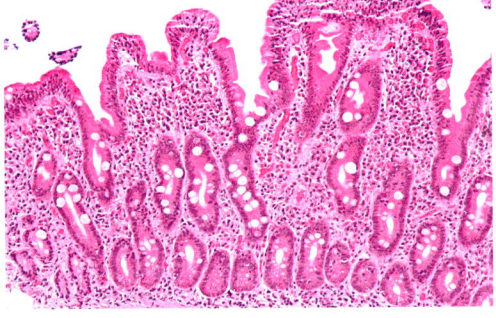

Fig. 3.15 *Histology stain of a duodenal biopsy from a patient with coeliac disease.*

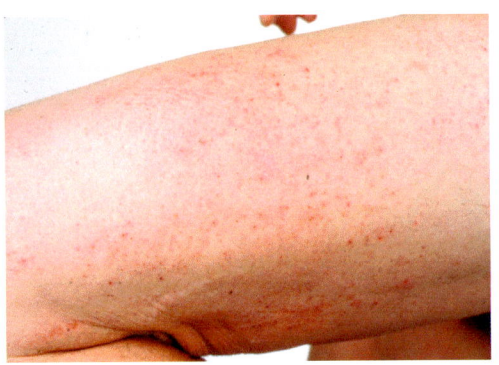

Fig. 3.14 *Dermatitis herpetiformis.*

P ≫ The stimulation of T-helper cells, as part of the immune response, results in the production of anti-endomysial, anti-gliadin and anti-tissue transglutaminase (tTG) IgA auto-antibodies; these form the basis of coeliac disease's serological testing.

E ≫ Classic histological findings of coeliac disease include:
- Sub-total villous atrophy (loss of finger-like projections)
- Crypt hyperplasia
- Inflammatory infiltration of the lamina propria, primarily comprising lymphocytes.

Investigations

Investigations should be undertaken in the following order.

Stepwise plan (NICE 2015, NG20):

The diagnosis of coeliac disease is dependent on a positive histological biopsy and serological confirmation.

1 Arrange serological testing
- Total IgA and IgA anti-tTG are usually raised and are first-line options. IgA anti-endomysial and IgG anti-gliadin may be used as alternatives. Serological testing should not be offered to infants.

3 Arrange other tests
- Routine FBC may reveal a microcytic/macrocytic anaemia (secondary to iron, B12 or folate deficiency)
- Electrolyte imbalance – ↓Ca, ↓Mg, ↓albumin
- HLA genetic testing may be considered if the diagnosis is unclear, despite serological and histological testing

Stepwise management of coeliac disease (NICE 2015, NG20)

The principles of treatment of coeliac disease constitute good dietary advice, correction of malabsorption and management of complications.

1 Strict lifelong gluten-free diet
- Good specialist advice on specific food avoidance and strategies to prevent cross-contamination within the household as well as accidental gluten ingestion

> **E** ≫ Foods containing wheat, rye and barley should be avoided. It is important to emphasise that rice, soya and maize-based products are safe.

2 Referral to external resources
- Referral to resources such as coeliac disease support groups and dietitians should also be offered to increase compliance

> **W** ≫ A higher incidence of psychological conditions, such as depression and anxiety, has been linked to coeliac disease. It is therefore important to be aware of these mental health issues and offer patients support and appropriate therapies.

3 Offer vitamin and mineral supplements
- These will commonly include vitamin B, D and calcium supplements; advise patients to seek specialist advice before purchasing over-the-counter supplements

4 Offer 12-monthly reviews to assess:
- Symptom control, including annual BMI monitoring
- Gluten-free diet adherence and consider appropriate dietitian referral
- The need for further investigations (e.g. DXA scan for osteoporosis)

5 Consider prednisolone
- Consider prednisolone in patients with refractory disease and seek urgent specialist advice

A proportion of patients develop persistent symptoms despite gluten-avoidance therapy. This is usually due to underlying complications, such as small intestinal bacterial overgrowth, irritable bowel disease or inflammatory bowel disease (see *Sections 3.4, 3.4.3.2* and *3.4.6*).

3.4.3.2 Small intestine bacterial overgrowth (SIBO)

Definition: SIBO is also sometimes known as blind loop syndrome. This condition is primarily characterised by an increase in the number of bacteria

in the small bowel. In normal circumstances, the small bowel contains less than 10^4/ml of organisms, the majority of which are anaerobic bacteria (e.g. *E. coli*, *Bacteroides*). The increase in bacterial proliferation is caused by several factors (see *Table 3.5*).

Table 3.5 *Factors affecting gut bacterial growth*

Reduced gastric acidity	Long-standing PPI therapy, post-gastrectomy
Reduced gut motility	Scleroderma, diabetic gastroparesis
Structural abnormalities	Post-small bowel resections (blind loops), small bowel diverticulosis, small bowel obstruction

Patients normally present with malabsorption symptoms (predominantly diarrhoea and steatorrhoea). The diagnosis of SIBO can be confirmed with a hydrogen breath test. The underlying cause should be treated if possible. Otherwise, a cyclical antibiotic regime (typically consisting of doxycycline, rifaximin and metronidazole) is used.

> **W** ≫ Bacteria readily metabolise glucose and convert it to hydrogen. This forms the basis of the hydrogen breath test. The test involves measuring the hydrogen levels in breath samples after ingesting a glucose meal.

3.4.3.3 Tropical sprue

This is a condition of acquired, progressive malabsorption, which is characterised by chronic diarrhoea and nutritional deficiencies. The condition mainly occurs in the Far East and South America (tropical areas that are near the equator). The exact cause is unclear; however, an infectious cause is likely. Histopathologically, changes are similar to those seen in coeliac disease. Patients often improve after leaving the tropical area. A prolonged course of tetracyclines for 4 weeks may be considered.

3.4.3.4 Whipple disease

Whipple disease is a rare, chronic infectious disease caused by the Gram-positive bacterium, *Tropheryma whipplei*. This disease occurs generally in middle-aged Caucasian men. Presentation is multi-systemic and affects virtually any organ. Patients usually first present with arthralgia and progressive unexplained weight loss. GI symptoms (e.g. diarrhoea) are often a late manifestation. Neurological symptoms (dementia, myoclonus) may occasionally be prevalent.

3

> E >> Diagnosis is made on biopsy, classically revealing the presence of periodic acid–Schiff (PAS) positive macrophages.

Treatment involves intravenous antibiotics for the first 2 weeks, followed by oral co-trimoxazole for at least a further year.

3.4.3.5 Short bowel syndrome

This syndrome refers to extensive bowel failure, most commonly due to massive surgical resections (>50%, usually for Crohn's disease or strictures), ischaemic injury or congenital abnormalities. Presentation and complications depend on the site and extent of injury or resection (see *Table 3.6*). Diarrhoea and malabsorption are major symptoms, with most patients having micronutrient deficiencies.

Table 3.6 *Various presentations of short bowel syndrome based on site of resection*

Proximal bowel	Distal ileum	Colon
• Iron deficiency • Micronutrient deficiency	• B12 deficiency • Interrupts bile salt absorption • Increased colonic oxalate re-uptake	• Water and sodium loss • Loss of fatty acid absorption

3.4.4 Tumours of the small bowel

The small bowel is a relatively uncommon site for neoplasia development, accounting for less than 4% of all GI cancers.

3.4.4.1 Benign tumours

Adenomas, hamartomas, lipomas and stromal tumours (GIST, see *Section 3.3.5*) represent the majority of primary benign lesions. Adenomas occur as a result of familial adenomatous polyposis (FAP), whereas hamartomatous polyps in the small bowel are common with Peutz–Jeghers syndrome. They are mostly asymptomatic and rarely cause problems.

3.4.4.2 Malignant tumours

Adenocarcinomas

These lesions account for more than 50% of all small bowel cancers. They usually arise in the peri-ampullary region of the descending duodenum and occur as a result of FAP or Crohn's disease. Capsule endoscopy or CT imaging may be used to identify the lesions. Surgical resection is the management of choice.

Lymphomas

In contrast to adenocarcinomas, lymphomas (non-Hodgkin) tend to arise in the ileum. They occur more commonly in immunocompromised patients (e.g. HIV) and patients with coeliac disease. Other subtypes include MALTomas and Burkitt. Abdominal pain and obstructive symptoms are the predominant features. Treatment involves surgical resection and chemoradiotherapy.

> P >> MALTomas are tumours that arise in the mucosa-associated lymphoid tissue, commonly situated in the sub-mucosa of the stomach and small intestines. They usually originate from the B-cell germ line, and play an important role in regulating mucosal immunity.

Carcinoid tumours

Also known as neuroendocrine tumours, these slow-growing tumours arise from the enterochromaffin cells of the intestine. They represent approximately 10% of all small bowel tumours, commonly developing in the terminal ileum and appendix. Patients typically present with obstructive symptoms and may occasionally present with systemic symptoms as a result of ectopic hormone production. This is known as carcinoid syndrome.

> E >> Carcinoid syndrome occurs in fewer than 10% of patients with carcinoid tumours, and usually only in the presence of liver metastasis. The ectopic secretion of serotonin (5-HT) and other vasoactive substances (e.g. prostaglandins, kinins, substance P, etc.) result in facial flushing, chronic diarrhoea, wheezing, palpitations and abdominal pain.

The mainstay treatment for carcinoid tumours of the intestine is surgical resection. Somatostatin analogues, octreotide and lanreotide may be used for symptomatic control of carcinoid syndrome.

3.4.5 Inflammatory bowel disease

3.4.5.1 Ulcerative colitis (UC)

Definition: the most common form of chronic inflammatory bowel disease with a relapsing and remitting course, that typically affects the rectum and extends proximally.

Epidemiology:
- Consistent incidence of 10 per 100,000
- May affect any age group but has a bimodal distribution – first peak at 15–30 and the second at 55–65
- Equal gender preponderance

Clinical features:
- Frequently presents with bloody diarrhoea
- Colicky abdominal pain and tenesmus may also be present
- Localised rectal disease may present with fresh PR bleeding and/or constipation
- For extra-abdominal manifestations of UC, see *Table 3.8*

Investigations
Investigations should be undertaken in the following order.

Stepwise plan:

The diagnosis of UC can be made using a combination of clinical evaluation, biochemical, radiological or histological evidence.

1   Arrange blood tests
- FBC (↓Hb, ↑WCC), LFTs (↓albumin is an important marker of severity), inflammatory markers (↑CRP/ESR)

2   Arrange stool testing
- Stool MC&S should be performed on all patients to exclude an infective cause. The use of faecal calprotectin is gaining favour in clinical practice
- NICE (2013, DG11) advocates the use of **faecal calprotectin** as an option to support the diagnosis of IBD. However, this should only be done when a cancer diagnosis has been excluded or is no longer suspected.

3   Obtain radiological imaging
- A simple film (AXR) ± an erect CXR should be obtained to assess for the presence of complications (e.g. megacolon, perforation) (see *Figs 3.16* and *3.17*)

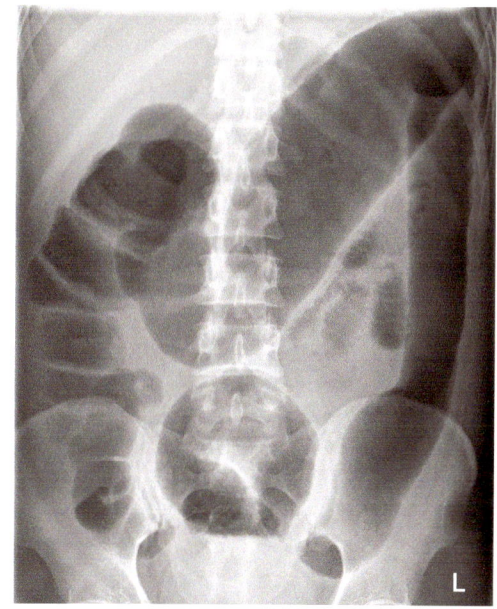

Fig. 3.16 *An AXR showing toxic megacolon of the transverse colon and lead-piping of the descending colon.*

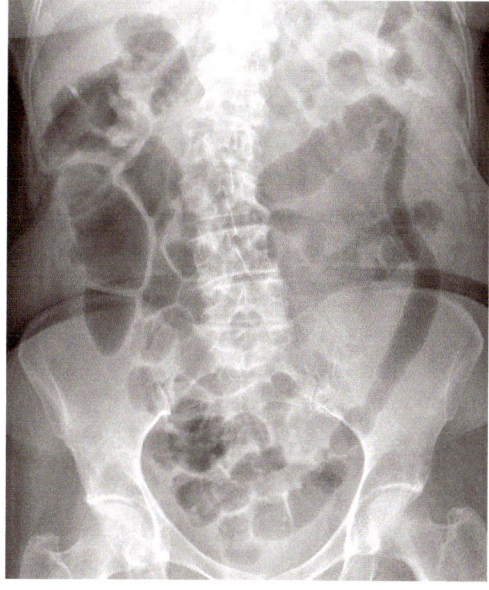

Fig. 3.17 *AXR showing classic thumbprinting of the colon.*

4   Arrange an endoscopy
- A full colonoscopy, with biopsies at a minimum of 5 sites, is regarded as the best modality in diagnosing UC. The pathological findings of UC are discussed in *Table 3.9*

> **E** ≫ Colonoscopy is contraindicated in acute colitis, as it is associated with a high risk of perforation. In such cases, a flexible sigmoidoscopy may be performed instead to confirm the diagnosis.

The Truelove and Witts criteria may be useful in evaluating the severity of an acute exacerbation of ulcerative colitis.

Table 3.7 *Truelove and Witts criteria*

	Mild	Moderate	Severe
Movements (/day)	<4	4–6	>6
Bleeding	Small	Moderate	Large
Pyrexia (T >37.8°C)	No	No	Yes
Pulse (HR >90)	No	No	Yes
Anaemia (Hb <10)	No	No	Yes
ESR (>30)	No	No	Yes

Management
The aim of UC treatment is to induce remission and subsequently maintain it. Management is based on severity.

Stepwise management of ulcerative colitis (NICE 2013, CG166)

Inducing remission in severe disease
1 **Urgent hospital admission**
- Ideally with both gastroenterology and colorectal services

2 **IV corticosteroids or cyclosporin**
- If steroids are contraindicated

3 **Offer VTE prophylaxis**
- Patients are pro-coagulopathic

4 **Add on IV cyclosporin if unresponsive to corticosteroids after 72 hours**
- Consider infliximab if cyclosporin is contraindicated

5 **Consider urgent surgery**
- In patients with acute complications (e.g. megacolon, perforation) or if they have failed to respond to medical therapy

Inducing remission in mild/moderate disease
1 **Aminosalicylates (e.g. mesalazine) are preferred over steroids as first-line agents**
- Topical forms (i.e. suppositories, enemas) may be useful in patients with distal disease (protosigmoiditis)

2 **Consider oral corticosteroids**
- In patients in whom aminosalicylates are contraindicated or as an add-on agent in patients who show no improvement after 4 weeks with aminosalicylates

3 **Tacrolimus may be added to corticosteroids**
- In the event of inadequate response

4 **Consider adalimumab, golimumab and vedolizumab**
- As alternative agents to the conventional therapy

Maintaining remission
1 **Oral or topical aminosalicylates are recommended first-line agents**
- These may be taken daily or as intermittent regimes

2 **Consider azathioprine or mercaptopurine (6-MP)**
- In patients who have >2 severe exacerbations in a year, requiring corticosteroid therapy, or who are unresponsive to oral aminosalicylates

3 **Consider elective surgery**
- Elective surgery may be offered to patients who are chronically symptomatic and fail to respond to medical therapy. Patients should be given adequate advice with regards to diet, psychological support and stoma care pre- and post-op

3.4.5.2 Crohn's disease (CD)

Definition: Crohn's is another form of chronic inflammatory bowel disease of unknown aetiology, characterised by transmural involvement and may affect any part of the GI tract.

Epidemiology:
- Increasing incidence of 6–7 per 100,000
- May affect any age group but has a bimodal distribution – first peak 15–20 and the second at 60–80
- Slight female preponderance

Clinical features:

- Diarrhoea is a common symptom; often not bloody
- Abdominal discomfort, weight loss may also be present
- Aphthous ulcers, glossitis and fistulae are common manifestations
- For extra-abdominal manifestations of CD, see *Table 3.8*

Investigations

Similarly, the diagnosis of CD is based on clinical suspicion, in combination with biochemical, radiological or histological evidence.

Stepwise plan:

1 **Arrange blood tests**
- FBC (↓Hb, ↑WCC, ↑platelets), LFTs (↓albumin), ↑CRP/ESR, haematinics (may show ↓Fe, B12, folate secondary to malabsorption depending on the site of disease)

2 **Arrange stool testing**
- Stool MC&S to rule out infections
- Faecal calprotectin is recommended

> ≫ Calprotectin is a dimer of calcium-binding protein. It contains up to 60% of neutrophilic cytosol material, and elevated levels may indicate high levels of neutrophils in the intestinal mucosa. It is therefore used as a surrogate marker of inflammation in the GI tract.

3 **Obtain radiological imaging**
- AXR ± erect CXR to look for complications (e.g. obstruction secondary to strictures, perforation)
- MRI pelvis is useful in perianal disease to evaluate the extent of disease and look for fistulae
- MRI enterography (see *Fig. 3.18*) or capsule endoscopy (see *Fig. 3.19*) may be used to assess for small bowel disease

4 **Arrange endoscopy**
- Ileocolonoscopy with visualisation of the terminal ileum and biopsies is recommended to establish a histological diagnosis
- An upper GI endoscopy may also be warranted in patients with UGI symptoms
- Histopathological findings of CD are discussed in *Table 3.9*

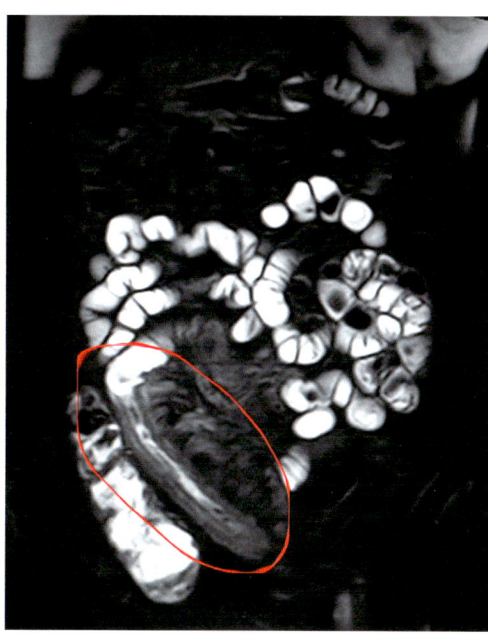

Fig. 3.18 *T2-weighted MRI enterography showing active terminal ileum disease.*

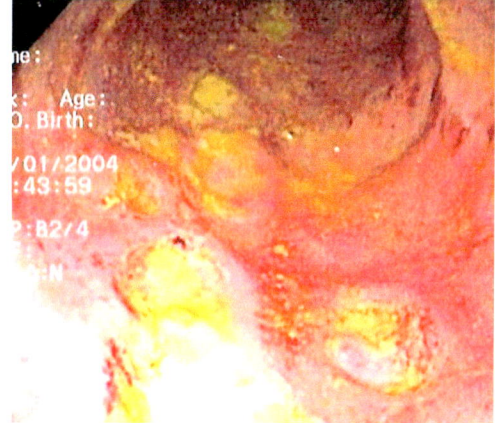

Fig. 3.19 *Endoscopic image showing deep ulcerations of the sigmoid colon.*

Management

The aims of CD management are similar to that of UC – inducing remission and maintaining it.

Stepwise management of Crohn's disease (NICE 2012, CG152)

Inducing remission

1 **Offer oral or IV corticosteroids as first-line agents**

3

2   Consider budesonide or 5-ASA therapy
- In patients with distal ileal or right-sided colonic disease as an alternative to steroids
- However, these agents should not be used in severe episodes

3   Azathioprine or 6-MP may be used as add-on therapy in resistive cases (>2 exacerbations/year)
- Methotrexate may be considered as an alternative to azathioprine if contraindicated or intolerant

> **E »** TPMT (thiopurine methyltransferase) levels should always be checked before starting azathioprine or 6-MP. This is because up to 10% of people have a lowered TPMT activity and as a result are more susceptible to thiopurine toxicity. Adverse effects include hypersensitivity reactions, marrow suppression and pancreatitis. Therefore, regular monitoring for neutropenia is recommended.

4   Consider biologic agents
- Biologic agents such as infliximab and adalimumab may be offered to patients who are unresponsive to conventional therapy

5   Consider surgery
- Consider surgery as an alternative to medical therapy in patients with localised distal ileal disease

Maintaining remission

1   Smoking cessation and lifestyle advice

2   Consider azathioprine or 6-MP as first-line agents
- These should also be offered post-surgery in patients with poorer prognosis
- Long-term steroids should never be used to maintain remission

3   Methotrexate may be offered as an alternative

4   Stricture management
- Balloon dilatation via colonoscopy may be offered to relieve short strictures
- However, surgery might be needed in more extensive disease

5   Monitoring
- Assessment for osteopenia/-porosis should be performed and appropriate treatment offered
- Colonoscopic surveillance for colorectal cancer should be offered to patients whose symptoms started 10 years ago

Management of perianal disease

1   Consider oral antibiotics
- Oral antibiotics (such as metronidazole or ciprofloxacin) may be used first-line in patients with simple perianal disease

2   Consider immunosuppression
- Azathioprine ± infliximab may be useful in fistula healing

3   Consider surgery
- Examination under anaesthesia (EUA), abscess drainage or seton insertion (for fistulae healing) may be necessary

3.4.5.3 Microscopic colitis

Microscopic colitis is a form of inflammatory bowel disease that only affects the colon and rectum. There are two subtypes:
- Lymphocytic colitis (see *Fig. 3.20*)
- Collagenous colitis (see *Fig. 3.21*)

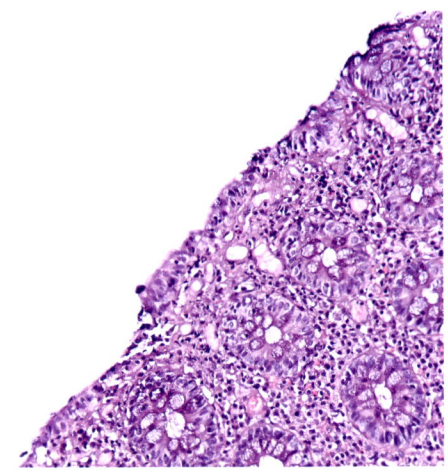

Fig. 3.20 *Lymphocytic colitis indicated by the increased number of lymphocytes within the mucosa.*

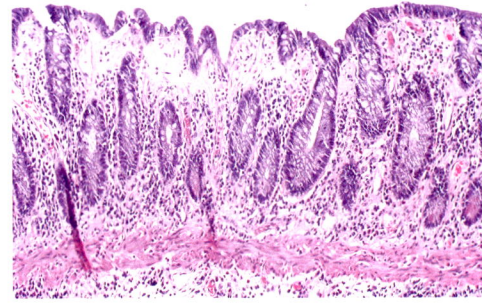

Fig. 3.21 *Collagenous colitis. Note the band of sub-mucosal collagen deposition (pink stain).*

Table 3.8 *Extra-abdominal manifestations of UC and Crohn's disease*

Extra-abdominal manifestations

Dermatological		

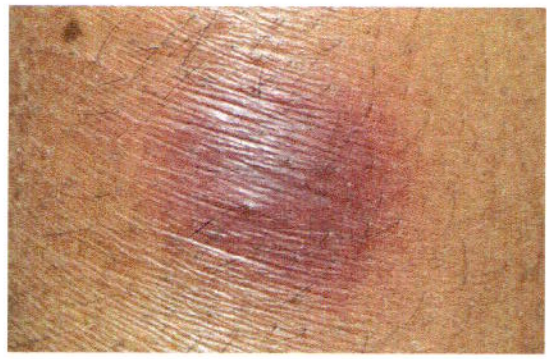

Fig. 3.22 *Erythema nodosum.*

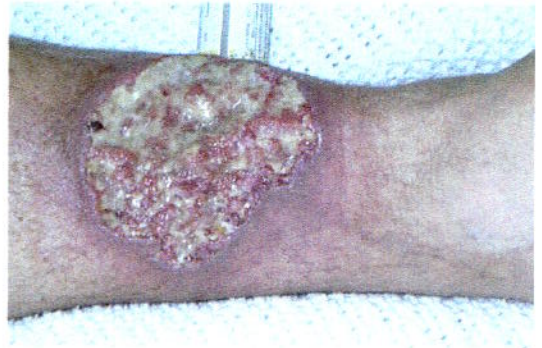

Fig. 3.23 *Pyoderma gangrenosum.*

Eyes		

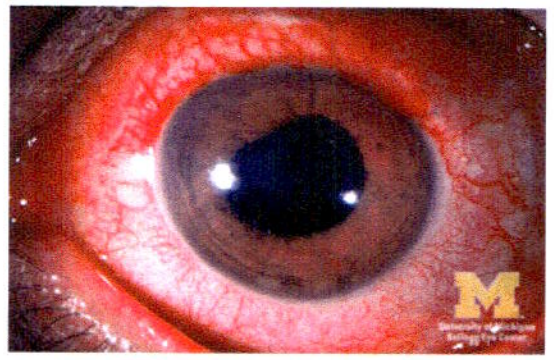

Fig. 3.24 *Anterior uveitis.*

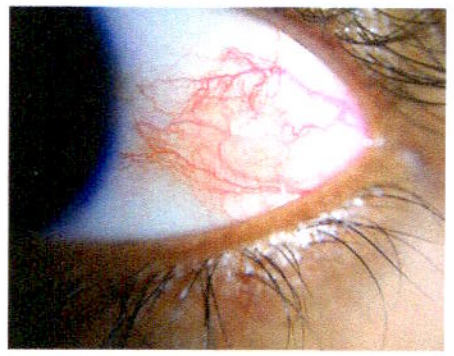

Fig. 3.25 *Episcleritis.*

Joints
- Arthritis
- Ankylosing spondylitis

Liver
- Gallstones (more common in Crohn's)
- PSC, cholangiocarcinoma (more common in UC)

Others
- Renal stones (oxalate – more common in Crohn's), amyloidosis

Table 3.9 *Comparison between the pathological findings of UC and Crohn's disease*

Pathology	Ulcerative colitis	Crohn's disease
Macroscopic		
Distribution	Continuous	Skip lesions, cobblestone pattern
Site	Rectum extending proximally to the ascending colon. May occasionally affect the TI (backwash ileitis)	Anywhere between the mouth and anus. Commonly affecting the TI and ascending colon
Stricture formation	No	Yes
Microscopic		
Inflammation	Confined to the mucosa. Crypt abscesses and goblet cell dysplasia are common	Transmural involvement. Extensive fibrosis with fissuring
Granuloma formation	Rare	Common (non-caseating)
Fistula formation	None	Yes

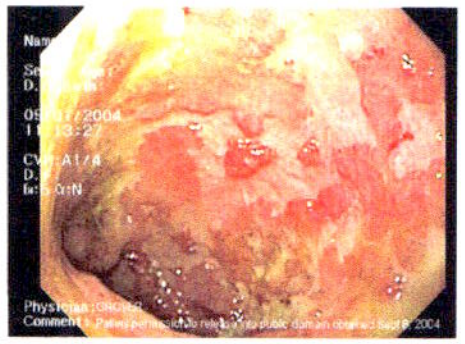

Fig. 3.26 *Endoscopic image of UC.*

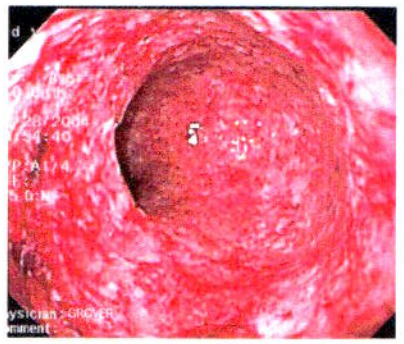

Fig. 3.27 *Endoscopic image of CD.*

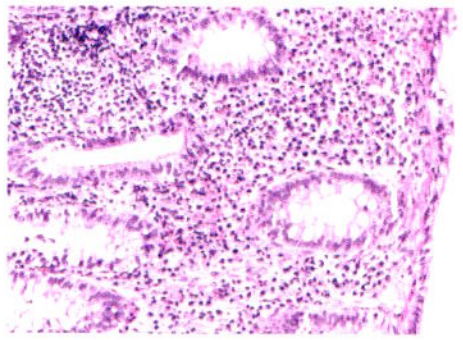

Fig. 3.28 *Histological image of UC.*

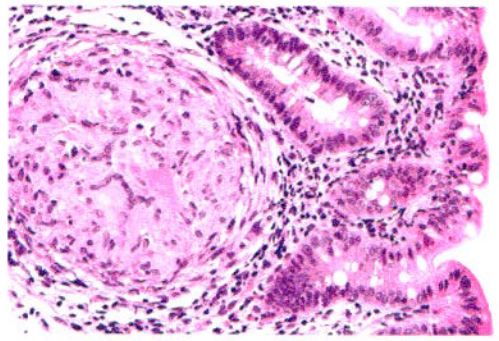

Fig. 3.29 *Histological image of CD.*

3

These are histopathological diagnoses, based on the type of inflammatory infiltrate. Associations have been observed with other conditions (such as coeliac disease and rheumatoid arthritis) as well as the use of NSAIDs and PPIs. Presentation of both the subtypes is very similar and patients usually present with chronic watery diarrhoea. Steroids are usually effective in these patients.

3.4.6 Irritable bowel syndrome (IBS)

Definition: The World Gastroenterology Organisation defines IBS as a functional bowel disorder in which abdominal pain or discomfort is associated with defecation and/or a change in bowel habit in the absence of an organic cause.

Epidemiology:
- More common in women and the younger population (20–30)
- Worldwide prevalence of 10–20%

Clinical features:
Patients usually present with at least a 6-month history of:
- Abdominal pain or discomfort
- Bloating
- Change in bowel habit
- Annual incidence of 1–2% per 100,000

Pathophysiology:
Altered gastrointestinal sensitivity towards stimuli. This may be triggered by environmental factors (including both physiological and psychological stress), as well as other factors (such as certain foods and bacteria overgrowth).

Diagnosis
IBS is **not** a diagnosis of exclusion and should be made positively on symptom-based criteria.

> **Stepwise plan:**
>
> **1   Elicit red flag signs and symptoms requiring urgent secondary care referral**
> - Unintentional weight loss
> - Rectal mass/bleeding
> - Family history of bowel/ovarian cancer
> - Aged over 60 with >6 weeks of altered bowel habit
>
> **2   Use the Rome criteria to aid the diagnosis of IBS:**

Table 3.10 *Rome criteria*

Abdominal discomfort/pain for ≥12 weeks associated with 2 or 3 of the following features:
- Relieved by defecation - Onset associated with change of bowel frequency - Onset associated with change of bowel form
Other supportive symptoms (at least 2):
- Altered stool passage - Other abdominal symptoms (bloating, distension, etc.) - Prandial association - Mucus discharge per rectum

> **P** >> IBS can be divided to either **diarrhoea-predominant** or **constipation-predominant**, based on the patient's symptoms.

Management
The treatment of IBS involves good patient education regarding lifestyle and dietary modifications, combined with pharmacological and psychological support.

> **Stepwise management of irritable bowel disease (NICE 2015, CG61)**
>
> **1   Lifestyle changes**
> - Encourage physical activity and leisure time
>
> **2   Dietary changes**
> - Encourage regular meals and adequate hydration, avoid high-fibre/starch, caffeinated and carbonated food/drinks
> - NICE advocates a single food avoidance diet (e.g. low FODMAP diet), fermentable oligosaccharides, disaccharides, monosaccharides and polyols)
>
> **3   Consider pharmacological therapy**
> - Based on the predominant symptom: anti-spasmodics, laxatives or antimotility (loperamide)
> - Amitriptyline may be used as a second-line agent
>
> **4   Consider psychological therapy**
> - CBT, psychotherapy or hypnotherapy should be considered for patients who are refractory to medical therapy

3.4.7 Ischaemic bowel disease

This umbrella term encompasses a group of disorders, the main three of which are acute mesenteric ischaemia, chronic mesenteric ischaemia (intestinal angina) and ischaemic colitis. They have hugely similar and overlapping aetiologies ranging from:

- Occlusive disease, e.g. primary atherosclerosis, distal embolism (**particular association with atrial fibrillation**), vasculitis, extrinsic compression
- To non-occlusive diseases, to septic shock, hypoperfusion

Patients generally present with very severe, constant colicky abdominal pain. Signs of peritonism may only develop in the later stages. There may be a post-prandial association in chronic mesenteric ischaemia, much like the exertional component of angina.

The investigation modality of choice is a CT angiogram, allowing localisation and visualisation of any potential occlusive (embolic or thrombus) cause (see *Fig. 3.30*).

E ≫ An urgent ABG with lactate analysis should always be performed if bowel ischaemia is suspected. A high lactate is consistent with cell hypoxia (ischaemia).

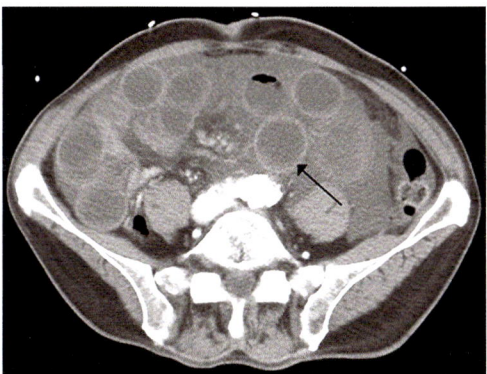

Fig. 3.30 *CT abdomen showing dilated small bowel loops with thickened walls suggestive of ischaemic bowel.*

Stepwise management of ischaemic bowel disease

1 **Active fluid resuscitation and supportive measures**

2 **Empirical antibiotics**

3 **Anticoagulation if indicated**

4 **Urgent angioplasty, embolectomy/thrombectomy or exploratory surgery if severe**

5 **Bypass surgery recommended in chronic disease**

3.4.8 Diverticular disease and diverticulitis

Definition: a diverticulum refers to an out-pouching of the mucosa through the muscular wall with the peritoneum still intact. Diverticulitis refers to the inflammation of these diverticula.

P ≫ Colonic diverticula are pseudo-/false diverticula because only the mucosa and sub-mucosa are involved.

Epidemiology:
- Affects up to 50% of people by the age of 50, and 70% by 80
- Slight female preponderance in the elderly cohort
- Left-sided disease (i.e. descending and sigmoid colon) is more common in the western population, whereas right-sided disease is more prevalent in Asian populations

W ≫ The sigmoid is most commonly affected because of its smaller diameter, which makes it susceptible to more strain and pressure.

Clinical features:
- Most patients are asymptomatic
- Altered bowel habit is usually present
- Diverticulitis typically presents with left iliac fossa (LIF) pain and pyrexia
- Abrupt intermittent perirectal (PR) bleeding may occasionally occur
- Annual incidence of 1–2% per 100,000

Pathophysiology:
- A low-fibre dietary intake has been implicated as an important factor that predisposes a patient to diverticular formation
- Low fibre in the stool increases intestinal transit time, eventually reducing the stool volume
- A smaller stool volume requires a higher intra-luminal pressure to allow passage of the stools
- As a result, weakened areas (particularly between the tenia coli where the vasa recti penetrate the wall) become susceptible to herniation and diverticula formation

3

- Diverticulitis occurs when a faecolith becomes impacted against the diverticulum and an infection subsequently ensues

Investigations

Investigations should be undertaken in the following order.

Stepwise plan:

1 **Arrange blood tests**
- ↑WCC, CRP may be present in diverticulitis

2 **Obtain imaging**
- A plain AXR ± erect CXR may show pneumoperitoneum
- Contrast-enhanced CT is the best modality of choice to look for abscess formation or active inflammation

3 **Arrange endoscopy**
- Flexible sigmoidoscopy may be necessary to exclude a more sinister cause (e.g. colorectal cancer)

E ≫ There is an increased risk of perforation of diverticula if enemas or colonoscopy is carried out in the acute setting. This should be avoided as far as possible.

Stepwise management of diverticular disease

Asymptomatic diverticular disease

1 **Encourage a high-fibre diet**

2 **Relieve constipation with laxatives**

Mild diverticulitis

1 **Encourage oral hydration and bowel rest**

2 **7-day course of oral co-amoxiclav and metronidazole**

Severe diverticulitis

1 **Patients should be admitted and made NBM from admission**

2 **IV fluids, analgesia and supportive therapy should be offered**

3 **Commence IV antibiotics promptly (based on local guidelines)**

4 **Consider surgery if indicated**

Management of complications

1 **Perforation – urgent surgical resection**

2 **Major haemorrhage – radiologically guided embolisation**

3 **Abscess – IV antibiotics and US/CT-guided drainage**

4 **Strictures – surgical resection or stent insertion**

3.4.9 Colonic polyps and polyposis syndromes

Polyps are abnormal growths that protrude from a membranous surface. They may occur anywhere in the body that has a mucosal membrane, from the nasal cavity or uterine cavity to the colon. Colonic polyps are relatively common – present in up to 50% of the western population over the age of 60. They can be sessile (see *Fig. 3.31*) or pedunculated (see *Fig. 3.32*). There are many histological types that may arise in the colon, but by far the most common are of the adenoma subtype.

3.4.9.1 Adenomas

Definition: adenomas are composed of benign, dysplastic tissue and arise from columnar epithelium or glandular tissue. They can be sub-divided, based on their glandular morphology, into tubular, tubulovillous and villous subtypes.

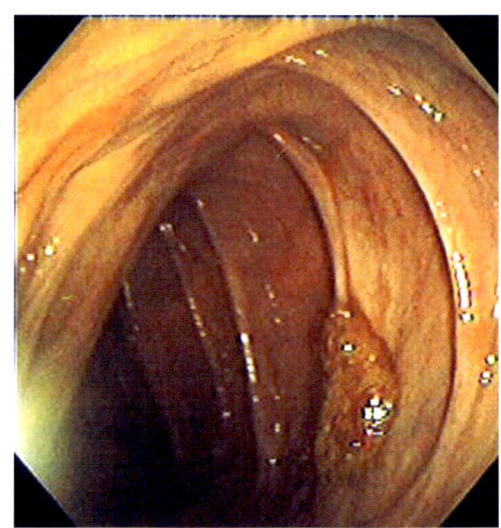

Fig. 3.31 *Sessile polyp.*

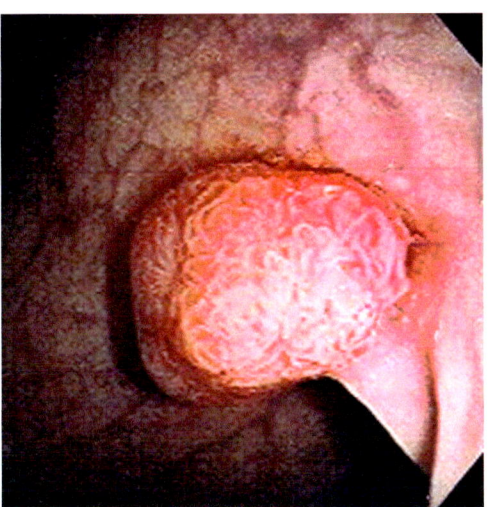

Fig. 3.32 Pedunculated polyp.

Pathology:
- Most adenomas occur sporadically and are asymptomatic
- However, they may occasionally develop as a result of an inherited polyposis syndrome

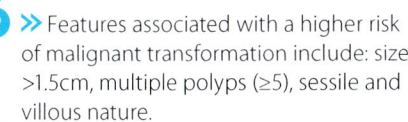
P >> Features associated with a higher risk of malignant transformation include: size >1.5cm, multiple polyps (≥5), sessile and villous nature.

- Most polyps are detected incidentally on colonoscopy and should be removed to reduce the risk of colorectal cancer development

Management
NICE (2011, CG118) recommends regular colonoscopic surveillance after the initial polypectomy.

Frequency of follow-up is guided by the number and size of the polyps:
- Annually: ≥5 polyps or ≥3 with at least one >1cm
- Every 3 years: >3 polyps or at least one >1cm
- Every 5 years: 1–2 polyps, all of which <1cm

3.4.9.2 Inherited polyposis syndromes
Familial adenomatous polyposis (FAP)

Epidemiology:
- 1 in 10,000, mean age of onset of 15 years
- Inheritance: autosomal dominant
- Genetics: APC gene on chromosome 5

Clinical features:
- Presents with hundreds to thousands of adenomas, which develop predominantly in the colon and rectum (see *Fig. 3.33*)
- They can also arise in the small bowel and stomach

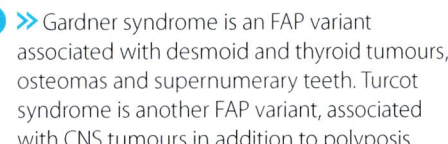
P >> Gardner syndrome is an FAP variant associated with desmoid and thyroid tumours, osteomas and supernumerary teeth. Turcot syndrome is another FAP variant, associated with CNS tumours in addition to polyposis.

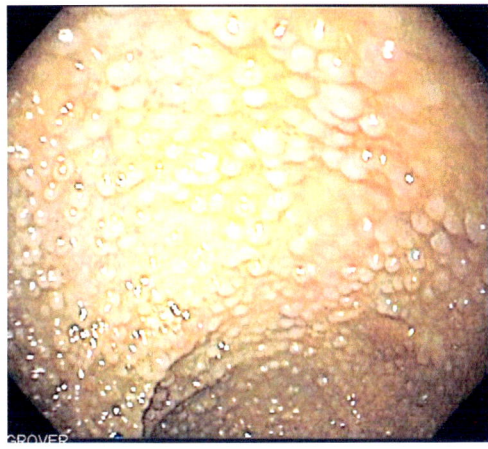

Fig. 3.33 Widespread colonic polyps seen on sigmoidoscopy in a patient with FAP.

Management
- 90% of patients with FAP will eventually develop cancer if untreated
- Early prophylactic colectomy and lifelong follow-up is the best treatment option to prevent cancer development
- First-degree relatives should be offered genetic testing

Hereditary non-polyposis colon cancer (HNPCC)

E >> This condition was historically known as Lynch syndrome. It is a misnomer, as colonic polyps are seen in this disease. The terminology 'non-polyposis' is used to distinguish the syndrome from FAP.

Epidemiology:
- 1 in 5000
- Mean age of onset is 40
- Inheritance: autosomal dominant

- Genetics: micro-satellite sequence instability due to hMSH2, hMLH1 DNA mismatch repair gene mutations

Clinical features:
- Adenomas tend to affect the right side of the colon
- Concurrent tumours affecting the breast, ovaries, bladder, stomach and endometrium may also be seen

> **P** ≫ The **Amsterdam Criteria** list is helpful in diagnosing HNPCC. Its criteria can be remembered using the '3,2,1 rule'.
> - ≥3 family members affected with ≥1 a first-degree relative
> - ≥2 generations are affected
> - ≥1 member <50 years is diagnosed with colon cancer
> - FAP must be excluded.

Peutz-Jeghers syndrome (PJS)

Epidemiology:
- 1 in 50,000
- Inheritance: autosomal dominant
- Genetics: serine threonine kinase (STK11) gene on chromosome 19

Clinical features:
- Multiple hamartomatous polyps affecting mainly the small bowel
- May also affect the stomach and colon
- Mucocutaneous pigmentation (lip, hands, feet; see *Fig. 3.34*)
- May be complicated by bleeding, obstruction and intussusception
- Associated with other cancers affecting the pancreas, breast, ovaries, endometrium, testicular tissue and lungs

Management
- Endoscopic polypectomy
- Regular endoscopic surveillance and screening of other cancers

Juvenile polyposis
An autosomal dominant condition, characterised by the development of tens to hundreds of hamartomatous polyps in the colon and rectum. This condition occurs mainly in children and adolescents, with up to 20% developing colon cancer by the age of 40. Management involves regular colonoscopic surveillance and polypectomy.

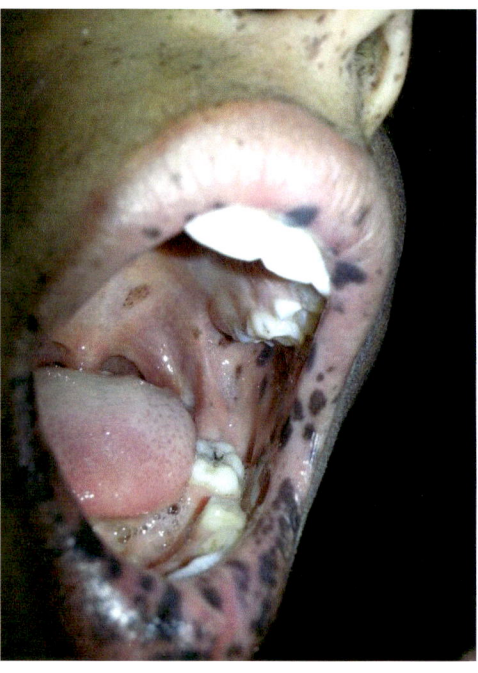

Fig. 3.34 *Lip pigmentation seen in PJS.*

3.4.10 Colorectal cancer

Definition: colorectal cancer (CRC) refers to a carcinoma that arises from the mucosa of the colon or rectum. About two-thirds of CRCs occur in the colon and the remaining third in the rectum. The majority are adenocarcinomas (95%), typically developing from a polyp.

Epidemiology:
- Third most common cancer worldwide
- Annual incidence of 50 in 100,000 and lifetime risk of 2%
- Slight male preponderance, especially rectal cancer
- Usually presents in the sixth decade
- Lower incidence in Africa and Asia

Risk factors:
- Family history of CRC or inherited polyposis syndromes
- Diet consisting of ↑red meat and saturated fat, ↓fibre
- Sedentary lifestyle: smoking, obesity, alcohol excess
- Inflammatory bowel disease
- Radiation exposure
- Annual incidence of 1–2% per 100,000

W ≫ Red meat contains high haem content, which is broken down to N-nitroso compounds in the gut. These compounds have been observed to cause DNA damage in the mucosal intestinal lining. Saturated fat, on the other hand, has been linked to inactivation of anticarcinogenic prostaglandins in the bowel.

Pathophysiology:
- The complex interplay between genetic and environmental factors seems to be at the centre of colonic carcinogenesis.
- It follows a stepwise progression regulated by accumulation of a number of genetic mutations.
- The classic, **two-hit hypothesis** model is often used to explain the development of CRC. The model describes multiple mutations in the progression of the carcinoma sequence. For example, mutations of the APC gene leading to adenoma formation can be considered as the 'first-hit'. Further mutations of tumour suppressor genes (e.g. *k-ras, p53*), i.e. 'second-hit', will eventually result in carcinoma development
- However, it is important to note that only 5% of all CRC arises from single gene mutations (e.g. FAP, HNPCC). The majority are triggered by an initial environmental cause (most commonly diet and lifestyle factors), resulting in sporadic genetic mutations. These mutations usually arise as a consequence of chromosomal or microsatellite instability.

P ≫ Chromosomal instability refers to the loss of heterozygosity and inactivation of tumour suppressor genes as a result of sporadic mutations and deletions on specific portions of the chromosome. Microsatellite instability, on the other hand, refers to inadequate repair of DNA mismatch sequences (i.e. microsatellites) as a result of DNA repair gene mutations.

Clinical features
- Presentation of CRC is dependent on the site of the lesion (see *Table 3.11*)
- Occasionally, patients may present as an emergency with acute bowel obstruction

Table 3.11 *Comparison of presentations of right-sided and left-sided CRC*

Right-sided lesion	Left-sided lesion
• Occult bleeding, anaemia	• Fresh PR bleeding
• Constipation	• Loose stools
• Late obstruction	• Early obstruction
• Colicky abdominal pain and weight loss	

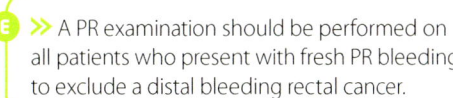

E ≫ A PR examination should be performed on all patients who present with fresh PR bleeding, to exclude a distal bleeding rectal cancer.

NICE (2014, CG131) has suggested urgent (2 weeks) secondary care referral for patients >40 with unexplained weight loss, >50 with unexplained PR bleeding and >60 with iron-deficiency anaemia or altered bowel habits.

Investigations
NICE (2014, CG131) recommends the following approach for investigation of patients with possible CRC.

Stepwise plan:

1 Arrange a formal colonoscopy
- This is the best first-line investigation for patients without significant comorbidities; this enables direct visualisation and biopsies to be obtained (see *Fig. 3.35*)
- Flexible sigmoidoscopy or CT colonogram may be used as alternatives in patients who are unable to undergo a colonoscopy due to their comorbidities

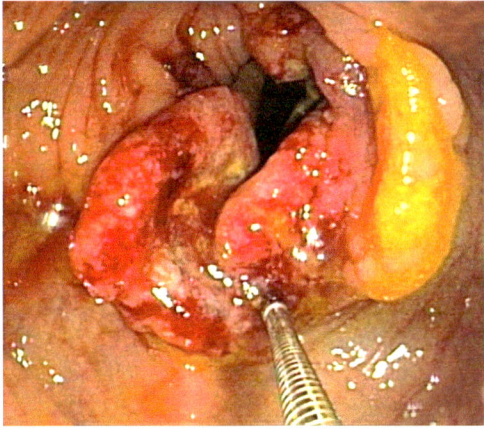

Fig. 3.35 *Colon cancer on endoscopy.*

2   Arrange staging imaging
- Offer a contrast-enhanced CT chest/abdo/ pelvis to evaluate tumour size, extent and spread (see *Fig. 3.36*)
- PET scans may be used to detect distal metastasis

3   Obtain further imaging
- Pelvic MRI for better assessment of rectal disease
- MRI liver may be indicated to identify liver mets

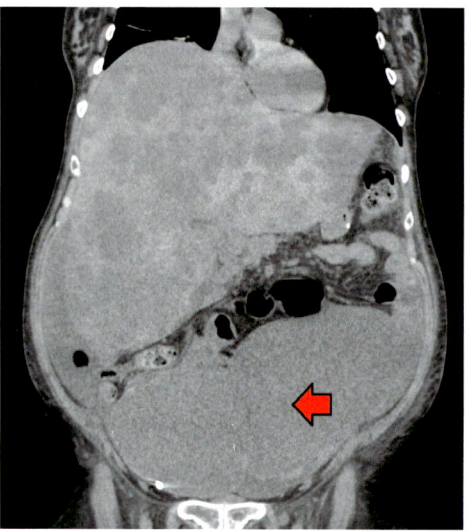

Fig. 3.36   *CT abdomen showing a bulky sigmoid cancer with extensive liver mets.*

4   Tumour marker
- The use of serum carcinoembryonic antigen (CEA) in diagnosis is limited; however, it is often used to monitor treatment response and follow-up

Both TNM and Duke classification can be used to stage CRC (see *Table 3.12*).

Table 3.12   *CRC staging*

Stage	Duke	Extent	% 5-yr S.
0	–	Carcinoma *in situ*	–
1	A	Confined within bowel wall	90
2	B	Local invasion without LN involvement	60
3	C	Spread to regional LNs	30
4	D	Distal metastasis	<10

Management

The management of colorectal cancer depends on staging, the patient's nutritional status and other comorbidities, requiring a multidisciplinary approach.

> **Stepwise management of colorectal cancer (NICE 2014, CG131)**

Localised rectal disease

1   Neoadjuvant radiotherapy may be offered to reduce recurrence

2   Offer laparoscopic surgical resection or low-energy contact X-ray brachytherapy (for early disease)

3   Adjuvant chemotherapy should be offered to patients with high-risk stage 2 disease and above

Localised colonic disease

1   Consider pre-operative chemoradiotherapy if indicated

2   Offer laparoscopic surgical resection

3   Offer adjuvant chemotherapy (capecitabine or oxaliplatin) to patients with high-risk stage 2 or 3 disease

Advanced or metastatic disease

1   Consider surgical resection if both primary and metastatic tumours are resectable

2   Offer chemotherapy in combination with biologics (e.g. bevacizumab or cetuximab) in patients with unresectable disease

3   Management of extra-hepatic metastasis
- Consider radiofrequency ablation (RFA) of lung metastasis
- Denosumab is recommended for prevention of pathological fractures secondary to bony metastasis

4   Management of hepatic metastasis
- Consider surgical resection or RFA if suitable
- Otherwise, offer chemotherapy in combination with cetuximab

5   Provide palliative care

3.5 Anorectal conditions

3.5.1 Haemorrhoids

Definition: haemorrhoidal cushions are vascular mucosal cushions that line the anal canal and function to help with the control of stool passage. These cushions may become dilated, enlarged and may eventually protrude through the anus. These are colloquially known as piles.

Aetiology:
- Usually caused by straining secondary to constipation
- Can also be caused by increased intra-abdominal pressures (e.g. pregnancy, abdominal mass)

> **E** ›› Classification is based on the extent of prolapse and reducibility.
> - First-degree – no prolapse
> - Second-degree – prolapse on straining but reduces spontaneously
> - Third-degree – prolapse but manually reducible
> - Fourth-degree – permanently prolapsed.

Clinical features:
- Patients frequently present with fresh PR bleeding
- They may occasionally have severe perianal pain associated with thrombosis as a result of strangulated haemorrhoids

Management
Management mainly involves pain relief and the treatment of constipation.
- Dietary advice (↑dietary fibre) and stool softeners may be useful
- Interventions such as injection sclerotherapy and band ligation may also be considered
- Surgical haemorrhoidectomy is reserved for resistant cases

3.5.2 Anal fissure

Definition: an anal fissure is a break in the mucosal squamous epithelium of lower anal canal. This condition affects up to 0.3% of adults. It is usually caused by excessive straining and trauma secondary to the passage of hard stools.

Clinical features:
- Patients tend to present with very severe anal pain and fresh PR bleeding
- PR examination is almost impossible due to the pain

Management
- Conservative measures (such as good anal hygiene and a warm bath) may provide some relief
- Laxatives (especially stool softeners) may be useful
- Topical GTN or calcium channel blockers provide resolution in up to 70% of patients

> **W** ›› Topical CCBs work by inhibiting the influx of calcium into the smooth muscle cells of the anal sphincter and thus reduce its hypertonicity.

- Surgical sphincterotomy may be considered in resistant cases

3.5.3 Anorectal abscess and fistulae

Definition: an abscess is the infection of soft tissue resulting in the accumulation of pus within its walled-off cavity. Anorectal abscesses commonly affect three main sites:
- Perianal – in close proximity to the anal verge
- Intersphincteric – in between the internal and external sphincters
- Ischiorectal – lateral to the sphincters and in the ischiorectal fossa

Clinical features:
- Patients present with extreme pain, often unable even to sit
- Anal/perianal discharge and occasionally systemic upset (pyrexia)
- Spontaneous rupture of these abscesses may predispose to fistulae formation (30%)

Management
Management often requires surgical drainage and healing with secondary intention. Antibiotics may have a role to play in very early disease.

3.6 Hepatobiliary medicine

Approach to jaundice and abnormal LFTs

Jaundice refers to yellow discoloration of the skin and sclera as a result of bilirubin (Br) accumulation within the tissues. It is usually only clinically noticeable at serum bilirubin levels >40µmol/L. The causes of jaundice can be divided into pre-hepatic, hepatic and cholestatic jaundice (see *Fig. 3.37*). They have distinct clinical presentations as well as distinct investigation findings (see *Table 3.13*).

3.6.1 Congenital hyperbilirubinaemias

3.6.1.1 Gilbert syndrome

Definition: this is an autosomal recessive inherited disorder of non-haemolytic, unconjugated hyperbilirubinaemia. It affects 5–10% of people in the western world. The syndrome is caused by a mutation that regulates the production of the uridine-diphosphoglucuronate

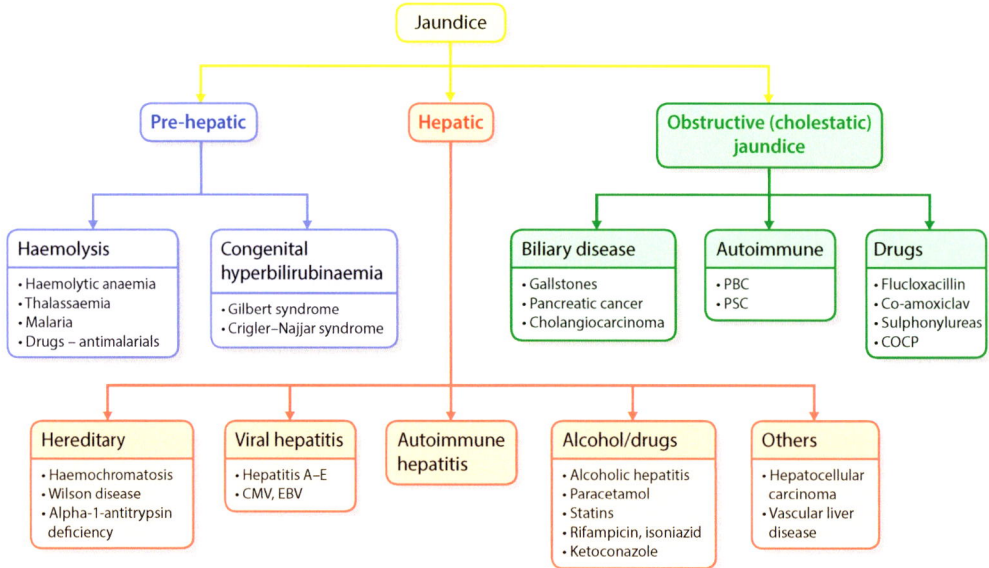

Fig. 3.37 *Causes of jaundice.*

Table 3.13 *Investigation of jaundice*

	Pre-hepatic	Hepatic	Cholestatic
Urine	• No bilirubin • ↑urobilinogen	• ↑bilirubin • ↑urobilinogen	• ↑bilirubin • No urobilinogen
LFTs	• ↑unconjugated Br • ↑LDH (haemolysis)	• ↑conjugated Br • Hepatic picture (↑↑AST/ALT) • ALT >1000 (likely viral, drug cause) • ↑GGT (alcohol) • ↑PT, ↓albumin	• ↑↑conjugated Br • Cholestasis picture • ↑↑ALP, GGT • ↑ALT/AST
Other tests	• Coombs test *(see Chapter 6)* • Blood film	• Liver screen – autoimmune profile, immunoglobulins, iron studies, viral screen, caeruloplasmin • Liver biopsy	• Autoimmune screen • Abdo USS • ERCP/MRCP

glucuronosyltransferase (UDPGT) enzyme responsible for the conjugation of bilirubin. This results in a **partial** (60–70%) **reduction** in conjugation activity.

Clinical features:

- Patients tend to present with intermittent jaundice that is associated with precipitating factors such as unusual physical activity, lack of sleep and fasting
- Certain medications (e.g. anti-cancer agents) may precipitate the condition
- LFTs tend to be entirely normal, apart from a high bilirubin

> **E** ≫ It is important to check the reticulocyte count to exclude any evidence of haemolytic causes.

Management
Patient education is important and no medical treatment is required.

3.6.1.2 Crigler-Najjar syndrome

This is an extremely rare congenital condition of unconjugated hyperbilirubinaemia. Mutations in chromosome 2 result in the impaired production of the UDPGT enzyme. The syndrome can be classified into two subtypes: Type 1 (absent UDPGT activity); and Type 2 (Arias syndrome, impaired UDPGT activity).

Type 1 Crigler-Najjar syndrome
Type 1 patients present in infancy with persistent jaundice and ultimately kernicterus if left untreated. Emergency plasma transfusion and phototherapy is necessary to prevent progression to kernicterus. Liver transplantation is the only definitive treatment.

Type 2 Crigler-Najjar syndrome
Type 2 Crigler–Najjar syndrome, unlike all other causes of inherited hyperbilirubinaemia, is **autosomal dominant** in inheritance. Unlike Type 1, there is some UDPGT activity. Apart from yellow skin, patients are largely asymptomatic.

> **P** ≫ Dubin–Johnson syndrome and Rotor syndrome are autosomal recessive disorders causing hyperbilirubinaemia. Both groups of patients remain largely asymptomatic.

> **E** ≫ Memory aid:

Crigler–Najjar Type 1	• Absent UDPGT (neonatal jaundice, fatal)
Crigler–Najjar Type 2	• Mild UDPGT activity (generally asymptomatic)
Gilbert syndrome	• Better (approximately 30% activity, compared to Type 2 Crigler–Najjar syndrome) UDPGT activity • Largely asymptomatic
Dubin–Johnson syndrome	• Isolated increase in conjugated bilirubin • Production of a melanin-like pigment contributes to blackening of the liver • Patients are largely asymptomatic
Rotor syndrome	• Increased conjugated bilirubin • Normal liver appearance • Largely asymptomatic

All these conditions present with autosomal recessive inheritance, apart from Type 2 Crigler–Najjar syndrome, which is autosomal dominant.

3.6.2 Acute liver injury (hepatitis)

Acute hepatitis can be caused by many pathologies. These include viruses, alcohol, toxins and other causes.

3.6.2.1 Viral hepatitis

Viral hepatitis is most commonly caused by hepatitis (A–E). However, other viruses (such as CMV, EBV and HSV) may also cause hepatitis and should be screened in patients who present with acutely deranged LFTs.

(Hepatitis A, B, C and E are discussed in *Table 3.16*. CMV and EBV are covered in *Chapter 9*.)

HBV serology testing is a quick and effective way to differentiate a patient's disease state (see *Table 3.14*).

3

Table 3.14 *Results of HBV serology in different disease states*

HBV serology	HBsAg	Anti-HBs	Anti-HBc IgM	Anti-HBc IgG
Acute infection	+	–	+	±
Chronic	+	–	–	+
Vaccinated	–	+	–	–
Previous	±	+	–	+

P ≫ Hepatitis D (delta virus) is an incomplete RNA virus that is dependent on concurrent HBV infection for replication. It has a blood-borne mode of transmission. Co-infection exacerbates the severity of acute hepatitis as well as increasing the risk of cirrhotic progression. There is no treatment for hepatitis D so effective management of HBV is important.

3.6.2.2 Drug-induced hepatitis

Numerous drugs have the potential to cause an acute liver injury. The pathophysiological mechanisms of drug-induced hepatitis are similar to those of viral hepatitis, in which there is acute liver parenchymal destruction. Various patterns of liver injury can occur. Some of the common drug-induced patterns are listed below.

Table 3.15 *Common patterns of drug-induced liver injury*

Liver injury pattern	Drugs
Hepatitis	Statins, ketoconazole, anti-TB drugs (e.g. rifampicin, isoniazid)
Cholestasis	Co-amoxiclav, flucloxacillin, chlor-promazine, NSAIDs, sulphonylureas, COCP
Fibrosis	Methotrexate
Necrosis	Paracetamol, NSAIDs

3.6.2.3 Alcoholic hepatitis

Definition: inflammation of the liver due to significant alcohol consumption. This represents an early stage in alcoholic liver disease, commonly associated with fatty deposition in the liver (steatosis).

W ≫ The pathophysiology of alcoholic liver injury involves the release of oxygen-free radicals during ethanol metabolism, ultimately resulting in mitochondrial damage and lipid perioxidation. Alcohol also increases gut wall permeability, resulting in endotoxin absorption. A cascade of pro-inflammatory cytokine release may induce hepatitis.

Clinical features:
- Patients usually present feeling generally unwell, occasionally with a fever and jaundice
- They may also have hepatomegaly due to steatosis
- Hepatic encephalopathy may also be present, though this is a poor prognostic indicator
- A **high MCV and GGT** often reflects excess alcohol intake

Management:
- Alcohol cessation in the first instance with withdrawal prevention
- Vitamin B1 replacement – Pabrinex (IV) then oral thiamine to prevent progression to Wernicke encephalopathy
- Nutritional supplementation
- Assess severity (30d mortality) using Maddrey score (discriminant factor, DF) and offer corticosteroids to patients with DF >32

P ≫ Maddrey discriminant factor (DF) can be calculated by:

DF = (4.6 × prothrombin time) + bilirubin (in mg/dl)

Alcoholism

Alcohol excess/misuse is a major problem in the UK. It affects up to 4% of the population between the ages of 16 and 65. It also accounts for a significant proportion of hospital admissions.

The current UK guidelines recommend a maximum of 14 units of alcohol per week for both men and women.

E ≫ Alcohol units = Alcohol by volume, ABV (%) * Volume (ml)/1000

Excessive alcohol consumption has a number of detrimental effects on the human body (see *Table 3.17*).

Table 3.16 *Viral hepatitis*

Viral hepatitis	Hepatitis A (HAV)	Hepatitis B (HBV)	Hepatitis C (HCV)	Hepatitis E (HEV)
Epidemiology	• Prevalence decreasing	• Most common cause of hepatitis • Chronically affects 350 million worldwide	• Affects 180 million worldwide	• Prevalence increasing
Virus	• Picornavirus (RNA)	• DNA virus	• RNA flavivirus	• RNA virus
Spread	• Faecal–oral	• Blood-borne • Vertical, sexual	• Blood-borne (IVDU, blood transfusion) • Sexual	• Faecal–oral • Main reservoir in pigs • Vertical
Clinical features	• Usually asymptomatic • Self-limiting illness	• Flu-like illness, general malaise • Jaundice (30–50%)	• Usually asymptomatic • May present with malaise, jaundice	• Usually asymptomatic • Self-limiting illness
Serology	• **Anti-HAV IgM** (acute infection) • **Anti-HAV IgG** (immunity/past infection)	• **HBV surface antigen** – *acute* infection, if persistent for >6 months (chronic) • **HBV surface antigen antibody (Anti-HBs)** (appears 3–6 months post-infection) – shows previous infection or vaccination • **HBV core antigen antibody (Anti-HBc)** (remains persistent): **IgM** (acute infection) **IgG** (past infection or chronicity) • **HBV envelope antigen** – active viral replication • **HBV DNA** represents viral load (used to monitor treatment)	• **HCV antibody (anti-HCV)** (6–12 weeks post-acute) • The presence of **HCV RNA** and **anti-HCV** represents *active infection* • **Genotyping** – 6 genotypes; Type 1 is the most common but most difficult to eradicate	• **HEV antibody (Anti-HEV IgM)** – *active infection*
Management	• Supportive	• Acute – supportive • Chronic – PEGinterferon ± antivirals (tenofovir/entecavir)	• Acute – symptomatic • Chronic – PEGinterferon ± ribavirin ± antivirals	• Supportive
Vaccination	• Yes	• Yes	• No	• No
Chronicity	• No	• Yes (5%)	• Yes (60–80%)	• No
Complications	• Cholestasis	• Cirrhosis (8–20% without treatment) • Hepatocellular carcinoma (HCC)	• Cirrhosis (25% after 20 years) • HCC	• 25% mortality in pregnant women

3

3

Table 3.17 *Effects of alcohol excess on various body systems*

System	Effects
Liver	Alcoholic hepatitis, alcoholic liver disease, cirrhosis
GI	Gastritis, oesophagitis, pancreatitis, cancer
CVS	Cardiomyopathy, arrhythmias
CNS	Brain damage, Wernicke encephalopathy, Korsakoff syndrome, alcohol-related seizures, peripheral neuropathy
Haem	Megaloblastic anaemia, folate deficiency

Alcohol withdrawal

This can be defined as a syndrome that occurs following an abrupt cessation of alcohol intake. Withdrawal symptoms usually appear 4–12 hours post-consumption and manifest as coarse tremors, tachycardia, hypotension, confusion and occasional hallucinations (delirium tremens, see *Chapter 4*) as well as seizures.

W ≫ Excessive alcohol intake results in adaptive neuronal changes. The neurotransmitters responsible for alcohol tolerance and withdrawal are glutamate, GABA, dopamine and serotonin. Sudden cessation of alcohol produces an imbalance in the interactive effects of these chemicals, resulting in increased activity of the excitatory pathways.

The Clinical Institute Withdrawal Assessment for Alcohol (CIWA) is a frequently used scale used to assess the severity of withdrawal and guide management. It comprises 10 items, each of which can be scored on a scale of 0 to 7. See Appendix for full CIWA protocol.

The treatment for alcohol withdrawal is with benzodiazepines (diazepam), and the dose and frequency are guided by the CIWA protocol. This often involves the use of benzodiazepines in the acute setting. All patients should also be given IV thiamine replacement to prevent progression to Wernicke encephalopathy.

Wernicke encephalopathy

This condition refers to a neuropsychiatric emergency resulting from long-standing thiamine (B1) deficiency.

E ≫ This condition classically presents with the triad of acute confusion, ataxia and ophthalmoplegia (nystagmus, lateral rectus palsy).

W ≫ Thiamine deficiency causes primary neurological injury as a result of oxidative stress and mitochondrial injury, eventually leading to apoptosis.

Intravenous thiamine replacement is effective if treated early, with improvement in symptoms in 24–48 hours. Other nutritional deficiencies should also be corrected.

Korsakoff syndrome

Korsakoff psychosis should be considered as a continuum of Wernicke encephalopathy at the later stages, if not treated adequately. This condition is characterised by anterograde and retrograde amnesia as well as confabulation. Treatment with IV thiamine should be given. However, not all patients may respond; and, in most cases, the memory impairment is irreversible.

3.6.3 Chronic liver disease

3.6.3.1 Cirrhosis

Definition: cirrhosis refers to irreversible damage and fibrosis of normal liver architecture. It remains one of the leading causes of hospitalisation and death, with an annual mortality of 13 per 100,000 population. Cirrhosis can be thought of as the last-stage progression of most chronic liver diseases.

Aetiology:
- Alcoholic liver disease
- Non-alcoholic fatty liver disease/non-alcoholic steatohepatitis
- Viral – chronic hepatitis B or C
- Hereditary – haemochromatosis, Wilson disease
- Autoimmune – primary biliary cirrhosis, primary sclerosing cholangitis
- Cryptogenic

Clinical features:
- Hands – palmar erythema, leuconychia (hypoalbuminaemia), Dupuytren contracture
- Face – jaundice, xanthelasma (PBC), parotid enlargement (alcohol excess), Kayser–Fleischer ring (Wilson)
- Trunk – spider naevi, loss of hair, gynaecomastia
- Abdomen – caput medusa, striae, hepatosplenomegaly, ascites

Child–Pugh Grading

This scoring system functions to assess the severity of chronic liver disease, cirrhosis in particular. It is often used to predict mortality as well as guide the management of patients with hepatocellular carcinoma.

E >> The mnemonic **'ABCDE'** is often used as an aide-memoire for the components in the scoring system.

Table 3.18 *Child–Pugh Grading score*

Component	1 point	2 points	3 points
Albumin	>35	28–35	<28
Bilirubin	<34	34–50	>50
Clotting (PT)	<4.0	4.0–6.0	>6.0
Distension (ascites)	None	Mild	Mod–Severe
Encephalopathy	None	Grade I–II	Grade III–IV

Classification is based on the total number of points:
- Class A: 5–6 points (1yrS 100%)
- Class B: 7–9 points (1yrS 81%)
- Class C: 10–15 points (1yrS 45%)

Diagnosis

Although cirrhosis may be suspected on ultrasound imaging, cirrhosis remains a histological diagnosis (see *Fig. 3.38*). Liver biopsy is the gold standard means of diagnosis.

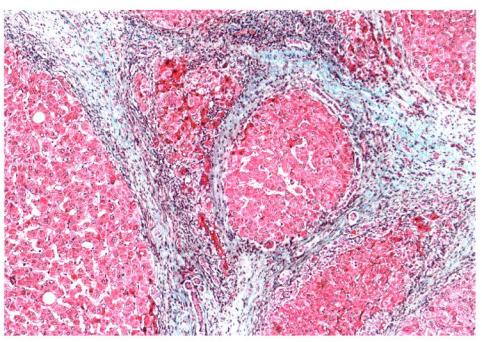

Fig. 3.38 *Micrograph of a cirrhotic liver. Notice the disruption of normal liver architecture with (blue-stained) fibrotic streaks and formation of cirrhotic nodules.*

3.6.3.2 Portal hypertension

As mentioned earlier, the liver has a dual blood supply, and most of the blood originates from the portal venous system. This unique system ensures that venous blood from most of the alimentary system gets transported through the liver (see *Fig. 3.39*). As such, the hepatic portal vein (black) is formed by the confluence of the superior mesenteric vein (blue) and splenic vein (orange).

Portal hypertension occurs when the pressure in the hepatic portal vein rises to pathological levels (>12mmHg). The aetiology of portal hypertension can be divided according to the site of venous obstruction.

P >> Pressures of higher than 12mmHg are associated with higher risk of variceal bleeds.

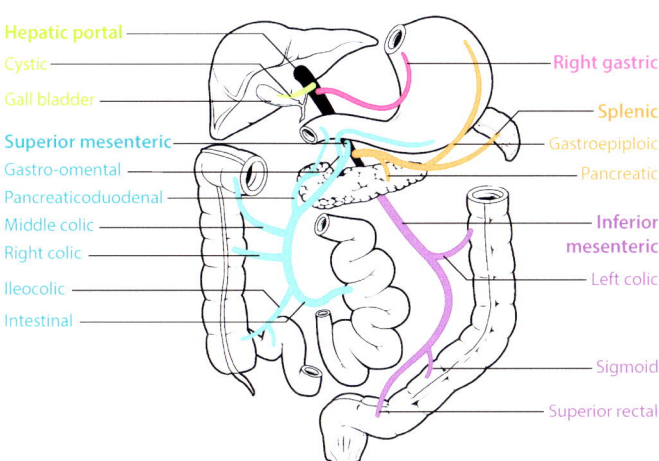

Fig. 3.39 *Hepatic portal venous system.*

- **Pre-hepatic** – portal vein thrombosis
- **Hepatic** – cirrhosis (most common), schistosomiasis, metastatic disease, sarcoidosis
- **Post-hepatic** – Budd–Chiari disease, veno-occlusive disease, right heart failure (venous congestion), constrictive pericarditis

Varices

Varices can be defined as abnormally dilated blood vessels, usually caused by abnormal blood flow. They are a common complication of portal hypertension. Increased vascular resistance of the portal venous circulation eventually results in the development of collateral vessels (varices) at porto-systemic anastomoses at the oesophagogastric junction, umbilicus (caput medusa/prominent abdominal wall veins) and rectum (haemorrhoids). These varices may enlarge and eventually bleed.

> **Stepwise management of oesophageal variceal haemorrhage**
>
> **1 Provide initial resuscitation**
> - As per upper GI bleeding (see *Chapter 12*)
>
> **2 Offer terlipressin and antibiotic therapy on admission**
> - NICE (2016, CG141) recommends offering **terlipressin** and **prophylactic antibiotic therapy** on admission to patients with suspected variceal bleeding
> - Somatostatin is an alternative agent
>
> **3 Arrange urgent upper GI endoscopy**
> - This is required to visualise the source of haemorrhage
> - **Band ligation** is the therapeutic modality of choice
>
> **4 Arrange temporary balloon tamponade**
> - A temporary balloon tamponade with a **Sengstaken–Blakemore tube** may be used in a life-threatening haemorrhage, if emergency OGD is not available or was unsuccessful
>
> **5 Consider transjugular intrahepatic porto-systemic shunting (TIPSS)**
> - If the variceal bleeding is not controlled endoscopically

E ≫ TIPSS involves placing a stent between the portal vein and hepatic vein within the liver under radiological guidance, percutaneously via the jugular vein. This creates a porto-systemic shunt, decompressing the portal venous system and resolving portal hypertension.

Prevention of variceal bleeding

Regular screening with upper GI endoscopy for varices should be offered to patients with cirrhosis. If non-bleeding varices are seen on OGD, a prophylactic beta blocker (e.g. carvedilol, propranolol) should be started. These are effective in reducing portal venous pressure and preventing variceal haemorrhage.

Hepatic encephalopathy

Hepatic encephalopathy is a neuropsychiatric condition caused by severe liver dysfunction. It commonly occurs in patients with chronic liver disease, as a result of accumulation of neurotoxins, which are normally metabolised by the liver.

This condition may be precipitated by:
- Drugs and substances – sedatives, benzodiazepines, alcohol
- Electrolyte disturbance – dehydration, low K, low Na
- GI bleeding
- Infection
- Constipation

Symptoms of hepatic encephalopathy range from fluctuating confusion (mainly inattention and impaired decision making), neglect and personality disturbances to reduced levels of consciousness at the extreme.

Grading of hepatic encephalopathy

The West Haven criteria are used to grade the severity of encephalopathy.

Table 3.19 *West Haven criteria*

Grade 0	Subclinical, minimal changes in memory, otherwise normal
Grade 1	Mild confusion, inattention, slowness in performing tasks
Grade 2	Lethargy, drowsiness, personality changes, inappropriate behaviour, gross deficit in performing tasks
Grade 3	Semi-stupor but rousable, gross disorientation, amnesia
Grade 4	Coma

Diagnosis

A routine liver function test as well as synthetic function (coagulation screen) will confirm the presence of underlying liver disease. An elevated serum ammonia increases the likelihood of hepatic encephalopathy, especially in patients in a coma.

Management

The management of patients with hepatic encephalopathy revolves around supportive care and removal of neurotoxins.

> **Stepwise management of hepatic encephalopathy**

1 Look for precipitating factors
- These may include electrolyte disturbances, dehydration or infection
- Routine bloods (including FBC, U&Es, LFTs) and a septic screen are useful
- Consider sending off plasma ammonia

2 Clear neurotoxins
- Regular bowel movements (twice daily) are recommended
- **Lactulose** is the first-line choice of laxative
- **Enemas** may often be useful in inducing bowel clearance

> **W** >> Lactulose is an osmotic laxative that works by retaining water in the digestive tract, resulting in softer stools. It is also metabolised by gut flora into short chain fatty acids, decreasing the pH of the colon and ultimately facilitating the breakdown of ammonia into its non-absorbable ionic form (NH_4^+).

3 Administer antibiotic prophylaxis
- NICE (2015, TA337) recommends the use of rifaximin in preventing recurrence of hepatic encephalopathy
- Rifaximin exerts its effects by eradicating ammonia-producing bacteria in the gut

Hepatorenal syndrome

A complication of advanced chronic liver disease characterised by the development of renal failure without any underlying renal pathology. This occurs as a result of splanchnic and systemic vasodilation, leading to sympathetic-induced vasoconstriction of the afferent arterioles and renal hypoperfusion. It is important to note that hepatorenal syndrome (HRS) is a diagnosis of exclusion.

There are two types of HRS:
- Type 1 – rapidly progressing renal failure with doubling of the creatinine in <2 weeks
  - Often triggered by a precipitating event (e.g. sepsis, upper GI bleed)
- Type 2 – gradual onset, often associated with diuretic-resistant ascites

Management involves strict fluid balance and fluid replacement with volume expanders (IV albumin). Nephrotoxic drugs (i.e. diuretics) should be stopped. Terlipressin may be effective in some patients. Liver transplantation is the best possible curative treatment.

Ascites

Ascites refers to accumulation of fluid in the abdominal cavity. This is a common complication of chronic liver disease as portal hypertension exerts an increased hydrostatic pressure, resulting in the transudation of fluid into the abdominal cavity. This is further exacerbated by a low plasma oncotic pressure due to low albumin synthesis.

Patients typically present with abdominal distension/discomfort, nausea, vomiting and – in severe cases – dyspnoea as a result of a hydrothorax or splinting of diaphragm but very tense ascites.

> **E** >> Serum–ascites albumin gradient (SAAG) is often used to determine the aetiology of the ascites. It can be calculated by (serum albumin – albumin in the ascetic fluid) with a cut-off of 1.1g/dl. The causes are shown in *Table 3.20*.

Table 3.20 *Causes of ascites based on SAAG*

High gradient (SAAG >1.1)	Low gradient (SAAG <1.1)
Caused by portal hypertension	Not associated with portal hypertension
• Cirrhosis	• Nephrotic syndrome
• Heart failure	• Malignancy
• Budd–Chiari syndrome	• Pancreatitis
• Constrictive pericarditis	• Tuberculosis

> **Stepwise management of ascites**

1 Offer patient education and dietary advice
- Salt (sodium) restriction is an effective way of helping to prevent ascites

2 Prescribe diuretics
- Spironolactone is the best first-line option
- Loop diuretics (e.g. furosemide) may be used to aid renal sodium excretion
- Caution: there is a risk of hyponatraemia

3 Offer therapeutic paracentesis
- Patients with large volume or resistant ascites may benefit from a drain
- Ascitic fluid should be sent off for microscopy, culture and biochemical analysis

4   Consider TIPSS
- In patients with refractory ascites who require very frequent paracentesis

Spontaneous bacterial peritonitis (SBP)

This represents a specific condition or complication of ascites. The ascitic fluid becomes infected, most commonly by *Escherichia coli* (~60%). Patients are often unwell, feverish and complain of severe abdominal pain. A diagnostic ascitic tap is usually performed. The cloudy and sometimes blood-stained appearance of the fluid may increase the probability of SBP. Fluid microscopy with a polymorph/neutrophil count of >250×10^6/L is diagnostic.

Patients are initially treated with broad-spectrum IV antibiotics until sensitivities guide further treatment. Albumin replacement is also indicated as per local protocol.

Antibiotic prophylaxis (oral ciprofloxacin) may be indicated in patients with a total protein of less than 15g/L in the ascitic fluid.

3.6.3.3 Non-alcoholic fatty liver disease

Definition: non-alcoholic fatty liver disease (NAFLD) is a histopathological condition characterised by excess of fat accumulating in the liver, in the absence of excessive alcohol consumption or any other underlying liver disease.

Epidemiology:
- Affects 20 to 30% of the population
- Increasing prevalence in younger people
- Equal gender preponderance

Clinical features:
- Mostly asymptomatic
- Hepatomegaly may sometimes be present
- Presence of risk factors similar to those in metabolic syndrome

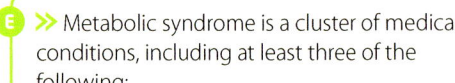

E ≫ Metabolic syndrome is a cluster of medical conditions, including at least three of the following:
- Truncal (central) obesity
- Hypertension
- Hypertriglyceridaemia
- Low high-density lipoprotein (HDL)
- Hyperglycaemia secondary to insulin resistance
- Annual incidence of 1–2% per 100,000

Pathophysiology
- The exact pathophysiology of NAFLD is still unclear but a 'two-hit hypothesis' has been postulated in the development of the disease
- Insulin resistance has been implicated as the 'first hit', responsible for fatty acid deposition in the liver (hepatic steatosis; see *Fig. 3.40a*)
- Further oxidative stress sets off the 'second hit'; and immune-mediated inflammation ensues, resulting in steatohepatitis (NASH; see *Fig. 3.40b*)
- Chronic hepatocellular injury eventually progresses to stellate cell activation and fibrosis (cirrhosis)

Investigations
Investigations should be undertaken in the following order.

> **Stepwise plan:**

NICE (2016, NG49) recommends the following in assessing patients with suspected NAFLD.

1   Identify risk factors and calculate fatty liver index (FLI)
- FLI comprises weight, height, waist circumference, serum GGT and triglyceride
- NICE advises against using just routine LFTs to rule out/diagnose NAFLD

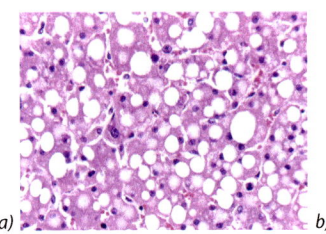 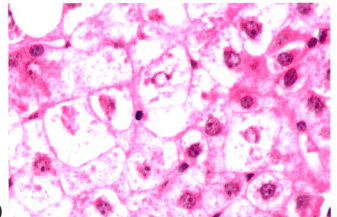 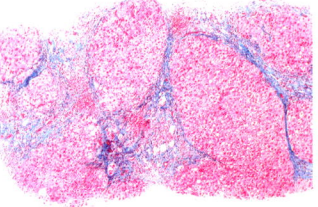

a)   b)   c)

Fig. 3.40 *(a) Steatosis indicated by numerous large-vacuoled cells (fatty deposition); (b) Progression to steatohepatitis is shown by leucocytic infiltration (purple nuclei) and presence of Mallory bodies (twisted rope shape); (c) Trichrome-stained specimen showing collagen deposition (blue streaks) and disorganisation of hepatic architecture.*

2 Diagnose NAFLD if FLI >60
- Liver ultrasound is often used to visualise fatty infiltration

3 Offer re-testing (FLI) every 5 years if FLI <60

4 Perform enhanced liver fibrosis (ELF) testing
- Allows quantification of fibrosis severity
- ELF involves analysis of serum immunoassays (e.g. hyaluronic acid, procollagen III amino terminal peptide) to generate an ELF score
- Advanced liver fibrosis is defined as an ELF >10.51

5 Arrange liver biopsy
- This is the gold standard investigation

Management
NAFLD treatment largely involves lifestyle modi-fication. However, pharmacological interventions may be beneficial in patients with advanced fibrosis.

> **Stepwise management of NAFLD (NICE 2016, NG49)**

1 Offer lifestyle advice
- Weight reduction and obesity advice as per NICE obesity guidelines
- Exercise has been shown to reduce fatty content in the liver
- Offer alcohol advice

2 Risk factor modification
- Good blood pressure and glycaemic control reduces oxidative liver injury, as well as decreasing cardiovascular risk

3 Offer pharmacological interventions
- Consider starting pioglitazone or vitamin E supplements in patients with advanced liver fibrosis, with or without diabetes mellitus
- Repeat ELF testing 2 years after treatment, to assess effectiveness of intervention

W ≫ Pioglitazone is a PPAR agonist (peroxisome proliferator activated receptor gamma) which functions to increase insulin sensitivity of the liver and ultimately reduce insulin resistance. However, it is contraindicated in patients with heart failure and pre-existing bladder cancer, as it is known to cause fluid retention and is associated with an increased risk of bladder cancer.

P ≫ Statins are not contraindicated in patients with NAFLD and should be continued, as they are effective in reducing cardiovascular risk. However, they should be stopped in the event of doubling of baseline LFTs over a period of 3 months.

3.6.4 Inherited liver disease
3.6.4.1 Hereditary haemochromatosis

Definition: an autosomal recessive genetic disorder characterised by excess iron deposition throughout the body.

Epidemiology:
- Most prevalent in people of northern European descent
- More common in men

Clinical features:
- Symptoms only present at the age of 40–60
- Early disease – non-specific symptoms of fatigue, abdominal pain, arthralgia and erectile dysfunction
- Advanced disease
  - Endocrine – diabetes mellitus, hypogonadism
  - Cardiac – arrhythmias, cardiomyopathy
  - Hepatic – hepatomegaly, cirrhosis
  - MSK – bronze complexion, arthralgia affecting second/third MCP joints
  - Neurological – mood disturbances, memory impairment
- Annual incidence of 1–2% per 100,000

E ≫ Patients with hereditary haemochromatosis (HHC) are often referred to as 'bronze diabetics'. Type 1 diabetes mellitus is highly associated with HHC, due to decreased insulin secretion as a result of iron deposition in pancreatic beta islet cells.

W ≫ Bronzing of the skin is an important and common dermatological manifestation of HHC. This occurs as a combined effect of excess haemosiderin deposition within the dermis as well as haemosiderin-induced melanocyte activation.

3

Pathophysiology:
- Mutation of the HFE gene (C282Y) on chromosome 6 results in a reduced production of an iron-modulating hormone known as hepcidin
- Hepcidin is responsible for regulating iron absorption in the gut
- It exerts its effects by inhibiting iron channels (ferroportin) of gut enterocytes
- Down-regulation of hepcidin increases gut absorption of iron, causing excess iron to accumulate in multiple organ systems

Investigations
Investigations should be undertaken in the following order.

Stepwise plan:

1 **Perform iron studies**
- Significantly elevated transferrin saturation (>45%) and ferritin are suggestive of HHC

P ≫ Ferritin is an acute phase protein and may be raised in chronic inflammatory conditions, excess alcohol, viral illness, liver disease as well as metabolic syndrome.

2 **Offer HFE genetic testing**
- To identify exact polymorphism and genotype (homozygous/heterozygous)
- Heterozygous forms of HCC rarely cause clinical symptoms

3 **Offer other tests**
- LFTs (may be deranged), random glucose may be elevated, ECG ± echocardiogram
- Liver MRI ± biopsy

Management
Patients who are asymptomatic without any evidence of excess iron may be treated with a 'watchful waiting' approach and appropriate advice.

Stepwise management of hereditary haemochromatosis

1 **Offer dietary advice**
- Low iron diet, avoid tea, vitamin C, alcohol

2 **Arrange regular venesection**
- Removal of blood will stimulate the bone marrow to produce new RBC, utilising iron stores

3 **Arrange chelation therapy**
- IV desferrioxamine may be considered in patients who are intolerant/contraindicated to venesection

4 **Offer genetic counselling**
- First-degree relatives should be screened

5 **Consider liver transplantation**
- In end-stage disease

3.6.4.2 Wilson disease

Definition: Wilson disease, sometimes referred to as hepatolenticular degeneration, is an autosomal recessive disorder characterised by an error in copper metabolism and accumulation.

Epidemiology:
- Global incidence of 30 per million
- Equal gender and ethnic preponderance

Clinical features:
- Symptom onset usually occurs around 20–30 years
- Children and young adults tend to present with liver symptoms whereas older adults are likely to have neuropsychiatric problems
- Annual incidence of 1–2% per 100,000

Table 3.21 *Systemic manifestations of Wilson disease*

System	Presentation
Liver	• Ranges from acute liver injury, cirrhosis and eventually fulminant liver failure
Ophthalmology	• Kayser–Fleischer rings (95% of patients; see *Fig. 3.41*) • May also have sunflower cataracts
Neuropsychiatric	• Movement disorders – tremors, dyskinesia, ataxia • Depression, psychosis (±hallucinations), dementia
Renal	• Associated with Fanconi syndrome (see *Chapter 7*)
Rheumatology	• Arthritis, chondrocalcinosis and osteopenia

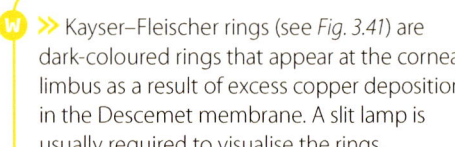

W ≫ Kayser–Fleischer rings (see *Fig. 3.41*) are dark-coloured rings that appear at the corneal limbus as a result of excess copper deposition in the Descemet membrane. A slit lamp is usually required to visualise the rings.

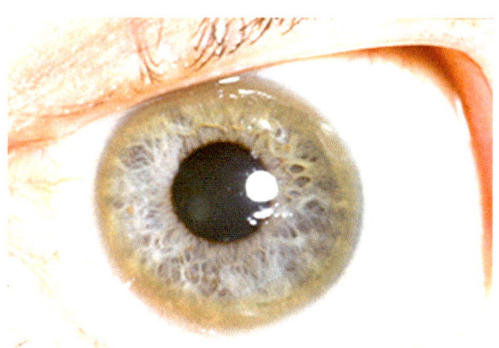

Fig. 3.41 *Kayser–Fleischer rings.*

Pathophysiology:
- Copper absorbed by the small intestine is transported to the liver to be stored and processed
- In normal circumstances, copper is then metabolised into caeruloplasmin and excreted in bile. However, in Wilson disease, mutations in the ATP7B (located on chromosome 13) result in a defective transporter protein, known as P-type adenosine triphosphatase (ATPase), usually responsible for intra-membrane passage of copper within hepatocytes
- This leads to abnormal excretion and accumulation of copper

Investigations
A diagnosis can be made with the presence of Kayser–Fleischer rings with a low caeruloplasmin or neurological symptoms.

Stepwise plan:

1 Check serum caeruloplasmin
- Reduced levels may be diagnostic
- It is important to note that, like ferritin, caeruloplasmin is an acute-phase protein and will be elevated during infections and inflammatory states

2 Check 24-hour urinary copper excretion
- Levels of >100mcg are suggestive

3 Arrange other blood tests
- LFTs are normally deranged with or without the presence of anaemia

4 Consider liver biopsy
- This is only performed if diagnosis is uncertain

Management
Wilson disease is a treatable condition and the principles of therapy involves patient education and removal of excess copper.

Stepwise management of Wilson disease

1 Offer dietary advice
- Avoidance of food with high copper content

2 Chelating agents
- Lifelong penicillamine ± zinc ± trientine

E » Side effects of penicillamine include nausea, rash, bone marrow suppression and lupus-mimicking symptoms.

3 Consider liver transplantation
- In severe liver disease

3.6.4.3 Alpha 1-antitrypsin deficiency

Definition: an autosomal co-dominant genetic disorder characterised by defective production of the enzyme alpha 1-antitrypsin (A1AT), a serine protease inhibitor (Pi) that is primarily synthesised by the liver.

Epidemiology:
- One of the most common inherited disorders in Caucasians
- Prevalence of 20–30 per 100,000

Clinical features:
- Respiratory symptoms (dyspnoea, wheeze) tend to present in the third and fourth decade of life
- Not all patients will develop liver disease; many adults present with deranged LFTs, with some eventually developing hepatitis and cirrhosis
- A1AT deficiency should be suspected in neonates with jaundice and in children/young adults with severe COPD
- Annual incidence of 1–2% per 100,000

Pathophysiology:
- A1AT deficiency is caused by mutations of the SERPINA 1 gene located on chromosome 14
- Defective forms of A1AT produced in the liver cannot be exported out of the liver and therefore accumulate
- A1AT is responsible for regulating the concentration of elastase in the lungs, and decreased serum A1AT results in uncontrolled elastin breakdown; this contributes to the development of emphysema
- Congestion of A1AT in hepatocytes eventually leads to cell apoptosis and precipitates liver failure

3

> **P** >> A1AT deficiency causes **panacinar** emphysema, a disease predominantly affecting the alveoli of the lower segments of the lungs. In contrast, smoking causes **centriacinar** emphysema – a bronchiolar disease mainly affecting the upper segments of the lungs.

Investigations

> **Stepwise plan:**

In a patient with suspected A1AT deficiency:

1 Measure serum A1AT levels
- Low levels (<10µmol/L)

2 Perform PFTs and CXR
- Spirometry will reveal an obstructive picture
- CXR may show evidence of emphysema

3 Obtain liver biopsy
- PAS positive globules may be visualised

4 Carry out genetic testing
- Genotyping/phenotyping

Management
Supportive care and prevention of complications are the main considerations in the management of patients with A1AT deficiency.

> **Stepwise management of A1AT deficiency**

1 Offer advice on lifestyle modification
- Smoking cessation and alcohol avoidance prevent disease progression and complications

2 Treat symptoms of respiratory disease
- Treat in accordance with COPD guidelines

3 Consider monitoring and management of liver disease
- HCC surveillance and liver transplantation in advanced disease

Augmentation therapy with IV recombinant A1AT was initially thought to have some benefits in patients with COPD but, due to the lack of substantial evidence and cost-effectiveness issues, NICE (2015) does not recommend its use at present.

3.6.5 Autoimmune liver disease

3.6.5.1 Autoimmune hepatitis

Definition: autoimmune hepatitis (AIH) is a chronic inflammatory liver disease of unknown aetiology, characterised by the presence of auto-antibodies.

Epidemiology:
- Has a strong female preponderance
- Bimodal age distribution, first peak in the 20s and the second during the peri-/postmenopausal period
- Annual incidence of 1 per 100,000 in the western population

Clinical features:
- Insidious onset of vague symptoms of fatigue, nausea, myalgia and occasionally upper abdominal discomfort
- Younger women may also present with amenorrhoea
- May also present as an acute hepatitis (up to 25% of cases) with persistently high liver enzymes; clinical jaundice and hepatomegaly are often present in these patients

> **E** >> Autoimmune hepatitis is associated with the following conditions:
> - Hashimoto thyroiditis
> - Rheumatoid arthritis
> - Graves thyrotoxicosis
> - Inflammatory bowel disease
> - Pleurisy
> - Urticaria
> - Proliferative glomerulonephritis
> - Autoimmune haemolytic anaemia

Pathophysiology:
- As with many other autoimmune conditions, the exact aetiology and pathogenesis is unclear
- The central dogma of these diseases is that an environment trigger (e.g. viral illness) often sets off an inflammatory cascade towards oneself in immunogenetically susceptible patients
- Many subtypes of the HLA, in particular HLA-DR3 and DR4, have been associated with AIH

> **P** >> The traditional classification of AIH, based on the auto-antibodies present, has now fallen out of fashion.

Investigations

AIH is a diagnosis of exclusion and requires a combination of the presence of auto-antibodies and histopathological evidence, as well as exclusion of other causes of hepatitis.

Stepwise plan:

1 Autoimmune profile
- Anti-nuclear antibody (**ANA**) and anti-smooth muscle antibody (**SMA**) are usually present

2 Protein electrophoresis
- High titres of IgG are suggestive of AIH, but they can be normal in some patients

3 Arrange other blood tests
- FBC may reveal anaemia
- LFTs will be deranged (hepatitis picture with elevated aminotransferases)

4 Consider liver biopsy
- Diagnostic showing interface hepatitis and plasma cell infiltration with or without cirrhosis

Management

The main modality of AIH treatment involves immunosuppression.

Stepwise management of autoimmune hepatitis

1 Observation
- 'Watchful waiting' approach may be used in asymptomatic, pre-cirrhotic patients

2 Immunosuppression
- High-dose oral prednisolone (40mg) is the first-line agent of choice in acute episodes
- This is normally tapered down over weeks, and azathioprine may be added if long-term therapy is required
- Remission is monitored by measuring ALT/AST and IgG levels post-therapy

3 Liver transplantation is indicated in very advanced disease

3.6.5.2 Primary biliary cirrhosis (PBC)

Definition: a chronic autoimmune disease characterised by progressive destruction of **small intrahepatic** bile ducts, resulting in cirrhosis.

Epidemiology:
- Female preponderance (9:1)
- Annual incidence in the UK is around 13 per 100,000
- Patients tend to present in their fourth and fifth decade
- More common amongst smokers

Clinical features:
- Fatigue and pruritus are the earliest symptoms
- Jaundice tends to present late
- Hepatosplenomegaly, facial hyperpigmentation and xanthelasmas may be present
- 25% of patients are asymptomatic and are diagnosed based on biochemical and immunological evidence

> **W** » Dietary cholesterol is metabolised in the liver and excreted in the bile as bile salts. In PBC, fibrosis of the biliary tracts results in cholestasis. As a result, cholesterol accumulates and commonly becomes deposited around the eyes and tendons as xanthelasmas (see *Fig. 3.42*) and xanthomas (see *Fig. 3.43*).

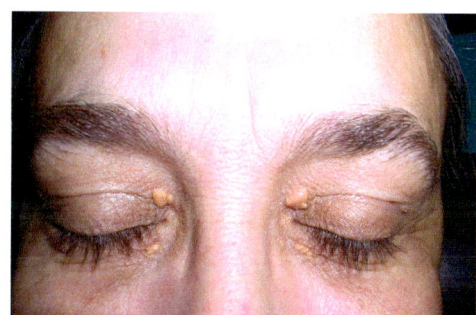

Fig. 3.42 *Xanthelasma.*

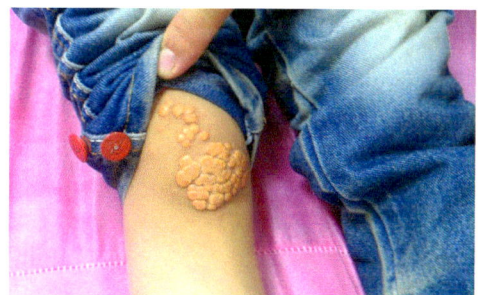

Fig. 3.43 *Xanthoma.*

Pathophysiology:

- The presence of AMA (anti-mitochondrial antibodies) in the majority of patients is highly suggestive of an underlying autoimmune process
- Chronic inflammation of the intra-hepatic bile ducts results in progressive ductal damage, leading to cholestasis and eventually liver failure

> **E** »» PBC is strongly associated with other autoimmune conditions such as thyroid disease, systemic sclerosis and coeliac disease.

Investigations

Investigations should be undertaken in the following order.

Stepwise plan:

1 Arrange liver function tests
- Predominantly a cholestatic picture (high ALP and GGT) but ALT/AST may be raised in late stages

2 Obtain autoimmune profile and immunoglobulin electrophoresis
- AMA (present in 95% of patients)
- High levels of IgM are indicative

3 Arrange imaging
- Extrahepatic biliary obstruction (i.e. gallstone) should be excluded by either USS or MRCP

4 Consider liver biopsy
- Only indicated if diagnosis is unclear
- May show lymphocytic infiltration with granulomatous changes

Stepwise management of primary biliary cirrhosis

1 Prescribe ursodeoxycholic acid (UDCA)
- Regarded as the best first-line therapy as it improves LFTs and may slow disease progression

> **W** »» UDCA has a membrane-stabilising effect on the biliary epithelium, protecting it from recurrent injury. It also increases biliary clearance preventing toxic bile acid in the liver.

2 Offer symptomatic treatment
- Pruritus – cholestyramine may be beneficial
- Rifampicin and naloxone are used as second-line agents

- Malabsorption – fat-soluble vitamin replacements, calcium supplements and bisphosphates should be offered

3 Consider liver transplantation
- Effective treatment for advanced disease but disease may recur in 30% of patients after 10 years

3.6.5.3 Primary sclerosing cholangitis (PSC)

Definition: a chronic inflammatory condition characterised by progressive sclerosis and fibrosis of the **extrahepatic** and/or **intrahepatic** bile ducts, resulting in multifocal biliary stricture formation.

Epidemiology:

- Male preponderance (2:1)
- Prevalence in the UK is 0.2 per 100,000
- Commonly presents in the third decade

Clinical features:

- Most patients tend to be asymptomatic and often the earliest presentation is deranged LFTs
- Intermittent jaundice and pruritus are common symptoms
- Other signs and symptoms include right upper quadrant pain, fatigue and hepatomegaly

Pathophysiology:

- The aetiology of PSC is unclear but overexpression of specific haplotypes suggests that it is an immunologically mediated disease
- The condition is also very closely linked with inflammatory bowel disease, especially **ulcerative colitis**
- Chronic inflammatory changes of the bile ducts result in biliary fibrosis and stricture formation
- Altered biliary flow leads to cholestasis and predisposes to episodes of bacterial cholangitis
- Ongoing injury will eventually result in cirrhosis

> **P** »» 80% of patients with PSC have co-existing ulcerative colitis and about 5–10% of ulcerative colitis patients have concurrent PSC. The presence of ANCA in both these conditions suggests an immune-mediated component.

Investigations

Stepwise plan:

The approach to investigating a patient with suspected PSC is similar to that of PBC:

1   Obtain liver function tests
- These will reveal a cholestatic picture with a high ALP and bilirubin
- Note that these values may fluctuate during the course of the disease progression

2   Arrange autoimmune profiling
- In contrast to PBC, AMA is absent in patients with PSC
- pANCA may be present in 60% of patients

3   Obtain imaging
- Magnetic resonance cholangio-pancreatography (MRCP) is the modality of choice to visualise the intra- and extrahepatic ducts
- Multifocal stricturing is commonly seen (see *Fig. 3.44*)
- ERCP is the second-line option, as it is more invasive

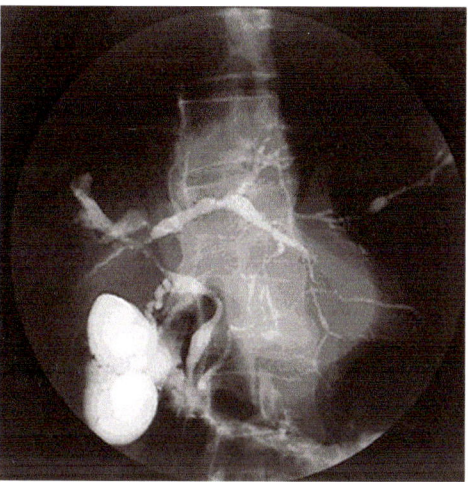

Fig. 3.44 *MRCP showing multifocal intra- and extrahepatic stricturing.*

4   Consider liver biopsy
- Rarely used but, if performed, the characteristic periductal 'onion skin' fibrosis may be present

Management
The principles of PSC treatment involve management of symptoms, cholestasis and its complications.

> **Stepwise management of primary sclerosing cholangitis**

1   Provide symptomatic relief
- Cholestyramine, a bile acid sequestrant, is considered to be the best first-line agent

2   Consider prescribing ursodeoxycholic acid (UDCA)
- This is widely used as it improves liver biochemistry, though there is still inconclusive evidence for its clinical benefits

3   Offer prophylactic antibiotics
- A cyclical regime (most commonly comprising three antibiotics alternating every few weeks) may be used to prevent episodes of acute bacterial cholangitis

4   Consider surgery
- ERCP with balloon dilatation and stenting are effective in specific patients
- Liver transplantation is indicated in patients with end-stage liver disease

3.6.6 Vascular liver disease
3.6.6.1 Portal venous thrombosis

Portal venous thrombosis (PVT) refers to the obstruction of blood flow in the portal venous circulation as a result of a blood clot. It rarely occurs as a primary event; however, it can occur in any pro-thrombotic condition.

> **E** ≫ As discussed previously, PVT is an important cause of **pre-hepatic** portal hypertension.

Recognised causes of PVT include pancreatitis, pancreatic malignancy, post-splenectomy and cirrhosis. As such, PVT can present either acutely or sub-acutely. Acute PVT typically presents with abdominal pain and diarrhoea, whereas patients with sub-acute PVT are asymptomatic and may eventually develop portal hypertension and its sequelae.

> **P** ≫ A PVT may also occur as a secondary event in patients with established cirrhotic liver disease. As such, PVT can precipitate decompensation.

PVT is best investigated with Doppler ultrasound studies. Treatment involves anticoagulation and patients are normally put on long-term maintenance therapy. However, the risks and benefits should first be considered, especially in cirrhotic patients who have higher bleeding risks.

3.6.6.2 Budd-Chiari syndrome

This is a rare hepatic outflow tract obstructive condition, occurring anywhere from the small hepatic veins to the inferior vena cava.

The aetiology for Budd–Chiari syndrome (BCS) is unknown in up to one-third of patients; however, BCS is associated with hypercoagulability conditions as a predisposing factor. Associations include those listed in *Table 3.22*.

Table 3.22 *Associations of Budd–Chiari syndrome*

Hereditary	Acquired
• Myelodysplasia • Polycythaemia rubra vera • Thrombophilia – factor V Leiden, protein C/S deficiency • Antiphospholipid syndrome	• COCP and HRT use • Pregnancy • Acquired polycythaemia • Surgery • Chronic infections

Clinical features:
- Presentation may be acute, with symptoms of upper abdominal pain, ascites, jaundice, tender hepatomegaly and acute liver injury
- Presentation may also be insidious, with progressively worsening ascites

Investigations

Stepwise plan:

1 Arrange blood tests
- May show normal/mildly deranged LFTs
- Also note that the prothrombin time may be elevated, reflecting the underlying liver disease as oppose to the hypercoagulable state

2 Arrange thrombophilia and haematological screening

3 Obtain ascitic fluid analysis
- Usually contains high protein

4 Obtain imaging
- USS ± Doppler, CT or MRI may be useful

P ≫ The caudate lobe of the liver is spared in BCS as it has a separate blood supply and venous drainage system.

Management
The predisposing condition should be treated in the first instance.

Stepwise management of Budd–Chiari syndrome

1 Arrange thrombolysis
- Alteplase may be utilised in acute situations, where a thrombus is visualised on imaging

2 Provide lifelong anticoagulation
- Recommended to prevent further episodes

3 Provide ascites management
- Medical therapy with a trial of diuretics and salt restriction
- Paracentesis may be used in resistant cases

4 Consider TIPSS and liver transplantation

3.6.7 Liver tumours

3.6.7.1 Benign tumours

These include hepatic adenomas, cystic liver disease (often associated with polycystic kidney disease) and haemangiomas, which are – by and large – the most common benign tumour. These lesions are often incidentally picked up on imaging.

3.6.7.2 Hepatocellular carcinoma (HCC)

Definition: the most common primary cancer arising from liver hepatocytes.

Epidemiology:
- Male preponderance (4:1)
- Fifth most common cancer worldwide
- Mean age of diagnosis is 60 years

Aetiology:
- Chronic HBV (most common worldwide) and HCV (most common in the UK)
- Cirrhosis – ALD, HHC, PBC
- Fungal infection – alfatoxin from *Aspergillus flavus, A. parasiticus*
- Also associated with PSC, androgenic steroids and COCP use

Clinical features:
- Patients usually have underlying cirrhosis and present with decompensated symptoms and worsening LFTs
- Weight loss, RUQ pain and hepatomegaly may also be present

Investigations
The diagnosis of HCC requires a combination of biochemical, radiological and histopathological evidence.

Stepwise plan:

1 Obtain imaging
- A liver ultrasound is often the first-line modality in HCC screening. However, it is only sensitive in detecting tumours up to 2cm in size

- CT chest/abdomen/pelvis is often performed to assess for distant metastases
- A liver MRI offers better-quality images and may be used if there is diagnostic uncertainty

2   Consider a liver biopsy
- Consider the balance between risk and benefit before performing this

P   » As there is a risk of tumour seeding along the needle tract, biopsies should be avoided in patients where resection or transplantation is being considered. This will minimise the risk of recurrence post-procedure.

3   Tumour marker
- Alpha-fetaprotein (AFP), used in combination with AUSS, provides a good screening tool for patients with cirrhosis
- Regular 6-monthly follow-up is recommended

Management
The treatment of HCC depends on the stage of the disease, the Child–Pugh score and the patient's performance status. The following are some of the treatment modalities.

Stepwise management of hepatocellular carcinoma

1   Perform hepatic resection
- First-line treatment for non-cirrhotic patients

2   Consider liver transplantation
- Single nodule <5cm or <3 nodules <3cm without underlying disease or cirrhosis

3   Consider radio-frequency ablation

4   Consider trans-arterial chemo-embolisation
- May be used in multinodular, intermediate disease

5   Consider chemotherapy
- Sorafenib is a multikinase inhibitor that targets VEGF and PDGF signalling
- Can be considered in advanced disease

6   Provide palliative care in end-stage disease

3.7 Diseases of the biliary tract

3.7.1 Gallstone disease

Definition: gallstones, also known as **cholelithiasis**, refer to solid, calculi formations that are formed from bile products within the gall bladder. When stones migrate out of the gall bladder and become lodged in the common bile duct (CBD), the condition is known as **choledocho-lithiasis**.

Epidemiology:
- Prevalence of 10% in the western population
- Female preponderance of 3:1
- Usually occurs in the fourth decade of life

E   » The adage of 'fat, forty, female, fair and fertile' is commonly used as an aide-memoire for the risk factors of gallstone disease.

Clinical features:
Around 70% of patients with gallstones are asymptomatic. Symptomatic stones present in one of a few ways:
- Biliary colic
- Acute cholecystitis (see *Section 3.7.2*)
- Pancreatitis (see *Section 3.8.1*)
- Obstructive jaundice (caused by a CBD stone)

Biliary colic occurs when the gallstone becomes impacted in the cystic duct. Patients usually present:
- Initially, with upper abdominal pain which later becomes localised to right upper quadrant (RUQ) pain. This can also radiate round the back and sometimes into the inter-scapular area
- Post-prandial association and occasionally nausea and vomiting

E   » Biliary colic is a misnomer, as (contrary to its name) it causes a constant sharp pain that usually lasts for between 15 minutes and 24 hours.

W   » Inter-scapular pain in patients with biliary colic is caused by diaphragmatic irritation. The phrenic nerve (C3–5) is responsible for the innervation of the diaphragm. As a result, pain stimuli are often referred to other somatic regions – in this case, the scapular tip.

3

Pathophysiology

- Gallstones can be classified according to their composition. Most gallstones are made up of cholesterol (~80%) and the rest are pigment stones, composed of calcium salts (black) or occurring as the result of an infection (brown, <5%)
- In clinical practice, gallstones tend to have a mixed composition
- The formation of cholesterol gallstones is dependent on an important triad of factors (see *Table 3.23*)

Table 3.23 *Factors predisposing to gallstone formation*

Factors	Mechanism
Cholesterol synthesis	Increased HMG Co-A reductase activity in the liver leads to increased cholesterol synthesis. Supersaturation of cholesterol relative to other bile content (bile salts, phospholipids, etc.), predisposes to crystallisation.
Composition of bile salt pool	Nucleating agents (e.g. mucin and fatty acids) are responsible for the crystallisation of cholesterol. The balance between cholesterol saturation and these factors determines whether or not crystals are formed.
Gall bladder motility	Stasis of bile facilitates microcrystals to aggregate and form cross-links with mucin, resulting in gallstone formation.

P ⟫ Cholesterol stones are often large and radio-opaque. In contrast, black pigment stones are smaller, more fragile and radio-opaque. However, brown pigment stones are radiolucent.

Investigations

NICE (2014, CG188) recommends the following approach in investigating patients with suspected gallstone disease.

Stepwise plan:

1 **Perform liver function tests**
- Bilirubin, ALP and GGT may be elevated in patients with CBD stones

2 **Offer abdominal ultrasound imaging**
- This is the best technique to detect stones (90% sensitive)

3 **Consider a magnetic resonance cholangio-pancreatogram (MRCP; see *Fig. 3.45*)**
- This will allow better visualisation of the CBD if US shows dilated bile ducts and abnormal LFTs

4 **Consider endoscopic ultrasound (EUS)**
- If the diagnosis is inconclusive on MRCP

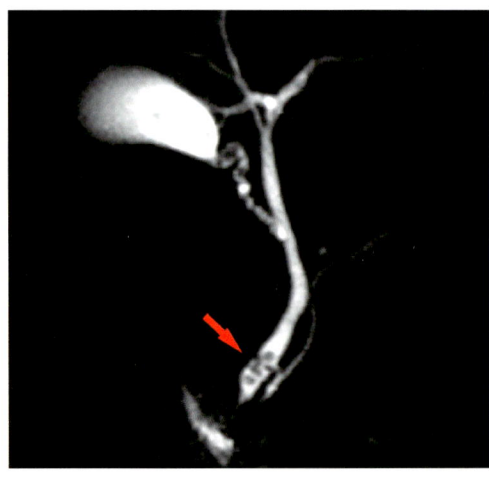

Fig. 3.45 *MRCP showing a large CBD stone.*

P ⟫ MRCP is a non-invasive imaging technique that heavily utilises T2-weighted magnetic resonance sequences. Interestingly, no contrast material is used and the technique exploits existing fluid (bile) in the biliary system to acquire the images. This allows MRCP to be used safely, even in patients with renal impairment.

Stepwise management of gallstone disease

The treatment of gallstone disease depends on whether the patient is symptomatic and the site of the stone. NICE (2014, CG188) recommends:

1 **Offer dietary advice**
- Avoid food and drinks (especially those with high fat content) that may trigger symptoms

Gall bladder stones

1 **Offer reassurance**
- If patients are asymptomatic

2 Offer symptomatic patients laparoscopic cholecystectomy
- This can be usually performed as an elective (day-case) procedure if patients are well, removing the need for an inpatient stay

Common bile duct stones

1 Perform an endoscopic retrograde cholangiopancreatogram (ERCP) for biliary clearance
- This should be done urgently (within 72 hours) if the patient is jaundiced (see *Fig. 3.46*)

2 Consider temporary biliary stenting
- If biliary clearance is not achievable with ERCP

3 Laparoscopic cholecystectomy is the definitive treatment

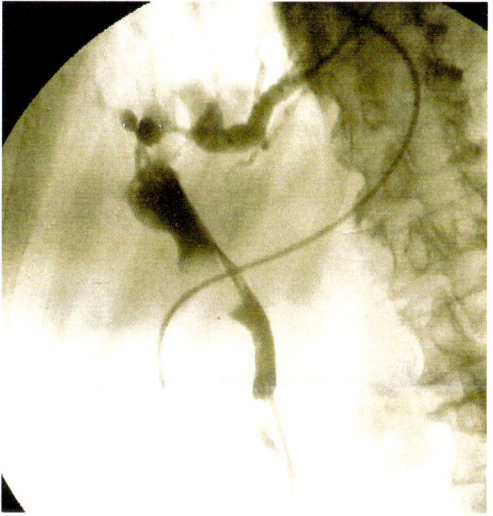

Fig. 3.46 *Basket retrieval of distal CBD stone with ERCP.*

> **P** ≫ Compared to MRCP, ERCP is a more invasive procedure but it has both diagnostic and therapeutic value. The procedure involves two stages – **endoscopy** and **fluoroscopy**. Firstly, an upper GI endoscope is passed to the level of the descending segment of the duodenum. At this stage, the ampulla of Vater is cannulated and contrast material is injected into the biliary tract. The outline of the system can then be visualised via fluoroscopy.

> **E** ≫ Occasionally, contrast material injected into the pancreatic duct may induce pancreatitis. The rates of post-ERCP pancreatitis are around 5%.

3.7.2 Cholecystitis

Definition: acute cholecystitis refers to acute inflammation of the gall bladder and represents a common complication of gallstone disease. Repeated episodes of cholecystitis over a prolonged period result in chronic cholecystitis.

Epidemiology:
- Female preponderance of 3:1 up to the age of 50
- Complicates up to 10% of symptomatic patients with gallstones

Clinical features:
- The initial stage of cholecystitis is similar to that of biliary colic, with epigastric pain later localising to the RUQ
- The key difference is the inflammatory component, with evidence of localised peritonitis, more severe and prolonged pain and the presence of a fever and leucocytosis
- Patients are commonly Murphy sign positive

> **W** ≫ The Murphy sign can be elicited by palpating the RUQ and instructing the patient to take a deep breath. During inspiration, the diaphragm is flattened and the tender gall bladder (which is pushed downwards) catches against the fingers. The test is positive if the inspiration is abruptly terminated and the same response is not elicited on the left side.

Pathophysiology:
- Gallstone obstruction at the neck of the gall bladder or cystic duct causes bile retention in the gall bladder, leading to progressive distension and initiation of an inflammatory response
- Acalculous cholecystitis may occur in 5–10% of cases, resulting from biliary stasis (due to sepsis, trauma or extrinsic compression) or biliary sludge

> **E** ≫ Mirizzi syndrome is a rare complication of gallstone disease, whereby multiple small gallstones or one large gallstone become impacted in the Hartmann pouch of the gall bladder and extrinsically compress the common bile duct, leading to obstructive jaundice. A fistula between the gall bladder and the CBD may occasionally occur.

3

Investigations

Stepwise plan:

1 Arrange blood tests
- Elevated WCC and CRP are usually present
- LFTs may be mildly deranged
- Amylase should be performed to rule out concurrent/underlying pancreatitis

2 Obtain abdominal USS
- This is the imaging modality of choice, with a high positive predictive value
- It may show a thickened, distended gall bladder, with pericholecystic fluid diagnostic of cholecystitis

3 Obtain CT abdomen
- This may sometimes be considered if an empyema or perforation is suspected

Management

The treatment of acute cholecystitis can be divided into initial medical therapy followed by further surgical intervention.

Stepwise management of cholecystitis

1 Provide medical therapy
- Offer opioid analgesia and anti-emetic therapy
- IV fluid resuscitation
- IV antibiotics (as per local hospital policy)

2 Consider surgical intervention (NICE 2014, CG188)
- Laparoscopic cholecystectomy (lap chole) may be performed within 1 week, or delayed until 6–12 weeks later
- Most episodes of cholecystitis settle enough, with antibiotic therapy, for lap choles to be performed 6–12 weeks later
- In cases where the condition is refractory to medical therapy, surgery should be performed immediately

3.7.3 Cholangitis

This condition is historically known as acute ascending cholangitis, as it primarily refers to bacterial seeding in the biliary tree, with the infection ascending into the gall bladder. The common organisms responsible in the UK are *Klebsiella* spp., *E. coli*, enterococci and streptococci.

It is most commonly caused by bile stasis as a result of an obstructing CBD stone. Other aetiologies include post-ERCP, biliary stricturing (e.g. PSC) or cancer.

E ≫ Patients are usually unwell and typically present with:

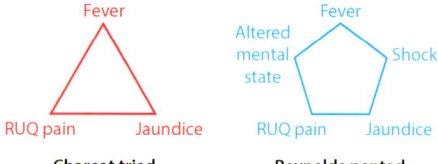

Fig. 3.47 *Charcot triad and Reynolds pentad.*

Patients with suspected cholangitis should be treated promptly, as progression to systemic sepsis (i.e. septicaemia) occurs rapidly. As a result, the condition is associated with high mortality and morbidity.

Stepwise management of acute cholangitis

1 Carry out initial resuscitation
- Septic shock should be treated appropriately with oxygenation and IV fluid resuscitation

2 Intravenous antibiotics (usually broad spectrum, based on local hospital policy) should be commenced
- Blood cultures should be taken to guide anti-microbial therapy

3 Biliary drainage
- ERCP with stone retrieval ± sphincterotomy ± stenting is recommended
- Percutaneous transhepatic biliary drainage is an alternative to ERCP in difficult cases

3.7.4 Cholangiocarcinoma

Definition: cholangiocarcinomas are rare cancers arising from the epithelial cells of anywhere in the biliary system. These account for around 1% of all cancers.

P ≫ They occur most often (approximately 60%) peri-hilarly at the bifurcation of the right and left hepatic ducts. These are classically known as Klatskin tumours.

Aetiology:

The cause of these cancers is unknown. However, a number of associations have been identified:
- **Inflammatory conditions of the biliary system,** such as PSC, are associated with a high

risk of developing cholangiocarcinomas, with a prevalence of up to 20% in PSC patients
- **Infections** with the liver flukes *Clonorchis sinensis* or *Opisthorchis viverrini* have been implicated. This explains the higher disease incidence in the Far East (particularly Thailand)
- **Gallstone disease**
- **Caroli disease** – a rare inherited condition characterised by intrahepatic duct dilatation associated with autosomal recessive polycystic kidney disease

Clinical features:
- The initial presenting complaint is typically jaundice
- Occasionally there is abdominal pain, with some evidence of weight loss

Investigations:
- Diagnosis is made on imaging – CT or MRCP
- The serum cancer marker CA 19–9 may be elevated
- Histological sampling via EUS with fine needle aspiration (FNA) may be utilised in the case of biliary obstruction

Management:
- Surgery is the mainstay treatment modality
- Radical surgical excision, with or without partial hepatic resection, may be considered in 20% of patients with early localised disease
- A palliative biliary stent may be inserted in malignant disease
- More recently, chemotherapy in association with endoscopic phototherapy has shown some benefit

3.8 Diseases of the pancreas

3.8.1 Acute pancreatitis

Definition: a medical and surgical condition characterised by acute inflammation of the exocrine pancreas as a result of an acute insult. Pancreatitis varies widely in its severity, from mild oedema to extensive necrosis. It is a potentially life-threatening condition which carries a mortality of 10%.

Epidemiology:
- Accounts for 1% of all surgical admissions and up to 3% of the causes of abdominal pain cases
- Annual incidence of 15–40 per 100,000 and is steadily rising
- Mean age of onset in the sixth decade

Aetiology:
- There are various causes of acute pancreatitis, but gallstone disease and alcohol account for the majority of cases (80–90%)

> **E** >> The mnemonic '**GET SMASHED**' is frequently used as an aide-memoire.
>
> | | |
> |---|---|
> | **G**allstones | **S**teroids |
> | **E**thanol | **M**umps and infections (e.g. Coxsackie B) |
> | **T**rauma | **A**utoimmune |
> | | **S**corpion venom |
> | | **H**yperlipidaemia, hypercalcaemia |
> | | **E**RCP-induced |
> | | **D**rugs – azathioprine, diuretics, valproate |

Pathophysiology:
- Premature intra-pancreatic activation of digestive enzymes (trypsinogen in particular) remains the central mechanism of pathogenesis
- This ultimately leads to autodigestion of the pancreas itself

Clinical features:
- Severe epigastric pain is the most common initial symptom
- Patients often describe pain radiating/penetrating through the back and occasionally as a tight band-like pain encircling the upper abdomen
- Nausea and vomiting are commonly associated symptoms
- Patients are often unwell, presenting with tachycardia, pyrexia and hypoxia

> **W** >> The Cullen sign (peri-umbilical discoloration; see *Fig. 3.48*) and the Grey Turner sign (flank discoloration; see *Fig. 3.49*) may be present in severe cases. This is indicative of pancreatic necrosis. The discoloration is a result of digestion of the subcutaneous blood vessels, forming methaemalbumin, which is responsible for its brownish appearance.

Investigations
The diagnosis of pancreatitis is based on clinical, biochemical and radiological evidence. In patients with suspected pancreatitis, investigation should be carried out as follows.

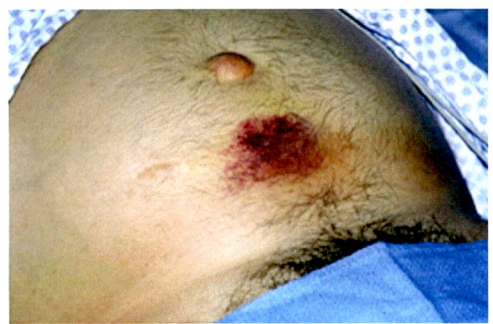

Fig. 3.48 *Cullen sign.*

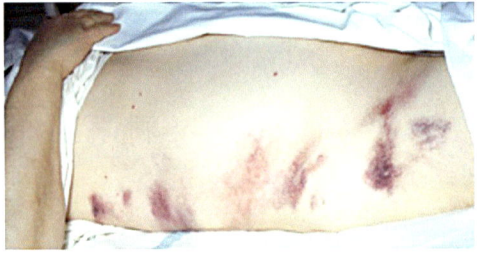

Fig. 3.49 *Grey Turner sign.*

Stepwise plan:

1   **Arrange blood tests including amylase/ lipase**
- Elevated amylase or lipase (usually 3x the upper limit)
- FBC (elevated WCC), CRP (daily to monitor progress)
- U&Es including glucose, calcium and albumin
- LFTs (cholestatic picture secondary to gallstones)
- ABG (may show hypoxia secondary to ARDS/ effusions)

W ≫ Serum amylase is an extremely sensitive test if measured within the first 24–48 hours of symptom onset, as it is readily excreted by the kidneys. Amylase is normally produced in the pancreas. During acute pancreatitis, these enzymes are released into the blood.

P ≫ However, it is important to note that an elevated serum amylase is also associated with a number of other abdominal conditions and this may occasionally confuse the diagnosis. The level of amylase does not correlate with the severity of pancreatitis.

2   **Obtain radiological imaging**
- Erect abdominal film to rule out any evidence of perforation in the first instance. May reveal pancreatic calcification
- Abdo USS – may be diagnostic in early disease and useful to screen for gallstones as a possible cause. In later stages, it may be more difficult to visualise the pancreas due to swelling
- CT abdomen with contrast (see *Fig. 3.50*) – usually performed at least 72 hours after admission to assess the extent of necrosis. Serial CTs may be necessary to look for later complications

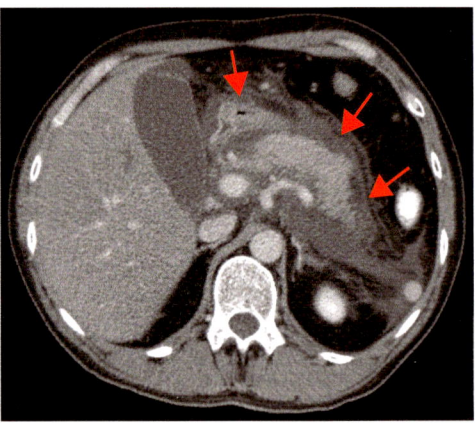

Fig. 3.50 *Axial view on a contrast-enhanced CT showing extensive fat stranding surrounding the pancreas and exudative fluid streaks indicative of acute pancreatitis.*

Glasgow prognostic score

The severity and prognosis of acute pancreatitis can be assessed using the Glasgow score. A serum CRP of >150 after 48 hours of symptom onset is in keeping with severe pancreatitis.

E ≫ The components of the score can be recalled using the mnemonic '**PANCREAS**'. A score of ≥3 indicates a severe event.

PaO$_2$ <8.0kPa	**R**enal function – urea >16mmol/L
Age >55 years	**E**nzymes – AST >200 or LDH >600
Neutrophils >15x10^9/L	**A**lbumin <32g/L
Calcium <2.0mmol/L	**S**ugar – glucose >10mmol/L

Management

The aims of pancreatitis management are: initial resuscitation, treatment of the underlying cause and monitoring for complications.

3

Stepwise management of acute pancreatitis

Initial resuscitation

1 Adequate oxygenation should be given
- To prevent hypoxia

2 All patients should be kept nil by mouth (NBM) initially while a decision is made on feeding strategy (preferably an early feeding strategy should be instituted)
- If an ileus is present, a nasogastric (NG) tube should be inserted, to help offload and rest the pancreas

3 Appropriate analgesia and anti-emetics should be given

4 Aggressive IV fluid replacement is the single most important medical therapy
- Isotonic crystalloid fluids are favoured

> **W** ≫ Activation of pro-inflammatory mediators leads to systemic vasoconstriction and increased cell permeability. This results in loss of fluid into the third space and, ultimately, shock may ensue.

5 Strict fluid balance with hourly volumes should be measured
- Unwell patients should be catheterised

6 VTE prophylaxis should be considered
- As patients with pancreatitis are pro-coagulopathic

7 Blood capillary glucose should be monitored
- And hyperglycaemia should be corrected with insulin

8 Enteral feeding should be considered
- In the event of prolonged fasting

9 Escalate care to ITU/HDU
- **If patient is not responding to initial treatment or if there is evidence of multi-organ failure**

> **P** ≫ The use of antibiotics is contentious, as prophylactic use has not been shown to improve mortality or disease progression. However, the use of meropenem or imipenem in cases of severe infected necrotising pancreatitis has been shown to be beneficial.

Interventional management of gallstone pancreatitis

1 Emergency ERCP with stone extraction and sphincterotomy
- Should be performed within 24 hours (NICE 2014, CG188) in patients with severe disease

2 Routine MRCP or EUS in the first instance
- To look for residual stones in less severe cases
- Followed by an ERCP

3 Urgent laparoscopic cholecystectomy with intra-operative cholangiogram
- Should be performed within 2 weeks of the acute event (preferably during the same hospitalisation) to prevent further episodes
- If left untreated, recurrence rates are up to 80%

Complications

The systemic inflammatory response that occurs as a result of pancreatitis is responsible for most of the early complications of the condition. These usually occur within the first 7 days and include:
- Respiratory – ARDS, pleural effusions
- Cardiovascular – hypovolaemic shock
- Disseminated intravascular coagulopathy
- Renal failure

Late complications (>1 week) tend to reflect local effects of pancreatic necrosis (see *Table 3.24*).

3.8.2 Chronic pancreatitis

Definition: chronic inflammation of the pancreas characterised by recurrent abdominal pain and progressive destruction of the exocrine pancreas. In contrast to acute pancreatitis, which is often self-limiting, chronic pancreatitis results in irreversible injury.

Epidemiology:
- UK prevalence of 3 in 100,000 and rising due to alcohol-related pancreatic damage
- Underdiagnosed condition due to its vague presentation

Aetiology:
The majority of cases are related to **alcohol** abuse (around 80%). The rest of the cases may be:
- Idiopathic
- Genetic – hereditary pancreatitis, cystic fibrosis
- Autoimmune
- Associated with malnutrition, dietary toxins

3

Table 3.24 *Late complications of pancreatitis*

Complications	Description
Pancreatic necrosis	• Extensive inflammation eventually progresses to necrosis • Superimposing infections are common • Urgent surgical necrosectomy is required • This is associated with high mortality
Pancreatic abscess	• A collection of pus adjacent to the pancreas • Tends to develop months after the acute event • Open or percutaneous drainage may be indicated
Fluid collection	• Rupture of the pancreatic duct and accumulation of fluid may develop in the adjacent lesser sac
Pancreatic pseudocyst	• Fluid collection in the lesser sac encapsulated by granulation/fibrotic tissue • Tends to develop 4–6 weeks post-attack • Smaller pseudocysts (<6cm) are typically asymptomatic and self-resolving • Larger pseudocysts (>6cm) may become infected or compress surrounding structures (e.g. duodenum, CBD). These require drainage, either percutaneously or endoscopically, at an interval of 6 weeks to allow maturation of the endocapsule

Clinical features:
- Intermittent upper abdominal pain radiating to the back
- Associated nausea and vomiting
- Malabsorption symptoms due to **exocrine pancreatic insufficiency**
  - Steatorrhoea or diarrhoea
  - Decreased appetite
  - Weight loss
- Glycaemic dysfunction secondary to **endocrine pancreatic insufficiency**

Investigations
The diagnosis of chronic pancreatitis is made primarily by imaging. Additional tests are performed to assess pancreatic function.

Stepwise plan:

1 **Obtain radiological imaging of the pancreas**
- CT pancreas with contrast is the best first-line modality; it usually reveals pancreatic calcification (see *Fig. 3.51*) or atrophy, and may also detect potential complications such as a pseudocyst (see *Fig. 3.52*)
- MRCP or EUS may be used if CT is contraindicated

2 **Assess pancreatic function**
- Serum glucose – may be elevated due to endocrine pancreatic insufficiency
- Faecal elastase – will be reduced in most cases

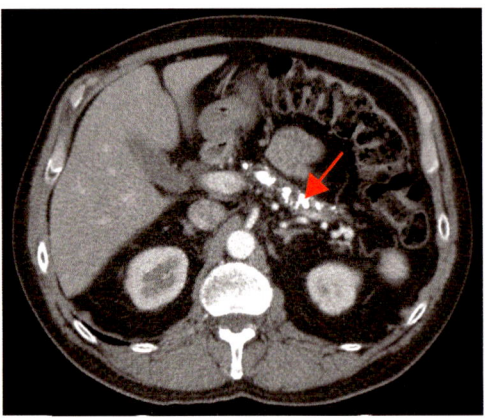

Fig. 3.51 *CT scan showing extensive pancreatic calcification (high attenuations).*

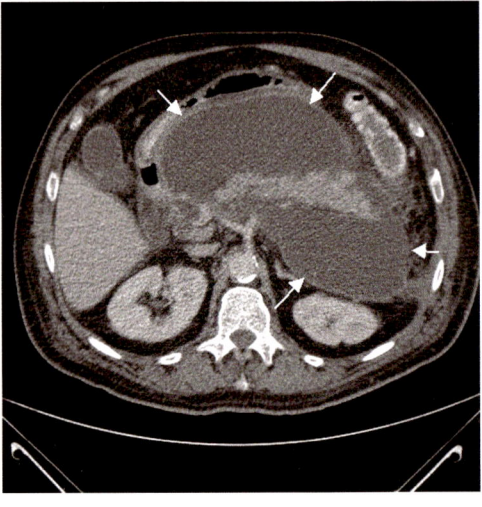

Fig. 3.52 *CT scan showing a large pseudocyst.*

Management

The treatment of chronic pancreatitis is mainly symptomatic.

Stepwise management of chronic pancreatitis

1 Offer dietary advice
- Alcohol cessation and low-fat diet

2 Provide analgesia
- NSAIDs are a good first-line option, but patients often require opiates in the later stages

3 Offer enzyme and vitamin supplements
- Creon and vitamin A, D, E and K should be replaced appropriately to reduce malabsorption

4 Consider PPI therapy
- To reduce malabsorption

5 Glycaemic control
- See management of diabetes mellitus (*Chapter 4, Section 4.4*)

3.8.3 Pancreatic cancer

Definition: pancreatic cancer primarily refers to a ductal adenocarcinoma affecting the exocrine gland of the pancreas. This represents 90% of all pancreatic tumours. These cancers are notorious for presenting late, a feature that is responsible for poor survival rates.

Epidemiology:
- Fifth most common cause of cancer deaths in the UK
- Annual incidence of 9 per 100,000
- Male preponderance of 2:1
- Peak incidence in the seventh decade

Clinical features:
- Initial symptoms are often vague – epigastric/ simple back pain and unexplained weight loss
- Painless jaundice and a palpable gall bladder may be present in tumours involving the head of the pancreas

> **E** ≫ The Courvoisier Law states that in the presence of a non-tender palpable gall bladder and jaundice, gallstones are unlikely to be the cause and an underlying malignancy should be suspected. The exception is in the event of a double gallstone, one in the gall bladder and the other in the CBD.

Risk factors
- Smoking has been implicated as the most important risk factor, as it is associated with a two-fold increase
- Other risk factors include chronic pancreatitis, alcohol, diabetes mellitus and genetic predisposition

> ≫ Pancreatic cancer is associated with a number of familial neoplastic syndromes. These include HNPCC, PJS, MEN-1 and breast cancer.

Pathophysiology:
- Most tumours (~60%) arise in the head of the pancreas, developing from premalignant intra-epithelial neoplasia, and eventually progressing to invasive carcinoma
- Local and regional lymphatic spread is common in early disease, with subsequent liver metastasis in the later stages

Investigations

Stepwise plan:

1 Arrange abdominal ultrasound
- This is often the initial imaging modality, looking for benign biliary pathology
- Duct dilatation, liver mets and head of pancreas mass may be seen on scanning

2 Obtain contrast-enhanced CT
- This offers a more detailed evaluation (see *Fig. 3.53*), allowing staging (TNM) and surgical assessment

3 Consider EUS
- Increasingly used to confirm a histological diagnosis

4 Look for tumour markers
- CA19-9 may be useful in guiding treatment

3

3

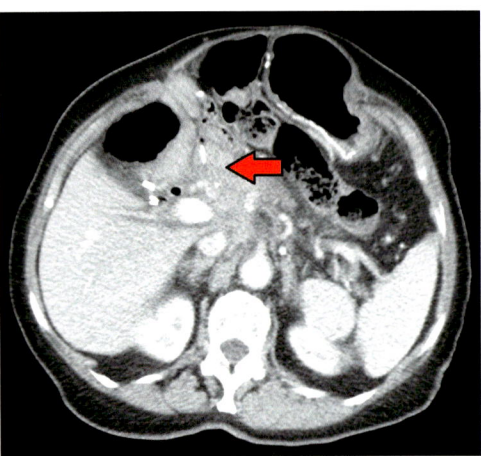

Fig. 3.53 *Axial view of a contrast-enhanced CT scan showing a bulky head of pancreas tumour.*

Management

Treatment is guided by a multi-disciplinary team and is based on staging.

Stepwise management of pancreatic cancer

1 Resectable disease (5–10%)
- Whipple procedure with adjuvant chemotherapy

2 Palliative chemotherapy
- NICE (2015, TA476) recommends paclitaxel or gemcitabine as first-line agents in metastatic disease

3 Palliative stent insertion and symptomatic control

Chapter 4
Endocrinology

Amar Vaswani and *Kelsey Wai Jan Wong*

Basic principles

Endocrinology refers to a branch of medicine that deals with the study of ductless glands, with a particular emphasis on the hormones secreted by these glands.

The body's endocrine system (see *Fig. 4.1*) works in tandem with the neurological system, via hormones and neurotransmitters, to maintain homeostasis.

Bridge to clinical medicine

- A hormone is defined as a regulatory substance that is produced and secreted by a gland, then transported in tissue fluid to stimulate specific cells or tissues into action
- A gland is defined as a cell (or group of cells) that secretes a chemical substance for discharge into surrounding structures

> **E** ≫ Endocrine glands are not the same as exocrine glands, the majority of which secrete substances through ducts.

- Endocrine signalling can also be accomplished via an **autocrine** (a substance that prompts a response in the very same cell that secreted it) or a **paracrine** (a substance that is secreted by a cell in order to achieve a local effect)
- Hormones can also be broadly classified into two groups based on their chemical structure – **peptide** hormones and **steroid** hormones

- Peptide hormones, such as adrenaline, are typically short-acting, act via second-messenger systems and G-protein action, and bind to receptors on the surface of a cell
- Steroid hormones, on the other hand, are generally longer-acting and bind directly to receptors in the cytoplasm of a cell. The receptor–hormone complex then migrates to the nucleus to achieve its effect. Examples of steroid hormones include cortisol and androgens.

> **P** ≫ Thyroxine, a hormone released by the thyroid gland, is an important exception. Structurally, thyroxine is a peptide hormone, but it acts on intracellular receptors, in much the same way as steroid hormones.

- Other cells in the body have a secondary endocrine function, and are not limited to the organs shown above (e.g. adipose tissue)

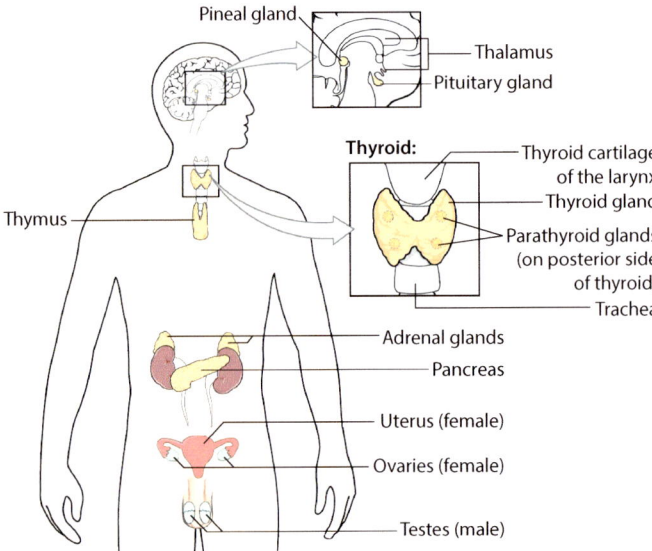

Fig. 4.1 *Overview of the endocrine system.*

4.1 The hypothalamus and pituitary gland

The hypothalamus is an almond-sized structure in the diencephalon of the brain that is located inferior to the thalamus. It has many important regulatory functions. It is linked to the pituitary gland (also known as the hypophysis) and interconnects with it to regulate the release of various hormones in the body.

- The pituitary gland is connected to the hypothalamus by the pituitary stalk (or infundibulum). It is anatomically divided into two lobes: the anterior lobe (adenohypophysis) and the posterior lobe (neurohypophysis) (see *Fig. 4.2*).
- The anterior lobe is derived from embryonic tissue from the developing mouth (known as the Rathke pouch), and is primarily composed of glandular tissue. The posterior lobe is an extension of the neural tissue of the hypothalamus. The pituitary gland itself sits in the sella turcica of the sphenoid.

E >> The anterior pituitary produces **and** stores hormones but the posterior pituitary only stores hormones. This is because the hormones associated with the posterior pituitary (ADH and oxytocin) are produced in the hypothalamus.

- A number of pathological processes connected to endocrine disorders are linked to hypo- or hyper-functioning of a gland, and a good understanding of the anatomy and physiology of each gland will therefore help underpin the knowledge base of each disorder.
- The anterior pituitary is made up of three parts: the pars distalis anteriorly; the pars intermedia (detailed above); and the pars tuberalis (a sheath enveloping the infundibulum). Unlike the posterior pituitary, the anterior pituitary does produce hormones, and stores them as well.

W >> The region between the anterior and posterior lobes of the pituitary is known as the intermediate lobe (or pars intermedia), and is home to cells that produce melanocyte-stimulating hormone (MSH). The effects of this hormone are not completely delineated, as the intermediate lobe is small and hormone production is significantly decreased in adulthood. One notable exception is during pregnancy, when MSH is said to account for the darkening of the labia and areola in women. Note that darkening of the skin is an example of a localised melanin response to UV radiation, **not** a by-product of MSH stimulation. One need only look at tan lines!

P >> The pineal gland, located in the epithalamic area of the brain, produces melatonin, a hormone associated with sleep regulation.

- The hormones produced by the anterior pituitary are released in response to hormones produced by the hypothalamus. This connection is established by the hypophyseal portal system.
- The hypothalamus releases several hormones, including GHRH and GHIH (aka somatostatin) (growth hormone-releasing and -inhibiting, respectively). GHIH regulates growth hormone (GH) production; CRH (corticotropin-releasing hormone) regulates ACTH (adrenocorticotropic hormone); and GnRH (gonadotropin-releasing hormone) initiates puberty and regulates FSH (follicle-stimulating hormone) and LH (luteinising hormone) (see *Fig. 4.3*).

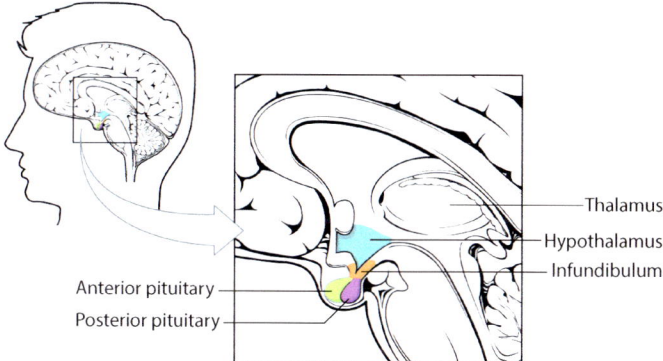

Thalamus
Hypothalamus
Infundibulum

Anterior pituitary
Posterior pituitary

Fig. 4.2 The hypothalamus–pituitary complex.

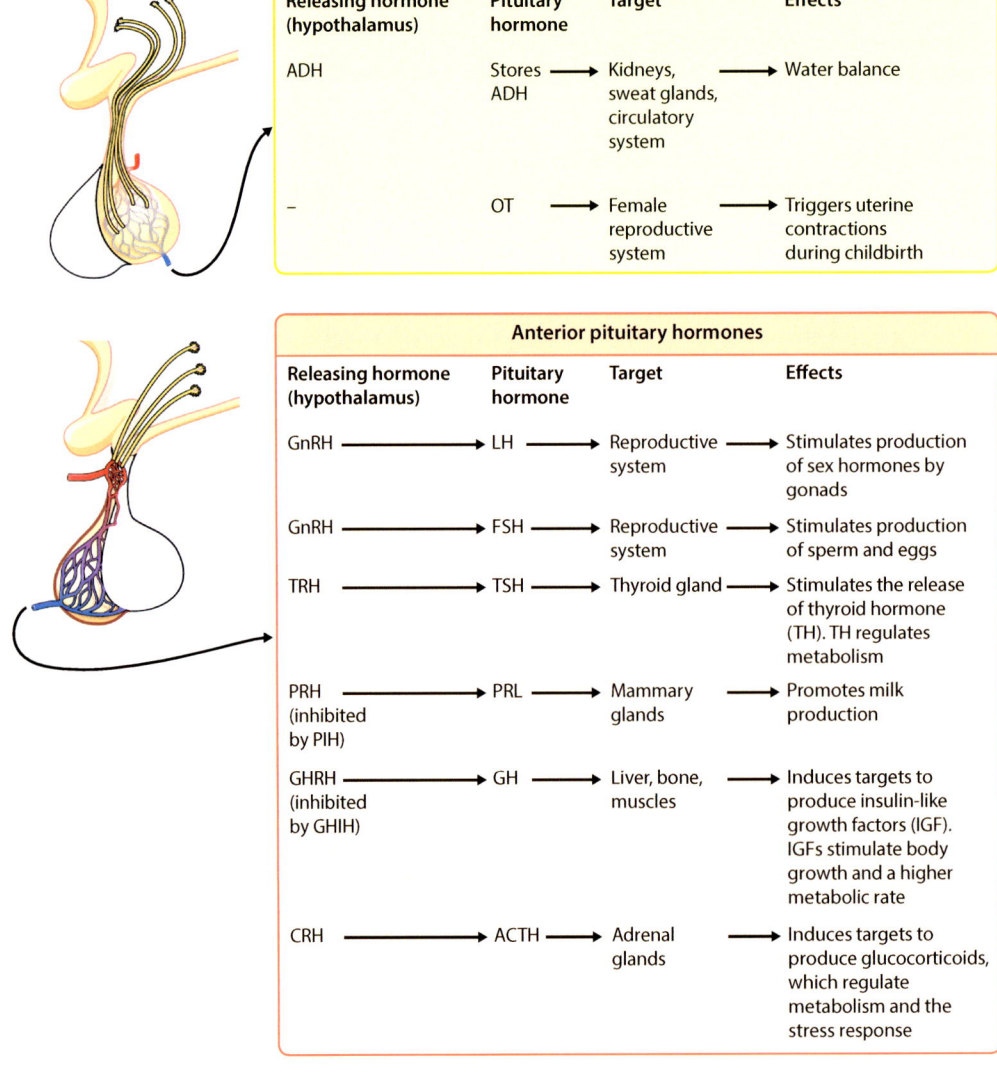

Posterior pituitary hormones			
Releasing hormone (hypothalamus)	Pituitary hormone	Target	Effects
ADH	Stores ADH →	Kidneys, sweat glands, circulatory system →	Water balance
–	OT →	Female reproductive system →	Triggers uterine contractions during childbirth

Anterior pituitary hormones			
Releasing hormone (hypothalamus)	Pituitary hormone	Target	Effects
GnRH →	LH →	Reproductive system →	Stimulates production of sex hormones by gonads
GnRH →	FSH →	Reproductive system →	Stimulates production of sperm and eggs
TRH →	TSH →	Thyroid gland →	Stimulates the release of thyroid hormone (TH). TH regulates metabolism
PRH (inhibited by PIH) →	PRL →	Mammary glands →	Promotes milk production
GHRH (inhibited by GHIH) →	GH →	Liver, bone, muscles →	Induces targets to produce insulin-like growth factors (IGF). IGFs stimulate body growth and a higher metabolic rate
CRH →	ACTH →	Adrenal glands →	Induces targets to produce glucocorticoids, which regulate metabolism and the stress response

Fig. 4.3 *The major pituitary hormones, their site of action and effect.*

The hypothalamus also secretes TRH (thyrotropin-releasing hormone), which regulates thyroid hormone release as well.

E ≫ Note that oxytocin is released by the paraventricular nuclei of the posterior pituitary, and that ADH is released by the supraoptic nuclei.

P ≫ GnRH is released in a pulsatile fashion, beginning at puberty, and has very low serum levels in childhood.

Regulation of hormones

Hormone regulation can be thought of as a feedback loop with three components: the hypothalamus, the pituitary and the endocrine gland. Examples include feedback loops involving the thyroid, adrenal glands and the gonads. *Figure 4.4* illustrates the hypothalamic–pituitary–adrenal–gonadotropic (HPAG) axis.

The regulation of FSH and LH here is visibly demonstrated, showing that hormone regulation is a dynamic process along this axis, exemplified by the positive and negative feedback loops.

Note that the HPAG axis only represents one part of hormone regulation, as there are other mechanisms that alter hormone concentration at any given time.

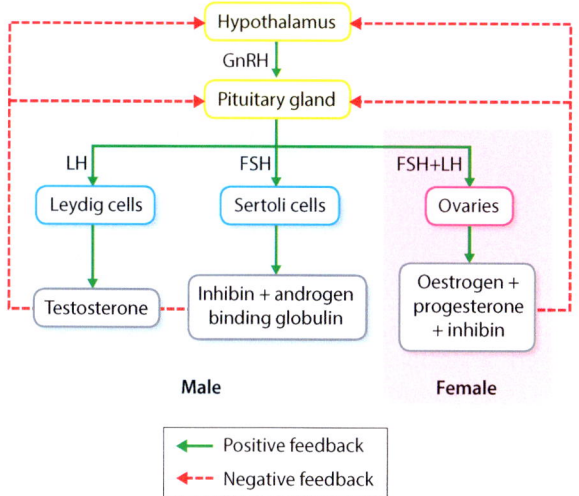

Fig. 4.4 *Hypothalamic–pituitary–adrenal–gonadotropic (HPAG) axis.*

For instance, growth hormone spikes after sleep, and cortisol is at its highest in the early morning (or the hours before waking).

Regulation of hunger and thirst

Sensations that involve hunger and thirst, while related to hormone secretion, are also multifactorial. Hunger, for example, with respect to endocrinology, is under the control of two hormones, leptin and ghrelin.

E ≫ Ghrelin makes your stomach **G**hrowl. Leptin is released when there are plenty of **L**eptovers.

W ≫ Ghrelin is a hormone produced by the stomach and stimulates hunger. When an individual has eaten a meal, adipocytes then release leptin, decreasing hunger pangs and inducing a sensation of satiety. The satiety centre of the body is in the ventromedial nucleus of the hypothalamus. Animal studies have demonstrated that removal of this area causes overfeeding and an inability to recognise satiety. Other mechanisms in the feeling of hunger include psychological stimulation (seeing food, thinking about food), blood levels of glucose, amino acids and fatty acids, and gut hormones (such as cholecystokinin) which depress hunger pangs.

Thirst, on the other hand, is inextricably linked to fluid and electrolyte balance within the body. Thirst beyond normal limits (polydipsia) is seen in conditions such as diabetes mellitus and diabetes insipidus. Osmoreceptors sense the solute concentration of the interstitial fluid, which is primarily altered by hypovolaemia or an increase in sodium in the diet. Osmolality is also affected by processes such as respiration, urination and perspiration. Polydipsia (seen in diabetes mellitus) occurs secondary to a high concentration of glucose in the blood, increasing osmolarity and stimulating thirst.

P ≫ Psychogenic polydipsia is characterised by unregulated thirst associated with mental illness. This may be life-threatening, as it causes a dilutional hyponatraemia and the associated low sodium may predispose the individual to seizures.

4.1.1 Acromegaly

Definition: acromegaly is primarily characterised by a growth of the extremities and associated features, in most cases caused by a GH-secreting pituitary adenoma. It is also associated with multi-system morbidity and early mortality.

Epidemiology:
- Pituitary adenomas may occur in approximately 15–20% of individuals, some only discovered on autopsy
- Only an estimated 2% are functioning GH adenoma
- This condition affects men and women equally

E ≫ Conditions such as acromegaly and hyperprolactinaemia are often caused by the presence of a pituitary tumour known as an adenoma. The tumour can cause symptoms related to hypersecretion of the hormone in question and a localised 'mass effect' that may compress nearby structures (such as the optic chiasm), leading to a bitemporal hemianopia.

4

P ≫ The most common types of adenomas are non-functioning adenomas, followed by prolactinomas and then by GH-secreting adenomas.

Aetiology/pathophysiology:
- Concomitant secretion of prolactin alongside a GH secretion (a mixed adenoma) may also be seen in certain cases
- Pituitary tumours may be associated with multiple endocrine neoplasia (MEN) type I
- Characteristic growth observed in acromegaly occurs as a result of disruption of normal hormonal feedback mechanisms, due to oversecretion of GH by the tumour

Clinical features:
- Local 'mass effect' of the tumour causes headaches and visual field defects, typically bitemporal hemianopia

- Growth of internal and external body structures: enlargement of upper and lower extremities (classic clinical vignettes focus on rings or shoes that no longer fit), prognathism, or a pronounced jaw (see *Fig. 4.5*), frontal bossing and enlargement of the nose
- Separation of the teeth, deepening of the voice and hyperhidrosis (excessive sweating) may also be noted
- Associated macroglossia (enlargement of the tongue) may predispose to obstructive sleep apnoea, so a dry mouth or extreme tiredness may be an associated symptom
- Associated with multi-system disorders, such as impaired glucose tolerance, hypertension, diabetes mellitus and osteoarthritis
- May also be associated with organomegaly, and this may be clinically evident if organs such as the heart, thyroid and prostate are involved

P ≫ Patients with acromegaly often have a cardiac cause of death, with arrhythmias and cardiomyopathy being complications. Carpal tunnel syndrome is another associated feature, and occurs due to nerve entrapment. There is also an increased risk of colorectal cancer, and the British Society of Gastroenterology recommends screening with colonoscopy at the age of 40.

E ≫ GH-producing adenomas result in gigantism in children, and acromegaly in adults.

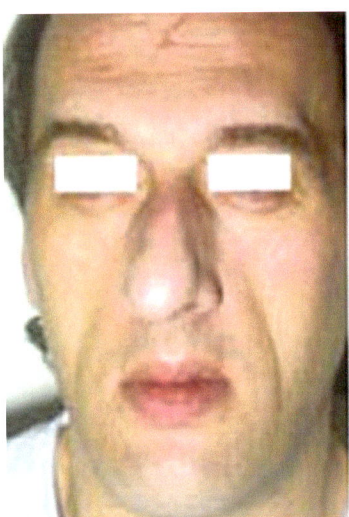
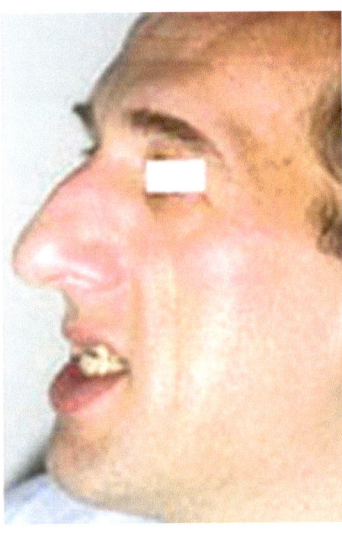

Fig. 4.5 Prognathism and maxillary widening, seen in patient with acromegaly.

Investigations

It may be difficult (for both patients and clinicians) to notice the physical changes associated with acromegaly until they have become irreversible, or until complications have occurred. The time frame for these changes spans years, and so the clinical course may be indolent.

Stepwise plan:

1   **Look for characteristic features from history and physical examination**

2   **Assess visual fields**

3   **Obtain IGF-1 levels**

W ≫ IGF-1, or insulin-like growth factor 1 (somatomedin C), is a growth factor produced in response to GH release. As a result, IGF-1 levels correlate to disease activity and are a useful initial screening tool.

4   **Perform an oral glucose tolerance test**

W ≫ Levels of serum growth hormone are not measured, and an oral glucose tolerance test is used instead. This is because growth hormone levels by themselves vary throughout the day and are unreliable in making the diagnosis. Normally, GH levels are suppressed by a glucose load. Thus, the patient is given a small glucose load, and serial GH measurements are obtained. In patients with acromegaly, the glucose load fails to suppress the excessive GH, thus confirming the diagnosis.

5   **Perform pituitary function tests**
- Prolactin, adrenal hormones, sex hormones and thyroid function tests

6   **Obtain an MRI scan of the pituitary**
- To localise the tumour – perform after biochemical studies have been conducted (see *Fig. 4.6*)

7   **Assess cardiovascular function (ECG, echocardiogram)**
- And monitor patient for impaired glucose tolerance or diabetes mellitus

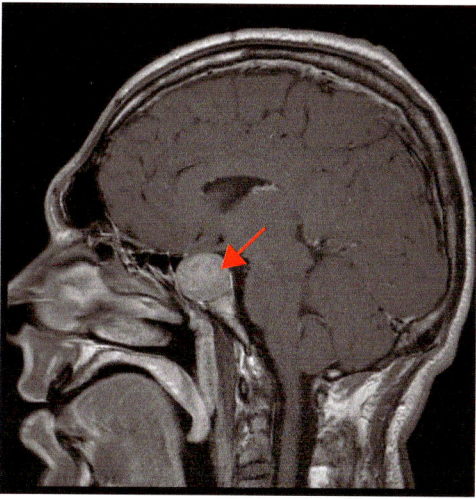

Fig. 4.6 *Pituitary adenoma seen on a brain MRI.*

Management

Stepwise management of acromegaly

1   **Surgery, particularly removal of the adenoma via a trans-sphenoidal resection, is the first-line treatment**
- Hypopituitarism may occur as a complication in some patients

2   **Somatostatin analogues, such as octreotide, mimic the action of GHIH**
- These are indicated in patients who are unfit for surgery or as adjuvant therapy

3   **Consider prescribing pegvisomant, a GH receptor antagonist**
- This a viable medical treatment option in patients with acromegaly

P ≫ Note that medical therapy does not shrink the tumour, and symptoms related to the 'mass effect' may still occur.

4   **Consider radiotherapy**
- This is an option for patients who are unsuitable surgical candidates or those who do not respond to medical treatment
- Hypopituitarism is also a complication

4

>> Note that pituitary carcinomas are rare, accounting for less than 1% of all pituitary tumours. Treatment modalities include surgery, radiotherapy and chemotherapy, but treatment is effectively palliative in nature.

4.1.2 GH deficiency

Definition: GH deficiency occurs when the pituitary gland is unable to produce sufficient GH for optimum growth of the body.

Epidemiology/clinical features:
- GH deficiency is very rare, and may present in childhood or adulthood (where it may be congenital or acquired)
- Features (especially in children) include diminished growth, decreased lean body mass, poor bone growth, loss of stamina and psychological symptoms such as depression

Aetiology/pathophysiology:
- GH deficiency may also occur as a result of a pituitary tumour
- Can also be caused by infiltrative or infectious agents
- Or may occur as a post-radiotherapy complication

Investigations

Stepwise plan:

1 **Skeletal X-rays of the wrist**
- Looking for skeletal age
- IGF-1 levels (will be low)

2 **GH provocation tests**

>> Suboptimal increase in GH levels after inducing with either arginine-L-dopa, arginine-GHRH or insulin-induced hypoglycaemia can confirm the diagnosis of GH deficiency.

3 **Obtain MRI brain scan**

4 **Carry out pituitary function tests**

Management

Stepwise management of GH deficiency

1 **Administer recombinant human growth hormone**

2 **Treat other pituitary hormone deficiencies**

3 **Treat underlying cause (if applicable)**

4.1.3 Hyperprolactinaemia

Definition: hyperprolactinaemia refers to a condition in which there is an elevated level of prolactin in the blood. This may be physiological (e.g. during breastfeeding) or pathological – in most cases due to a pituitary adenoma (prolactinoma).

Epidemiology:
- Prolactinomas are the most common type of pituitary adenoma, accounting for up to 40% of cases
- Affects significantly more women than men

Aetiology/pathophysiology:
- Prolactinomas are the most common cause of pathological hyperprolactinaemia, and may be co-secreted with a GH adenoma
- May be caused by hypothyroidism
- May be drug-induced; caused by antipsychotic medication

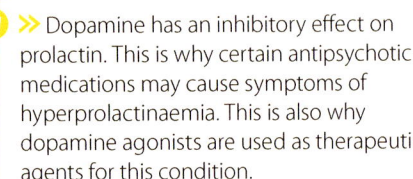>> Dopamine has an inhibitory effect on prolactin. This is why certain antipsychotic medications may cause symptoms of hyperprolactinaemia. This is also why dopamine agonists are used as therapeutic agents for this condition.

Clinical features:
- Local 'mass effect' of the tumour causes headaches and visual field defects, typically bitemporal hemianopia (seen in both)
- In men: reduced libido, erectile dysfunction, gynaecomastia, infertility
- In women: amenorrhoea, galactorrhoea, osteopenia

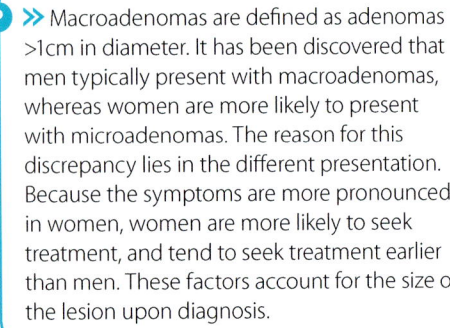>> Macroadenomas are defined as adenomas >1cm in diameter. It has been discovered that men typically present with macroadenomas, whereas women are more likely to present with microadenomas. The reason for this discrepancy lies in the different presentation. Because the symptoms are more pronounced in women, women are more likely to seek treatment, and tend to seek treatment earlier than men. These factors account for the size of the lesion upon diagnosis.

Investigations

Stepwise plan:

1   **Exclude pregnancy, assess visual fields**

2   **Obtain thyroid function tests**

> **W** ≫ Recall that hypothyroidism may be a cause of hyperprolactinaemia. Inappropriate TRH secretion may overcome normal inhibitory feedback, and prolactin is thus secreted excessively.

3   **Obtain serum prolactin level**
- Very high levels are diagnostic

4   **Obtain MRI brain scan**
- To visualise adenoma (see *Fig. 4.6*)

Management
Management involves treating the underlying cause.

Stepwise management of hyperprolactinaemia

1   **Dopamine agonists (cabergoline, bromocriptine) are used first line**
- Check cardiorespiratory function, as these drugs may cause cardiorespiratory fibrosis
- Cabergoline has a better side effect profile

> **E** ≫ Unlike acromegaly, medical treatment in this case does shrink the tumour.

2   **Trans-sphenoidal resection**
- If caused by a prolactinoma

4.1.4 Hypopituitarism

Definition: hypopituitarism refers to a state in which one or more of the pituitary hormones is deficient. While there is usually a mixture of pituitary hormone deficiencies, in rare cases this is characterised by a deficiency of all pituitary hormones.

Aetiology
- The most common cause of panhypopituitarism is compression and subsequent trauma to the pituitary by a tumour, or surgery
- Other causes include infection and radiotherapy

> **W** ≫ Several hormones may be deficient in hypopituitarism, and they are typically lost in a particular order. Generally, GH and the gonadotropins (FSH and LH) are lost first, in the course of the disease, and thyroid hormones and cortisol are the last ones to be lost. An easy way to remember this is to think of hormones being lost in order to 'promote survival'. The body 'would prefer' to lose reproductive capacity and growth first, followed by hormones required for regulatory and stress reaction purposes (such as thyroid hormone and cortisol).

Investigations
Hypopituitarism can be investigated with pituitary function tests. Symptoms observed correspond to the hormone deficiency seen, e.g. infertility and impotence (seen in gonadotropin deficiency); or fatigue, weight gain and cold intolerance (seen in hypothyroidism).

Management
Management involves treating the underlying cause and replacing the hormones in question.

4.1.5 Pituitary apoplexy
Pituitary apoplexy (acute pituitary failure) is a medical emergency, and refers to an acute haemorrhagic infarction of the pituitary gland. Symptoms include a headache of sudden onset, nausea and vomiting and drowsiness, often progressing to coma. Prompt administration of hydrocortisone can be lifesaving. The condition has a high mortality rate and may be difficult to diagnose, because of a wide differential diagnosis that can include meningitis and a subarachnoid haemorrhage.

> **P** ≫ Sheehan syndrome (postpartum pituitary necrosis) is a form of acute pituitary necrosis that occurs due to hypotension or peri-/postpartum haemorrhage. It presents initially with failure to lactate, and is characterised by pituitary hormone deficiency and amenorrhoea later in the course of the disease. This condition is rare, and is more likely to occur in regions without access to adequate obstetric care.

4

4.1.6 Empty sella syndrome

Empty sella syndrome is a benign condition that may cause the patient to present with headaches. It is typified by the inability to visualise the pituitary gland on MRI. Endocrine abnormalities are uncommon, and appropriate reassurance should be given to patients.

4.1.7 Craniopharyngioma

Definition: craniopharyngiomas are benign tumours that arise from the remnants of the Rathke pouch.

Epidemiology:
- More common in children, and may account for up to 10% of childhood brain tumours
- Accounts for 1–3% of adult brain tumours
- No particular gender preponderance

Aetiology/pathophysiology:
- Pathogenesis is incompletely understood, but is thought to involve neoplastic change of the Rathke pouch
- Most commonly found in the sellar or supra-sellar region

Clinical features:
- Local 'mass effect' of the tumour causes headaches and visual field defects, typically bitemporal hemianopia
- Pituitary hormone dysfunction
- Because of their location, craniopharyngiomas may also cause hydrocephalus as a result of blockage to CSF flow at the third ventricle

Investigations

> **Stepwise plan:**

> 1 **Pituitary function tests**
> - To assess visual fields
>
> 2 **Obtain MRI of the brain**
> - To visualise the lesion (see *Fig. 4.7*)

Management

Management primarily involves surgical resection of the tumour and subsequent radiotherapy. Despite what may appear to be total resection, craniopharyngiomas are likely to recur. The recurrence rate is reduced in patients who receive radiotherapy.

P ≫ Note that surgical resection in children is associated with a mortality rate as high as 10%. Complications (such as seizures, visual field abnormalities and pituitary hormone deficiency) may also occur.

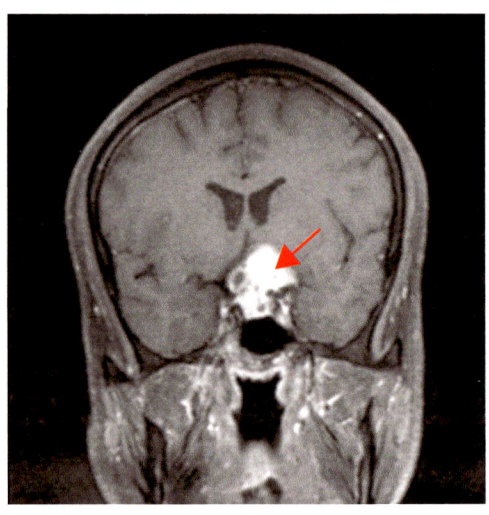

Fig. 4.7 *MRI brain showing a large craniopharyngioma.*

4.1.8 Syndrome of inappropriate ADH secretion (SIADH)

Definition: SIADH refers to a condition in which hyponatraemia, hyperosmolar urine and plasma hypo-osmolarity occur, in the absence of other endocrine abnormalities, as a result of excess secretion of ADH.

Epidemiology:
- Excessive hydration (particularly via IV infusion) is a far more common cause of hyponatraemia than SIADH

Aetiology/pathophysiology:
- SIADH may be caused by a number of pathological processes
- These include, but are not limited to, malignancy (ectopic ADH production by neoplastic cells, commonly associated with small cell lung cancer), drugs, meningitis and surgery

Clinical features:
- SIADH results in water retention and hyponatraemia, which is often the first abnormality detected after routine bloods have been performed
- Note that this water retention is not accompanied by oedema because of urinary excretion of sodium

E ≫ Signs of extensive hyponatraemia, e.g. confusion, drowsiness and a lowered GCS should be watched for and treated accordingly. Patients with mild hyponatraemia are usually asymptomatic.

- High urine osmolality and a high urinary sodium – be sure to assess and rule out other endocrine causes before considering SIADH

Investigations

Stepwise plan:

1 **Obtain serum sodium levels**
- Low serum sodium <135mmol/L is often an incidental finding

2 **Exclude other causes of hyponatraemia before attempting to investigate SIADH further**
- See *Chapter 7* for management of hyponatraemia

3 **Obtain urine osmolality (elevated) and urinary sodium (>40mmol/L)**

4 **Exclude other causes of hyponatraemia secondary to endocrine dysfunction**
- e.g. thyroid disorders or adrenal insufficiency

Management

Stepwise management of SIADH

1 **Treat any underlying cause**

2 **Appropriately restrict fluid**
- This will help correct hyponatraemia by increasing serum sodium

3 **If patients do not improve, consider using demeclocycline**

> **W** >> Although demeclocycline is an antibiotic, it is sometimes used to treat SIADH because it reliably reduces the efficacy of ADH (vasopressin) at the collecting duct as a side effect.

4 **Consider V2 receptor antagonists**
- Severe cases merit consideration of V2 receptor antagonists at the collecting duct, e.g. conivaptan

4.1.9 Diabetes insipidus

Definition: the term 'diabetes' has its roots in Latin and Greek, meaning both 'to straddle' and 'siphon', alluding to the 'siphoning' of urine (polyuria) from the 'straddle area'. *Insipidus* is Latin for 'lacking taste', which is, of course, a comparison with diabetes mellitus (glycosuria).

Aetiology/pathophysiology:

- While SIADH has to do with excess ADH stimulation, diabetes insipidus (DI) has to do with direct or relative ADH deficiency (see yellow *Why?* box below).
- There are two principal classifications of DI: neurogenic (cranial/central) DI and nephrogenic DI. These vary both in pathophysiology and treatment strategy
- The development of neurogenic or central DI is primarily associated with insults to the pituitary or CNS lesions. Central DI has numerous causes, most notably pituitary surgery, meningitis and head trauma.
- Nephrogenic DI, on the other hand, may be congenital in origin (affecting the V2 receptor or aquaporin channel mutations). It can also occur secondary to electrolyte disturbances.

> **E** >> An important cause of nephrogenic DI is the use of medications. Lithium use, in particular, is a common cause of nephrogenic DI. Use of demeclocycline, which is a treatment for SIADH, may also cause DI.

> **W** >> More specifically, central DI occurs as a result of insufficient production of ADH by the pituitary gland as a result of disease processes which damage the pituitary or CNS. Nephrogenic DI occurs secondary to decreased responsiveness to ADH by receptors at the collecting duct.

Clinical features:

- Polydipsia, polyuria (>3L/day; nocturia may also be common).
- Both forms of DI result in the excretion of dilute urine, which can lead to hypernatraemia, which may present as excessive thirst. If left untreated, hypernatraemia is potentially fatal (see *Chapter 7*). Note that life-threatening hypernatraemia is uncommon in patients with DI because thirst regulation ensures an adequate intake of water.

Investigations

Stepwise plan:

1 **Assess urea and electrolytes**
- Serum sodium may be normal or elevated

2 **Assess urine osmolality**
- DI will correspond with low urine osmolality (<300mol/kg)

4

3   **A water deprivation test helps confirm the diagnosis**
- A patient with suspected DI is deprived of water for up to 8 hours
- In patients without DI, there will be low urine volume and an increased urine osmolality (more concentrated urine)
- Patients with DI have a high urine volume and a low urine osmolality (dilute urine despite fluid deprivation)

4   **Give an injection of desmopressin (a synthetic analogue of ADH) after water deprivation to distinguish between central and nephrogenic DI**
- If urine osmolality increases after the injection, the diagnosis is most likely central DI
- If urine fails to concentrate after the injection, the patient is most likely unresponsive to ADH and has nephrogenic DI

Management

The management of DI is related to the type of DI identified.

Stepwise management of diabetes insipidus

Central DI

1   **Treatment involves replacing the deficient hormone**
- The drug of choice is desmopressin; this may be given IV in the acute setting or intranasally for regular use

2   **Long-term management involves measuring sodium levels at regular intervals**

- Patients are advised to miss one dose of desmopressin per week to prevent hyponatraemia developing

Nephrogenic DI

1   **Nephrogenic DI may be more difficult to treat**
- Unlike central DI, which involves replacing a deficient hormone, nephrogenic DI does not respond to desmopressin and treatment may be more difficult

2   **Identify the underlying cause**
- Identification of any underlying cause (particularly drugs) is important
- Note that DI associated with lithium use may be irreversible

3   **Patients should be advised to drink enough fluid**
- Alternatively, a low-sodium diet may be attempted

4   **Consider thiazide diuretics**
- Consider using thiazide diuretics, such as hydrochlorothiazide or chlorthalidone, as treatment options

W ≫ The use of diuretics as a treatment modality for DI may seem paradoxical at first – why would we prescribe diuretics to a patient who is already excreting so much fluid? However, diuretics actually improve the overall clinical picture by increasing fluid resorption at the proximal tubule, helping fluid and electrolyte balance altogether, producing a net benefit.

4.2 The thyroid gland

The thyroid gland is a major endocrine gland situated just anterior to the trachea. It has two opposing lobes joined by a central isthmus (see *Fig. 4.8*).

- Thyroid follicles within the thyroid gland are rich in **colloid**, a viscous fluid in which thyroid hormone production takes place
- Thyroid hormone is produced when TSH (released by the anterior pituitary) binds to receptors on thyroid follicles, stimulating entry of **iodide ions** (I^-) into the follicle. Iodine is primarily obtained from dietary sources
- Oxidation and bonding of iodide ions with a glycoprotein called **thyroglobulin** within the

colloid produces **triiodothyronine** (T_3) and **tetraiodothyronine** (T_4), also known as **thyroxine**

E ≫ Less than 1% of circulating T_3 and T_4 are unbound. The majority of thyroid hormones is bound to protein (such as thyroid-binding globulin, or TBG) to prevent uptake. T_3 is more metabolically active than T_4. Most T_3 is produced by enzymatic removal of iodide from T_4 peripherally, e.g. in the liver.

- Thyroid hormone regulation is exerted via a negative feedback mechanism (see *Fig. 4.9*)

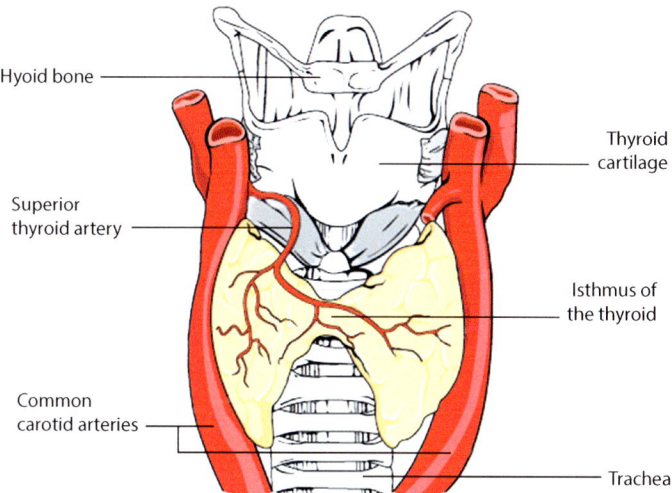

Fig. 4.8 *Gross anatomy of the thyroid gland.*

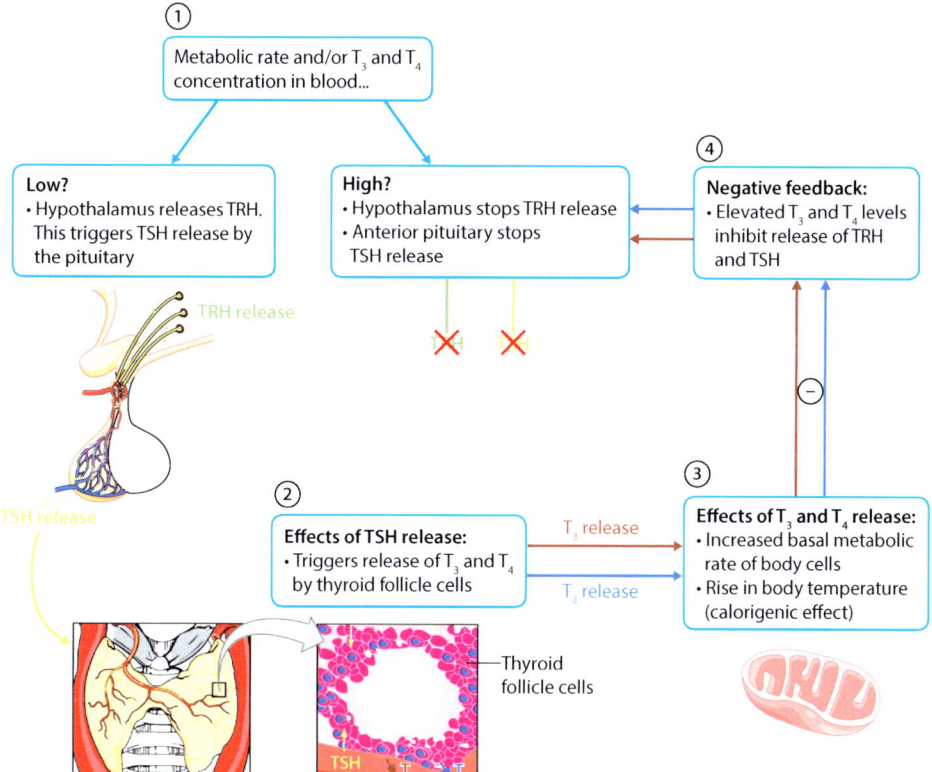

Fig. 4.9 *Hypothalamus–pituitary–thyroid (HPT) axis.*

Thyroid hormones have widespread regulatory and metabolic effects throughout the body. Hypo- or hyper-functioning states (detailed later in this chapter) can have serious consequences, affecting metabolism, growth and reproductive capacity.

Cells interspersed between the follicles of the thyroid gland are called parafollicular (or C) cells. These secrete the hormone **calcitonin**, which is produced in response to elevated serum calcium. Calcitonin mediates its effects by decreasing

4

osteoclastic activity while promoting osteoblasts. It is not thought to have a prominent role in calcium homeostasis.

- It is important to note that enlargement of the thyroid gland in response to disease (**goitre**) does not indicate a hyper- or hypo-functioning state; further investigation is warranted

4.2.1 Hyperthyroidism (thyrotoxicosis)

Definition: hyperthyroidism is characterised by an elevated level of thyroid hormone in the body that occurs as result of thyroid gland overactivity.

Aetiology/pathophysiology:

 Graves disease is the most common cause of thyrotoxicosis, accounting for a reported 60% of cases. Graves disease is classically characterised by hyperthyroidism associated with ophthalmopathy (exophthalmos) and dermopathy (thyroid acropachy and pretibial myxoedema). Graves disease occurs as a result of autoimmune activity against the TSH receptor.

 Eye signs, while often emphasised in Graves disease, may only be seen in 40% of patients. Exophthalmos (see *Fig. 4.10*) in Graves disease is said to occur as a result of lymphocytic infiltration and production of mucopolysaccharides by surrounding fibroblasts. This, in turn, promotes oedema of orbital structures, forcing the eye forward. Smoking and the use of radio-iodine therapy are also associated with an increased risk of developing ophthalmopathy. Pretibial myxoedema is also caused by mucopolysaccharide deposition.

- Ophthalmopathy and dermopathy seen in Graves disease may be treated with steroids
- Other causes of thyrotoxicosis include toxic multinodular goitre, thyroiditis, exogenous use of thyroid hormone supplements (**factitious thyrotoxicosis**) and some medications
- A rare form of teratoma, known as struma ovarii (not exclusively related to the ovary) is a benign ectopic thyroid-producing tumour that may lead to hyperthyroidism

 The development of Graves disease is also associated with other autoimmune conditions such as Addison disease, type 1 diabetes and vitiligo. Graves disease is also far more likely to affect women than men.

Clinical features:

- A vast array of symptoms can accompany thyrotoxicosis; these include weight loss, palpitations (secondary to **atrial fibrillation**), diarrhoea, heat intolerance, loss of libido, oligo- or amenorrhoea and proximal muscle weakness
- Clinically apparent signs may include lid lag, sweaty palms, a fine tremor, goitre (see *Fig. 4.12*), pretibial myxoedema (see *Fig. 4.11*) and thin, brittle hair

 Patients with undiagnosed or untreated hyperthyroidism may unfortunately progress to, or present with, thyroid storm (also known as a thyrotoxic crisis). This is a medical emergency, and is usually triggered by a precipitating event such as surgery, infection or trauma. Patients with thyroid storm are hyperthermic, have altered mental status and are vulnerable to life-threatening arrhythmias.

Thyroid storm

Thyroid storm is a medical emergency – it commonly presents with hyperpyrexia, tachycardia, atrial fibrillation and altered mental state. Patients may complain of nausea, vomiting, diarrhoea and abdominal pain. It is usually precipitated by acute illness, trauma, or stress.

If a thyroid storm is suspected, treat promptly as follows:
- Provide adequate hydration and cooling
- Initiate beta blockers (propranolol)
- Administer antithyroid agent such as propylthiouracil
- Iodine (Lugol solution) 4 hours after antithyroid treatment

 Thyroid storm is a medical emergency – treatment involves adequate hydration and cooling, followed by prompt administration of antithyroid agents (propylthiouracil). This is followed by giving the patient iodine, which at first may seem counter-intuitive. Iodine effectively inhibits further thyroid hormone production. This approach may be thought of as 'feeding the factory', while the antithyroid medications shut it down. Beta blockers (propranolol) and steroids are also used to treat thyroid storm.

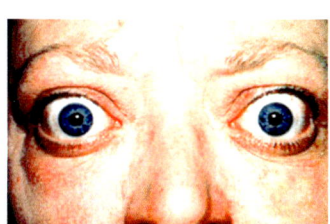

Fig. 4.10 Exophthalmos.

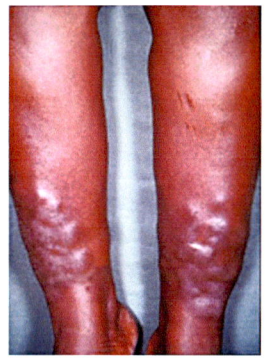

Fig. 4.11 Pretibial myxoedema.

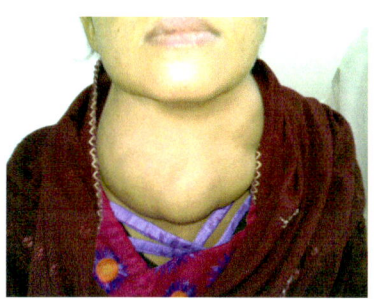

Fig. 4.12 Goitre.

4

P ≫ Thyrotoxic period paralysis is another complication of thyrotoxicosis, in which a patient experiences episodes of muscle weakness, pain or cramping secondary to **hypokalaemia**. This may prove to be life-threatening if respiratory muscle weakness occurs. The episodes usually involve symmetrical symptoms, and may be provoked by exercise, alcohol or high-carbohydrate meals. Treating the hyperthyroidism and ensuring adequate potassium replacement are the mainstays of therapy.

Investigations

Stepwise plan:

1 **Obtain thyroid function tests (TFTs)**
- These will likely show elevated T_3 and T_4 levels but a decreased TSH

2 **Auto-antibody testing will help distinguish Graves disease from other causes of hyperthyroidism**
- Anti-TSH receptor antibodies have the highest sensitivity and specificity, approaching 99%
- Anti-thyroid peroxidase and anti-thyroglobulin antibodies may also point towards Graves disease, though these are less specific

3 **Radio-iodine uptake scans may help identify 'hot' or 'cold' regions, determining level of over- or under-activity**
- Uptake scans will demonstrate **diffuse** uptake in Graves disease

4 **Arrange other investigations**
- Fine needle aspiration cytology (if needed)
- ECG (treat any associated AF)

Management

Before starting treatment, an assessment of the patient beyond basic biochemistry should be carried out. If the patient is severely unwell or has atrial fibrillation, referral to secondary care is warranted. In addition, if the patient has risk factors for a more sinister cause of hyperthyroidism, such as a localised, growing lump or hoarseness without an attributable cause, they should be referred urgently.

Stepwise management of hyperthyroidism

1 **Anti-thyroid medication is the first-line treatment**
- Carbimazole and methimazole are the most widely used agents
- Two major approaches to anti-thyroid treatment are used: 'block and replace' and 'titration'
- The block and replace method involves prescribing anti-thyroid medication, along with thyroxine replacement, to achieve a stable euthyroid state – titration involves titrating drug doses until the lowest possible dose of anti-thyroid medication achieves a euthyroid state

P ≫ Anti-thyroid medication may take some time to exert its effect. Beta blockers may be given in the interim.

E ≫ Carbimazole and methimazole are teratogenic drugs, and should never be prescribed to pregnant patients. In this case, propylthiouracil is used instead. Patients taking anti-thyroid medication also have a 1% risk of agranulocytosis, and should be advised to return should they feel ill, experience flu-like symptoms or have a sore throat.

2   Consider using radioactive iodine
- Radioactive iodine may be used as a treatment in refractory cases or in Graves disease that is not sufficiently controlled with anti-thyroid therapy. This may predispose to hypothyroidism or **worsen ophthalmopathy**.

> **E** ≫ Radio-iodine therapy is contraindicated in pregnancy and breastfeeding.

3   Consider surgical treatment
- A sub-total or total thyroidectomy may be carried out if the above therapies fail

4.2.2 Hypothyroidism

Definition: hypothyroidism is characterised by a decreased level of thyroid hormone in the body, which occurs as result of thyroid gland underactivity.

Aetiology/pathophysiology:
- Hypothyroidism, like most endocrine pathology, can be primary or secondary. One of the major causes of primary hypothyroidism is autoimmunity (Hashimoto thyroiditis and atrophic thyroiditis), particularly in developed regions.
- Hashimoto thyroiditis and atrophic thyroiditis differ in that Hashimoto's may have a variable presentation, in which patients present with a painless goitre, but may be clinically euthyroid or slightly hypothyroid. Patients with atrophic thyroiditis are usually grossly hypothyroid as a result of immune-mediated disease.

> **E** ≫ Hypothyroidism is significantly more common in women, and the most common cause of hypothyroidism worldwide is a lack of dietary iodine. Low levels of thyroid hormone are also seen in any major illness. Measurement of TFTs when the patient is ill may therefore prove to be unreliable.

> **W** ≫ Congenital iodine deficiency syndrome (previously known as cretinism), which presents with a hypothyroid state at birth, usually occurs a result of maternal or dietary iodine deficiency. Symptoms vary significantly from primary adult hypothyroidism, with the majority of infants presenting with lethargy and reduced muscle tone. If left untreated, this condition can cause growth failure and reduced intellectual capacity.

- Other causes of hypothyroidism include sarcoidosis, thyroidectomies, radiotherapy and certain drugs, such as amiodarone and lithium

Clinical features:
- Patients with hypothyroidism generally feel tired and intolerant of cold
- As with thyrotoxicosis, there are a number of signs and symptoms
- In contrast, many of the body's processes are slowed down; hypothyroid patients may experience constipation, a reduced libido, dry skin, hair loss and weight gain

> **P** ≫ One important (seemingly paradoxical) symptomatic difference between thyrotoxicosis and hypothyroidism occurs with regard to menstrual irregularity. Patients with hyper-thyroidism typically present with amenorrhoea, whereas patients with hypothyroidism are more likely to experience menorrhagia.

> **E** ≫ Patients with undiagnosed or insufficiently treated hypothyroidism may unfortunately progress to, or present with, a myxoedema coma. This is a life-threatening medical emergency, and is usually set off by a stressful event, such as surgery, infection or trauma. Patients present acutely with hypothermia and a reduced mental status and may sometimes experience seizures. Treatment involves prompt administration of IV levothyroxine and steroids, as well as ensuring that the patient is adequately warmed.

> **W** ≫ Subclinical hypothyroidism will present with an elevated TSH and a normal thyroid hormone level. This is because TSH increases the amount of T_4 available. Patients should be treated if they become symptomatic, or if the TSH level is inappropriately high.

Investigations

Stepwise plan:

1   Obtain thyroid function tests (TFTs)
- These will likely show decreased T_3 and T_4 levels but an increased TSH – patients with secondary hypothyroidism will have low levels of TSH and low levels of T_3 and T_4

2 Arrange auto-antibody testing
- Auto-antibody testing, particularly with anti-thyroid peroxidase antibodies, may help point to an immune-mediated cause, such as Hashimoto thyroiditis

3 Carry out other investigations
- Other useful investigations include a serum cholesterol (which may be elevated), a fasting blood glucose and a creatine kinase, both of which may be elevated as well

Management
Measurement and monitoring of the TSH level is an important principle in managing hypothyroidism. Patients generally notice a marked improvement in symptoms as their TSH level normalises.

Stepwise management of hypothyroidism

1 Offer levothyroxine first line
- Start at a dose of 50mcg and adjust accordingly, using 25-mcg increments

2 Patients with cardiovascular comorbidities should be started at a dose of 25mcg

E » Patients should be warned that symptoms may take weeks to months to improve.

Overt hypothyroidism (NICE CKS 2011)

1 Treat overt hypothyroidism with levothyroxine

2 Do not use triiodothyronine (T₃) in combination with levothyroxine

3 All patients who are stable on levothyroxine require at least annual measurement of serum thyroid-stimulating hormone:
- To check adherence
- To ensure that the dosage of levothyroxine is still correct

4 In addition, NICE also recommends:
- All women with subclinical hypothyroidism who are pregnant or planning a pregnancy and are not receiving levothyroxine treatment should be started on levothyroxine therapy while waiting for referral to a specialist

4.2.3 Benign thyroid disease

Interpretation of thyroid function tests
TSH is the most useful biochemical marker in the evaluation of thyroid status, where no concomitant pituitary lesion exists. After looking at TSH, consider T_3 and T_4 levels in order to make a diagnosis (see *Tables 4.1* and *4.2*).

Table 4.1 *Patterns of TFTs with low TSH and their corresponding diagnoses*

Low TSH			
TFTs	**Potential diagnoses**	**Features**	**Management**
High T_3/T_4	1. Thyrotoxicosis 2. Toxic multinodular goitre	See *Section 4.2.1* Toxic multinodular goitres present with thyrotoxicosis and 'hot nodules' on radio-iodine uptake scan	See *Section 4.2.1* Anti-thyroid drugs and surgical removal
Low T_3/T_4	1. Pituitary dysfunction 2. Sick euthyroid syndrome (non-thyroidal illness)	Systemic illness depresses thyroid function	Treat underlying cause

Table 4.2 *Patterns of TFTs with high TSH and their corresponding diagnoses*

High TSH			
TFTs	**Potential diagnoses**	**Features**	**Management**
Normal T_3/T_4	Subclinical hypo-thyroidism	Common in elderly May also be caused by poor adherence to treatment	Levothyroxine
Low T_3/T_4	Hypothyroidism	See *Section 4.2.2*	See *Section 4.2.2*
High T_3/T_4	Ectopic thyroid hormone	Seen in various malignancies, struma ovarii	Treat underlying cause

4

Other forms of thyroiditis:

- De Quervain thyroiditis: a self-limiting clinical progression, from initially hyperthyroid to hypothyroid and finally to euthyroid. Often preceded by viral illness. Hallmark feature is a diffuse, **painful** goitre.
- Riedel thyroiditis: patients are typically euthyroid, but may be hypothyroid secondary to autoimmune fibrosis of the thyroid. This disease typically causes **a wooden, hard** goitre that causes compression of local structures. Treat with prednisolone.
- Thyroid cyst: asymptomatic, or may cause localised compression. Treat with aspiration or excision.

4.2.4 Thyroid cancer

The majority of thyroid nodules are benign adenomas, and fewer than 10% of these nodules constitute neoplastic lesions. The various types of thyroid cancer are described in *Table 4.3*. Thyroid cancer rarely results in a clinically hyperthyroid state, and most often shows up as a 'cold nodule' on a radio-iodine uptake scan. Naturally, while a high index of suspicion is mandated for all neck and thyroid lumps, urgent referral is warranted if the patient presents with a painless neck lump and has symptoms indicating compression or obstruction, such as dysphagia, hoarseness or superior vena cava obstruction. Investigation often includes fine needle aspiration and biopsy.

Table 4.3 Types of thyroid cancer, their features and management

Lesion	Features	Management
Papillary thyroid carcinoma	• Most common thyroid neoplasm; approximately 70% of all thyroid cancer • History of head and neck radiation is also a risk factor • Lymphatic spread is more likely than haematogenous spread	• Total thyroidectomy • Radio-iodine to ensure removal of neoplastic cells • Annual assessment with thyroglobulin levels to assess for recurrence • Excellent prognosis
Follicular thyroid carcinoma	• 15% of thyroid cancer • Haematogenous spread	• Total thyroidectomy • Radio-iodine to ensure removal of neoplastic cells • Annual assessment with thyroglobulin levels to assess for recurrence • Excellent prognosis
Medullary carcinoma of the thyroid	• May be part of multiple endocrine neoplasia (MEN) type 2 syndrome • Arises from parafollicular cells, calcitonin may be elevated	• Screen for MEN 2 • Total thyroidectomy • Radio-iodine to ensure removal of neoplastic cells
Anaplastic carcinoma of the thyroid	• Least common thyroid neoplasm • More likely to occur in women and the elderly	• Very poor prognosis • Treatment options are generally palliative

4.3 The parathyroid glands

The parathyroid glands are four small glands (see *Fig. 4.13*), located on the posterior aspect of the thyroid gland, which are primarily involved in calcium and phosphate homeostasis. They secrete parathyroid hormone (PTH). Disorders in calcium balance, namely hyper- or hypocalcaemia, may prove to be severely detrimental (see *Chapter 7*) if left unchecked.

The role of parathyroid hormone in the regulation of calcium

Fig 4.14 provides an overview of calcium homeostasis and the role of the parathyroid glands in maintaining this balance.

- A drop in the serum calcium concentration is detected by the parathyroid gland
- This stimulates the chief cells of the parathyroid gland to release PTH into the circulation
- PTH regulates serum calcium concentration by acting on:
  - **Bone** – inhibiting osteoblast and stimulates osteoclast, which increases bone resorption and, in turn, increases calcium concentration in the circulation
  - **Kidneys** – increasing renal reabsorption of calcium ions at the ascending loop of Henle, distal tubules and collecting ducts. In addition,

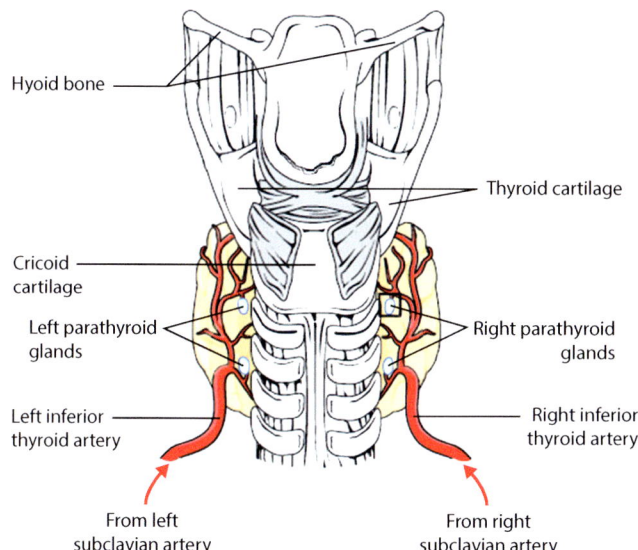

Fig. 4.13 *Gross anatomy of the parathyroid glands.*

4

PTH inhibits renal phosphate reabsorption at the proximal tubules
- **Intestines** – stimulating the absorption of calcium and phosphate ions from the intestinal lumen
- A negative feedback loop regulates the level of serum PTH
- In contrast, high levels of calcium are detected by the parafollicular cells of the thyroid gland which releases **calcitonin**. Calcitonin acts on bone to inhibit osteoclast activity, thereby reducing calcium concentration in the circulation
- This strict interplay between PTH and calcitonin maintains serum calcium concentration at homeostasis

4.3.1 Hyperparathyroidism

Definition: hyperparathyroidism refers to a clinical state in which there is an excess of PTH.

Epidemiology:
- Most common in women aged 50–60
- Primary hyperparathyroidism is the most common form
- Primary hyperparathyroidism and malignancy constitute the most common reasons for hypercalcaemia

Aetiology/pathophysiology:
Hyperparathyroidism may be said to exist in three forms:
1. **Primary**: one or more of the parathyroid glands contributes to increased PTH levels; also associated with multiple endocrine neoplasia

(see *Section 4.7*). Approximately 80% are caused by **adenomas**, 20% are due to gland hyperplasia, and less than 1% are due to parathyroid carcinoma.
2. **Secondary**: secondary hyperparathyroidism occurs as a result of **any condition that predisposes to hypocalcaemia**. These include chronic kidney disease (via decrease in formation of 1,25 dihydroxycholecalciferol), malabsorption syndromes and insufficient vitamin D.
3. **Tertiary**: prolonged secondary hyperparathyroidism leads to **hyperplasia** of the parathyroid glands, and excess PTH levels.

Clinical features:

> **E** ≫ Features of hypercalcaemia predominate – classically bone pain, nephrolithiasis, abdominal pain, pancreatitis and depression (bones, stones, moans and abdominal groans).

- Other features may include lethargy, myalgia, fatigue and a shortened QT interval

Investigations
Ensure that other causes of hypercalcaemia are excluded before considering a diagnosis of hyperparathyroidism. These include the use of certain calcium-sparing medications such as **thiazide diuretics.** Ensure that the patient has adequate renal function as well and does not consume an excess of dietary calcium.

4

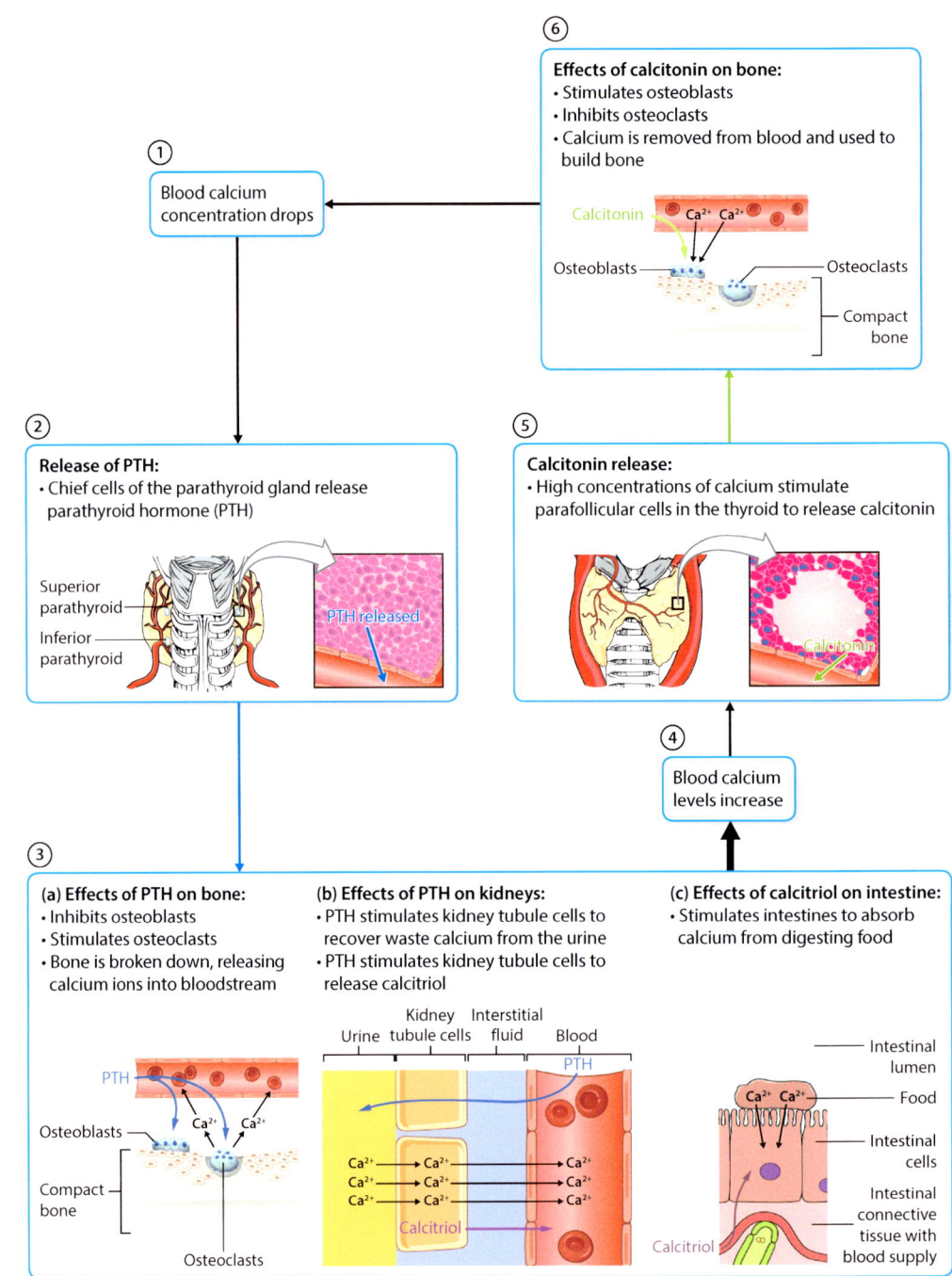

Fig. 4.14 *Role of PTH in calcium regulation.*

Stepwise plan:

1 **Check serum calcium, phosphate, PTH and alkaline phosphatase levels (see *Table 4.4*)**

2 **DXA scans and X-rays may demonstrate osteopenia**

Management
NICE (2007, TA117) only recommends cinacalcet in secondary hyperparathyroidism to patients on dialysis who are not improving with medical therapy or who are unfit for surgery. The management of the different forms of hyperparathyroidism is outlined in *Table 4.4*.

4.3.2 Hypoparathyroidism

Definition: hypoparathyroidism refers to the clinical state in which there is a decrease in the amount of PTH present within the body.

Aetiology/pathophysiology:
- The primary cause of hypoparathyroidism (in the **vast majority of cases) is iatrogenic** (neck surgery or radiation, including accidental or intentional removal of the parathyroid gland)
- Rarely it may be congenital (e.g. DiGeorge syndrome)
- Autoimmunity and destruction of parathyroid glands in systemic disease such as haemochromatosis may also be causes

W ≫ Pseudohypoparathyroidism refers to a clinical state in which hypocalcaemia is present, but PTH is elevated, primarily because of end organ receptor insensitivity to the effect of PTH.

Clinical features:
- Symptoms of hypocalcaemia predominate
- These include muscle twitching, lethargy, muscle spasms, psychosocial changes and a prolonged QT interval

E ≫ Twitching of the facial muscles on tapping the cheek (Chvostek sign – fairly common) and spasm of the muscles of the hand on application of a BP cuff (Trousseau sign – rare) may be exam findings.

Investigations:
- Obtain serum calcium, phosphate, PTH and alkaline phosphatase
- These typically demonstrate a decreased Ca, elevated PO_4^-, decreased PTH and a normal ALP

P ≫ Hypomagnesaemia may also be a potential cause of hypocalcaemia and should be excluded.

Management

Stepwise management of hypoparathyroidism

1 **Administer IV calcium gluconate**
- If there is severe hypocalcaemia, prompt administration of IV calcium gluconate is indicated

2 **Administer calcium and vitamin D replacement**
- The mainstay of treatment outside the emergency setting is calcium and vitamin D replacement

P ≫ Recombinant PTH has recently been approved in the USA. At the moment it remains an effective but expensive treatment.

Table 4.4 *Management of hyperparathyroidism*

Type	Ca	PO$_4$	ALP	PTH	Management
Primary hyperparathyroidism	↑	↓	↑	↑/=	• Screen for MEN • **Surgical removal** of parathyroid glands is **first line** • If patients are unfit for surgery, medical therapy with alendronate and cinacalcet (calcimimetic agent that lowers calcium and PTH) may be attempted
Secondary hyperparathyroidism	↓	↑/↓	↑	↑	• **Medical therapy** is **first line** – treat underlying cause • Treatment with CKD: 1. Phosphate binders such as sevelamer 2. Calcium supplementation 3. Vit D replacement
Tertiary hyperparathyroidism	↑	↓/=	↑	↑	• **Surgical removal** of the gland is **first line** • Cinacalcet may be used as adjunctive therapy

4

4

4.4 Diabetes mellitus

Definition: diabetes mellitus refers to a metabolic condition characterised by hyperglycaemia and vascular complications secondary to an absolute deficiency or insensitivity to insulin. The Latin word *mellitus* means 'sweet' or 'containing honey'.

Aetiology/pathophysiology:
- The regulation of blood glucose level is described in *Fig. 4.15*
- There are several types of diabetes mellitus – these include type 1 and type 2 diabetes mellitus, maturity onset diabetes of the young (MODY), latent autoimmune diabetes of adulthood and gestational diabetes
- Type 1 diabetes occurs as a result of autoimmune or idiopathic destruction of pancreatic beta islet cells. This usually takes place in childhood or around the time of puberty. In some cases, auto-antibodies may be present at an early age. Type 1 diabetes, previously known as insulin-dependent diabetes mellitus (IDDM), also does not demonstrate a high genetic concordance in twin studies.
- Type 2 diabetes, on the other hand, occurs as a result of insulin resistance and typically presents in older patients. The onset of the disease is gradual and is linked to obesity, a poor diet and a sedentary lifestyle. Individuals with this disease often have a strong family history, and genetic concordance in twin studies tends to be high.

> **P** ≫ MODY refers to an inherited (autosomal dominant) form of type 2 diabetes that tends to be seen in patients below the age of 25. These patients often have a strong family history of diabetes mellitus, and therapy should be commenced as early as possible.

> **W** ≫ LADA is a variant of type 1 diabetes that occurs post-puberty, with a more gradual onset. It is often misdiagnosed as type 2 diabetes. Auto-antibody tests, lower C-peptide levels and a lower BMI may help point towards the diagnosis. Treatment with type 2 medications helps initially, but patients require insulin as definitive therapy.

- Gestational diabetes is not uncommon in pregnancy, and may predispose to foetal macrosomia or frank development of type 2 diabetes later in life

> **E** ≫ A **glucagonoma**, a tumour of the alpha cells of the pancreas, characterised by high levels of serum glucagon, disrupts the insulin–glucagon balance and may predispose to diabetes mellitus. In 70% of cases, it is accompanied by crusting and rupturing of a red vesicular rash that spreads along various parts of the body, known as a **necrolytic migratory erythema**. The only curative therapy is surgical resection.

> **P** ≫ Wolfram syndrome is a rare, genetic disorder caused by a mutation in the wolframin gene, causing endoplasmic reticulum pathology. This condition is also known as DIDMOAD, which stands for **d**iabetes **i**nsipidus, **d**iabetes **m**ellitus, **o**ptic **a**trophy and **d**eafness. There is no specific cure, and treatment involves managing the presenting diseases and their complications.

Epidemiology:
- Type 1 diabetes is thought to be triggered by infection, physical trauma, diet, environment or stress; it accounts for less than 10% of all patients with diabetes mellitus. Type 1 diabetes is most likely to be seen in Caucasians and Europeans
- Type 2 diabetes accounts for the vast majority of cases of diabetes mellitus (up to 90%); South Asian and Afro-Caribbean populations tend to be more affected
- The incidence of type 2 diabetes appears to be increasing worldwide

Clinical features:

> **E** ≫ Patients with any form of diabetes typically present with polyuria, polydipsia, lethargy and hyperglycaemia.

- Cutaneous manifestations may also be present in many cases; these include acanthosis nigricans (skin hyperpigmentation, see *Fig. 4.16*), fungal infections and necrobiosis lipoidica (a rare granulomatous erythematous disease that typically affects the shins of diabetic patients, see *Fig. 4.17*)

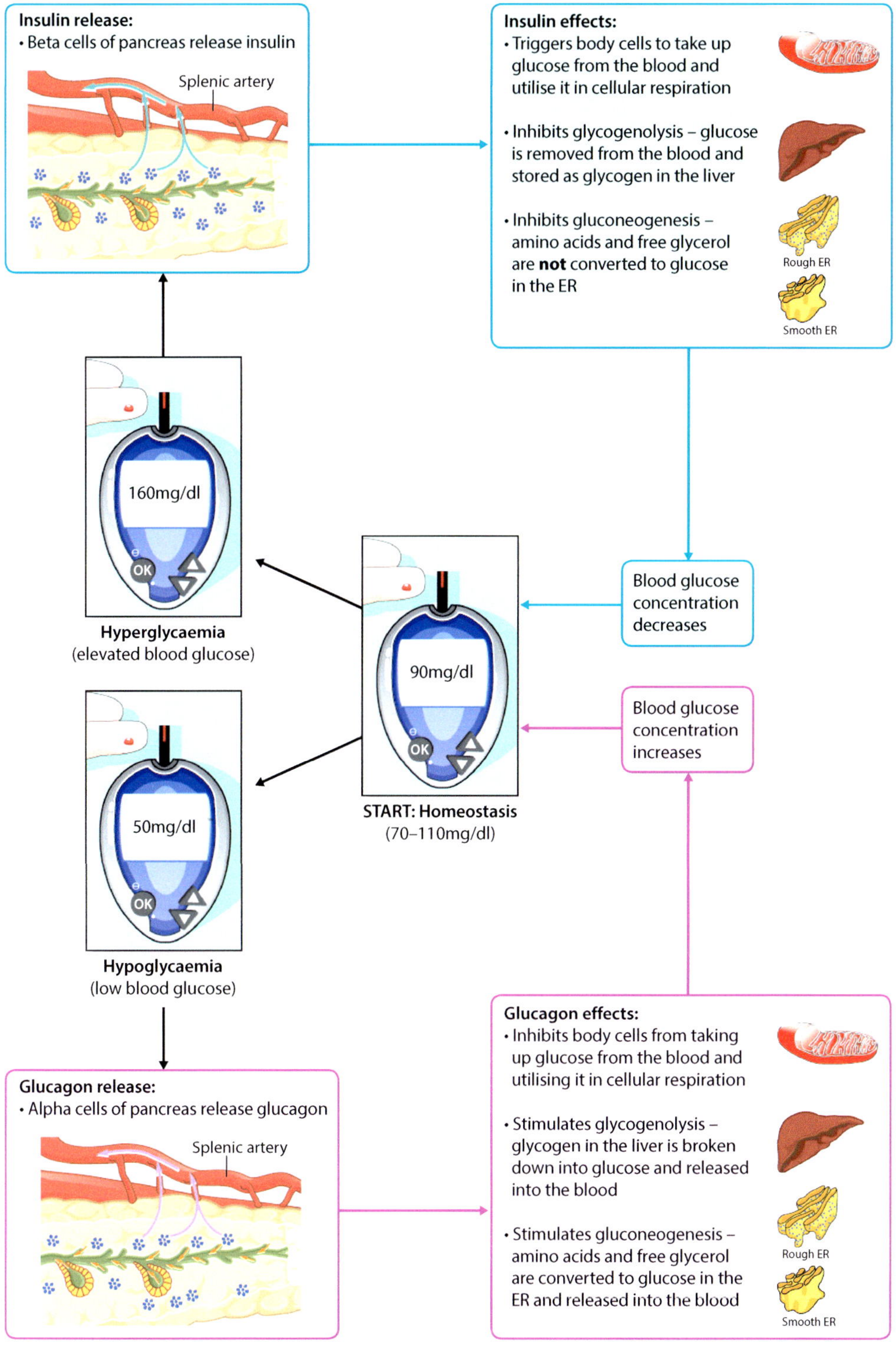

4

Insulin release:
- Beta cells of pancreas release insulin

Splenic artery

Insulin effects:
- Triggers body cells to take up glucose from the blood and utilise it in cellular respiration
- Inhibits glycogenolysis – glucose is removed from the blood and stored as glycogen in the liver
- Inhibits gluconeogenesis – amino acids and free glycerol are **not** converted to glucose in the ER

Rough ER

Smooth ER

160mg/dl

OK

Hyperglycaemia
(elevated blood glucose)

Blood glucose concentration decreases

90mg/dl

OK

START: Homeostasis
(70–110mg/dl)

Blood glucose concentration increases

50mg/dl

OK

Hypoglycaemia
(low blood glucose)

Glucagon release:
- Alpha cells of pancreas release glucagon

Splenic artery

Glucagon effects:
- Inhibits body cells from taking up glucose from the blood and utilising it in cellular respiration
- Stimulates glycogenolysis – glycogen in the liver is broken down into glucose and released into the blood
- Stimulates gluconeogenesis – amino acids and free glycerol are converted to glucose in the ER and released into the blood

Rough ER

Smooth ER

Fig. 4.15 *Regulation of blood glucose levels.*

4

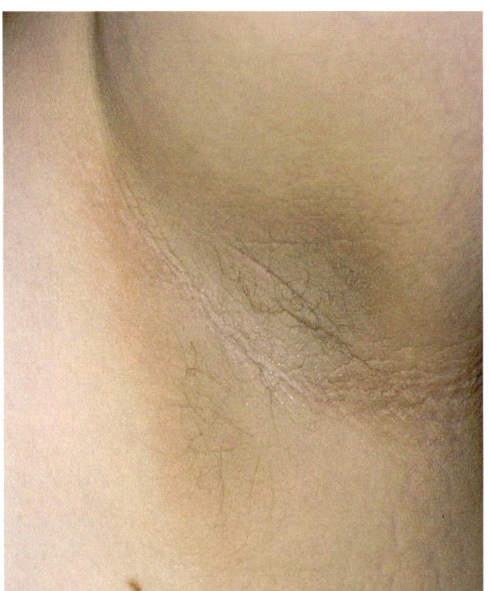

Fig. 4.16 *Acanthosis nigricans of the axilla.*

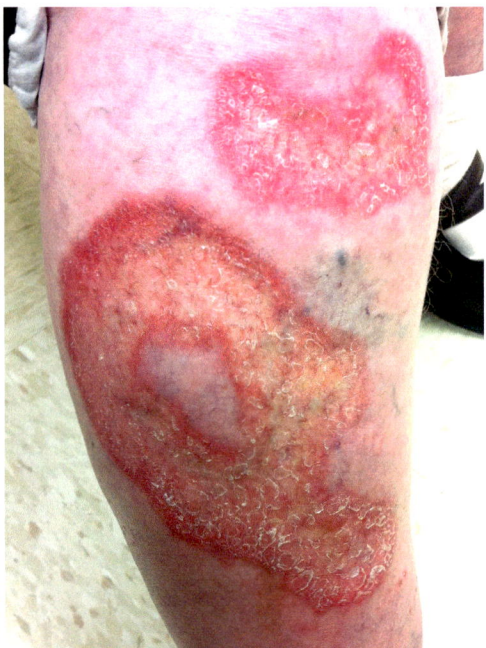

Fig. 4.17 *Necrobiosis lipoidica.*

- Patients with type 1 diabetes may also present acutely with **diabetic ketoacidosis**, (see *Section 4.4.3*)
- Patients with diabetes (particularly types 1 and 2) are at risk of microvascular complications (e.g. retinopathy, nephropathy) and macrovascular complications (e.g. stroke and myocardial infarcts)

Investigations

Stepwise plan:

Type 1 diabetes mellitus (NICE 2015, NG17, NG18)

1. **Diagnose type 1 diabetes on clinical grounds in adults presenting with hyperglycaemia, bearing in mind that people with type 1 diabetes typically (but not always) have one or more of:**
- Ketosis
- Rapid weight loss
- Age of onset below 50 years
- BMI below 25kg/m^2
- Personal and/or family history of autoimmune disease

2. **C-peptide and diabetes auto-antibodies should not specifically be measured to confirm the diagnosis**

3. **Admit for emergency treatment if clinical features of diabetic ketoacidosis (DKA) are present**
- Arrange urgent specialist referral if patients do not have ketonuria
- If ketonuria is present, arrange a same-day referral

4. **Measure urine albumin excretion (looking for microalbuminuria), renal function, serum cholesterol**
- Rule out coeliac disease if weight loss is a presenting feature

5. **Guidelines do not recommend screening for type 1 DM during the asymptomatic phase**
- There is currently no appreciable evidence that screening and early treatment prevent progression

Type 2 diabetes mellitus

1. **Assess the patient for symptoms**
- Diagnosing type 2 DM requires an assessment of the patient, considering whether they are symptomatic or asymptomatic

2. **Evaluate blood pressure, risk factors, family history, lipid levels and consider referrals for multi-disciplinary team management**
- Endocrinologist, cardiologist, ophthalmologist, specialist nurse, dietitian and podiatrist

Confirming diabetes mellitus (WHO)

Because of the nature of the clinical course of the disease, patients with type 2 diabetes are **often**

diagnosed on routine screening, whereas young people with type 1 diabetes **are likely to present with symptoms**.

The following parameters are therefore **more helpful in confirming a diagnosis of type 2 DM**, although the criteria may also be applied to type 1 DM.

WHO criteria for diagnosing diabetes (2006, 2011)

If the patient is **symptomatic** (i.e. polydipsia, polyuria and unexplained weight loss in type 1 diabetics):

1. A **random** venous plasma glucose concentration ≥11.1mmol/L **or** a fasting plasma glucose concentration ≥7.0mmol/L
2. **Or** a 2-hour plasma glucose concentration ≥11.1mmol/L **2 hours after** 75g anhydrous glucose in an oral glucose tolerance test (OGTT)
3. Glycated haemoglobin (HbA1c) may also be used in diagnosing diabetes mellitus; a HbA1c of ≥48mmol/mol (6.5%) is diagnostic

If the patient is **asymptomatic**, the above criteria must be **applied on two separate occasions**.

> E ≫ Note that a HbA1c of less than 48mmol/mol (6.5%) does not exclude DM, and in certain cases (e.g. haemoglobinopathies such as sickle cell disease and diseases such as HIV) HbA1c levels are unreliable in clinching the diagnosis.

Impaired fasting glucose (IFG)

Impaired fasting glucose (**note that impaired fasting glucose and impaired glucose tolerance are known as 'prediabetes' in layman's terms**) refers to the clinical state in which the fasting blood sugar levels are reproducibly elevated, but not high enough to be classed as frank diabetes. Patients with IFG have some degree of insulin resistance and are at risk for cardiovascular complications.

> **WHO criteria: fasting plasma glucose level from 6.1mmol/L to 6.9mmol/L**

Impaired glucose tolerance (IGT)

Impaired glucose tolerance presents a much greater risk, in terms of developing type 2 DM and experiencing cardiovascular complications, than IFG.

> **WHO criteria: 2-hour glucose levels between 7.8 and 11.0mmol/L after a 75g OGTT**

Management

> **Stepwise management of type 1 diabetes**

1 Offer lifestyle advice:
- Advise patients about the importance of diet and regular exercise, as well as the importance of ensuring that they have insulin available at all times

2 Treat with insulin
- Partner with patient to achieve treatment goals and to ensure best possible outcome (see *Section 4.4.1* for further information on insulin regimens)

3 Review patient's glycaemic control annually
- A HbA1c of <48mmol/mol (<6.5%) is ideal

4 Patients should also be followed up for:
- Eye complications (diabetic retinopathy)
- Diabetic neuropathy and diabetic foot
- Lipid panel and blood pressure
- Review of injection sites, observing for lipoatrophy

Table 4.5 *Diabetes diagnostic summary*

	Normal	IFG prediabetes	IGT prediabetes	Diabetes mellitus
Fasting plasma glucose	<6.1mmol/L	6.1–6.9mmol/L		≥7.0mmol/L (symptomatic, otherwise needs 2 measurements)
After 75g OGTT	<7.8mmol/L		7.8–11mmol/L	>11.1mmol/L (symptomatic, otherwise needs 2 measurements)
Random plasma glucose				>11.1mmol/L (symptomatic, otherwise needs 2 measurements)
HbA1c		42–47mmol/mol (6.0–6.4%)	42–47mmol/mol (6.0–6.4%)	>48mmol/mol (6.5%)

Stepwise management of type 2 diabetes (NICE 2015, NG28)

The NICE guidelines have recently been updated to reflect several changes in the management of type 2 DM. The guidelines no longer espouse strict targets. Instead, the focus is now on **individualised care and flexibility**.

1 Adopt an individualised care plan
- The care plan must be tailored to the needs and circumstances of the patient, taking into consideration personal preferences, comorbidities and polypharmacy

2 Offer lifestyle advice
- Refer patients to dietitians for individualised attention and for dietary guidance
- Set a target for weight loss of 5–10% of body weight if the patient is obese
- NICE advises against the consumption of food specifically marketed to diabetics
- Advise patients to reduce overall glycaemic load and carbohydrate consumption

3 Take measures to control blood pressure
- Blood pressure targets for diabetics are 140/90 and 130/80 if end organ damage is present (retinopathy, nephropathy, cerebrovascular accidents, etc.)
- ACE inhibitors are used first line in diabetics
- Do not combine ACE inhibitors and ARBs to treat hypertension
- Follow the hypertension treatment guidance given in *Chapter 1* (see *Section 1.4*) to optimise blood pressure control
- Do not offer antiplatelet therapy to diabetics unless cardiovascular complications have occurred. Statins should only be used for primary prevention (NICE recommends atorvastatin 20mg) if QRISK2 score >10%
- NICE recommends atorvastatin 80mg to patients for secondary prevention of cardiovascular disease

4 Discuss and agree HBA1c targets with individual patients
- NICE advises that we should offer patients encouragement and support to meet those targets. In adults with type 2 diabetes, measure HbA1c levels at:
  - 3–6 monthly intervals (tailored to individual needs), until the HbA1c is stable on unchanging therapy
  - 6-monthly intervals once the HbA1c level and blood glucose lowering therapy are stable

5 Follow guidelines for targets, including:
- Lifestyle control only: 48mmol/mol (6.5%)
- Lifestyle and metformin only: 48mmol/mol (6.5%)
- Lifestyle and a drug with associated hypoglycaemia, e.g. a sulphonylurea: 53mmol/mol (7.0%)
- If HbA1c reaches 58mmol/mol (7.5%) on a lifestyle and a single drug, reinforce lifestyle advice and aim for 53mmol/mol (7.0%)
- Do keep in mind that targets should be considered on a case by case basis

6 Start medication
- Metformin is the first-line treatment

> **E** » Metformin is contraindicated in renal disease. It may also cause GI upset and worsen lactic acidosis.

- Two major pathways exist in terms of drug therapy, depending whether or not metformin is tolerated
- If metformin is **tolerated**:
  - Reinforce **lifestyle change** and titrate dose of metformin
  - If HbA1c reaches 58mmol/mol (7.5%), a combination of metformin and a second agent may be used. Combinations include:
    - Metformin + pioglitazone
    - Metformin + sulphonylurea
    - Metformin + gliptin
    - Metformin + SGLT-2 inhibitor
  - If control is inadequate, and HbA1C remains at 58mmol/mol (7.5%) or higher, offer a third agent as part of triple therapy, or consider the use of insulin
- If metformin is **contraindicated or not tolerated**:
  - Reinforce lifestyle changes, and start initial therapy if HbA1C reaches 48mmol/mol (6.5%) on lifestyle modification alone
  - Initial therapy includes pioglitazone, a sulphonylurea or a gliptin first line if metformin is contraindicated
  - If the HbA1c remains at 58mmol/mol (7.5%), add a second medication
  - If control remains inadequate, offer insulin for better control

P ▶▶ The evidence suggests that low-carbohydrate (and, in some cases, ketogenic) diets may improve diabetic control more effectively than reduced-calorie diets. But bear in mind that both strategies are effective for weight loss, and that patient adherence to lifestyle changes is a far more effective approach than dietary change that produces a greater benefit but is far less sustainable.

E ▶▶ Medications used in diabetes mellitus
- Metformin
  - This is a biguanide, which exerts its effect by increasing insulin sensitivity
  - Offer standard release initially, consider modified release if standard release is not tolerated
  - Has a lower incidence of hypoglycaemia; not particularly associated with weight gain
  - Major side effect is GI disturbance
  - Review drug if eGFR <45ml/min/1.73^2, **stop metformin** if eGFR <30ml/min/1.73^2
- Sulphonylureas
  - These act by stimulating islet cells
  - The main side effects of sulphonylureas are weight gain and hypoglycaemia
  - Short-acting agents (e.g. gliclazide) are preferable to long-acting agents (e.g. glibenclamide) in the elderly
- Thiazolidinediones
  - Pioglitazone
  - PPAR gamma agonist
  - Side effects of pioglitazone include weight gain, liver dysfunction and oedema. These are contraindicated in heart failure
  - Pioglitazone used for longer than a year may increase the risk of **bladder cancer**
  - NICE recommends only continuing the medication if there is a >0.5% decrease in HbA1c in 6 months
  - These have recently fallen out of favour due to their adverse side effect profile
- DPP-4 inhibitors (gliptins)
  - Improve insulin secretion and inhibit glucagon
- GLP-1 agonists (e.g. exenatide)
  - Subcutaneous therapy, once weekly
  - May cause GI upset or pancreatitis

- SGLT-2 inhibitors
  - e.g. canagliflozin and empagliflozin
  - Inhibit renal reabsorption of glucose in the PCT
  - Should not be prescribed in patients with frequent UTIs or genital candidiasis.

W ▶▶ Patients who fast, e.g. those attempting to lose weight via methods such as intermittent fasting, or Muslim patients during Ramadan, should be offered appropriate advice if they have diabetes mellitus.
- Patients should be advised to monitor glucose
- If patients are on metformin, guidance recommends splitting the dose, taking a smaller dose in the morning and a larger dose at night
- Switch oral hypoglycaemic medications to once-daily at night-time.

4.4.1 Insulin regimens

Insulin prescriptions should be tailored to each individual patient according to their needs and lifestyle preferences. Patients and their partners and families should be advised appropriately.

Human insulin, produced by recombinant DNA technology, is used in preference to animal insulin. Insulin may be broadly classified in terms of 1) duration of action and 2) type of regimen (see *Fig. 4.18*).

W ▶▶ Insulin injections are given subcutaneously and are rotationally injected at various sites in the body. These include (but are not limited to) the arms, quadriceps, abdomen and gluteal region. Disposable pens are available, and the needle should be changed daily.

Lipodystrophy (degeneration of the adipose tissue) is a complication of insulin injection use, and may be observed if one site is repeatedly injected. Adequate rotation of injection sites can help minimise the risk, and patients should be advised to administer insulin in this way.

4

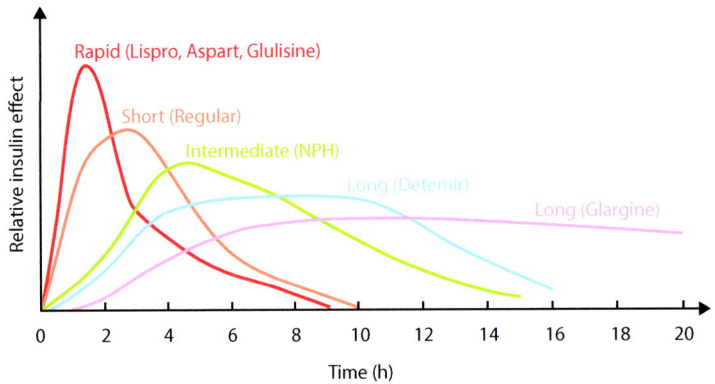

Fig. 4.18 *Types of insulin and their duration of action.*

4

Types of insulin
- **Short-acting**
  - Aims to mimic natural insulin release by the body around mealtime
  - Give 15–30 minutes before meals
  - Types include **soluble insulin** or **rapid-acting** analogues
  - Can be given IV for emergencies; rapid-acting analogues act within 15 minutes
  - Peak onset between 2 and 4 hours
- **Intermediate-acting**
  - Mimics basal insulin release throughout the day
  - Isophane insulin recommended by NICE
  - Peak onset 4–10 hours
- **Long-acting**
  - Insulin glargine or detemir
  - Can be given in a once-daily regimen at bedtime
- **Biphasic preparation**
  - Premixed solution containing short-acting insulin (which shuttles glucose from meals) and an intermediate-acting insulin (providing basal cover)

Regimens
A variety of regimens may be used, depending on the patient's needs.
- **Once a day**
  - Usually long-acting agents before bedtime
  - Suitable for type 2 diabetics (regimen of choice after oral therapy) or if dependent on carers
- **Twice a day**
  - Biphasic insulin given before morning and evening meal
  - Steady control may be difficult; may predispose to fasting hyperglycaemia or nocturnal hypoglycaemia
- **Basal bolus**
  - Long or intermediate insulin at bedtime for overnight control
  - Short-acting insulin at mealtimes

- **Continuous subcutaneous insulin infusion (CSII)/insulin pump**
  - Adjustable rate given by an indwelling catheter worn under clothes
  - Predictable glucose levels, used for type 1 diabetics who are children or with erratic lifestyles and recurrent hypoglycaemic episodes
  - Not recommended for type 2 diabetics

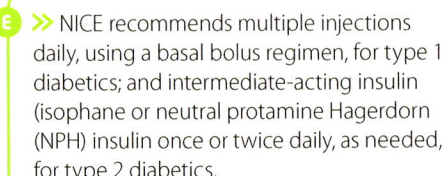 **E** ➤➤ NICE recommends multiple injections daily, using a basal bolus regimen, for type 1 diabetics; and intermediate-acting insulin (isophane or neutral protamine Hagerdorn (NPH) insulin once or twice daily, as needed, for type 2 diabetics.

P ➤➤ Two causes of morning hyperglycaemia in diabetics

Dawn phenomenon
- Abnormal early-morning hyperglycaemia (usually type 1 diabetics)
- Caused by release of hormones (such as GH, cortisol and glucagon) during sleep, which cause glucose release from the liver
- Reflects possible inadequacy of night-time insulin dosage
- Patients should avoid high-carbohydrate meals at night

Somogyi effect
- Similarly, if a patient does not eat enough at night, nocturnal hypoglycaemia causes hormone release to increase glucose levels
- In diabetics, this may reflect a higher than required dose of insulin the previous night, which contributes to nocturnal hypoglycaemia.

4.4.2 Complications of diabetes mellitus

There are numerous complications associated with diabetes mellitus. Ensuring **tight glycaemic control** will help reduce these complications, particularly those that are microvascular in nature. Lifestyle advice should be continually reinforced, while also providing support for smoking cessation and lipid management.

Acute complications
- DKA (see *Section 4.4.3*)
- Hyperosmolar hyperglycaemic state (HHS/HONK) (see *Section 4.4.4*)
- Hypoglycaemia (see *Section 4.4.5*)

Gastroparesis
NICE (2015, NG28) recommends considering a diagnosis of gastroparesis in adults with type 2 diabetes if they have erratic blood glucose control or unexplained gastric bloating or vomiting. **Metoclopramide** or **domperidone** are recommended agents.

Cardiovascular complications
Patients with diabetes are much more likely to experience cardiovascular and cerebrovascular events (e.g. ACS, angina, peripheral arterial disease and stroke – see *Chapter 1* and *Chapter 5*).

Patients with diabetes are **four** times more likely to have an MI, and **twice as likely** to have a stroke. They are also more likely to have peripheral vascular disease.

P ≫ Erectile dysfunction is a common complication associated with diabetes mellitus and this is important to keep in mind, as treatment can be offered.

Diabetic nephropathy
Diabetic nephropathy comes on insidiously, and may predispose to papillary necrosis, renal failure and UTI.

Nephropathy may be diffuse or nodular, with the latter having **Kimmelstein–Wilson** lesions on microscopy (PIC).

Monitor **annually** for:
- Microalbuminuria
  - Small increase in albumin excretion by the kidneys
  - Independent risk factor for complications and all-cause mortality
  - Use an early morning albumin:creatinine ratio (ACR) to assess
    - ACR >2.5 in men
    - ACR >3.5 in women

- Proteinuria
  - ACR ≥30mg/mmol
  - If chronic kidney disease is present, or if ACR >70mg/mmol, refer for specialist assessment

Manage by optimising risk factors, and offer **ACE inhibitor therapy** to all patients with nephropathy, proteinuria and microalbuminuria, and those who are type 1 diabetics.

Diabetic eye disease

W ≫ The exact pathogenesis is incompletely understood, but is thought to occur as sequelae to microvascular retinal disease. This in turn causes retinal ischaemia and new vessel formation (probably driven by vascular endothelial growth factor (VEGF) production).

E ≫ Diabetic eye disease is the most common cause of blindness in developed nations.

May result in:
- **Retinopathy (treat with photocoagulation)**
  - Non-proliferative
    - (Mild)
      - ≥1 microaneurysm
    - (Moderate)
      - Microaneurysms, blot haemorrhages and hard exudates with cotton wool spots and venous beading/looping
    - (Severe)
      - Widespread blot haemorrhages, microaneurysms and venous beading
      - Severe intraretinal microvascular abnormalities
  - Proliferative retinopathy (see *Fig. 4.19*)
    - Neovascularisation
    - More common in type 1 diabetics
- **Maculopathy**
  - Decrease in visual acuity
  - If **clinically significant**, macular oedema (see *Fig. 4.20*), retinal thickening and hard exudates within one disc width of the macula are present
- **Cataracts**
- **Rubeosis iridis and glaucoma**

P ≫ Rubeosis iridis refers to neovascularisation that occurs in severe ischaemia, causing vessels to proliferate over the iris, making it appear red. If they cause obstruction of aqueous drainage, this may lead to glaucoma.

4

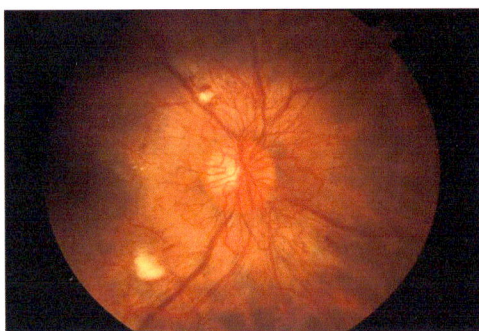

Fig. 4.19 *Proliferative retinopathy.*

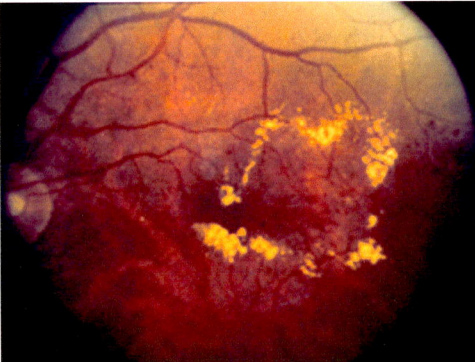

Fig. 4.20 *Macular oedema.*

Diabetic neuropathy

Diabetic neuropathy is a major cause of foot ulcer development and the most common cause of peripheral neuropathy worldwide.

> **W** ≫ Microvascular damage and ischaemia to the vasa vasorum (blood vessels that supply the nerves) and toxic metabolite accumulation are implicated in its development.

> **E** ≫ NICE recommends choosing between amitriptyline, duloxetine, gabapentin or pregabalin as therapy for neuropathic pain.

May present with:
- **Peripheral sensorimotor neuropathy**
  - Classic glove and stocking distribution
  - Loss of ankle reflexes; and, later, knee reflexes
- **Painful neuritis**
- **Diabetic amyotrophy**
  - Severe proximal lower limb muscle weakness and muscle wasting

- **Autonomic neuropathy**
  - Postural hypotension
  - Asymptomatic myocardial ischaemia (**silent MI**)
  - Gastroparesis
  - Urinary incontinence
- **Mononeuropathy**
  - Cranial nerves III, IV and VI are common
  - Mononeuritis multiplex (more than one nerve sometimes affected)

Diabetic foot care

Loss of sensory input causes patients to be less careful about foot trauma. In addition, peripheral vascular disease may lead to ischaemia. Both vascular disease and neuropathy may cause foot disease and ulcers (see *Fig. 4.21*).

Once damage occurs, healing also is made more difficult, both intrinsically because of vascular disease, and extrinsically because of pathogens, e.g. leading to osteomyelitis in complicated cases.
- Feet may be painful or deformed (Charcot joint)
- Diabetic neuropathic ulcers are likely to be painless and located on the **plantar** surface of the foot

> **Stepwise management of diabetic foot disease**
>
> 1 **Daily foot inspection**
>
> 2 **Treat infection**
>   - Usually with long-term antibiotics
>
> 3 **Manage neuropathy**
>
> 4 **Assess vascular status**

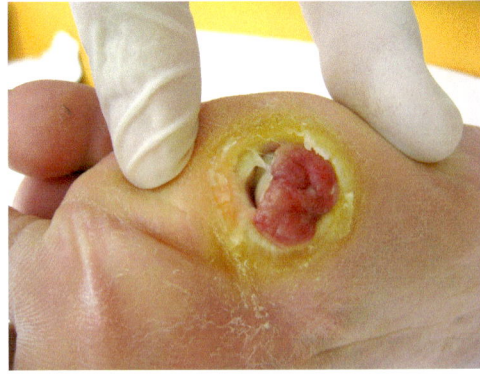

Fig. 4.21 *Diabetic foot ulcer.*

4.4.3 Diabetic ketoacidosis (DKA)

Definition: DKA is a medical emergency secondary to absolute insulin deficiency or resistance, presenting with a triad of hyperglycaemia, ketonaemia and acidaemia.

Epidemiology:

- More commonly seen in the younger and undiagnosed patient groups

Aetiology/pathophysiology:

- Several trigger factors may provoke an episode of DKA; these include poor adherence to treatment, infection, trauma, illness, cardiovascular or cerebrovascular incidents

Clinical features:

- Rapid onset (symptoms usually present within 24 hours)
- Patients have abdominal pain and vomiting with a 'fruity' breath secondary to ketosis
- Often have reduced level of consciousness with Kussmaul respiration (deep, laboured breathing)

Investigations

Various guidelines differ on diagnostic criteria, but as a general rule:

1. **Acidosis**: pH <7.3
2. **Hyperglycaemia**: glucose >11.1mmol/L or known diabetes
3. **Ketonaemia**: ketones >3mmol or ++ on dipstick
4. In addition, obtain FBC, U&Es, blood cultures, lactate and a CXR to screen for presence of infection

Management

Management of DKA involves correction of hyperglycaemia, return of normal acid–base balance, and restoring electrolyte balance, particularly with regard to potassium and avoiding hypoglycaemia.

> **Stepwise management of diabetic ketoacidosis**

1   Start a fluid replacement regimen

- **IV 0.9% sodium chlorine 1L for the first hour**, 1L for the next two, the following two, the subsequent four and six hours

E ≫ A helpful way to remember the fluid replacement regimen is to initially resuscitate with 1L for the first one hour, then remember it as if it were a locker code –122446, ergo, 1L for the subsequent 2, then 2, then 4, then 4, then 6 hours each. This is a sample regimen for quick reference. The goal is fluid replacement to achieve normalisation of corrected sodium levels. When this occurs, one should replace fluids at 0.45% normal saline and at a slower infusion rate.

2   Administer insulin safely

- To reduce hyperglycaemia, while avoiding potential hypoglycaemia and hypokalaemia

3   Add 50 units Actrapid insulin to 50ml 0.9% sodium chloride

- Then infuse, using a syringe driver

4   Administer IV Actrapid insulin at 0.1 units/kg bodyweight/hour

- If no bodyweight is obtainable, 6 units is recommended per hour
- **Switch to 3 units per hour after blood glucose is ≤14mmol/L**

5   Administer potassium replacement

>5.5mmol/L	No replacement indicated
3.5–5.5mmol/L	40mmol/L (maintain K^+ levels between 4.0 and 5.5)
<3.5	Request senior assistance (HDU/ITU)

W ≫ Insulin shuttles potassium back into cells, and hypokalaemia may occur as a result. Administration of potassium replacement is therefore an important treatment goal.

6   Monitor sodium levels

- **When plasma glucose reaches 14mmol/L, offer 5% dextrose alongside 0.9% saline to prevent hypoglycaemia**

7   Set treatment goals

- Monitor venous blood gas 2-hourly, electrolytes 4-hourly, glucose and ketones hourly
- Aims:
  - Decrease serum ketones <0.5mmol/L per hour
  - Decrease capillary blood glucose by 3mmol/L per hour
  - Increase bicarbonate by 3mmol/L per hour
  - Maintain K^+ between 4.0 and 5.5mmol/L

P ≫ If the pH is <6.9, consider IV administration of sodium bicarbonate.

8   Consider prescribing broad-spectrum antibiotics if an infective aetiology is suspected

9   Resolution:

- Maintain on sliding scale insulin if not eating; transfer to subcutaneous insulin if eating and drinking

- Ensure administration of long-acting insulin the night before transferring to subcutaneous insulin
- Ensure that subcutaneous insulin is started at least 30 minutes before stopping IV insulin (short half-life of 2.5 mins)
- Educate patient about condition and advise preventative measures

4.4.4 Hyperosmolar hyperglycaemic state (HHS)

Definition: also known as hyperosmolar hyperglycaemic non-ketotic coma (HONK), this condition involves:

1. Dehydration and profound hyperglycaemia (>33.3mmol/L)
2. Hyperosmolality (≥320mmol/kg)
3. Hypovolaemia in the absence of significant ketoacidosis

> **E** ≫ Mortality rates in HONK are much higher than those of DKA. Unlike DKA, however, pH usually remains above 7.3, and ketones are generally absent/low.

Aetiology/pathophysiology:

- Typically occurs as a complication of type 2 diabetes, often precipitated by a disease state or concomitant illness (e.g. MI, CVA, infection or poor adherence to diabetic medication)
- May also occur as a first presentation of diabetes mellitus

Clinical features:

- Patients typically have muscle cramps and may present with confusion
- They usually have profound weakness, weight loss, polydipsia and polyuria in the time span leading up to admission
- Despite the nomenclature, patients rarely present in a comatose state on admission

> **P** ≫ [Serum plasma osmolality = 2 (Na + K) + urea + glucose]
>
> From the above equation, we can deduce that hyperglycaemia causes a hyperosmolar state, which results in an osmotic shift of water into the intravascular compartment. The end result is intracellular dehydration. Ketosis does not occur as basal insulin secretion is enough to prevent ketogenesis, yet insufficient to lower blood glucose levels.

Investigations

> **Stepwise plan:**

1 Measure blood glucose
- Blood glucose often shows marked hyperglycaemia (>33mmol/L)

2 Check for glycosuria
- Urine dipstick will demonstrate glycosuria with low or absent ketones

3 Serum osmolality (will be markedly elevated)

4 Look for a precipitating cause
- Obtain FBC, U&Es, LFTs, CXR, ECG, troponin, blood cultures

Management

The aims of treatment are to restore fluid, electrolyte and acid–base balance, and determine if there is an underlying precipitating event. In many cases, step-up care to ITU is warranted.

> **Stepwise management of hyperosmolar hyperglycaemic states**

1 Monitor osmolality
- In order to assess response to treatment

2 IV 0.9% sodium chloride initially
- Switch to 10% dextrose when blood glucose falls below 15mmol/L

3 IV Actrapid insulin should be started at a lower dose (0.05 units/kg bodyweight or 3 units/hr

4 Potassium replacement:

>5.5mmol/L	No replacement indicated
3.5–5.5mmol/L	40mmol/L (maintain K$^+$ levels between 4.0 and 5.5)
<3.5	Request senior assistance

5 Look for and treat any underlying precipitants

6 Resolution:
- Glucose <16.7mmol/L
- Plasma osmolality <315mmol/kg
- Improvement in mental status and vital signs
- Remember to administer subcutaneous insulin before weaning the patient off IV insulin to allow for effective insulin cover

4.4.5 Hypoglycaemia

Hypoglycaemia refers to a clinical state in which low plasma glucose occurs (<3.0mmol/L). It has three criteria (the Whipple triad) for diagnosis:

1. Hypoglycaemia
2. Symptoms indicative of hypoglycaemia
3. Resolution of symptoms after treating hypoglycaemia

Symptoms typically exist on a spectrum, with symptoms such as giddiness, sweating, hunger and tingling typically predominating at a glucose level of 2.5–4.0mmol/L, and more neurological symptoms predominating at a blood glucose level of <2.5mmol/L, such as confusion, drowsiness and seizures.

P ≫ An **insulinoma**, a **benign** tumour of pancreatic beta cells, has suboptimal secretion of insulin in response to glucose, and may cause a fasting hypoglycaemia. This may be detected with elevated insulin, proinsulin and C-peptide levels in the setting of hypoglycaemia.

Patients with suspected insulinoma should undergo a 72-hour fast as a first-line treatment. Insulin levels should fall as the patient becomes hypoglycaemic, but in insulinomas the level stays the same or is increased compared to baseline. In contrast, patients with high insulin and low C-peptide are likely to have taken exogenous insulin, as insulin from outside the body does not have C-peptide present. Surgery for insulinoma is curative.

Management

Measure plasma glucose levels, and assess response to treatment. Further investigations include measurement of insulin, proinsulin and C-peptide, as well as a 72-hour fast (gold standard for diagnosis of insulinoma). If the patient is diabetic, assessing glucose control may help prevent further complications in the future.

Stepwise management of hypoglycaemia

1. **If patient is alert, offer an oral or liquid source of glucose**
   - e.g. a sugary drink or a meal

2. **If the patient is drowsy but has an intact swallow, buccal Glucogel may be offered**

3. **If the patient is unconscious, or has impaired swallow, obtain prompt IV access and treat with 125ml of 20% dextrose or 250ml of 10% dextrose**
   - Alternatively, **1mg of glucagon** may be used as an intramuscular injection

E ≫ Note that glucagon has poor efficacy in patients with hypoglycaemia who also have a background of liver disease or alcohol excess. In addition, it is important to provide oral carbohydrate intake within 30 minutes of glucagon administration to ensure that hypoglycaemia does not recur.

4.5 The adrenal gland

The adrenal glands, with their rich vascular supply, have both gland and neuroendocrine tissues in their **cortex** and **medulla** (see *Fig. 4.22*). The adrenal cortex is divided into three major regions – the zona glomerulosa, zona fasciculata and zona reticularis, all of which secrete particular hormones.

The main mineralocorticoid produced by the zona glomerulosa is aldosterone. Aldosterone is involved in the regulation of sodium and potassium in the body, and plays an important role in the renin–angiotensin–aldosterone system (see *Chapter 7*). The zona fasciculata produces glucocorticoids, which mainly downregulate the immune system to reduce inflammation, and the zona reticularis primarily

produces a **small amount** of androgens (the bulk is produced by the gonads).

The adrenal medulla, on the other hand, is composed of neuroendocrine tissue that secretes the catecholamines epinephrine and norepinephrine. These cause peripheral vasoconstriction and stimulate breakdown of liver glycogen, increasing glucose levels in response to stress.

4.5.1 Cushing syndrome

Definition: Cushing syndrome refers to a clinical state in which there is pathological overproduction of cortisol.

4

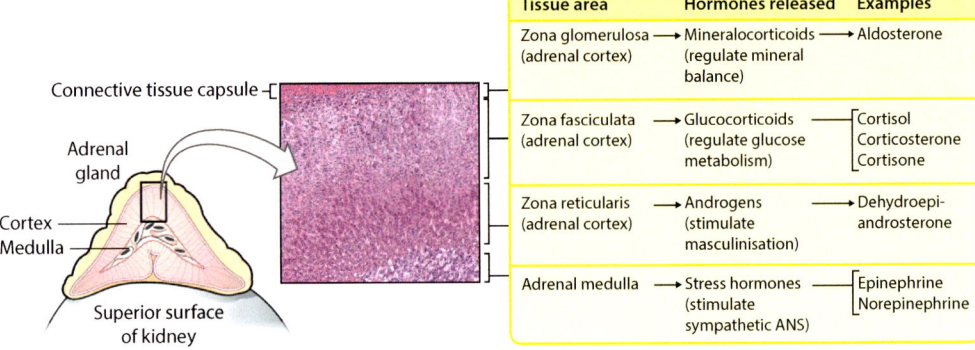

Connective tissue capsule

Adrenal gland

Cortex
Medulla

Superior surface
of kidney

Tissue area	Hormones released	Examples
Zona glomerulosa (adrenal cortex)	→ Mineralocorticoids (regulate mineral balance)	→ Aldosterone
Zona fasciculata (adrenal cortex)	→ Glucocorticoids (regulate glucose metabolism)	Cortisol Corticosterone Cortisone
Zona reticularis (adrenal cortex)	→ Androgens (stimulate masculinisation)	→ Dehydroepi-androsterone
Adrenal medulla	→ Stress hormones (stimulate sympathetic ANS)	Epinephrine Norepinephrine

Fig. 4.22 The adrenal gland.

Epidemiology:
- The condition is fairly uncommon, with a greater incidence in patients with concomitant diabetes, hypertension or osteoporosis
- It is more commonly seen in women

Aetiology/pathophysiology:

E ≫ **Cushing disease**, characterised by a **pituitary adenoma** secreting an excess amount of ACTH, accounts for up to 80% of cases and is the most common cause, apart from steroid therapy.

- Approximately 10% of cases are caused by a cortisol-secreting adrenal adenoma, and less than 1% are caused by an adrenal carcinoma
- Recall that ACTH-secreting tumours may also be a cause of Cushing syndrome (most often associated with small cell lung cancer)

Clinical features:

P ≫ Apart from the classic features of Cushing disease (e.g. suprascapular fat pads, abdominal striae, depression, truncal obesity and easy bruising), an iatrogenic cause, particularly inadequately titrated glucocorticoid medication, may contribute to symptoms.

- Cushing syndrome is a multi-system condition and, as such, has a vast array of presentations (see *Fig. 4.23*)

Investigations
When investigating Cushing syndrome, first confirm the diagnosis, and second localise the source of the disease.

Stepwise plan:

1 **Confirm Cushing syndrome, primarily using:**
- **1mg overnight dexamethasone suppression test**
  - Given at 11pm, cortisol levels are measured at 8am
  - Normally, cortisol will be suppressed (<100nmol/L)
  - Failure to suppress indicates Cushing syndrome of **any aetiology**
- **OR 24h free urinary cortisol**, ideally three collections
  - Less convenient than overnight dexamethasone suppression testing

W ≫ Dexamethasone, a steroid hormone, is used as a suppressive agent and provides negative feedback to the pituitary gland to decrease ACTH production. A patient with Cushing syndrome will fail to suppress cortisol, and the levels will remain elevated in the morning. A higher dose (8mg) can suppress cortisol if the source of overproduction is the pituitary, thus distinguishing between a pituitary adenoma (Cushing disease) and an ectopic source.

2 **Localise the lesion, primarily using:**
- ACTH levels
  - If low, adrenal pathology is likely

E ≫ In adrenal tumours, ACTH is low, and cortisol is high. In ectopic ACTH, both ACTH and cortisol are high.

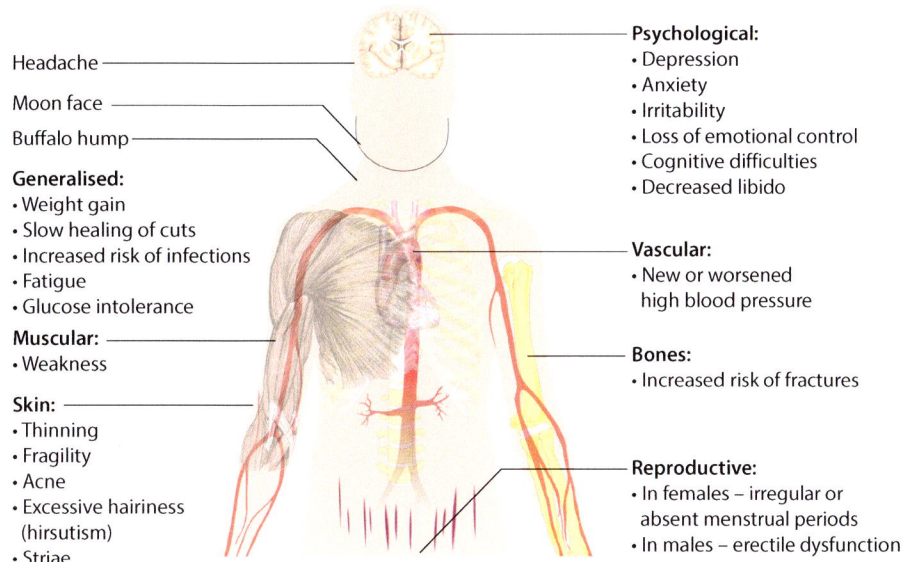

Headache

Moon face

Buffalo hump

Generalised:
• Weight gain
• Slow healing of cuts
• Increased risk of infections
• Fatigue
• Glucose intolerance

Muscular:
• Weakness

Skin:
• Thinning
• Fragility
• Acne
• Excessive hairiness
  (hirsutism)
• Striae

Psychological:
• Depression
• Anxiety
• Irritability
• Loss of emotional control
• Cognitive difficulties
• Decreased libido

Vascular:
• New or worsened
  high blood pressure

Bones:
• Increased risk of fractures

Reproductive:
• In females – irregular or
  absent menstrual periods
• In males – erectile dysfunction

Fig. 4.23 *Signs and symptoms of Cushing syndrome.*

• If high:
  – 8mg high-dose dexamethasone suppression test
  – If there is >50% suppression, the diagnosis is Cushing disease (pituitary source)
  – If there is <50% suppression, an ectopic ACTH-secreting tumour is more likely

Management

Stepwise management of Cushing syndrome

1 If the cause is a pituitary adenoma (Cushing disease)
• Offer **trans-sphenoidal surgical resection first line** and glucocorticoid support

2 If the cause is an ectopic tumour, such as an adrenal adenoma, or bilateral adrenal hyperplasia
• **Surgical adrenalectomy is the first-line treatment,** with adequate glucocorticoid support postoperatively

3 Lastly, mifepristone, a steroidogenesis inhibitor, may be used pre-operatively or in cases where a patient is unwilling or unable to go through with surgery
• Medical therapy is far less effective, however, and surgical therapy remains the first-line treatment in the majority of cases

P ≫ Nelson syndrome refers to the development of a large, corticotrophic pituitary adenoma that occurs after bilateral adrenalectomy. While rare, this condition is not uncommon in patients undergoing bilateral removal of their adrenal glands.

E ≫ Remember to assess and treat complications of Cushing syndrome, e.g. optimising risk factors, monitoring steroid doses, mood disorders and osteoporosis.

4.5.2 Adrenal insufficiency (Addison disease)

Definition: adrenal insufficiency refers to the underproduction of hormones of the adrenal cortex, particularly mineralocorticoids and glucocorticoids.

Epidemiology:
• Approximately 5 million cases worldwide annually

Aetiology/pathophysiology:
Classically divided into primary adrenal insufficiency (Addison disease), and secondary adrenal insufficiency.
• Primary insufficiency (Addison's) refers to the inability of the adrenal glands to produce hormones, usually secondary to autoimmune destruction of the gland

4

- Secondary insufficiency usually occurs as a result of pituitary or hypothalamic failure

E ≫ Autoimmunity is the most common cause of Addison disease in the developed world, but tuberculosis is the most common cause worldwide. The use of steroid medication is the most common cause of secondary insufficiency.

Clinical features:
- Adrenal insufficiency may present acutely or in a chronic form.
- Acute presentations include an addisonian crisis, in which a patient, usually with known Addison disease or on long-term steroid medications, has a precipitating event (e.g. illness, surgery, infection) which causes an increase in the demand for mineralocorticoids and glucocorticoids. These patients present with clinical features of shock and hypoglycaemia. **Treatment is with high-dose IV hydrocortisone**.

P ≫ Waterhouse–Friderichsen syndrome is also another cause of acute adrenal insufficiency, caused by bilateral adrenal haemorrhage usually secondary to a meningococcal infection.

- Symptoms of chronic adrenal insufficiency include fatigue, weight loss and depression, and may be insidious
- Addison disease also has an association with other autoimmune conditions such as vitiligo, pernicious anaemia and Hashimoto thyroiditis

E ≫ Signs include hyperpigmentation, particularly of the buccal mucosa and the palmar creases (see *Fig. 4.24*).

Investigations
In some patients, electrolyte abnormalities can also help point towards the diagnosis. Patients with adrenal insufficiency may have **hypo**natraemia, **hypo**glycaemia and **hypo**calcaemia, and may also have associated **hyperkalaemia**.

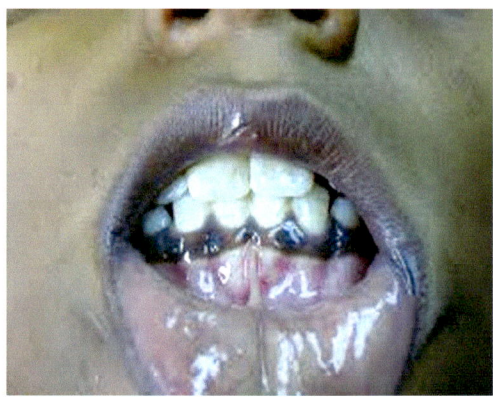

Fig. 4.24 *Hyperpigmentation of the buccal mucosa seen in Addison disease.*

Stepwise plan:

1 **Measure baseline U&Es, check for electrolyte abnormalities**
- Note that classic hyponatraemia and hypokalaemia are seen in Addison (primary) disease, and that electrolytes are usually normal in secondary disease

2 **Measure early morning serum cortisol**
- <100–500nmol/L warrants further investigation, >500nmol/L points away from a diagnosis of adrenal insufficiency

3 **The best confirmatory test is the short Synacthen test**
- Synacthen is an analogue of ACTH
- Serum cortisol is measured shortly before and after administration of synacthen
- In adrenal insufficiency, **cortisol levels do not rise** in response to this

P ≫ In the short Synacthen test, 250mcg of ACTH is given IV or IM. Serum cortisol is measured initially and at 30 minutes.

4 **Next, perform plasma ACTH**
- ACTH levels are high in Addison disease, cortisol is low

5 **Carry out other investigations:**
- Screen for other autoimmune disorders
- Thyroid function tests
- Other aetiologies include tuberculosis, haemochromatosis, amyloidosis and malignancy

Management

Stepwise management of adrenal insufficiency

1. **Ensure adequate patient education and possibility of wearing a medic alert bracelet**
2. **Replacement of glucocorticoids and mineralocorticoids: hydrocortisone and fludrocortisone**

E ≫ Hydrocortisone doses should be increased up to 2–3 times IM or IV in minor illnesses or surgery to avoid precipitating crises.

4.5.3 Hyperaldosteronism (Conn syndrome)

Definition: hyperaldosteronism refers to a clinical state in which there is an overproduction of aldosterone.

Aetiology/pathophysiology:
- Hyperaldosteronism may be primary (Conn syndrome) or secondary
- Primary hyperaldosteronism (Conn syndrome)
  - Originally thought to be caused by adrenal adenomas
  - 70% of cases are due to bilateral adrenal hyperplasia
- Secondary hyperaldosteronism occurs as a result of an overproduction of renin, causing renin–angiotensin–aldosterone system overactivity (e.g. renin-producing tumour or renal ischaemia)

P ≫ Patients may also develop hyper-aldosteronism as a result of eating liquorice, which mimics the effects of aldosterone. Liquorice is a flavouring used in the manufacture of sweets and desserts.

Clinical features:
- Patients with hyperaldosteronism classically present with **hypernatraemia**, **hypokalaemia** and **hypertension**
- In some cases, potassium levels may be normal
- Patients may present with headaches, lethargy and muscle cramps

Investigations

Stepwise plan:

1. **Obtain urea and electrolytes**
- Hypernatraemia
- Hypokalaemia
- Alkalosis

2. **Obtain aldosterone:renin ratios**
- Renin is **low** and aldosterone is **high** in primary disease (Conn syndrome), exemplified by high aldosterone:renin ratio
- **Normal** ratio in secondary disease
- Spironolactone and diuretics should be stopped 6 weeks before testing
- Antihypertensive medications may affect measurement
- If control is necessary, opt for verapamil instead of nifedipine, for instance

W ≫ The principle behind the test is the decrease in plasma renin activity caused by negative feedback, as a result of high aldosterone concentrations. This helps differentiate between primary and secondary disease.

3. **Carry out other investigations**
- ECG may demonstrate electrolyte abnormalities
- CT adrenal glands

Management

Stepwise management of hyperaldosteronism

1. **In primary hyperaldosteronism (Conn syndrome), adrenalectomy is the first-line and definitive therapy**
- Medical therapy may be used prior to surgery

2. **If the cause of hyperaldosteronism is bilateral adrenal hyperplasia, first-line treatment is medical**
- Using aldosterone antagonists such as **spironolactone, eplerenone or amiloride**

3. **In secondary hyperaldosteronism, the mainstay of therapy is treating the underlying cause**

4.5.4 Phaeochromocytoma

A phaeochromocytoma is a rare, catecholamine-secreting tumour, usually of the adrenal medulla. It causes palpitations, sweating, hypertension and

4

arrhythmias that may prove fatal if the condition is left untreated. It follows the 'rule of 10s', where 10% of phaeochromocytomas are bilateral, 10% are malignant, 10% occur in children and 10% occur outside the adrenal medulla.

Phaeochromocytomas may also be part of multiple endocrine neoplasia (MEN) type II, neurofibromatosis or von Hippel–Lindau syndrome. Investigations involve screening for **urinary metanephrines**.

Surgical excision is definitive, but medical management with alpha blockers (such as phenoxybenzamine), followed by beta blockers, is required pre-operatively.

4.5.5 Congenital adrenal hyperplasia

Congenital adrenal hyperplasia (CAH) refers to an inherited deficiency of 21-hydroxylase in the vast majority of cases, causing androgen excess and cortisol deficiency. An 11-beta hydroxylase deficiency may also be causative. Mineralocorticoid deficiency may be present, and the condition may also be classified as salt-sparing and non-salt-sparing.

Boys with CAH are unlikely to present with anything other than hyperpigmentation, but girls may have indiscriminate genitalia and virilisation at birth. At puberty, both boys and girls may have early pubarche, and girls may also present with hirsutism and amenorrhoea. Treatment in a multi-disciplinary team involves replacing deficient hormones, offering psychological support and providing potential surgical correction of ambiguous genitalia.

4.6 The gonads and puberty

The gonads (namely the testes in males and the ovaries in females) are primarily involved in the production of gametes and sex hormones. The testes produce **testosterone**, which affects spermatogenesis and produces secondary sexual characteristics. The ovaries primarily secrete oestrogen and progesterone, which are involved in ovulation, regulation of the menstrual cycle and pregnancy.

The largest change in the regulation of these hormones occurs during puberty, a developmental stage characterised by rapid physical growth and sexual maturation (see *Fig. 4.25*).

4.6.1 Hypogonadism

Hypogonadism refers to a decrease in the functional activity of the gonads. This may lead to decreased sex hormone production and complete or partial infertility.

Hypogonadism may be:
- **Primary** (in that the primary abnormality is impaired gonadal response to pituitary hormones, also known as *hypergonadotrophic hypogonadism*)
  - May be congenital (e.g. Klinefelter syndrome) or acquired (gonadal torsion, trauma or surgery)
- **Secondary** (in which the defect lies with the pituitary or hypothalamus, also known as *hypogonadotrophic hypogonadism*), exemplified by conditions like Kallmann syndrome, or systemic disease

4.6.2 Polycystic ovarian syndrome (PCOS)

Polycystic ovarian syndrome (PCOS) refers to a condition in which numerous cysts within the ovaries produce a clinical triad of **infertility**, **hirsutism** and **oligomenorrhoea/amenorrhoea**. Patients may also suffer from acne, obesity and male pattern baldness. In addition, patients are likely to have insulin resistance and dyslipidaemia.

> **P** ≫ While an elevated LH, and a LH:FSH ratio >2, are classic findings, these are not included in the **Rotterdam criteria**, which are used to clinch the diagnosis:
> 1. Clinical or biochemical hyperandrogenism
> 2. Oligomenorrhoea
> 3. Polycystic ovaries, 12 or more follicles or ovarian volume >10cm^3

One of the mainstays of therapy is encouraging weight loss. This helps in a myriad of ways, decreasing the risk of cardiovascular sequelae, improving fertility and improving ovulation. No particular therapy treats the condition, and symptomatic control is necessary. Co-cyprindiol and eflornithine help treat hirsutism and acne, and metformin is used off-licence, while clomifene helps improve pregnancy rates by stimulating ovulation.

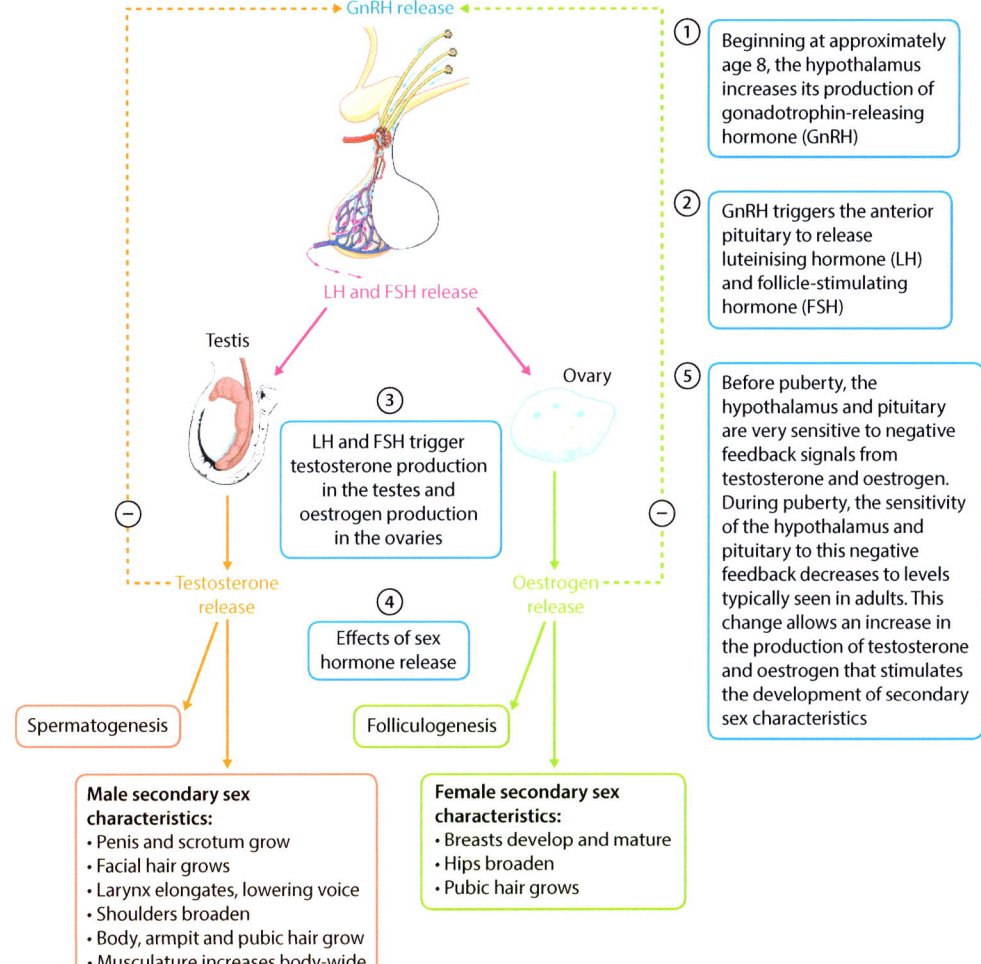

GnRH release

① Beginning at approximately age 8, the hypothalamus increases its production of gonadotrophin-releasing hormone (GnRH)

② GnRH triggers the anterior pituitary to release luteinising hormone (LH) and follicle-stimulating hormone (FSH)

LH and FSH release

Testis

Ovary

③ LH and FSH trigger testosterone production in the testes and oestrogen production in the ovaries

⑤ Before puberty, the hypothalamus and pituitary are very sensitive to negative feedback signals from testosterone and oestrogen. During puberty, the sensitivity of the hypothalamus and pituitary to this negative feedback decreases to levels typically seen in adults. This change allows an increase in the production of testosterone and oestrogen that stimulates the development of secondary sex characteristics

Testosterone release

④ Effects of sex hormone release

Oestrogen release

Spermatogenesis

Folliculogenesis

Male secondary sex characteristics:
• Penis and scrotum grow
• Facial hair grows
• Larynx elongates, lowering voice
• Shoulders broaden
• Body, armpit and pubic hair grow
• Musculature increases body-wide

Female secondary sex characteristics:
• Breasts develop and mature
• Hips broaden
• Pubic hair grows

Fig. 4.25 *Hormones of puberty.*

4.6.3 Precocious puberty

Precocious puberty refers to pubertal development that occurs at an abnormally young age.

> **E** ≫ This is defined as puberty in boys before the age of 9, and puberty in girls before the age of 8.

Types of precocious puberty
- Gonadotropin-dependent (central/true) precocious puberty
  - Generally idiopathic
  - More common in girls
  - Premature activation of HPG axis
- Gonadotropin-independent (pseudo) precocious puberty
  - 20% of cases
  - Caused by increased production of sex steroids, independent of HPG activation
  - e.g. congenital adrenal hyperplasia or McCune–Albright syndrome (see *Chapter 5, Section 5.17*)

Management
After carrying out relevant hormonal function tests, management involves resecting tumours (note that resecting central tumours does not reverse pubertal changes) and using GnRH agonists in gonadotropin-dependent precocious puberty.

4

4

W ≫ GnRH is released in a pulsatile fashion in normal physiology. Treatment with agonists causes excessive stimulation of the pituitary, thereby desensitising it to pulsatile releases. This decreases FSH and LH and can be resumed when the age for normal puberty arrives. This helps the child achieve their predicted adult height.

- Broad chest with wide-spaced nipples
- Coarctation of the aorta
- Bicuspid aortic valve
- Gonadal failure (fibrotic ovarian streaks, which should be removed)
- Metabolic disease and autoimmune disease

Management of the condition is lifelong, and requires monitoring of cardiovascular, urogenital and metabolic function, as well as psychosocial support.

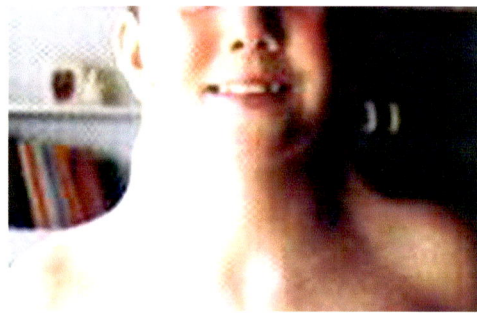

Fig. 4.26 *Webbed neck seen in a patient with Turner syndrome.*

4.6.4 Delayed puberty

Puberty may be delayed, in some cases, by congenital causes or acquired causes (such as excessive exercise, malnutrition, hypothyroidism and damage to the HPG axis or gonads prior to puberty).

P ≫ Kallmann syndrome is characterised by delayed or absent puberty and impaired olfaction (hyposmia or anosmia). Patients may be unaware of their inability to smell adequately and this is usually picked up on routine investigation. The condition is also associated with other congenital abnormalities, such as cleft palate and hearing loss, but these symptoms vary from patient to patient.

4.6.5 Turner syndrome

Turner syndrome is characterised by the chromosomal abnormality 45XO. Associations include:

- Short stature
- Webbed neck (appears in 20–25% of cases; see *Fig. 4.26*)

4.6.6 Klinefelter syndrome

Klinefelter syndrome is characterised by genotypically male patients with an extra X chromosome (commonly 47 XXY or 48 XXYY). Characteristics include:

- Tall, slender, long-limbed
- Infertility with small testes
- Decreased facial, pubic hair
- Learning disabilities

4.7 Disorders affecting multiple endocrine systems

4.7.1 Multiple endocrine neoplasia (MEN)

MEN refers to a group of syndromes characterised by tumours of the endocrine gland that present in a predictable pattern. *Table 4.6* summarises the most salient findings in each condition, but bear in mind that variations do exist. There are three major subtypes: MEN I, MEN IIa and MEN IIb.

P ≫ The gene implicated in the development of MEN I is the MEN 1 gene, whereas the RET oncogene is implicated in the development of both MEN IIa and MEN IIb.

4.7.2 Autoimmune polyendocrine syndrome

Autoimmune polyendocrine syndrome refers to a group of rare conditions characterised by autoimmune action against one or more of the endocrine glands.

Table 4.6 *MEN subtypes*

MEN I	Characterised by: **PPP**
	• **P**arathyroid (hyperparathyroidism)
	• **P**ituitary tumours
	• **P**ancreatic tumours
	   ○ Usually a gastrinoma (Zollinger–Ellison syndrome)
	   ○ May also be insulinoma or VIPoma

MEN IIa (Sipple syndrome)	Characterised by: **PPM** • **P**arathyroid (hyperparathyroidism) • **P**haeochromocytoma • **M**edullary carcinoma of the thyroid
MEN IIb	Characterised by: **PMMN** • **P**haeochromocytoma • **M**edullary carcinoma of the thyroid • **M**arfanoid body habitus • **N**euroma (particularly mucosal)

These are:

- Type I
  - Autosomal recessive inheritance, caused by a defect in the autoimmune regulator gene on chromosome 21
  - Mild immunodeficiency, e.g. with candida infections
  - Type I classically affects the parathyroid and adrenal glands, causing hyperparathyroidism and Addison disease
- Type II
  - Also known as Schmidt syndrome
  - Not linked to any one particular gene
  - Characterised by Addison disease, hypothyroidism, type 1 diabetes mellitus, pernicious anaemia and alopecia

4

Chapter 5
Neurology

Amar Vaswani, Samantha Jingyun Koh and ***Li Anne Ong***

Basic principles

The study of neurology focuses on understanding and managing disorders of the nervous system, which can be broadly divided into the central nervous system (CNS) and the peripheral nervous system (PNS). To arrive at an accurate diagnosis, the physician needs to use a combination of thorough history-taking, clinical examination (with the aim of localising the lesion if possible), appropriate imaging investigations, and a degree of pattern recognition.

Bridge to clinical medicine

The neuron and action potential

- The basic structural and functional unit of the nervous system is the **neuron**, a cell designed to transmit and receive chemical and electrical signals, allowing for rapid communication (see *Fig. 5.1*)
- Neurons are supported by **glia**; glial cells also have a role in signalling, but function primarily as supportive tissues that complement the role of neurons
- The human body contains a vast number of neurons – the human brain alone is said to contain approximately 85 billion neurons
- The neuron is similar to most other cells, in that it has a cell body (soma) and nucleus, endoplasmic reticulum and mitochondria; however, as a specialised signal-relaying cell, it also has features like **dendrites** and **axons** to help it fulfil this role
- **Dendrites** are branch-like structures that receive signals from other cells via a synapse, and transmit the signal to their neuron's cell body
- A **synapse** is the junction between neurons; neurotransmitters travel across synapses as part of signal transmission, to reach the recipient neuron's dendritic end
- The change in electrical potential associated with the transmission of an impulse is known as the **action potential** (see *Fig. 5.2*)
- The influx of sodium ions into the cell causes **depolarisation**, increasing the voltage of the neuron from its **resting membrane potential** of −70mV
- As the membrane potential of the cell becomes more positive and approaches +30mV, potassium efflux contributes to **repolarisation**
- At the height of depolarisation, voltage-gated sodium channels are inactivated; this means that no further propagation can occur for a period of time, known as the **refractory period**
- The refractory period may be **relative** (meaning that a stronger stimulus can further propagate an impulse), or **absolute** (meaning that no further impulse can occur, regardless of the strength of the stimulus)
- The transmission of a signal within the neuron itself takes place in the **axon**, a cylindrical structure that carries signals to axon terminals where they synapse

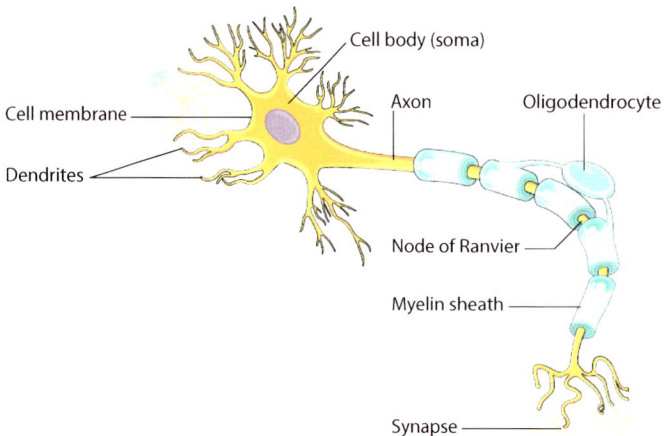

Fig. 5.1 Neuron.

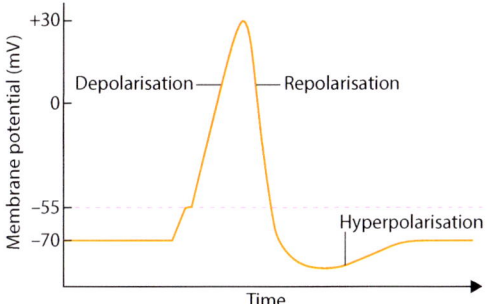

Fig. 5.2 *Action potential.*

> **W** ≫ Myelin, a lipid-rich substance, insulates the neuron, decreasing capacitance and electrical resistance, and making the impulse less likely to leave the axon. Each axon is myelinated in such a way that there are gaps between each myelinated area, known as **nodes of Ranvier**. The propagating impulse 'jumps' from node to node, increasing velocity in a process known as **saltatory conduction**. These properties make impulses that travel through myelinated axons much faster than those travelling through their unmyelinated counterparts.

- Some axons have a **myelin sheath**, which is produced by oligodendrocytes in the CNS and Schwann cells in the PNS
- Neurons may be unipolar, bipolar, pseudounipolar or multipolar; the majority of neurons are multipolar in nature

- Neuroglia include **astrocytes**, which connect neurons and blood capillaries, forming the blood–brain barrier in the CNS; **satellite cells** in the PNS, which provide neuronal support; **microglia**, which have immunological and phagocytic functions; **ependymal cells**, which line CSF-filled ventricles and the central canal of the spinal cord; and **oligodendrocytes** in the CNS and **Schwann cells** in the PNS, which are involved in the formation of myelin (see *Fig. 5.3*)

The central nervous system

- The central nervous system comprises the brain and spinal cord, enveloped by three protective layers: the **dura mater**, or 'tough mother'; the lattice-like **arachnoid mater**; and the **pia** (or soft) mater (see *Fig. 5.4*)
- Cerebrospinal fluid lies between the arachnoid and pia mater, and is produced by choroid plexuses in the ventricles
- The brain, broadly, encompasses the cerebral cortex and hemispheres, thalamus, hypothalamus, basal ganglia, brainstem and cerebellum
- The **cerebral cortex** is itself delineated by ridges (**gyri**) and grooves (**sulci**)
- The cerebral hemispheres are connected by the **corpus callosum**, a structure that allows the transmission of information
- Each hemisphere can be functionally and anatomically classified into specific territories, and grossly into various **lobes** (see *Fig. 5.5*)
- The **frontal lobe** refers to the part of the brain that contains the motor cortex and olfactory bulb; the motor cortex is responsible for planning and execution of actions, and the olfactory

5

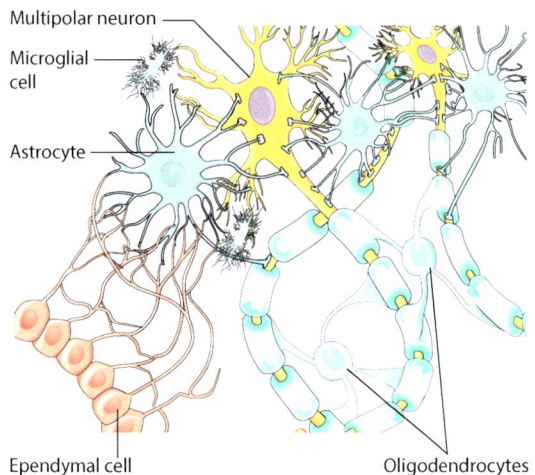

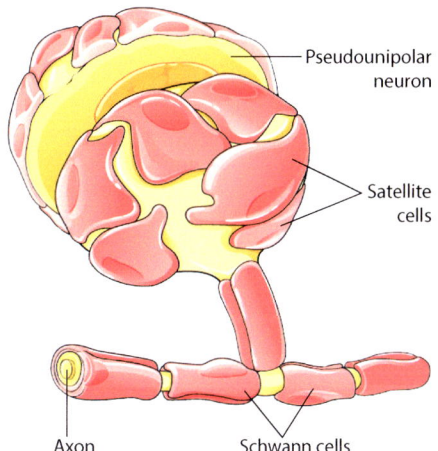

Fig. 5.3 *Glial cells of the nervous system.*

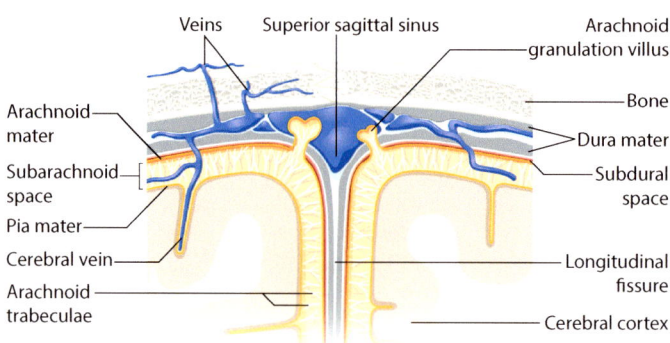

Fig. 5.4 *Layers of the central nervous system.*

bulb controls processing of smells, as well as behavioural regulation
- The dominant hemispheric frontal lobe also governs motor speech, exemplified by the **Broca area**

> **P** ≫ Neuronal connections here are also responsible for elements of cognition, and patients with frontal lobe damage are often prone to personality changes, lability, disinhibition and impaired appraisal of risk.

- The **parietal lobe**'s major functions are the processing of sensory stimuli, proprioception and orientation of the body in space
- The **temporal lobe** is primarily involved in auditory processing, but also contains the **hippocampus** (named for its seahorse-like shape), which is involved in memory formation. The **limbic system**, a neurally connected pathway between the thalamus, hypothalamus, **amygdala** and hippocampus, allows for regulation of emotions and behaviour
- The **occipital lobe** is primarily involved in the processing of visual stimuli

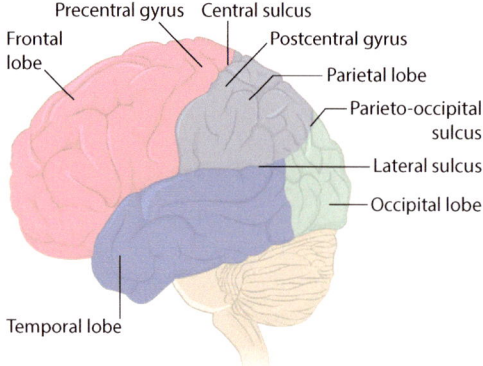

Fig. 5.5 *Lobes of the cerebral cortex.*

- The **thalamus** is often colloquially described as a 'relay station', and is involved with processing of sensorimotor input from the body, whilst regulating information from the cerebral cortex
- The roles of the **hypothalamus** and **epithalamus** have already been discussed (see *Chapter 4*)

The spinal cord
- The spinal cord is a long cylinder of nervous tissue extending from the brainstem, running through the skull's foramen magnum, descending into the protective bony vertebral column, giving off 31 pairs of spinal nerves: 8 cervical, 12 thoracic, 5 lumbar, 5 sacral and 1 coccygeal

> **P** ≫ Nerves C1–C7 exit above their corresponding vertebrae. Remaining nerves exit below their corresponding vertebrae.

- The spinal cord extends and terminates at L1–L2 in adults (as the conus medullaris, before terminating as the filum terminale), while the remaining spinal nerves extend further (as 'horse-tail'-like nerve fibres, or cauda equina), leaving the vertebral column at their appropriate vertebral levels

Sensory and motor pathways
- The spinal cord allows the body to perform motor, sensory and reflex functions, by way of various nerve pathways (see *Fig. 5.6*)
- The **motor pathways** carry signals from the brain, down the spinal cord, to affect various muscle groups; they are therefore (aptly) known as the corticospinal tracts. (Anterior and lateral CSTs are situated in their various positions in the spinal cord)
- The **sensory pathways** carry signals from recipient tissues, which travel up the spinal cord to the brain for interpretation; they can hence be thought of as **ascending tracts**

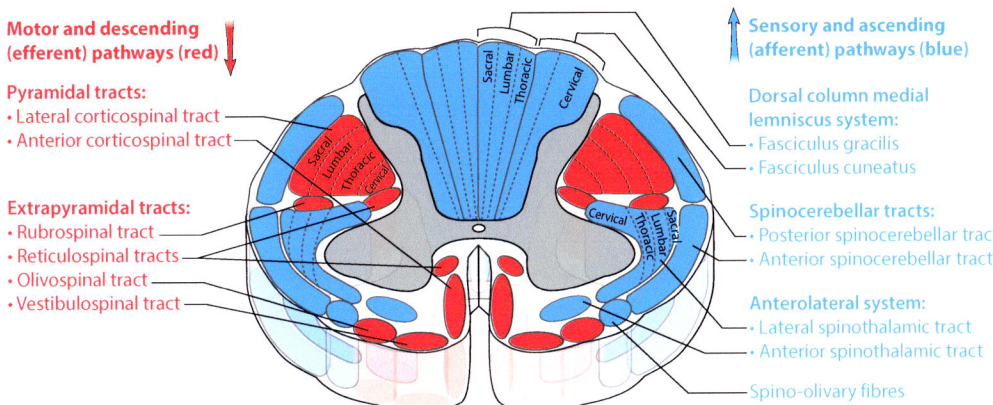

Fig. 5.6 *Sensory (blue) and motor (red) pathways of the spinal cord.*

5

- Ascending tracts can be divided into dorsal column, and the aptly named spinothalamic tracts, of which there are anterior and lateral branches
- The **dorsal column** fibres specialise in transmitting the sensations of touch, pressure, vibration and proprioception to the lower body and legs (via the fasciculus gracilis) and to the upper body and arms (via the fasciculus cuneatus)
- The **lateral spinothalamic tract** fibres specialise in transmitting the sensations of pain and temperature

> P >> The **anterior spinothalamic tract** fibres specialise in transmitting the sensations of crude touch and pressure.

Upper and lower motor neurons
- The descending motor pathways transmit information from the brain to the effector muscles by way of two motor neurons – firstly the upper motor neuron (UMN), and secondly the lower motor neuron (LMN)

- The motor signal travels from the brain down the upper motor neuron and then synapses with the lower motor neuron (in the spinal cord), travelling down the LMN to reach its intended spinal root, where efferent nerves carry the motor signal to the intended effector muscle
- Lesions that affect upper and lower motor neurons present with differing clinical signs, and are summarised in *Table 5.1*

MRC grading of muscle weakness
The Medical Research Council's grading of muscle weakness is a useful tool that clinicians use to determine the severity of a patient's muscle weakness by scoring the power of a muscle of interest. A score is given, ranging from 0 to 5, relative to the maximum effort expected for that muscle (see *Table 5.2*).

Cerebral and cerebellar circulation
- The blood supply of the cerebrum can be divided into two vascular networks – the anterior and the posterior cerebral circulation

E >> **Table 5.1** *Signs of upper and lower motor neuron lesions*

	UMN lesion signs	LMN lesion signs
Tone	Increased	Decreased
Fasciculations	Absent	May be present
Disuse atrophy	None	Severe
Muscle weakness	Generally affects flexors in lower limbs and extensors in upper limbs	Distal muscle weakness (flexors and extensors may be equally involved)
Reflexes	Hyper-reflexic	Hypo-reflexic or absent
Plantars	Up-going (Babinski sign)	Down-going

Table 5.2 *MRC grading of muscle weakness*

5	Normal power – muscle is able to withstand gravity and full resistance
4	Active movement against gravity and some resistance
3	Active movement against gravity
2	Active movement without gravity
1	Only a flicker of active movement
0	No movement

- These two networks are connected via interconnections of the circle of Willis, which runs along the floor of the cerebral vault (see *Fig. 5.7*)
- Three main cerebral arteries are involved – the anterior cerebral artery (ACA), middle cerebral artery (MCA) and posterior cerebral artery (PCA)
- The ACA and MCA arise from the internal carotid and are part of the anterior cerebral circulation, while the PCA (the terminal branch of the basilar artery) is part of the posterior cerebral circulation

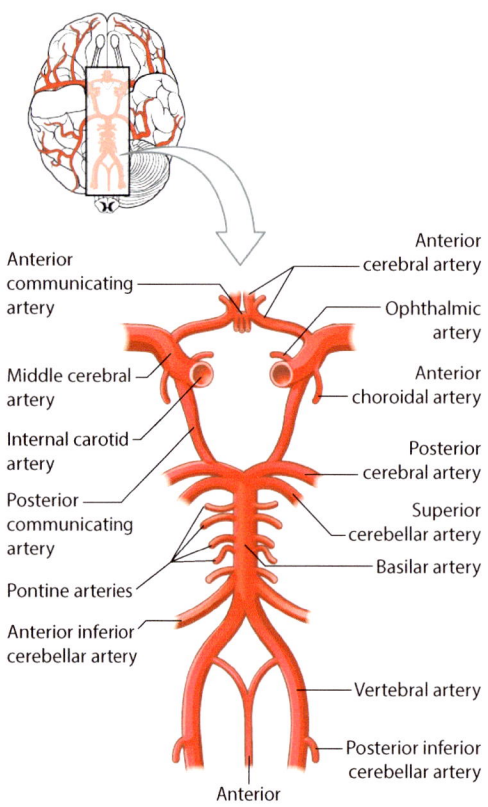

Anterior communicating artery
Anterior cerebral artery
Ophthalmic artery
Middle cerebral artery
Anterior choroidal artery
Internal carotid artery
Posterior cerebral artery
Posterior communicating artery
Superior cerebellar artery
Basilar artery
Pontine arteries
Anterior inferior cerebellar artery
Vertebral artery
Posterior inferior cerebellar artery
Anterior spinal artery

Fig. 5.7 *The circle of Willis.*

- Respective anterior communicating arteries connect the ACAs of either side, while posterior communicating arteries connect either side's ICA and PCA

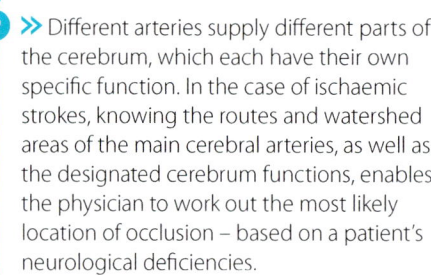

P ≫ Different arteries supply different parts of the cerebrum, which each have their own specific function. In the case of ischaemic strokes, knowing the routes and watershed areas of the main cerebral arteries, as well as the designated cerebrum functions, enables the physician to work out the most likely location of occlusion – based on a patient's neurological deficiencies.

- The ACA is mainly associated with the frontal lobe. Distributed on the orbital surface and the whole medial surface of each hemisphere, it curves back and over the roof of the corpus callosum, as far as the parieto-occipital sulcus. It supplies the superior frontal gyrus.
- ACA syndrome results from the occlusion of the ACA, leading to loss or reduction in function of the parts of the brain receiving blood supply from the ACA. This may cause:
  - Contralateral hemiparesis/hemiplegia
  - Contralateral sensory deficit
  - Apraxia
  - Anosmia
  - Urinary incontinence.
- The MCA is the **most direct branch of the internal carotid artery** and is therefore **most prone to embolism**. It travels in the lateral sulcus, supplying the insular cortex, posterior limb of the internal capsule and basal ganglia. It gives off branches supplying most of the lateral surface of each hemisphere, with some exceptions:
  - The superior frontal and parietal lobes, supplied by the ACA
  - The inferior part of the temporal and occipital lobe, supplied by the PCA.
- The PCA arises from the terminal bifurcation of the basilar artery, supplying inferior and lateral aspects of the occipital and temporal lobes, medial aspects of the occipital lobe and posterior two-thirds of the temporal lobe, the thalamus, subthalamic nucleus and brainstem

E ≫ Occlusion of the PCA causes contralateral (macular-sparing) hemianopia.

Peripheral nervous system

- The **PNS** comprises nerves outside the brain and spinal cord, which connect the CNS to effector organs
- It is divided into the somatic nervous system (**SNS**) and autonomic nervous system (**ANS**). The ANS (see *Table 5.3*) can be further categorised into sympathetic and parasympathetic nervous systems. In total, 12 pairs of cranial nerves, 31 pairs of spinal nerves and peripheral autonomic nerves make up the PNS.
- The ANS nerves supply muscles such as cardiac, smooth muscle, exocrine and endocrine glands, even adipose tissue – and are responsible for involuntary body functions. Each ANS nerve pathway comprises a preganglionic and postganglionic neuron.
- **Sympathetic fibres** arise from the thoracic and lumbar spinal cord. Their short preganglionic fibres synapse with long postganglionic neurons (in ganglia) in the sympathetic ganglion chain (alongside the spinal cord). Postganglionic fibres carry on from the ganglion chain until they reach their effector organ. They are famously involved in the **fight or flight response**, referring to the body's response to high stress (be it emotional, physical or environmental stressors). **Heart rate, respiratory rate and blood pressure increase, as does sweat gland activity. Pupils constrict and bowel function slows.**
- **Parasympathetic fibres** arise from the cranial and sacral spinal cord. Their longer preganglionic fibres synapse with shorter postganglionic fibres at a terminal ganglion, which lies close to the effector organ. The famous 'rest and digest' term summarises the parasympathetic fibres' role. They promote bodily activities that occur in relaxed situations, such as digestion.

> **E** ≫ Most organs are innervated with both sympathetic and parasympathetic nerves, or dual autonomic innervation. This allows more precise control of the organ's functioning activity.

- The somatic nervous system (**SoNS**) comprises efferent motor nerves for voluntary muscle movement, and afferent sensory neurons that transmit sensation from the body to the CNS. The SoNS is made up of spinal and cranial nerves:
  - **Spinal nerves** are peripheral nerves acting between the spinal cord and effector organs. Hence, they transmit sensory information from sensory organs to the spinal cord, as well as motor information from the spinal cord to the effector organ
  - **The cranial nerves** are 12 pairs of peripheral nerves acting between the brainstem and effector organs (see *Fig. 5.8*, summarised in *Table 5.4*).

The neuromuscular junction

- The neuromuscular junction (NMJ) is the area between a single motor neuron axon terminal and a muscle cell (the smallest unit of skeletal muscle fibre)
- As a motor neuron axon reaches the effector organ, each axon divides and gives rise to multiple axon terminals, each in close association with one muscle cell of the effector muscle/organ, by way of one NMJ

> **P** ≫ Each terminal axon further divides into terminal buttons, which lie in a shallow groove of the muscle cell, known as the motor end plate.

- The electrical nervous signal passes along the axon, triggering the opening of voltage-gated Ca^{2+} channels
- The influx of calcium at the terminal button triggers the release of the neurotransmitter, acetylcholine, from vesicles within the terminal buttons
- ACh diffuses across the NMJ to bind onto membrane receptor channels on the muscle cell,

Table 5.3 *Autonomic nervous system*

	Sympathetic		Parasympathetic	
	Preganglionic neuron	Postganglionic neuron	Preganglionic neuron	Postganglionic neuron
Length	Short	Long	Long	Short
Ganglion	Sympathetic ganglion chain (alongside spinal cord)		Terminal ganglia (near effector organ)	
Neurotransmitter	ACh (acetylcholine)	NA (noradrenaline)	ACh	ACh

5

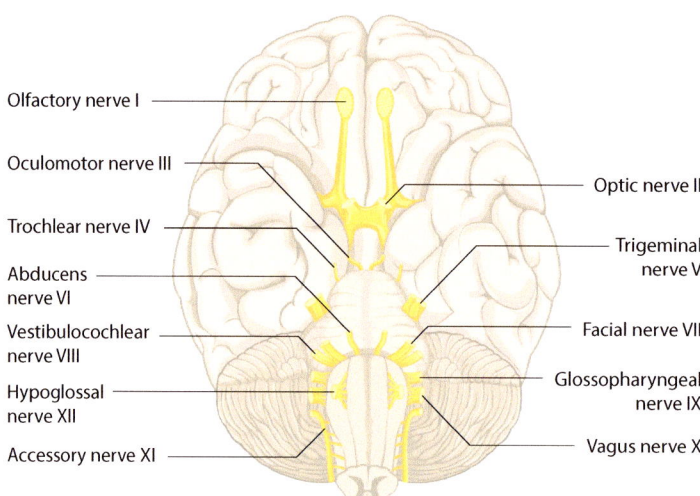

Fig. 5.8 *Cranial nerves.*

Table 5.4 *Cranial nerves and their functions*

Number	Name	Modality	Function
I	Olfactory	Sensory	• Smell
II	Optic	Sensory	• Vision
III	Oculomotor	Motor	• Elevates upper eyelid • Pupillary constriction, lens curvature • Eye movements
IV	Trochlear	Motor	• Moves eye down, inwards and laterally
V	Trigeminal	Sensory and motor	• Facial sensation • Muscles of mastication
VI	Abducens	Motor	• Moves eye laterally
VII	Facial	Sensory and motor	• Taste from anterior two-thirds of the tongue • Muscles of facial expression • Salivation and lacrimation
VIII	Vestibulocochlear	Sensory	• Hearing and balance
IX	Glossopharyngeal	Sensory and motor	• Taste from posterior one-third of the tongue • Carotid body innervation • Salivation
X	Vagus	Sensory and motor	• Sensation from larynx, pharynx, thoracic and abdominal viscera • Taste from epiglottis • Larynx/pharyngeal movements
XI	Accessory	Motor	• Neck movements
XII	Hypoglossal	Motor	• Tongue movements

opening them and allowing an influx of cations like Na^+, depolarising the motor end plate, resulting in an end plate potential
- ACh is later removed by acetylcholinesterase

P » Botulinum toxin paralyses muscles, by preventing them from responding to nerve impulses. It does so by preventing the release of ACh from the terminal end button and into the NMJ. Organophosphates inhibit AChE, preventing destruction of ACh. Muscles like the diaphragm remain depolarised, unable to return to their resting condition.

Dermatomes and myotomes
- Knowing one axon terminal associates with one muscle cell, by extension one postganglionic nerve fibre must associate with multiple cells
- If we keep tracing back to one nerve root, we find it supplies entire muscle groups; a muscle group that is supplied by one nerve root is known as a **myotome**
- Knowledge of the body's myotomes is extremely useful in clinical practice because it allows us to work backwards from a patient's clinical signs of muscle weakness to narrow down the possible location of a spinal lesion
- A **dermatome** (see *Fig. 5.9*) refers to the sensory area of skin each nerve root is distributed to

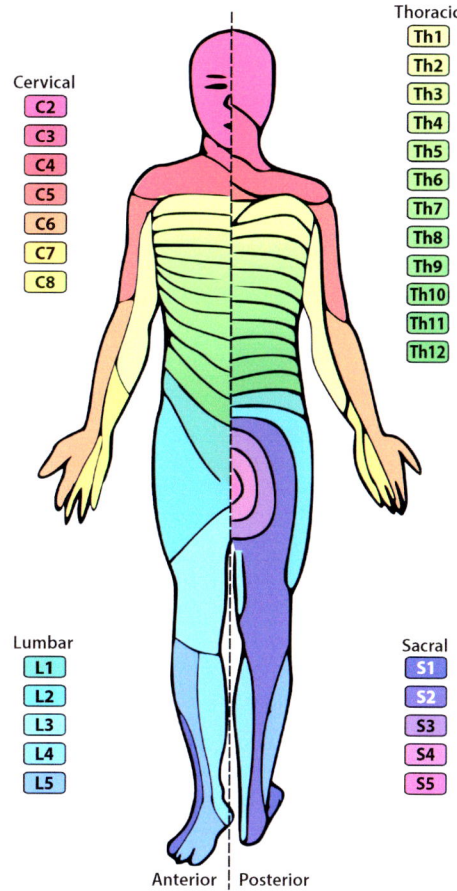

Fig. 5.9 *Dermatomes.*

5.1 Neuro-ophthalmology

5.1.1 Pupillary abnormalities

Common pupillary defects include:
- RAPD (relative afferent pupillary defect):
  - Caused by damage anywhere between the retinal ganglion cell layer to the lateral geniculate body
  - Result: when light is shone on the unaffected eye, both eyes constrict fully and symmetrically – if light is swung over to the affected eye, both pupils will still be constricting but to a lesser degree
- Miosis
  - Commonly associated with Horner syndrome, involving a lesion on the sympathetic chain between the hypothalamus and the eye (e.g. Pancoast tumour of the lung, trauma, thoracic aortic aneurysm)
  - To confirm Horner syndrome, drop 4% cocaine drops into the eye, which will dilate the unaffected eye but will leave the affected side undilated
- Fixed dilated pupil
  - Sphincter pupillae damage can result in a fixed dilated pupil, which is unable to contract in response to the appropriate stimuli
  - Third nerve palsy needs to be excluded if a pupil is not reacting to light or accommodating; other causes could include surgical or physical trauma affecting the sphincter pupillae, or a tumour or a posterior communicating artery aneurysm
  - **A unilateral enlarged pupil may be due to uncal herniation and is considered a neurosurgical emergency**

5.1.2 Papilloedema

Hydrocephalus causes an excessive accumulation of cerebrospinal fluid (CSF) in the brain, which results in an abnormal expansion of ventricles. This widening creates potentially harmful pressure on the tissues of the brain. Raised intracranial pressure will translate to the optic nerves as well, since the optic nerve sheath is also surrounded by CSF. The high pressure in the CSF reduces the ability of axons to perform axoplasmic flow and drain all nutrients away from the optic head. This will lead to swollen optic head with excessive axoplasm, resulting in papilloedema.

Investigations include:
- Blood pressure (DDX: malignant hypertension)
- Glucose, FBC and differential WCC, U&E, creatinine and ESR (DDX: infective/inflammatory processes)
- Neuroimaging (urgent CT brain, especially if there are signs such as headache, nausea)
- Lumbar puncture if MRI is normal and benign intracranial hypertension is suspected

5.1.3 Third (oculomotor) nerve palsy

Third cranial nerve palsy or oculomotor nerve palsy classically presents with a combination of ptosis, mydriasis and cycloplegia of the affected eye, accompanied by resting abduction, exotropia and hypotropia. Fixed dilated pupil and horizontal diplopia may be present in some cases.

Causes of oculomotor nerve palsy include:
- Idiopathic (25% of cases)
- Microvascular disease – DM, hypertension (often without pupillary involvement)
- Vascular causes – extradural haematoma (pupil-sparing third nerve palsy), posterior communicating artery aneurysm

W ≫ It is important to recall that the posterior communicating artery runs adjacent to the third nerve. Hence, any aneurysm of the artery can cause a third nerve palsy. Vasospasms are a common complication of aneurysms, which can make the aneurysm elusive and at times missed on MR angiography. A repeat MR angiogram may therefore be helpful in detecting the presence of third nerve palsy symptoms, and confirming a suspicion of posterior communicating artery aneurysm.

5.1.4 Fourth (trochlear) nerve palsy

The trochlear nerve innervates the superior oblique muscle of the eye which is responsible for abducting, depressing and internally rotating the eye. A fourth nerve palsy includes a combination of vertical diplopia and excyclotorsion, with an occasional presentation of compensatory head tilt/turning to the opposite side of the palsy.

E ≫ Bearing in mind the very long, slender and paratentorial course of the fourth nerve, it is easy to understand why trauma is one of the most common causes of fourth nerve palsy.

P ≫ The Bielschowsky test can be used to elicit a fourth nerve palsy. A patient with right fourth nerve palsy will demonstrate an increase in hyperdeviation (of the affected side) on ipsilateral head tilt. This hyperdeviation is absent when the head is tilted to the contralateral side (positive test).

5.1.5 Sixth (abducens) nerve palsy

The abducens nerve rightly supplies the abductor muscle of the eye, the lateral rectus muscle. Sixth nerve palsy results in esotropia of the affected side due to unopposed action of the medial rectus, and limited abduction of the affected eye, resulting in horizontal diplopia. Common causes of sixth nerve palsy include:
- Microvascular disease – DM, hypertension
- External compression – acoustic neuroma, raised intracranial pressure (see *Section 5.9*)

5.1.6 Visual pathways and field defects

Figure 5.10 illustrates the organisation of visual pathways and the visual field defects associated with the locations of particular injuries or lesions.
- Vision is generated through complex visual pathways, beginning at the photoreceptors in the retina – note that images from the right visual field are detected by the nasal retina of the right eye and the temporal retina of the left eye (blue lines in *Fig. 5.10*) and vice versa for the left visual field (red lines)

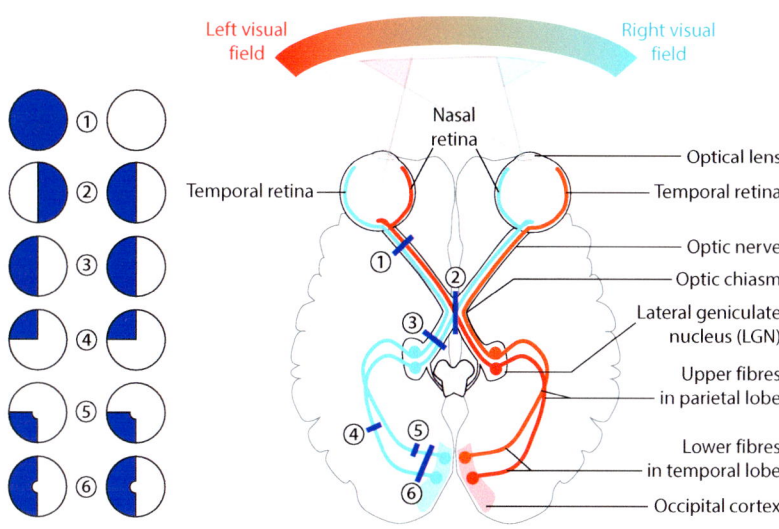

Fig. 5.10 *Visual pathways and defects.*

- Information from the retina leaves the eyes and travels to the brain via the optic nerve; at the optic chiasm, the nasal retina fibres decussate and enter the contralateral optic tracts, while the temporal retina fibres stay uncrossed and enter the ipsilateral optic tracts
- The optic chiasm is located between the temporal lobes, lying between the third ventricle (above) and the pituitary (below); it receives the two optic nerves anteriorly, which leave posteriorly as the optic tracts
- The optic tracts travel around the midbrain and synapses at the lateral geniculate nucleus (LGN) – fibres leave the LGN as optic radiations, with upper fibres travelling in the parietal lobe and lower fibres in the temporal lobe
- These fibres ultimately reach the primary visual cortex in the occipital lobe

Lesions at different points along the visual pathway will result in different visual field defects. These, along with their common aetiologies, are described in *Table 5.5*.

> **P** ≫ Parinaud syndrome (also known as dorsal midbrain syndrome) refers to a disease process characterised by vertical gaze palsy (impaired ability to look up or down), convergence nystagmus **or** diplopia. These phenomena occur because of the presence of a pineal gland tumour compressing the vertical gaze centre at the medial longitudinal fasciculus (MLF). Patients with multiple sclerosis are also at greater risk of developing Parinaud syndrome.

Table 5.5 *Visual field defects and their causative lesions (numbers in brackets correspond to their location on Fig. 5.10)*

Location	Causative lesion	Visual field defect
Optic nerve (1)	• Glaucomatous cupping • Vitamin B12 deficiency • Trauma • Optic neuritis	• Arcuate scotoma • Centrocecal scotoma • Complete unilateral loss of visual field
Chiasm (2)	• Pituitary tumour • Craniopharyngioma • Meningioma	• Bitemporal hemianopia
Optic tract (3)	• Tumour, MS	• Contralateral homonymous hemianopia
Temporal lobe fibres (4)	• Stroke	• Contralateral superior quadrantanopia
Parietal lobe fibres	• Tumour	• Contralateral inferior quadrantanopia
Macular fibres at the occipital cortex (6)	• MS	• Homonymous hemianopia (macular-sparing)

5.2 Vestibular disorders

Approach to vertigo

In clinical practice, it is important to ascertain whether an individual who presents with dizziness is lightheaded or presyncopal or if they have true vertigo. Vertigo itself implies a **false sense of motion or a spinning sensation**, as opposed to the sensation of being off-balance or blacking out.

Approximately 90% of patients who present with vertigo in the primary care setting have benign paroxysmal positional vertigo (BPPV), Ménière disease or vestibular neuronitis. A thorough history, including medication review, should be obtained. Helpful considerations include the presence of **hearing loss** as a symptom, as well as the **duration** of symptoms. Vertigo with hearing loss is more often caused by Ménière disease or labyrinthitis. Persistent vertigo may also point towards a diagnosis of labyrinthitis or vestibular neuronitis.

5.2.1 Benign paroxysmal positional vertigo (BPPV)

Definition: BPPV occurs as a result of inner ear dysfunction, in which otoliths are most commonly dislodged into the semicircular canals, producing the sensation of vertigo.

Epidemiology:
- Typically affects people above the age of 50
- Affects more women than men

Aetiology/pathophysiology:
- Most BPPV cases have idiopathic causes; however, attributable causes (such as head trauma) are more likely to cause the condition in younger people
- BPPV can also co-present with other vertiginous disorders such as Ménière disease and vestibular neuronitis

Clinical features:
- Symptoms typically occur in an episodic fashion, often **provoked by head movement**
- Symptoms may be worse when the head is moved to one side, or upon waking in the morning
- It is important to note that hearing loss or tinnitus is **not** a feature of BPPV, and episodes typically last under a minute and often resolve temporarily when the head is kept still

Investigations

Stepwise plan:

1 **Ask for any history of rheumatoid arthritis or neck or back pain, which may complicate further investigations**
- Examine the ear and the area around it

2 **Arrange a Dix–Hallpike test**

Management

Advise the patient not to drive or perform work that may be adversely affected by vertigo. Reassure patients that symptoms may resolve with time.

Stepwise management of benign paroxysmal positional vertigo (NICE CKS 2013)

1 **Discuss with patient if watchful waiting may be a suitable option**

2 **Consider a repositioning manoeuvre**
- Such as the Epley manoeuvre

3 **Consider Brandt–Daroff exercises**
- The patient can perform these at home if the Epley manoeuvre cannot be performed immediately or is inappropriate

P ≫ **Brandt–Daroff exercises**
Instruct the person on how to perform these exercises at home.

Advise them to:
- Sit on the edge of a bed or couch with their eyes closed
- Lie down sideways on one side with their eyes closed so that they are lying on their side with the lateral aspect of their occiput resting on the bed, with the head positioned as if they are looking towards the ceiling
- Rest in this position for at least 30 seconds, until any vertigo subsides
- Keeping the eyes closed, sit upright again, and remain in this position for 30 seconds
- Repeat on the other side
- Repeat the sequence 3–4 times until they are symptom-free
- Repeat 3–4 times a day until there have been two consecutive days without symptoms.

5.2.2 Ménière disease

Definition: Ménière disease refers to a condition in which there is extensive expansion of the membranous labyrinth, also known as endolymphatic hydrops, which gives rise to the sensation of vertigo and other associated symptoms described below.

Epidemiology:
- Generally affects people around the age of 40–50, but exact prevalence is unknown

Aetiology/pathophysiology:
- The aetiology of this disease is thought to be multi-factorial, involving a complex interplay of genetic, metabolic, vascular and infective factors; an exact pathogenesis is unknown
- Several theories have been put forward to describe the pathophysiology of Ménière disease, but most are based on implications of the disease post-mortem – the mechanism in this disease is thought to be overproduction or impaired absorption of endolymphatic fluid, accounting for pressure and damage to surrounding structures

Clinical features (NICE CKS 2012):
- **Ménière disease produces a classic triad of core symptoms** (vertigo, tinnitus and fluctuating hearing loss), although the symptom of aural fullness is increasingly acknowledged by many as a fourth core symptom
- The majority of people also have other symptoms (such as anxiety and depression)
- Acute attacks typically last from minutes to hours, most commonly 2–3 hours
- Acute episodes can occur in clusters, although remission may last several months

Investigations (NICE CKS 2012):
- **There are no specific clinical signs or diagnostic tests for Ménière disease**
- **A firm diagnosis of Ménière disease requires all three of the following criteria:**
  - Vertigo – at least two spontaneous episodes lasting at least 20 minutes within a single attack of Ménière disease
  - Tinnitus and/or perception of aural fullness
  - Hearing loss confirmed by audiometry to be sensorineural in nature

Management
Advise the patient not to drive (inform the DVLA) or perform work that may be adversely affected by vertigo. The diagnosis of Ménière disease should be confirmed by an ENT specialist.

> **Stepwise management of Ménière disease (NICE CKS 2012)**
>
> **1 If symptoms are severe, admit for IV labyrinthine sedatives**
> - And fluids, hydration and nutrition
>
> **2 For an acute attack, consider prescribing a 7-day course of prochlorperazine**
> - May be prescribed buccally or IM if symptoms are moderate
>
> **3 Consider a trial of betahistine**
> - To see if there is a preventative benefit

5.2.3 Labyrinthitis

Definition: labyrinthitis refers to an inflammatory condition that affects the inner ear.

> **W** ≫ The terms labyrinthitis and vestibular neuronitis have historically been used interchangeably, but some authorities suggest that the term vestibular neuronitis be used when there is vestibular neuropathy **only**, whereas the term labyrinthitis may be used more broadly – referring to both vestibular and labyrinth pathology.

Epidemiology:
- Actual incidence and prevalence remain unknown

Aetiology/pathophysiology:
- Most cases of labyrinthitis have a discernible inflammatory cause; these may be viral (half of which also have a prior upper respiratory tract infection) or due to bacterial agents
- Viral pathogens include varicella-zoster virus (VZV), cytomegalovirus (CMV), measles, mumps or rubella. Bacterial pathogens are often linked to otitis media or cholesteatomas, and may also arise as a complication of late-stage syphilis

> **E** ≫ Viral labyrinthitis is the most common cause of the disease, usually seen in adults between the ages of 30 and 60.

Clinical features:

- Patients with labyrinthitis typically have:
  - **Sudden** onset of severe vertigo with associated nausea and vomiting
  - Sensorineural hearing loss and tinnitus
  - Symptoms that may persist in the acute period for up to 72 hours

P » Patients with labyrinthitis are less likely to describe the feeling of aural fullness (than those with Ménière disease), and the tinnitus or hearing loss is often a presenting feature.

Investigations

Stepwise plan:

1 **Take a thorough history and perform a physical examination**
- With particular emphasis on examining the cranial nerves, gait and balance, and carrying out Weber and Rinne tests

2 **Examine the ear and obtain an audiogram**

Management
Advise patients to lie still with their eyes closed.

Stepwise management of labyrinthitis (NICE CKS 2011)

1 **Consider the use of prochlorperazine for 3 days regularly**

2 **Then prescribe as required**
- It may delay recovery by affecting the body's compensatory mechanism if taken for longer

P » The evidence does not suggest a role for antiviral medication or for benzodiazepines, despite some physicians choosing to use the latter.

5.3 Facial nerve palsy (including Bell palsy)

Definition: a facial nerve palsy refers to an upper or lower motor neuron lesion that causes weakness or paralysis of the facial muscles and symptoms, associated with diminished innervation of the facial nerve.

Epidemiology:

E » Bell palsy refers to an idiopathic unilateral palsy of unknown origin and sudden onset. Some have hypothesised a viral aetiology for the development of this condition. Bell palsy accounts for up to three-quarters of facial palsy. Remember that facial palsies that are bilateral, progressive or have an attributable cause are not diagnosed as Bell palsy.

- Affects men and women equally
- Bell (idiopathic) palsy is more common in pregnant women

Aetiology:
- Stroke
- Tumour compression
- Trauma (e.g. forceps delivery during birth)
- If facial palsies are recurrent or bilateral, consider a diagnosis of sarcoidosis, Lyme disease, Guillain–

Barré syndrome or HIV, particularly if additional features of these conditions are suspected

Clinical features:

W » It is important, particularly in unilateral palsies, to determine whether the lesion is due to an upper motor neuron (UMN) lesion or a lower motor neuron (LMN) lesion. A helpful way to remember this is that **upper** MN lesions **spare** the **upper face**. In lower motor neurons, the terminal neuronal tract is affected; whereas in UMN lesion, secondary pathways exist (so-called 'dual innervation'), allowing the patient to move and wrinkle their forehead, and delineating the type of lesion observed.

- Acute LMN lesion (Bell's is most common)
  - Sudden onset
  - Unilateral facial weakness (see *Fig. 5.11*)
  - Earache or preauricular pain
  - Eye dryness and inability to close eyes completely
  - **Bell sign** – eye rolls when patient attempts to close it
  - Hyperacusis (remember that the facial nerve innervates the stapedius)

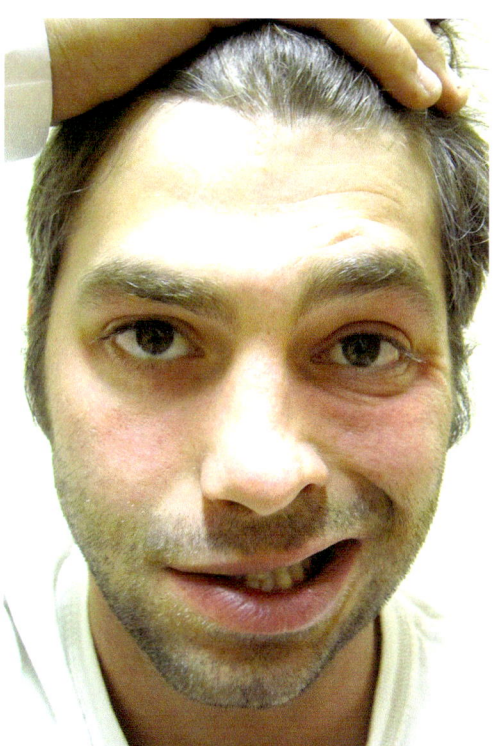

Fig. 5.11 *Bell palsy. Note the right facial paralysis (with upper face involvement) when the patient was asked to smile.*

Ramsay Hunt syndrome (NICE CKS 2012)

Severe pain might indicate Ramsay Hunt syndrome. This is caused by herpes zoster and is associated with a painful rash and herpetic vesicles.

Treatment for **Ramsay Hunt syndrome is with acyclovir and steroids. Note that this differs if the diagnosis is Bell palsy.**

Approach to Bell palsy (NICE CKS 2012)

Antiviral treatments are **not** recommended, alone or in combination with prednisolone, for the treatment of Bell palsy.

> **Stepwise management of Bell palsy**

1   Offer reassurance
- Patients should be reassured that most people recover from Bell palsy in 6–9 months
- Only a small number are left with permanent effects

2   Provide eye care
- Adequate eye lubrication with eye drops
- Taping the eye to protect it, particularly during sleep, should be encouraged

3   Prescribe prednisolone
- Within 72 hours of symptom onset
- 25mg BD for 10 days

5.4 Syncope

Approach to syncope

Syncope, as defined by the European Society of Cardiology (2009), refers to a **transient loss of consciousness** caused by global cerebral hypoperfusion, characterised by rapid onset, short duration and spontaneous complete recovery. Patients with syncope require thorough assessment in order to determine the underlying cause.

European Society of Cardiology (2009) classification of syncope:
- Reflex (neutrally mediated) syncope (see *Table 5.6*)
- Syncope due to orthostatic hypotension
  - After standing up
  - Relationship with introduction of new medication or alteration in medication dosage
  - Lying/standing BP first line

> **E** ⟫ Diagnosis of postural hypotension may be made if there is a change greater than 20/10 on lying/standing BP after standing for 3 minutes.

- Tilt-testing if uncertain or unconfirmed
- Eliminate offending drugs, **increase salt and water intake**
- If still refractory, consider using an alpha agonist (midodrine)
- Cardiac syncope
  - Arrhythmia
    - Bradycardia or tachycardias
    - Abnormal ECGs
    - Pacemaker or ICD malfunctions
    - Treat underlying cause
  - Structural heart disease
    - Investigate with echocardiography
    - Treat underlying cause

Table 5.6 *Type of reflex syncope*

Vasovagal	• Emotional distress or orthostatic stress (prolonged standing in hot, crowded areas) • Common in young adults/adolescents • Dizziness, nausea-associated, prior to faint • Recovery is rapid if patient falls, allowing blood to flow back to the brain • Benign condition – offer **reassurance**, emphasise trigger recognition and avoiding agents that lower BP
Situational	• Cough, sneezing, micturition, post-prandial • Recognise triggers
Carotid sinus hypersensitivity	• Abnormal sensitivity in up to one-third of patients • Carotid sinus massage may be helpful in assessment
Atypical	

Reflex/neutrally mediated syncope is the most common type. Asking for features of the syncopal event (including duration and associated symptoms), particularly from witnesses, is exceptionally helpful. It is also helpful to ask about relevant family history (e.g. of cardiac conditions) and review medications.

5.4.1 Seizures and epilepsy

One key distinction to make is what constitutes a seizure and what is meant by the term epilepsy.

SIGN diagnosis and management of epilepsy in adults (2015)

A seizure can be defined as a transient occurrence of signs and symptoms due to abnormal electrical activity in the brain. This manifests itself as a disturbance of consciousness, behaviour, emotion, motor function or sensation.

The International League Against Epilepsy (2014) defines **epilepsy** as a disease of the brain, defined by any of the following conditions:

• At least two unprovoked seizures occurring more than 24 hours apart
• One unprovoked seizure and a probability of further seizures similar to the general recurrence risk after two unprovoked seizures, occurring over the next 10 years
• Diagnosis of an epilepsy syndrome (various types)

Only one-third of patients are said to have an attributable cause. Patients with a positive family history, learning disabilities and previous neurological infections are at increased risk.

W ➤➤ Todd paresis refers to focal weakness of a body part post-ictally (after a seizure). It most commonly affects the upper or lower limbs and is consigned to either the left or right half of the body, but may also affect speech or vision. It usually resolves within 48 hours. The condition was observed by Robert Bentley Todd, a popular Irish-born London physician, in 1849. Dr Todd was a noted physiologist, who was also known for the 'Hot Toddy' (a concoction of warm brandy, cinnamon, sugar and water that he prescribed for his patients).

Status epilepticus is a continuous seizure for 30 minutes or longer, or recurrent seizures without regaining consciousness lasting 30 minutes or longer (see *Chapter 12*).

E ➤➤ Provoked seizures are **non-epileptic**, i.e. they are due to a discernible cause, e.g. metabolic, toxic, infectious, producing seizures.

Broadly, seizures may be grouped into:
• **Simple focal (partial)**
  – Focal motor or sensory symptoms
  – Usually arises from one region of the brain
  – Consciousness retained
  – Most common type of partial seizure arises from the temporal lobe – patients may describe an aura (vague gastric discomfort)
• **Complex focal (partial)**
  – May have preceding aura (unexpected tastes, smells, paraesthesias or a rising abdominal sensation) before loss of consciousness

- – Automatisms, e.g. lip-smacking, chewing
- – Usually unable to recall seizure
- **Focal (partial) seizures progressing to generalised tonic-clonic convulsions**
  - – Also known as secondarily generalised seizures
  - – Associated with unilateral jerks, unilateral head turning and Todd paresis

> **P** ➤➤ The terms 'simple' and 'complex' refer to the estimated state of consciousness and awareness. Broadly, 'simple' means no impaired consciousness, and 'complex' means impaired consciousness.

- **Absence seizures (petit mal)**
  - – Begin in childhood
  - – Sharp onset and offset; child stares for a few seconds
  - – Eyelid twitching
  - – Usually less than 30 seconds
  - – May occur dozens to hundreds of times daily
- **Myoclonic seizures**
  - – Seizures that cause brief, shock-like contraction of the limbs, without apparent impairment of consciousness
- **Tonic-clonic (grand mal) seizures**
  - – Stiffening, rhythmic limb-jerking
  - – Associated with tongue-biting; incontinence, loss of consciousness

NICE and the Joint Epilepsy Council (2011) advise that an individual with epilepsy who dies suddenly without an identifiable cause is said to have **Sudden Unexpected Death in Epilepsy (SUDEP)**, which correlates with the frequency and severity of seizures. Accidents related to seizure onset are also an important cause of mortality.

> **Stepwise management of a seizure (NICE CKS 2015)**
>
> **1 Stabilise the patient if they are having an active seizure**
> - See *Chapter 12*
>
> **2 Assess risk factors and history**
>
> **3 Arrange blood tests (FBC, U&Es, LFTs) and an ECG**
> - Treat any underlying abnormalities or reversible causes
>
> **4 Offer advice and referral**
> - Refer patient to a neurologist

- Advise patient to stop driving until they have specialist confirmation
- Advise family on management of seizures, and ask them to record any subsequent seizures if possible

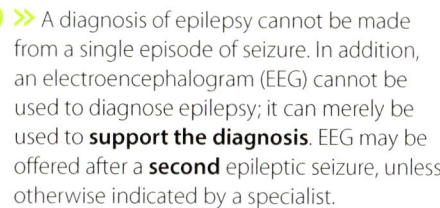

> **E** ➤➤ A diagnosis of epilepsy cannot be made from a single episode of seizure. In addition, an electroencephalogram (EEG) cannot be used to diagnose epilepsy; it can merely be used to **support the diagnosis**. EEG may be offered after a **second** epileptic seizure, unless otherwise indicated by a specialist.

5 Consider neuroimaging
- Neuroimaging (with MRI as first line) is recommended if patients have evidence of focal onset, or are refractory to first-line therapy

6 Initiation of anti-epileptic medication should follow risk–benefit assessment
- This is usually instituted after a second seizure, or once the diagnosis has been confirmed

Treatment

Generally, anti-epileptic drug treatment is classified into:
- Broad-spectrum anti-epileptic medication (e.g. levetiracetam, lamotrigine, sodium valproate, topiramate)
- Narrow-spectrum anti-epileptic medication (e.g. phenytoin, carbamazepine)

Bear in mind that there is no single best agent – the choice of pharmacologic therapy depends on the patient's comorbidities, socio-economic background and type of epilepsy.
- Of these, levetiracetam is a commonly used therapy, partly because it has the fewest interactions with other medications and is generally well tolerated (even in CKD or liver disease), but do bear in mind that it has reportedly been associated with an increased incidence of mood disorders, anxiety and suicidal ideation
- There is also good evidence for carbamazepine as a first-line agent in the context of focal (partial) epilepsy
- Another medication, ethosuximide, is largely used as an alternative agent in absence seizures

5

➤➤ Pregnant patients with diagnosed epilepsy should ideally aim to manage their epilepsy with one agent. **Lamotrigine** is the drug of choice in this case, as sodium valproate is associated with the development of neural tube defects.

➤➤ Patients may also present with a conversion disorder related to epilepsy, known as a **psychogenic non-epileptic seizure**. Patients with this condition have a variable presentation, may have relapsing jerking movements (sometimes related to pelvic movement) and may have a history of trauma or abuse. An inpatient video EEG is required to make the diagnosis.

5.5 Headache

Approach to headache

Headache is one of the most common presenting symptoms worldwide. It is more likely to affect women. The International Headache Society (2013) differentiates headaches into **primary** and **secondary** categories. A secondary headache usually has an attributable cause, and is likely to be of greater severity.

Reaching a diagnosis requires careful consideration of the type of pain described, duration of symptoms, associated precipitants or features and onset. The physician should also develop an appreciation of when to investigate and refer, as well as a knowledge of 'red flag' symptoms.

Headaches in over-12s: diagnosis and management (NICE 2012, CG150)
NICE recommends considering the need for further evaluation if these are present:
• Sudden-onset headache, reaching maximal intensity within 5 minutes
• Worsening headache with fever
• New-onset cognitive/behavioural dysfunction or neurological deficit
• Recent head trauma or change in characteristic of headache
• Features of acute glaucoma or giant cell arteritis

Primary headaches
• Tension-type headache
• Cluster headache
• Migraine
• Others:
  – Stabbing
  – Exertional
  – Post-coital
  – Valsalva
  – Persistent

 ➤➤ Exertional and post-coital headaches have a sudden onset and may peak at the point of maximal exertion (e.g. during orgasm in post-coital headaches). You should aim to exclude subarachnoid haemorrhages in these cases.

Secondary headaches
• Associated with an attributable cause, such as:
  – Trauma
  – Vascular event
  – Infection
  – Raised intracranial pressure
  – Space-occupying lesions
• Concomitant disorders that may exacerbate primary headache
  – Medication overuse headache

NICE recommends being alert to the possibility of medication overuse headache in people whose headache developed or worsened while they were taking the following drugs for 3 months or more:
• Triptans, opioids, ergots or combination analgesic medications on 10 days per month or more
• Paracetamol, aspirin or an NSAID, either alone or in any combination, on 15 days per month or more

5.5.1 Migraine

Definition: a migraine refers to an episodic primary headache disorder that may present with aura or prove to be chronic.

Epidemiology:
• Studies in the UK and USA estimate annual prevalence at 7% in men and 18% in women
• Nearly three times more common in women

Aetiology/pathophysiology:
- The condition is thought to be neurovascular
- Inflammation of trigeminal sensory neurons causes increased vascular permeability and platelet activation
- This is thought to increase the sensitivity of neuronal fibres, which then interpret normal arterial flow through meningeal arteries as painful; this is thought to account for the 'pulsatile' pain observed in migraine

 P ≫ The International Headache Society recognises various types of migraine. But – briefly – there are three major forms:
- Migraine with aura (classical)
- Migraine without aura
- Chronic migraine.

Approach to migraine
It is important to remember that the diagnosis of migraine is made clinically, but red flag symptoms should always be assessed and evaluated.

Migraine without aura:
- The diagnosis of migraine can be made precisely by following the International Headache Society Guideline
- Generally, the mnemonic 'POUND' is helpful, in that three or more of the criteria are highly suggestive of migraine:
  Pulsatile in nature
  One day's duration
  Unilateral (largely)
  Nausea or vomiting
  Disability (from work or from physical activity)
- **Migraine with aura** (British Association for the Study of Headache (BASH) guidelines)
  - Diagnosis is easier; affects one-third of migraine patients
  - Typical aura – progressive, onset usually 5–50 minutes prior to headache, with **transient hemianopic disturbances and a spreading scintillating scotoma**
  - Aura may also include paraesthesia and numbness of hand, face and upper limbs

P ≫ Migraines may also be associated with the onset of menstruation. In this case, migraine diaries may help with diagnosis.

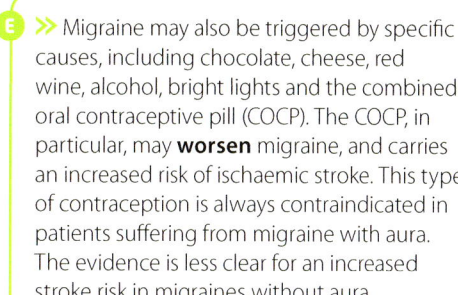 **E** ≫ Migraine may also be triggered by specific causes, including chocolate, cheese, red wine, alcohol, bright lights and the combined oral contraceptive pill (COCP). The COCP, in particular, may **worsen** migraine, and carries an increased risk of ischaemic stroke. This type of contraception is always contraindicated in patients suffering from migraine with aura. The evidence is less clear for an increased stroke risk in migraines without aura.

Stepwise management of migraine with or without aura

1   Acute treatment
- **Combination therapy**
  - Oral triptan + NSAID
  - **Or** oral triptan + paracetamol
  - If between 12 and 17 years of age, consider nasal triptan preferentially
  - Consider the use of an anti-emetic, even if there is no nausea or vomiting

2   Prophylaxis
- If >2 attacks a month
- Propranolol or topiramate
- **Topiramate is teratogenic**
- If both propranolol and topiramate are contraindicated, consider acupuncture
- Riboflavin and magnesium supplementation may help reduce frequency in some patients
- Lifestyle modification – reduce caffeine intake, avoid triggers (chocolate, cheese)

5.5.2 Tension-type headache

Tension-type headaches are episodic or chronic headaches related to stress or difficulty. They are classically described as feeling like 'a tight band around the head' and are more common in women. Tension headaches are sometimes bilateral, but usually not pulsatile.

Stepwise plan (NICE 2012, CG150):

1   Further investigations are usually unnecessary

2   Provide reassurance, as this condition is generally self-limiting

3   Provide first-line pharmacological management
- Paracetamol
- NSAIDs (ibuprofen 400mg first line)

5

5

4 **Prescribe medication for chronic recurrent tension-type headaches**
- Tricyclic antidepressants (amitriptyline)
- Titrate down over time
- NICE recommends acupuncture in this case, as a form of prophylaxis

5.5.3 Cluster headache

Cluster headaches refer to a specific type of headache associated with intense pain coming from within, around or behind the eye. Patients usually present with a headache and a red, watery eye, with or without nasal congestion. The condition is more common in men, and its aetiology is unknown.

Clinical features:
- The symptoms occur in 'clusters' of 4–12 weeks at a time
- Several times a day without aura
- Usually annually and during the same season each year
- The headaches also frequently occur at night
- They may last up to three hours and cause the patient to be uncomfortably restless

Stepwise plan:

1 **The diagnosis is made clinically**

2 **Encourage appropriate lifestyle changes**
- Smoking and alcohol can trigger cluster headaches

3 **Provide treatment for acute attacks**
- Treat with 100% oxygen and a subcutaneous or nasal triptan (e.g. sumatriptan)

E ≫ There are two other differentials when diagnosing cluster headache. These are:
- Chronic paroxysmal hemicranias
  - Occur several times a day
  - Responsive to indomethacin; symptoms of cluster headache will not be alleviated by this drug
- Short-lasting unilateral neuralgiform headaches with conjunctival injection and tearing (SUNCT)
  - Can occur up to hundreds of times in a 24-hour period
  - Difficult to treat; lamotrigine suggested as a potential therapeutic option.

4 **Provide prophylaxis**
- Prophylactic treatment with verapamil should be instituted before the season in which a 'cluster' will occur
- This will differ from patient to patient

5.5.4 Trigeminal neuralgia

Trigeminal neuralgia is a severe, disabling condition, characterised by painful episodes of sudden, sharp stabbing pain in the region of trigeminal nerve distribution (specifically the V2 and V3 branches). In most cases, trigeminal neuralgia occurs secondary to nerve compression by arteries or veins, and in a smaller number of cases secondary to compression by a tumour or arteriovenous malformation.

The episodes may occur several times a day, and are described like 'electric shocks'. They may sometimes be triggered by activities such as washing, shaving, brushing teeth or a cold draught.

The condition is most likely to occur in older patients, but younger individuals (particularly those with multiple sclerosis) are more likely to present at a younger age, and also have a higher incidence of the condition presenting bilaterally.

Stepwise plan:

1 **Diagnosis is clinical**
- MRI may help exclude secondary causes

2 **Carbamazepine is the first-line treatment**
- Second-line agents include baclofen or gabapentin

P ≫ Carbamazepine is effective in about half the cases of trigeminal neuralgia, but has several notable side effects (particularly dizziness or drowsiness and a small risk of agranulocytosis). A derivative of carbamazepine, oxcarbazepine, whilst being more expensive, has been reported to have fewer side effects.

3 **In patients who are unresponsive to medical therapy, consider surgical therapy**
- Options include:
  - Percutaneous radiofrequence coagulation or Gamma knife
  - Microvascular decompression or rhizotomy (use of electric current to dampen pain signals)

5.6 Infections of the nervous system

The nervous system (like other systems) is susceptible to infections. Some infections affect the layers of the central nervous system (for instance, infections of the meninges cause meningitis), whereas parenchymal infections result in encephalitis. Infections caused by other pathogens (such as helminths, prions, fungi and protozoa) are discussed in *Chapter 9*.

5.6.1 Meningitis

Definition: meningitis refers to inflammation of the meninges due to infective organisms such as viruses, bacteria or fungi, or (rarely) due to non-infective causes.

Epidemiology:
- More likely to affect infants, young people and older individuals
- Most common cause of death secondary to infectious disease in the young

Aetiology:
- Meningitis can present with predominantly meningitic symptoms (see classic features listed below), frank sepsis, or a combination of the two
- Most common aetiology is viral (Coxsackie, echoviruses)
- The incidence of bacterial meningitis has greatly decreased because of the introduction of the Men C (meningococcus), pneumococcal and Hib vaccines (*H. influenzae*)
- Patients with a history of spinal procedures (e.g. surgery, anaesthesia, lumbar puncture) or shunts are at greater risk of developing meningitis
- Proximity to other people in confined spaces, especially in young people (classically in universities and the military), is also often cited as a risk factor in the development of meningitis

Approach to meningitis

> **W** ≫ There are myriad causes for the development of meningitis. This is further complicated by the fact that the aetiological agent is not immediately recognisable at presentation. For instance, viral meningitis (despite being the most common cause of meningism) is clinically indistinguishable from bacterial meningitis. A high index of suspicion is therefore required, and all cases of suspected meningitis should be treated empirically as bacterial meningitis until proven otherwise.

- Classic features of meningitis include:
  - Fever
  - Headache
  - Neck stiffness
  - Photophobia
  - Non-blanching petechial rash in meningococcal meningitis
  - Altered mental status or seizures (see *Section 5.6.2*)
  - Shock

> **P** ≫ Research indicates that a large number of patients have at least two of these symptoms at presentation, but bear in mind that symptoms may be non-specific, particularly in children.

  - Kernig sign
    - Pain when hip is fully flexed and knee is extended
  - Brudzinski sign
    - Flexion of the neck produces reflex flexion of the hip and/or knee

> **E** ≫ In the Kernig sign, pain occurs due to stretching of the meninges due to movement. In the Brudzinski sign, reflex flexion occurs primarily to reduce meningeal irritation. However, in practice, the diagnostic value of these signs is fairly limited.

- One approach, when looking for a possible aetiological agent, is to consider age group and the potential risk factors associated with a particular patient (see *Table 5.7*).

> **P** ≫ Mollaret meningitis refers to a form of aseptic meningitis characterised by recurrent episodes of meningism interspersed with weeks of being symptom-free. The exact aetiological cause has yet to be confirmed, but *Herpes simplex* (HSV-2) has been implicated in the pathogenesis of this condition.

5

Table 5.7 *Common meningitis-causing pathogens*

Age/at-risk group	Features
Neonates and Infants	• Most common agent in neonates is **Group B streptococci** • Other agents include *E. coli* and *Listeria monocytogenes* • Neonates most at risk include those with low birth weight, transplacental infection or premature birth • **Non-specific symptoms** – irritability, difficulty feeding, pyrexia, respiratory difficulty
Children	• Most common agents are ***Neisseria meningitidis* (meningococcus)**, ***Strep. pneumoniae* (pneumococcus)** and ***Haem. influenzae*** (particularly if unimmunised) • A generalised purpuric rash with a fever, headache or other associated symptoms in a child warrants urgent antibiotic treatment (treat as meningococcal meningitis until proven otherwise)
Adults	• Most likely agents are *N. meningitidis* and *Strep. pneumoniae* • Consider appropriate risk factors – e.g. military background, crowded living conditions
Elderly	• Most common agent is *Strep. pneumoniae* • Other agents include *Listeria monocytogenes* and *N. meningitidis*
Immunocompromised	• Agents include *Listeria monocytogenes*, mycobacteria (including *M. tuberculosis*) and CMV
HIV/AIDS	• Cryptococcal meningitis should be considered in addition to other agents affecting immunocompromised individuals • Request cryptococcal antigen test

Investigations

Stepwise plan:

1 Provide empirical treatment immediately
• Treatment should proceed immediately, and should not be delayed while relevant investigations are carried out

2 Arrange lumbar puncture (LP)
• Carry out LP if no contraindications present (e.g. raised ICP, focal neurology)

• Normal CSF is clear in colour
• CSF is usually evaluated for glucose, protein, Gram stain, Ziehl–Neelsen stain (among others)

3 Arrange blood tests
• Blood cultures
• Viral/bacterial PCR
• ABG
• FBC, U&Es, coagulation screen, CRP, ESR

Lumbar puncture (LP) CSF analysis

Table 5.8 *LP analysis*

	Bacterial	Viral	Tuberculous	Fungal
Colour	Turbid/cloudy	Clear	Mildly turbid/cloudy	Varies
White cells	Predominantly polymorphs	Predominantly lymphocytes	Predominantly lymphocytes	Varies
Glucose	<40% serum glucose	>60% serum glucose	Lowered	Lowered
Protein	Elevated	Normal/mildly raised	Elevated	Elevated
CSF opening pressure	Elevated	Normal	Elevated	Elevated

Management

> **Stepwise management of meningitis (NICE 2010, CG102)**

1   Start initial empirical therapy
- Initial blind therapy for patients
  - IV ceftriaxone/cefotaxime for at least 10 days
- NICE (2010, CG102) advocates the use of IV cefotaxime in neonates and infants, as ceftriaxone may worsen jaundice or cause acidosis, particularly in newborns or premature babies
- If <3 months or >50 years old:
  - Add IV amoxicillin
  - Treat for at least 14 days
  - If allergic to penicillin, offer chloramphenicol

> **E** ≫ If the patient is in primary care or in the community setting, IM benzylpenicillin should be given in suspected meningococcal disease.

2   Provide additional therapy
- Offer concomitant IV acyclovir if HSV encephalitis or viral meningitis is suspected
- Offer dexamethasone 0.15mg/kg QDS (max dose 10mg) for 4 days in suspected or confirmed **bacterial meningitis**, as this reduces inflammation
- Resuscitate with fluids as appropriate
- NICE advises against the use of high-dose steroids in meningococcal septicaemia, and advises that dexamethasone, if appropriate, should be given within 4 hours of antibiotic therapy and no later than 12 hours after antibiotics have been administered
- Corticosteroids **should not** be used in infants who are less than 3 months old

3   Offer prophylaxis
- Household members and close contacts should be offered either rifampicin or ciprofloxacin
- Ciprofloxacin has largely replaced rifampicin as the prophylactic agent of choice

5.6.2 Encephalitis

Definition: refers to inflammation of the brain parenchyma, and is most often caused by viruses. Encephalitis can occur together with meningeal inflammation, producing meningoencephalitis.

Epidemiology:
- More likely to affect neonates, the elderly and the immunocompromised

Aetiology:
- Most frequent organism implicated is **herpes simplex (HSV-1)**, causing **herpes simplex encephalitis (HSE)**, which typically affects the temporal lobes, producing focal symptoms such as aphasia
- Bacteria, fungi and parasites (e.g. in toxoplasmosis) may also cause encephalitis

> **E** ≫ Encephalitis is classically associated with a triad of symptoms (fever, headache and altered mental status), which progress fairly rapidly.

Investigations
- Lumbar puncture (barring any contraindications)
- Blood tests (as in meningitis)
- Neuroimaging (CT/MRI), which may demonstrate pathology (see *Fig. 5.12*)

> **P** ≫ A ring-enhancing lesion on CT/MRI (see *Fig. 5.13*) should prompt consideration of several possible diagnoses, including cerebral abscesses, tumours, metastasis and demyelination. Most cases require neurosurgical referral. If a cerebral abscess is suspected, IV ceftriaxone should also be administered.

Management
- Prompt IV acyclovir (improves prognosis if given early in disease progression)
- Empirical treatment for meningitis
- Corticosteroids are **not** encouraged
- Judicious fluid therapy so as not to exacerbate possible cerebral oedema
- Monitoring and treatment of any accompanying seizure

5

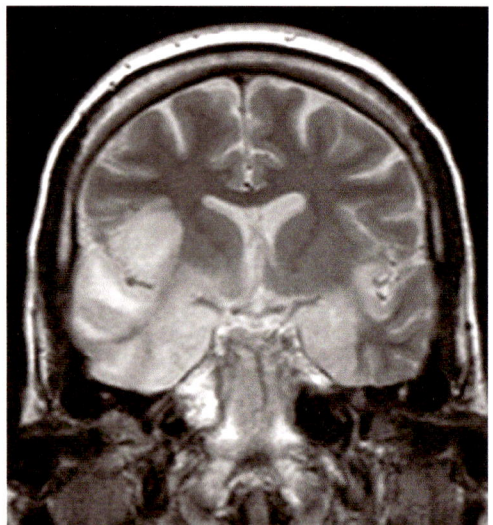

Fig. 5.12 *Large hyperintense right temporal lesion on MRI suggestive of cerebral oedema, caused by HSV encephalitis.*

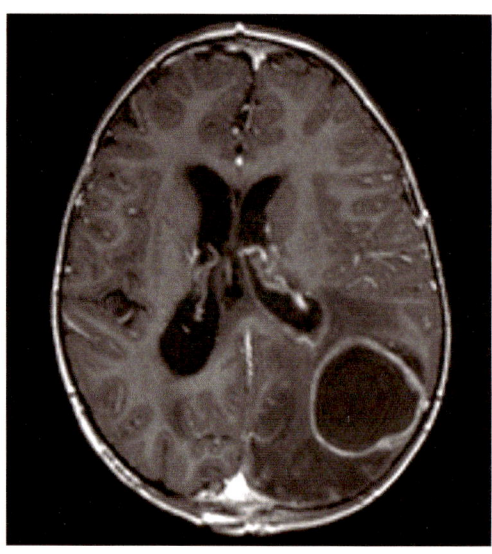

Fig. 5.13 *Ring-enhancing lesion on MRI brain scan, consistent with a cerebral abscess.*

5.7 Stroke

Definition: a stroke (cerebrovascular accident/CVA) is defined as an acute neurological event caused by cerebrovascular pathology.

Epidemiology:
- Annual incidence is 15 million people worldwide
- Higher in Afro-Caribbean populations
- Most common cause of long-term disability

> **E** ≫ Risk factors for the development of stroke include:
> - Hypertension (most important risk factor)
> - Smoking
> - Diabetes mellitus
> - Hypercoagulability
> - Hyperlipidaemia
> - COCP
> - Trauma
> - Atrial fibrillation (5 x increased risk)
> - Anticoagulation (increased risk of bleeding).

Aetiology/pathophysiology:
- Strokes are broadly divided into two groups:
  - **Ischaemic** (80%)
    - If less than 24 hours, it is considered a **transient ischaemic attack** (or mini-stroke,

in layman's terms), although this definition is currently being revised
  - Caused largely by atherothromboembolism
  - Embolic stroke may occur secondary to:
    - Atrial fibrillation
    - Septic emboli from infective endocarditis
    - Valvular heart disease (e.g. mitral stenosis)
    - Air embolus iatrogenically
    - Fat embolus in trauma, particularly long bone fracture
  - **Haemorrhagic** (20%)
    - Intracerebral spontaneous haemorrhage (primary)
    - Aneurysmal rupture, subarachnoid haemorrhage or vascular malformation (secondary)

> **W** ≫ The pathophysiology of an ischaemic stroke, regardless of how it might occur, is related to the degree of occlusion of the cerebral artery affected. A haemorrhagic stroke, on the other hand, may result in an expanding haematoma (caused by blood vessel rupture) that can provoke damage in three major ways: direct anatomical insult, compression of surrounding structures or raised ICP.

Table 5.9 Oxford/Bamford classification of stroke

Classification	Characteristics
TACS/TACI (total anterior circulation stroke/infarct)	• Greatest mortality at 1 year (>50%) • Large infarct, usually affects middle cerebral artery (MCA) or anterior cerebral artery (ACA) • All 3 criteria
PACS/PACI (partial anterior circulation stroke/infarct)	• Usually involves branches of MCA or ACA • 2 out of 3 of the criteria are present
LACS/LACI (lacunar stroke/infarct)	• Occlusion of small arteries around the thalamus, pons, basal ganglia and internal capsule • Variable presentation: pure motor, pure sensory, sensorimotor, ataxia or dysarthria • No higher cortical dysfunction or homonymous hemianopia present

POCS/POCI (posterior circulation stroke/infarct)	• Vertebrobasilar stroke
	• Any of:
	  – Cerebellar/brainstem dysfunction
	  – Loss of consciousness
	  – Homonymous hemianopia that occurs in isolation

Clinical features:

Stroke and transient ischaemic attack in over-16s: diagnosis and initial management (NICE 2008, CG68)

• Prompt recognition of symptoms improves outcomes:
  – Outside hospital
    ○ FAST (face, arm, speech test), looking for facial droop, arm weakness, slurred speech – refer immediately; this is a validated tool, with a positive predictive value of 75%
  – A&E
    ○ Validated scoring system (ROSIER – recognition of stroke in the emergency room)

• Formal classifications include:
  – Classification by clinical appraisal of the infarct, i.e. **Oxford/Bamford** classification
  – Classification by **anatomical territory**

Oxford/Bamford classification

Classification of stroke can be made according to syndrome or infarct, by replacing the last letter in the system. The last letter in the classification is switched from S (syndrome) to I (infarct), when the location has been confirmed on neuroimaging. Table 5.9 summarises this classification.

Classification by anatomical territory

Table 5.10 Stroke presentation based on anatomical territory

Anatomical site/presenting condition	Features
Anterior cerebral artery (ACA)	• Contralateral sensory and motor weakness • **Lower** limb symptoms predominate
Middle cerebral artery (MCA)	• Contralateral sensory and motor weakness • **Upper** limb symptoms predominate • Contralateral homonymous hemianopia • Aphasia
Posterior cerebral artery (PCA)	• Contralateral homonymous hemianopia • **Macular sparing**
Wallenberg syndrome (lateral medullary syndrome)	• Affects posterior inferior cerebellar artery (PICA) • **Ipsilateral:** loss of **facial** pain and temperature • **Contralateral** loss of **body** pain and temperature • **Cerebellar dysfunction**
Weber syndrome	• Ipsilateral third nerve palsy with contralateral hemiplegia • Midbrain infarct, caused by posterior cerebral artery infarction
Locked-in syndrome	• Patient is aware of surroundings • No impaired cognition • Complete paralysis apart from eye muscles • May be caused by basilar artery infarction

5

5

E ⟫ The following criteria are assessed:
- Contralateral hemiparesis, motor weakness with or without sensory loss
- Homonymous hemianopia
- Higher cortical dysfunction (e.g. speech disorder).

Investigations

Stepwise plan:

1 Arrange neuroimaging
- Urgent, best initial test
- CT or MRI
- CT recommended because of ease of access (see *Figs 5.14* and *5.15*)

E ⟫ Haemorrhagic stroke must be urgently excluded (using neuroimaging) before treatment for ischaemic stroke is initiated.

2 Arrange blood tests and check blood pressure
- FBC, U&Es, ESR
- Assess for presence of hypertension

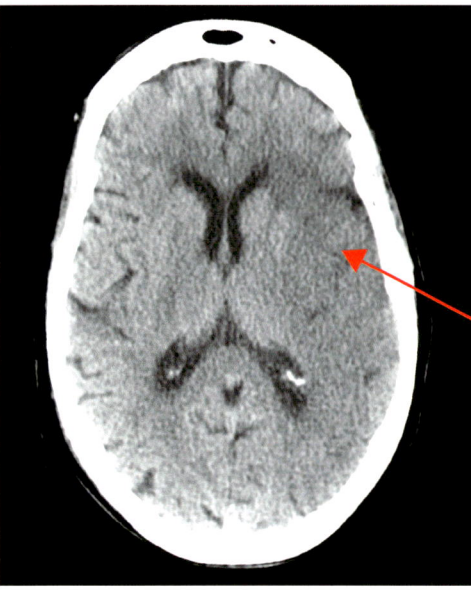

Fig. 5.14 CT brain showing a right MCA stroke. Note the hypoattenuated (darker) tissue, indicative of an infarct.

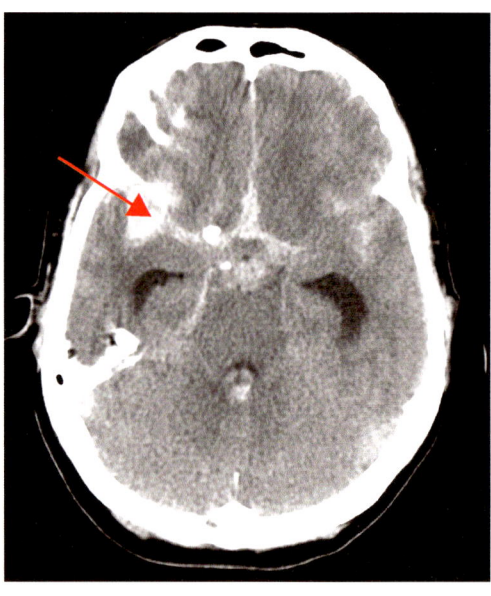

Fig. 5.15 CT brain showing a left temporal lobe subarachnoid haemorrhage.

3 Obtain speech and language (SALT) assessment
- Assess swallow

4 Perform cardiac assessment
- ECG (assess for AF)
- Echocardiography (emboli, valvular disease)

5 Carry out carotid artery assessment
- Carotid artery imaging (duplex ultrasound)

Management
Recognised stroke patients should be admitted to specialist stroke units. Treatment of stroke is urgent, and appropriate neuroimaging should be arranged as soon as possible.

Stepwise management of stroke (NICE 2008, CG68)

1 Exclude haemorrhage
- Exclude haemorrhage on neuroimaging

2 Consider thrombolysis
- Alteplase is the agent of choice (NICE)
- It should be administered by trained staff operating on a stroke service or in A&E
- **Give within 4.5 hours of symptom onset**
- **Ensure haemorrhage has been excluded**

3 Arrange nutrition and hydration
- **Urgently assess swallow by SALT**
- Keep patient NBM if swallow-impaired; consider NG tube

- Keep blood glucose between 4 and 11mmol/L; use sliding scale if there is a history of DM

E ➤➤ Aspiration pneumonia is a serious complication associated with stroke; swallow should always be assessed in patients presenting with stroke symptoms.

4 Prescribe aspirin
- 300mg orally once haemorrhage has been excluded
- Give rectally if swallow is impaired

5 Arrange surgical management
- Refer to neurosurgery if haemorrhage present
- Bleeding aneurysms may be coiled (refer to interventional radiology)
- **When stable**, patients should be considered for carotid endarterectomy if stenosis >50% (according to NASCET – North American Symptomatic Carotid Endarterectomy Trial) or >70% (according to ECST – European Carotid Surgery Trial)

6 Provide post-stroke management
- Early mobilisation
- If in AF, appropriate anticoagulation using CHADS scoring system should be commenced 2 or more weeks after the initial ischaemic stroke
- Risk factor optimisation; prescribe a statin if necessary; optimise blood pressure control after the patient has recovered
- **Aspirin given for 2 weeks, then switch to oral clopidogrel monotherapy 75mg once daily (aspirin + dipyridamole is an equally effective combination)**
- Refer for physiotherapy, occupational therapy and speech therapy assessment

5.7.1 Transient ischaemic attack (TIA)

A TIA, much like a stroke, is an acute neurological event secondary to cerebrovascular pathology, but **resolves within 24 hours**. Indeed, symptoms often resolve within minutes to hours. More recent definitions focus on the absence of detectable infarction on imaging modalities, irrespective of duration of symptoms.

E ➤➤ Patients who have had a suspected TIA are at much greater risk of subsequent stroke and should be assessed using the ABCD$_2$ scoring system.

Age ≥60 (1 point)
Blood pressure ≥140/90 (1 point)
Clinical features
- Unilateral weakness (2 points)
- Slurred speech, absence of motor weakness (1 point)

Duration of symptoms, DM
- >60 minutes (2 points)
- 10–59 minutes (1 point)

Diabetes mellitus (1 point).

Patients with an ABCD$_2$ score ≥4:
- 300mg daily aspirin immediately
- Specialist assessment and investigation within 24 hours

Patients with an ABCD$_2$ score 3 or lower:
- 300mg daily aspirin immediately
- Specialist assessment and investigation when possible, but no later than 1 week after the onset of symptoms

NICE (2008, CG68) advises that patients presenting with two or more TIAs within a week (known as 'crescendo TIA') should be treated as high risk, regardless of their ABCD$_2$ score.

P ➤➤ Patients presenting with a TIA should be offered 300mg aspirin for 2 weeks (much like those presenting with a stroke), and should be switched to aspirin and dipyridamole thereafter. Appropriate anticoagulation and risk factor optimisation should proceed accordingly.

W ➤➤ Amaurosis fugax (which means 'fleeting darkness'), refers to a form of painless **transient** visual loss that may be monocular or binocular. Patients classically describe the condition as 'a curtain coming down' on their vision. It is typically caused by emboli from the ipsilateral carotid artery and represents a non-hemispheric TIA. Patients should be assessed (using the ABCD$_2$ score) and managed accordingly. Carotid artery imaging should also be arranged.

5

5.8 Head injury

5.8.1 Subarachnoid haemorrhage

Definition: subarachnoid haemorrhage (SAH) refers to a medical emergency characterised by bleeding into the subarachnoid space.

Epidemiology:
- 6–9 per 100,000
- Affects more women than men

> **E** ≫ Risk factors for the development of SAH include:
> - Smoking
> - Hypertension
> - Alcohol
> - Cocaine
> - Connective tissue diseases (e.g. Ehlers–Danlos, Marfan's)
> - Family history.

Aetiology/pathophysiology:
- 80–85% of all SAHs are **caused by the rupture of berry aneurysms**
- The majority of berry aneurysms occur in the circle of Willis

> **W** ≫ The bleed is thought to be multifactorial in causative origin, with features such as genetic susceptibility of the arterial lamina, and size and number of aneurysms, and associated factors such as hypertension and smoking contributing to the development of a bleed.

> **P** ≫ Recall that berry aneurysms themselves are associated with other conditions, such as adult polycystic kidney disease, connective tissue disorders and coarctation of the aorta.

- Other causes include trauma, space-occupying lesions and arteriovenous malformations

Clinical features:
- Patients describe a **sudden** headache, usually occurring within **seconds to minutes,** classically a **thunderclap headache**
- May be described as 'the worst headache of their life'
- May present with seizures, vomiting and depressed level of consciousness, but these are non-specific features
- SAH should be suspected and investigated in sudden-onset headaches

> **P** ≫ In a smaller number of patients, headaches, dizziness and visual disturbances may precede SAH by 2–3 weeks. These warning symptoms are known as a **sentinel bleed**, and are thought to arise due to aneurysmal expansion. Prompt investigation and treatment should be carried out.

Investigations

Stepwise plan:

1 **Arrange CT scan without contrast as first-line investigation**
- Investigation of choice (see *Fig. 5.14*)
- Detects approximately 95% of SAH
- Angiography, particularly using a catheter, may help localise the bleed. Endovascular coiling can then be attempted

2 **Order lumbar puncture**
- If SAH is suspected, but the CT is **negative**
- Perform after 12h, allowing sufficient time for red cell lysis to occur
- Detection of xanthochromia (yellow discoloration of CSF) confirms the diagnosis

Management

Stepwise management of subarachnoid haemorrhage

1 **Arrange for endovascular coiling or neurosurgical clipping (urgent referral)**
- Endovascular coiling preferred, if possible

2 **Provide supportive therapy**
- Referral to neurosurgery
- Regular neurological observations
- Postoperative nimodipine (60mg 4-hourly) to reduce vasospasm, which may lead to ischaemia

3 Offer preventive measures
- Encourage lifestyle modification
- Screen first-degree relatives with genetic conditions

> **E** ≫ Rebleeding is the most common complication, followed by ischaemic injury and hydrocephalus. The condition still carries with it a 50% chance of mortality – even without the development of complications.

5.8.2 Subdural haematoma

A subdural haematoma refers to pooling of blood in the subdural space. It most commonly occurs secondary to rupture of bridging veins acutely.

> **P** ≫ Subdural haematomas are also associated with vigorous coup and counter-coup forces in non-accidental injuries in children, and are linked with 'shaken baby syndrome'.

Older individuals or alcoholics are also more likely to develop subdural haematomas as a result of cerebral atrophy.

Approach to subdural haematoma
Features in the history may include a fluctuating level of consciousness, drowsiness, headache or incontinence.

> **Stepwise plan:**

1 **Assess GCS level and obtain a non-contrast CT scan**
- Demonstrates a crescent-shaped haematoma (see *Fig. 5.16*)

2 **Arrange management, including:**
- Neurosurgical referral
- Evacuation of haematoma via burr hole craniostomy
- Alternatively, craniotomy (second-line treatment)

> **E** ≫ Patients treated with appropriate surgical management often demonstrate rapid improvement of symptoms.

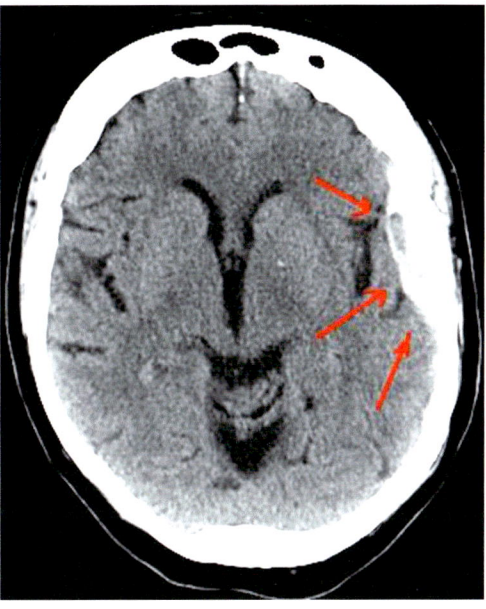

Fig. 5.16 *Subdural haematoma.*

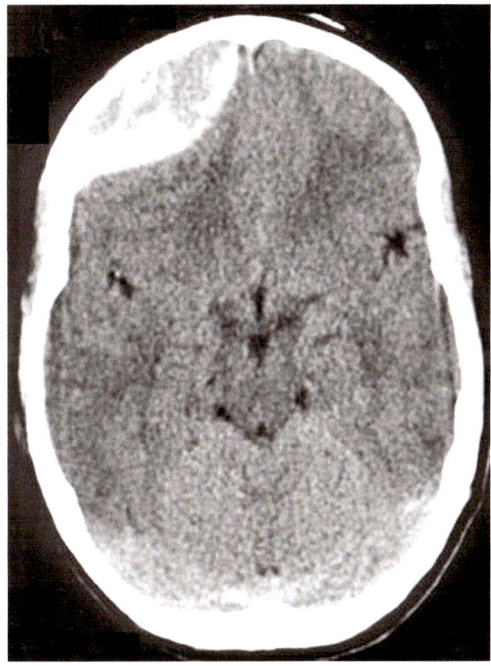

Fig. 5.17 *Extradural haematoma.*

5.8.3 Extradural haematoma

An extradural haematoma refers to a pooling of blood between the dura mater and the skull. It most commonly occurs as a result of trauma (coup/counter-coup), particularly middle meningeal artery rupture in the context of parietal or temporal bone fractures. Patients may present with a history of trauma, and this is classically (but not always) accompanied by a **lucid interval**, in which the patient's GCS deteriorates over hours to days, after initially improving following the injury. They may also present with features of raised intracranial pressure.

Approach to extradural haematoma

> **Stepwise plan:**

1 Arrange non-contrast CT scan
- May demonstrate skull fractures

- Classically associated with a lens-like haematoma (see *Fig. 5.17*)

2 Refer to neurosurgery for surgical management
- Urgent referral warranted, as there is excellent prognosis with evacuation of the haematoma

5 | 5.9 Raised intracranial pressure (ICP)

Approach to raised ICP

Intracranial pressure may be raised by a number of causes, and may occur acutely or over a period of time.

Aetiology:
- Space-occupying lesions in the brain
- Infections
- Intracranial thrombosis or disorders of CSF regulation (e.g. producing hydrocephalus)

Clinical features:
- **Headache**
  - Nocturnal or morning (usually upon waking)
  - Worse on coughing or straining
- **Nausea and vomiting**
- **Visual problems**
  - Ptosis
  - Cranial nerve (III and VI) palsies
  - Blurring of optic disc, hyperaemia and papilloedema

Hydrocephalus
Hydrocephalus refers to an increase in the circulating volume of CSF within the cerebral ventricles, beyond normal limits. Hydrocephalus is classified into four forms:
- Communicating
  - Impaired absorption of CSF
  - No obstruction to CSF flow within the ventricles
  - Causes include subarachnoid haemorrhage, meningitis (possibly increased CSF protein)
- Non-communicating (obstructive)
  - May be due to congenital abnormalities (Arnold–Chiari, Dandy–Walker malformations) or acquired (e.g. bleeding, infection, tumours)

E ❯❯ Patients who present with features of raised ICP (i.e. morning/nocturnal headaches, vomiting, pulsatile tinnitus and papilloedema), who are also young, obese or pregnant, may have a condition called idiopathic intracranial hypertension (previously known as pseudotumour cerebri or benign intracranial hypertension). Though the cause is generally unknown, some drugs (e.g. COCP) have been known to be associated with its development. An elevated CSF opening pressure (>25cm H_2O) is diagnostic of raised ICP, and in the case of idiopathic intracranial hypertension, appropriate neuroimaging should be carried out to exclude other causes. Conservative management for patients with the condition includes weight loss and medical therapy with acetazolamide and diuretics. Patients who are unresponsive to medical therapy may require lumbar-peritoneal or ventriculo-peritoneal shunting or repeat lumbar punctures to relieve the pressure. Regular ophthalmology follow-up is also recommended.

- Normal pressure hydrocephalus
  - Dilated cerebral ventricles
  - Normal to mildly elevated pressure
  - Triad of urinary incontinence, dementia and gait disturbances
  - Sometimes known as 'wet, wacky and wobbly'
  - Gait described as 'magnetic' – with feet seemingly stuck to the floor with smaller strides
  - Diagnosis made on MRI/CT (see *Fig. 5.18*)
  - Medical treatments rarely resolve the problem

- Lumbar punctures with large volume removal may provide short-term improvement
  - CSF shunting is definitive therapy
- Hydrocephalus *ex vacuo*
  - Compensatory dilation of ventricles and spaces in response to brain atrophy (e.g. in dementia)

Medical therapy mainly provides a stop-gap measure until definite surgical therapy (via a drain or shunt) can be initiated.

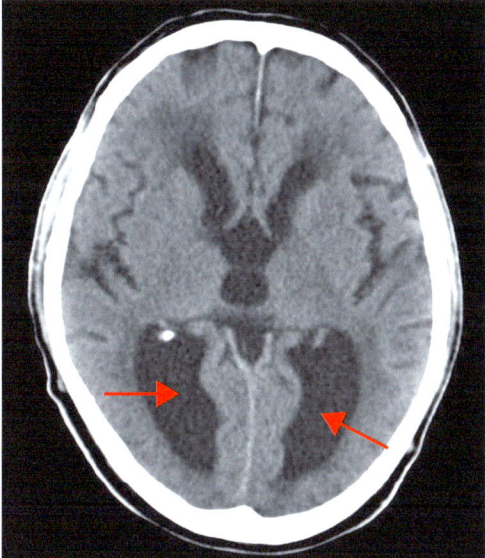

Fig. 5.18 *CT brain showing enlarged ventricles, in keeping with hydrocephalus.*

Management

> **Stepwise management of acute elevation of ICP**

1 Elevate head of bed (to improve drainage) and provide oxygen and ventilation
- Target PO_2: >13kPa
- Target PCO_2: 4.5kPa

2 Treat pyrexia or seizures (if present)

3 Prescribe mannitol or hypertonic saline
- Causes osmotic diuresis and initial reduction in CSF
- May later cause a rebound increase in ICP
- Give as a bolus, as opposed to continuous infusion

P ≫ Cerebral vein thrombosis may occur in some patients and present similarly to idiopathic intracranial hypertension. In other cases, it may present with more stroke-like features, particularly if there is occlusion of the cerebral veins or venous sinuses. Just under half of patients present with seizures early on in the disease process. The precise diagnosis can be made using a CT scan of the head or MRI. D-dimer levels and antiphospholipid antibodies should be requested where appropriate. Recommended treatments include therapeutic-dose anticoagulation, but one must bear in mind that the exclusion of haemorrhage is paramount before initiating treatment.

5.10 Space-occupying lesions of the brain

Space-occupying lesions affecting the brain are largely malignant in origin, although some lesions may be caused by haematomas, infiltration, infections or abscesses. Brain tumours may be primary or secondary cerebral metastases.

Symptoms may vary, depending on the site and size of the lesion. For example, there may be general symptoms of **raised ICP**, or insidious behavioural changes and anosmia if the frontal lobe is affected, or dysphasia if the temporal lobe is affected.

E ≫ If a patient, usually well into adulthood, presents with seizures, space-occupying lesions should be excluded as a potential cause.

Brain tumours
- Most brain tumours in adults (approximately two-thirds) are supratentorial; infratentorial tumours are more common in children
- Mobile phone use has been implicated in the development of brain tumours, but the evidence is unclear at this time
- Patients with specific inherited disorders, e.g. von Hippel–Lindau and neurofibromatosis, are at greater risk of developing brain tumours
- The **most common** brain tumours in adults are **metastatic**, with lung and breast cancer particularly likely to metastasise to the brain

5

P ⟫ Glial tumours (e.g. ependymomas, astrocytomas) along with meningiomas, make up the most common forms of primary brain tumours. One variant in particular, glioblastoma multiforme (GBM), is extremely malignant and aggressive. Surgery is the preferred treatment modality, with adjuvant chemoradiotherapy, but the prognosis is poor. Patients with GBM have an average survival rate of 1 year.

Approach to space-occupying lesions
1. **Arrange imaging**
   - CT (see *Fig. 5.19*) or MRI (MRI gives better visualisation)
2. **Treat underlying cause and raised ICP (if associated)**
3. **Tumours warrant neurosurgical excision, if at all possible**

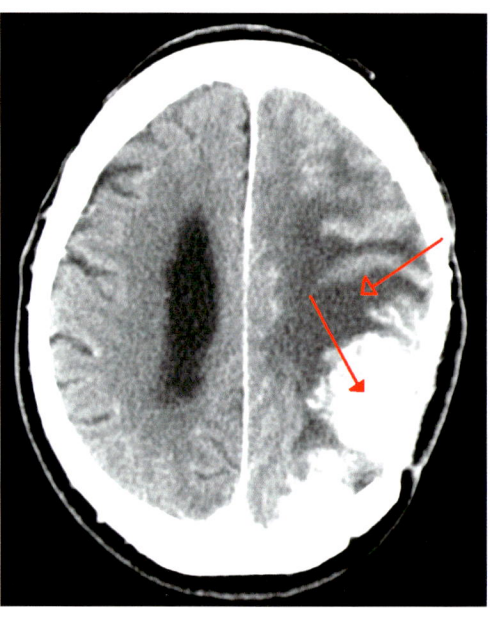

Fig. 5.19 *CT brain demonstrating a right-sided meningioma with surrounding cerebral oedema.*

5.11 Multiple sclerosis

Definition: multiple sclerosis refers to a chronic cell-mediated autoimmune demyelinating disorder of the central nervous system.

Epidemiology:
- More common in areas further from the equator, such as northern Europe, Australia and New Zealand; Scotland has the highest incidence and prevalence rates in the UK.
- Females are more commonly affected (3:1)
- Most people are diagnosed between 20 and 40 years of age

Aetiology:
- Genetic factors (such as HLA-DRB1) are linked to development of MS
- Environmental factors such as viral infections (EBV, CMV), lack of sunlight and vitamin D are thought to play a role too

Pathophysiology:
- Inflammation, demyelination and axonal degeneration are caused by CD4 cell-mediated destruction of oligodendrocytes, resulting in neuronal death
- Histological results show the presence of inflammatory cells such as macrophages, T and B cells

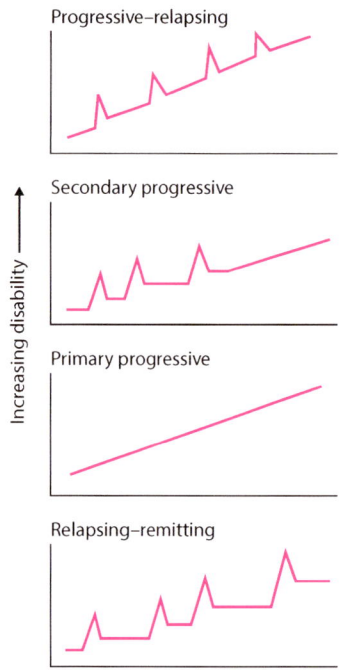

Fig. 5.20 *Types of presentation of MS.*

Clinical features:
- Multiple sclerosis can present in a number of ways because it can affect different areas of the CNS

- Classically, the first presentation occurs with optic neuritis, where patients complain of reduced visual acuity, a scotoma, colour desaturation and pain on eye movement
- The most common subtype of multiple sclerosis is the **relapsing-remitting** subtype, which accounts for about 80–85% of cases, with the rest representing more progressive forms of disease (see *Fig. 5.20*)
- Other presentations of MS are described in *Table 5.11*

E ≫ The Lhermitte phenomenon is described as an 'electric shock-like sensation' radiating down the trunk or limbs, triggered by neck flexion.

W ≫ The Uhthoff phenomenon refers to worsening neurological symptoms that occur with elevated body temperatures (e.g. with exercise or a hot bath), thought to be due to decreased neuronal conduction at these higher temperatures.

Internuclear ophthalmoplegia

Internuclear ophthalmoplegia (INO) is a lesion of the medial longitudinal fasciculus (MLF) in the brainstem that connects cranial nerve VI to III. The MLF is responsible for coordinated conjugate lateral gaze. As seen in *Fig. 5.21*, activation of the left lateral rectus via the left abducens nerve (VI) causes the left eye to abduct. Signals are concurrently sent to the contralateral oculomotor nucleus via the MLF, resulting in conjugated right eye adduction. However, in INO, this reflex/conjugate movement is disrupted. This results in nystagmus of the eye that abducts without any adduction in the contralateral eye during lateral gaze.

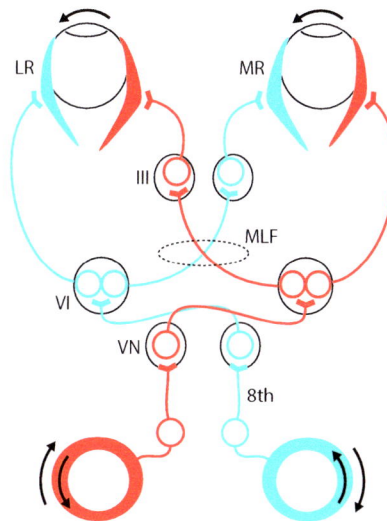

Fig. 5.21 *Pathway of the MLF.*

Table 5.11 *Clinical presentations of MS*

Visual	• Optic neuritis (often first presentation) • Ophthalmoplegia (can cause diplopia) • Bilateral internuclear ophthalmoplegia • Relative afferent pupillary defect (Marcus Gunn pupil) detected on swinging light test
Sensory **(most common initial feature of MS)**	• Spinothalamic tract – loss of pain and temperature sensation • Posterior column – loss of vibration, light touch and proprioception • Root lesion – radicular pain, usually in the lower thoracic and abdominal area • Trigeminal neuralgia • Tingling, tightness, twisting, burning and tearing sensations are often described by patients
Motor	• Upper motor neuron features such as spasticity (legs>arms), hypertonia, hyper-reflexia and extensor plantar responses • Transverse myelitis
Cerebellar	• Ataxia • Slurred speech • Nystagmus • Vertigo
Autonomic	• Loss of bladder and bower continence • Erectile dysfunction • Impotence • Increased sweating • Constipation
Others	• Fatigue, depression

Investigations

Clinical symptoms or MRI lesions have to be disseminated in time and space for MS to be diagnosed (refer to the McDonald criteria).

- MRI: MRI images taken 3 months apart showing gadolinium-enhanced lesions at different sites
- Lumbar puncture: IgG oligoclonal bands in cerebrospinal fluid
- Evoked potentials: demonstrates delayed response

Management

> **Stepwise management of multiple sclerosis (NICE 2014, CG186)**

Table 5.12 *Symptomatic management of MS*

Fatigue	Amantadine, cognitive behavioural therapy, supervised exercise programme
Balance	Vestibular rehabilitation
Spasticity	Baclofen or gabapentin as first-line treatment
Emotional lability	Amitriptyline
Neuropathic pain	Choice of amitriptyline, duloxetine, gabapentin or pregabalin
Bladder incontinence	May attempt intermittent self-catheterisation or anticholinergics (may worsen instead)

1 **For acute exacerbations (new symptoms or worsening of existing symptoms lasting more than 24 hours in the absence of infections or other causes)**
- Offer oral prednisolone or IV methylprednisolone (similar efficacy)
- Note that treatment does not alter prognosis
- Symptomatic management of MS is outlined in *Table 5.12*

2 **Prevent relapse using disease-modifying therapies**
- Interferon-beta SC reduces relapse by 30–40%
- Glatiramer acetate SC, an immunomodulating drug, reduces relapse by 30%
- Dimethyl fumarate, teriflunomide and alemtuzumab are also recommended by NICE for relapsing-remitting MS
- Natalizumab, a recombinant humanised monoclonal antibody, reduces relapse by 68%, but remember that an important side effect is progressive multifocal leukoencephalopathy caused by infection with the JC virus
- Oral fingolimod, a spingosine 1-phosphate receptor modulator, prevents lymphocytic movement across the blood–brain barrier, and reduces relapse by 50%

5.12 Spinal disorders

5.12.1 Lumbar spinal stenosis

Lumbar spinal stenosis refers to narrowing of the central spinal canal. This may be due to a number of causes, such as tumours or prolapsed discs, but is most commonly the result of a combination of degenerative changes.

> **W** ≫ Degenerative changes within the disc, facet joint osteoarthritis, formation of osteophytes and articular cartilage erosion all contribute to mechanical compression and narrowing of the spinal canal.

Patients may present with:
- Progressive back or lower limb pain, which is made worse by walking
- Some patients may also experience buttock pain, numbness and paraesthesia
- Pain may be eased by sitting, walking uphill or leaning forward (this causes flexion of the spine, enlarging the canal and temporarily relieving stenosis)

> **E** ≫ Patients with spinal stenosis present with the above-mentioned features of **neurogenic** claudication. It may difficult to distinguish these effects from the symptoms of arterial claudication observed in peripheral arterial disease. Some helpful clues that may point to a diagnosis include the nature of the pain – neurogenic pain in spinal stenosis is often positional, and the presence (or absence) of peripheral pulses.

Approach to lumbar spinal stenosis

Stepwise plan:

1 **MRI is the investigation of choice**

2 **Lifestyle modification**
 • Weight reduction

3 **NSAIDs and physiotherapy**

4 **If patients are unresponsive to medical management, consider a decompressive laminectomy**

5.12.2 Syringomyelia

Syringomyelia is characterised by the development of an expansile fluid-containing tubular cavitation within the spinal cord, usually affecting the cervical portion of the cord and compressing surrounding structures. If this condition occurs in the brainstem, it is termed syringobulbia. Syrinx is the root word for 'tube' in Greek.

P ≫ The most common cause of syringomyelia is anything that obstructs the flow of CSF. This is exemplified by the Arnold–Chiari malformation in just under half of cases, a congenital (or in fewer cases, acquired, usually through trauma) disorder involving cerebellar herniation through the foramen magnum. The Arnold–Chiari malformation has two major types – type I and type II. Syringomyelia is associated with type I Arnold–Chiari malformation, which is thought to be the result of improper development of the posterior fossa. Type II malformation is characterised by less severe herniation and the development of a myelomeningocele.

Patients with syringomyelia may present with:
 • Insidious onset, peak between 20 and 30 years of age
 • Rapid progression of symptoms; symptoms may differ from patient to patient, based on characteristics of individual syrinx
 • Classically, a **cape-like** loss of sensation over the chest, shoulders and upper limbs
 • Proprioception and vibration generally preserved, unless syrinx expands into dorsal columns
 • Muscle weakness in distal arms (expansion into anterior horn cells)

Approach to syringomyelia

Stepwise plan:

1 **MRI is the investigation of choice**

2 **Neurosurgical intervention is first line**
 • Treatment modalities include:
  – Shunt insertion
  – Syringotomy and drainage
  – Laminectomy
  – Surgical decompression of Arnold–Chiari malformation (where necessary)

5.12.3 Anterior spinal artery syndrome/vertebrobasilar occlusion

Anterior spinal artery syndrome, or Beck syndrome, refers to an ischaemic event (or frank infarction) that causes a decrease in blood supply to the anterior two-thirds of the spinal cord.

This condition causes loss of sensory input from the anterior cord (e.g. pain and temperature) but preserves vibration and proprioception sense because of sparing of the dorsal columns (see *Fig. 5.22*). It is commonly caused by aortic pathology (e.g. dissection, aneurysm).

Unfortunately, the treatment does not really alter the course of symptoms, and patients are generally paraplegic or quadriplegic, depending on the level of the injury.

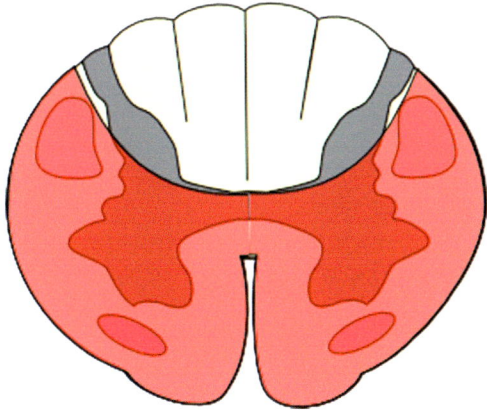

Fig. 5.22 *Anterior spinal artery syndrome; note sparing of the dorsal columns.*

5

5.12.4 Spondylosis and spondylolisthesis

- Spondylosis refers to age-related degeneration of the spinal cord, most commonly caused by osteoarthritis. Patients may experience pain or sensorimotor disturbances secondary to nerve root compression. Treatment is conservative, with physiotherapy and NSAIDs.
- Spondylolisthesis, on the other hand, refers to the anterior or posterior displacement of a vertebra. This is not the same pathological process as lumbar disc herniation.

5.12.5 Brown-Séquard syndrome

This condition is caused by an insult or injury to one lateral half of the spinal cord (see *Fig. 5.23*). As a result (because of the location of the lesion), there is ipsilateral loss of **proprioception and vibration sense at the level of the lesion**, as well as contralateral loss of pain and temperature below the level of the lesion.

> **E** ≫ While the aetiology is usually related to traumatic disruption or hemisection, the condition itself is fairly rare.

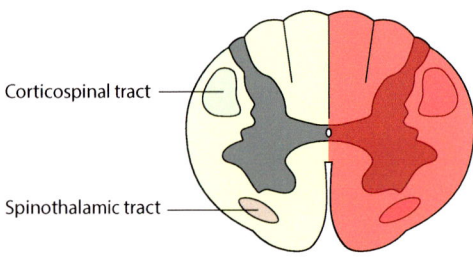

Corticospinal tract

Spinothalamic tract

Fig. 5.23 *Brown-Séquard syndrome.*

5.12.6 Prolapsed intervertebral disc

Also colloquially known as a 'slipped' disc, this condition is caused when damage to the outer fibrous ring of the intervertebral disc, known as the *annulus fibrosus*, causes bulging or herniation of the soft, inner layer, known as the *nucleus pulposus*. Patients with PID often have a history of sport, trauma, or heavy lifting prior to injury.

> **W** ≫ Tears and herniation almost always occur in a posterolateral fashion. This is because of the presence of the posterior longitudinal ligament, which prevents direct posterior displacement.

Approach to prolapsed intervertebral disc (PID)

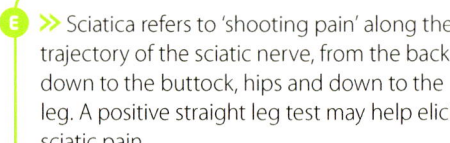

Stepwise plan:

1. **Consider presence of moderate to severe back pain with or without unilateral sciatica (depending on the degree of herniation observed)**

> **E** ≫ Sciatica refers to 'shooting pain' along the trajectory of the sciatic nerve, from the back down to the buttock, hips and down to the leg. A positive straight leg test may help elicit sciatic pain.

2. **Monitor for red flag symptoms**
- NICE (2016, NG59) advocates looking out for red flags relating to back pain, including:
  - Saddle anaesthesia
  - Bowel or bladder dysfunction or loss of control leading to incontinence
  - Trauma
  - Point tenderness or sudden onset (possible spinal fracture)
  - Pain at night; waking from sleep
  - Onset in under-25s or over-50s
  - History of malignancy
  - History of intravenous drug misuse, immunosuppression or infection
- The diagnosis is usually made clinically; investigation does not alter the course of management
- Should investigation be required in intractable cases, MRI is a suitable option
- Patients should be offered appropriate analgesia, encouraged to mobilise as much as possible without excessive strain and consider physiotherapy

> **P** ≫ If symptoms do not resolve in 6–8 weeks, further specialist assessment is necessary, and surgery may be required.

5.12.7 Subacute combined degeneration of the cord

Subacute combined degeneration of the cord refers to progressive demyelination of the dorsal columns of the spinal cord. Patients with pernicious anaemia, malabsorption disorders, vitamin B12 and vitamin E deficiency are most at risk. Uniform sensorimotor weakness occurs in a gradual pattern, with impairment of vibration and proprioception.

In cases of vitamin B12 deficiency, treatment with vitamin B12 (1mg IM every other day until symptoms improve, then 1mg every 2 months) may halt progression, or in some cases reverse symptoms. If progression is severe, neurodegeneration may unfortunately be irreversible.

>> Patients who are deficient in both vitamin B12 and folate should be assessed and treated for B12 deficiency with particular emphasis. NICE advises that treatment of folate deficiency may improve symptoms to the point of masking B12 deficiency to a significant degree, which may allow progression of neurodegeneration.

5.13 Movement disorders

Approach to tremors

A **tremor** is an involuntary, rhythmic oscillatory movement, and these may be described using various parameters, the most common of which is whether they occur on **action** or at **rest**. There are myriad causes for tremor, and carefully observing the type of tremor may provide clues as to the condition.

Tremors may be further described using frequency, basis of medical condition or even by type of medication. Tremors may also be a presenting feature indicating a more serious underlying pathology. A thorough history and physical examination help clinch the diagnosis, as there is no one particular test used to distinguish one tremor from another.

Tremors may also sometimes be described in the context of a clinical examination (**fine**, as with salbutamol use or thyroid disorders), **coarse**, or **flapping** (seen classically with carbon dioxide retention or liver impairment).

5.13.1 Essential tremor

Essential tremor is the most common type of tremor encountered. Essential tremor typically involves the upper limbs in 70% of patients, and may also involve speech and a tremor of the head (titubation).

A large number (up to half) of patients also have a positive family history of the condition. The diagnosis is largely clinical, with patients demonstrating marked improvement of the action tremor with alcohol or benzodiazepines. The tremor is worse when goal-oriented or when the arms are outstretched, and is rare at rest.

Treatment is usually instigated to alleviate dysfunction or embarrassment associated with the condition. Propranolol and primidone are first-line agents.

5.13.2 Parkinsonism

Parkinsonism is a broad term, encompassing hypokinetic conditions of various aetiologies that produce a clinical syndrome characterised primarily by a **resting tremor**, **bradykinesia** and **rigidity**.

Note that while this term derives its name from Parkinson disease, Parkinson disease is only one cause of parkinsonism. Parkinson disease, specifically, is a progressive neurodegenerative disorder.

Although Parkinson disease is the most common cause of parkinsonism, assessment of other causes in the differential diagnosis merit some consideration. These include:

- Parkinson plus syndromes (parkinsonism + other features)
  - Multi-system atrophy (Shy–Drager syndrome)
    - Parkinsonism + cerebellar signs + autonomic dysfunction (bladder atony, postural hypotension)
  - Progressive supranuclear palsy
    - Parkinsonism + speech disturbances + personality changes/dementia + vertical gaze palsy
  - Lewy body dementia
    - Parkinsonism + deteriorating cognitive ability + visual hallucinations
  - Corticobasilar degeneration
    - Parkinsonism + alien limb syndrome (limb movement without cognitive awareness of

5

actual movement) + apraxia (disorder of planned motor performance e.g. individual understands commands but has difficulty articulating words) + aphasia (impaired speech and language)
- Creutzfeldt–Jakob disease
- Vascular parkinsonism, usually secondary to ischaemic or haemorrhagic lesions
- Antipsychotic medication, metoclopramide, prochlorperazine
- Wilson disease
- Chronic traumatic encephalopathy (e.g. dementia pugilistica – repeated head trauma, commonly associated with boxers)

5.13.3 Parkinson disease

Definition: Parkinson disease is a neurodegenerative disorder characterised by a resting tremor, rigidity and bradykinesia.

Epidemiology:
- Affects 1–2% of people worldwide
- Typically affects older individuals, with average onset between 60 and 70 years of age

Aetiology/pathophysiology:
- Progressive degeneration and loss of dopaminergic neurons in the pars compacta of the **substantia nigra**
- Associated with accumulation of a protein, alpha-synuclein in the substantia nigra
- Linked to specific genes in a small proportion of patients, with environmental factors being implicated as well (e.g. pesticides)

Clinical features:
- Bradykinesia (slowness of movement) or hypokinesia (poverty of movement), e.g.:
  - Reduced facial expression, arm swing, or blinking
  - Slow, shuffling gait, difficulty turning in bed
  - Difficulty with fine movements, e.g. cramped handwriting (micrographia), buttoning clothes
- Stiffness or rigidity
  - Classic **lead-pipe** rigidity (constant resistance felt upon passive flexion of the limb)
  - Cogwheel rigidity (intermittent relaxation felt during passive flexion in the presence of tremor and increased tone)
- Rest tremor
  - Classically **pill-rolling**
  - Usually improves on moving
  - May be absent in 30% at onset
- Other features include:
  - Early
    - Reduced sense of smell
    - Depression, anxiety, sleep disturbances (including REM sleep disorders – in which patients may act out dreams, as physiological muscle paralysis during sleep is impaired)
- Late
  - Postural instability (tendency to fall backwards after a sharp pull), falls, postural hypotension
  - Dementia and psychosis

Approach to Parkinson disease (NICE 2017, NG71)
The diagnosis is made **clinically**. NICE recommends using the UK Parkinson's Disease Society Brain Bank Clinical Diagnostic Criteria (see *Table 5.13*).

NICE recommends the use of **SPECT** imaging when it is difficult to differentiate between parkinsonism and essential tremor. Other tests, such as PET, MR-spectroscopy and levodopa challenge tests, are **not** recommended.

Table 5.13 *UK Parkinson's Disease Society Brain Bank Clinical Diagnostic Criteria*

Step 1: Diagnosis of parkinsonism	Bradykinesia *plus at least one of the following* • Muscular rigidity • Fine rest tremor (4–6Hz) • Postural instability
Step 2: Exclusion criteria for Parkinson disease	• Previous history of CVAs, head injury, encephalitis, neuroleptic treatment, cerebral tumour, hydrocephalus, MPTP exposure • Positive family history with >1 relative affected • Symptoms of early severe autonomic involvement/dementia • Positive signs – supranuclear gaze palsy, Babinski, cerebellar signs, unilateral features after 3 years • Poor response to levodopa in the absence of malabsorption
Step 3: Supportive criteria for Parkinson disease	• Unilateral onset, persistently asymmetrical features • Rest tremor present • Progressive course of >10 years • Good response to levodopa

Management (NICE 2017, NG71)

Prompt referral to a specialist is required. If a drug is thought to be the cause, stop the offending agent. Consider providing support for ADLs and driving, as well as encouraging regular exercise. Screen for depression and assess disability using the Unified Parkinson Disease rating. A multi-disciplinary team approach (involving physiotherapist, occupational therapist, nutritionist and speech therapist) should be pursued. NICE divides management of Parkinson disease into treatment of motor and non-motor symptoms.

Stepwise management of motor symptoms

1 **Discuss the potential risk/benefits of the medications, and the patient's needs and goals, before commencing treatment**

2 **Consider prescribing medication**
- Levodopa is the first-line therapy for patients in the early stages of disease whose symptoms affect their quality of life
- Dopamine agonist (pramipexole or ropinirole) or monoamine oxidase B (MAO-B) inhibitors (selegiline or rasagiline) may be considered in patients whose symptoms do not impact their quality of life

3 **Consider adjuvant therapy**
- **First-line** – consider a non-ergot derived dopamine agonist, MAO-B or COMT inhibitors (entacapone, tolcapone) in patients who have developed motor fluctuations despite being on levodopa therapy
- **Second-line** – amantadine may be considered

- **Third-line** – intermittent SC apomorphine or SC apomorphine infusions

4 **Consider deep brain stimulation**
- This may be considered in patients with advanced disease that is not controlled by best medical therapy

Do not abruptly stop anti-Parkinsonian medications, as this may precipitate acute dyskinesia or neuroleptic malignant syndrome.

Dopa-decarboxylase inhibitors (e.g. carbidopa) are given, together with levodopa, to prevent peripheral metabolism of levodopa to dopamine, reducing peripheral side effects and increasing the effect of levodopa centrally.

Management of non-motor symptoms

Symptomatic management of non-motor symptoms of Parkinson disease is detailed in *Table 5.14*.

5.13.4 Motor neuron disease

Motor neuron disease refers to a group of neurodegenerative disorders that primarily affect, as the name suggests, motor neurons in the body, leading to worsening disability and eventual death. The diagnosis of these conditions is clinical, but, in some instances, electromyography or nerve conduction studies can be used to help with confirmation.

Amyotrophic lateral sclerosis (ALS) (Lou Gehrig's disease)
- Most common form of motor neuron disease
- Up to 10% attributed to familial causes, but the rest of cases are idiopathic

5

Table 5.14 *Management of non-motor symptoms of Parkinson disease*

Depression	Early recognition and referral to psychological team
Drooling of saliva	Speech and language therapy; consider glycopyrronium bromide
Impulse control disorder	Patient education; modify dopaminergic therapy upon specialist consultation; cognitive behavioural therapy may also be considered
Orthostatic hypotension	Medications review; modify anti-hypertensives and consider ceasing anticholinergics; midodrine or fludrocortisone may be used
Dementia	First-line treatment – cholinesterase inhibitor Second-line treatment – memantine
Psychosis	Medications review; modify anti-Parkinsonian medications as tolerated; offer quetiapine or clonidine; olanzapine should **not** be used
Daytime sleepiness	Consider modafinil with at least annual review
Restless legs and rapid eye movement sleep behaviour disorder	Medications review; clonazepam or melatonin may be offered

5

- Symptoms may progress rapidly or slowly, and classification is based on region of muscle weakness and atrophy
- Majority of patients present with 'limb onset' ALS, i.e. symptoms occur in the limbs, classically with lower motor neuron signs in the upper limbs and upper motor neuron signs in the lower limbs
- A smaller number of patients present with 'bulbar onset' ALS, in which facial muscles tend to be affected first
- In both cases the disease progresses to other regions of the body
- Up to 50% of patients may present with cognitive dysfunction, behavioural disturbances and emotional lability
- The goal of treatment is primarily supportive, given the fact that there is no cure at present – the medication **riluzole** (a glutamate antagonist) is thought to help extend lifespan by several months, but does not affect progression
- The leading cause of death in these patients is respiratory failure due to progressive muscle weakness and atrophy

Progressive bulbar palsy
- Neurodegeneration in nerves supplying bulbar muscles (patients may present with disability/weakness in swallowing, talking or chewing)
- The pathophysiology involves a lower motor neuron lesion in cranial nerves IX, X and XII, and may thus demonstrate wasting of tongue muscles, absent jaw jerk or gag reflex
- Patients are at high risk of aspiration pneumonia
- Treatment is largely supportive, as the disease progresses rapidly
- There is no cure for the disease at present

Pseudobulbar palsy
- Unlike progressive bulbar palsy, this involves an upper motor neuron lesion in cranial nerves IX, X and XII
- The tongue muscles (and consequently speech) are spastic, with jaw jerk and gag likely to be hyper-reflexic

Hereditary spastic paraplegia
- Group of genetic diseases that present with progressive muscle spasticity and disordered gait in the lower limbs
- Pathogenesis thought to involve axonal degeneration
- Patients with this condition have varying levels of disability but a normal life expectancy

5.13.5 Hemiballismus

Hemiballismus is a very rare disorder that causes **large-amplitude, involuntary, flinging** movements of one half of the body. The most common cause of hemiballismus is stroke contralateral to the lesion, but very few patients who have a stroke develop hemiballismus. Other causes include traumatic injury, neoplasia or ALS.

The condition is thought to occur secondary to insult to the subthalamic nucleus of the basal ganglia. It is generally self-limiting, with recovery occurring over several months. Dopamine antagonists may be used, should symptoms not settle.

5.13.6 Tourette syndrome

Tourette syndrome is a neuropsychiatric disorder characterised by multiple motor and vocal tics (sudden repetitive rhythmic motion) with a strong genetic association. The aetiology is thought to be multifactorial, and there are associations with attention deficit hyperactivity disorder (ADHD) and obsessive–compulsive disorder (OCD).

Patients typically present with **persistent**, multiple vocal or motor tics, usually over a year and before the age of 18. Other features may include echolalia, making obscene gestures and foul language (pathognomonic, but only appears in 10%). Treatment is supportive, with habit reforming encouraged.

5.13.7 Myoclonus

Myoclonus refers to sudden involuntary twitching or jerks of muscle that may cause functional impairment. There are many different causes of myoclonic jerks (e.g. epilepsy, CJD, multiple sclerosis, SLE, etc.).

One important differential to be aware of is **benign essential myoclonus**. Features include:
- Frequent myoclonic muscular contractions, up to 50 times a minute
- May be spontaneous or hereditary
- Presents in childhood or adolescence
- May respond to clonazepam or sodium valproate

5.13.8 Huntington disease

Huntington disease is an autosomal dominant disorder characterised by progressive neurodegeneration caused by cysteine-adenosine-guanine (CAG) triplet repetition found on the HTT (Huntingtin) gene located on chromosome 4. Features include:
- Onset of symptoms usually in mid-life (30–50 years of age)
- Behavioural problems and depression may precede neurological symptoms
- Chorea
- Poor coordination
- Dysarthria, dysphagia and jerky eye movements

- Progressive decline in cognition, followed by memory deficits
- Features of Parkinsonism and progression to dystonia (sustained muscle contraction, causing repetitive, twisting movements)

> **W** ➤ CAG trinucleotides affect the functioning of the Huntingtin protein, which interacts with a wide variety of cells and is responsible for a number of processes. On a molecular level, dysfunction is thought to occur because a mutant version of Huntingtin is produced, which interferes with cellular processes, aggregating to form inclusion bodies and causing cell death and affecting neurotransmitter release. Degeneration of neurons at the striatum of the basal ganglia is the most common variation, but this may progress to affect other areas as well.

There is no cure for the disease, and patients **have a reduced life expectancy** (estimated at 20 years after the onset of symptoms).

> **P** ➤ Treatment involves managing symptoms (e.g. benzodiazepines for chorea), and treating associated depression, both in the patient and in their loved ones. The disease process is difficult, both from a physical and emotional standpoint, and physicians should ensure that adequate support is available for patients and their families.

5.13.9 Friedreich ataxia

Friedreich ataxia is the most common inherited ataxia in the developed world, and is inherited in an autosomal recessive fashion.
- Patients with the condition have a mutation in the frataxin gene on chromosome 9, leading to impaired production of frataxin, a mitochondrial polypeptide

- Patients are generally in their teens and twenties, and experience progressive ataxia, weakness and loss of proprioception and joint position

> **E** ➤ Friedreich ataxia is also classically associated with pes cavus, hypertrophic cardiomyopathy, arrhythmia, scoliosis, visual disturbances and diabetes mellitus.

- Patients should be followed up with nerve conduction studies, demonstrating decreased or absent sensory impulses, neuroimaging, ECG and echocardiography
- Optimal management of the condition is best achieved through the involvement of a multi-disciplinary team

5.13.10 Ataxic telangiectasia

Ataxic telangiectasia is a rare, autosomal recessive condition typified by symptomatic presentation, usually in early childhood, which may consist of:
- Progressive cerebellar ataxia
- Basal ganglia dysfunction
- Immunodeficiency (specifically IgA deficiency, leading to recurrent infection)
- Increased risk of cancer, usually systemically in lymphoma or leukaemia earlier on in life, followed by the development of specific lesions, such as lumps seen in breast cancer
- Telangiectasia, which may develop anywhere on the body
- Patients with this condition are also highly likely to have elevated **alpha fetoprotein** levels

Treatment involves addressing symptoms, e.g. addressing neurological features, screening for and treating any associated malignancy, prescribing antibiotics where necessary in cases of infection. Multi-disciplinary team involvement is helpful, particularly with regard to physiotherapy, occupational therapy and speech and language assessment.

5.14 Peripheral neuropathy

Approach to peripheral neuropathy

There are numerous causes of a peripheral neuropathy, most of which involve systemic, metabolic or toxic aetiologies. A thorough history and examination, followed by appropriate laboratory investigations, may be helpful in making a diagnosis.

Neuropathy affecting a particular nerve is termed **mononeuropathy**. If it affects a number of nerves in a region of the body, it is termed a **polyneuropathy**. Should the neuropathy affect multiple nerves in differing locations in the body, the term used is **mononeuritis multiplex**.

5

E » Certain medications, such as isoniazid and vincristine/vinblastine, are associated with the development of peripheral neuropathy.

It is helpful to consider peripheral neuropathy in terms of **sensory deficits** or **motor deficits**.

Largely sensory deficits
- Classically described as a 'glove and stocking' distribution of tingling and numbness
- Reflexes may be diminished or absent
- Most common causes
  - **Diabetic neuropathy**
    - Thought to arise as a result of diabetic vascular injury to the small blood vessels supplying nerves (vasa vasorum)
    - May be **painful**
  - **Vitamin B12 deficiency**
    - May additionally present with glossitis, anaemia
    - Numerous causes, including pernicious anaemia, malabsorption, malnutrition, gastrectomy, infection/parasites
    - **May result in irreversible damage to the nervous system**
    - Associated with **subacute combined degeneration of the spinal cord** – gradual, progressive demyelination of the dorsal columns, leading to worsening paraesthesia and weakness
  - **Alcohol**
    - Peripheral neuropathy caused by direct effect of alcohol and impaired absorption of B vitamin group
- Other causes:
  - Leprosy
  - Vasculitis

Largely motor deficits
- Isolated or general weakness
- May have respiratory muscle weakness
- Causes
  - Guillain–Barré syndrome
  - Hereditary sensorimotor neuropathies
  - Lead poisoning

E » Patients with aetiologies causing peripheral neuropathy may also experience **autonomic neuropathy** (e.g. in diabetes or Guillain–Barré syndrome), affecting the autonomic nervous system, causing symptoms such as urinary retention, impotence, sweating, inappropriate tachycardia or bradycardia and GI disturbances.

5.14.1 Guillain-Barré syndrome

Definition: Guillain–Barré syndrome refers to an immune-mediated demyelinating neuropathy.

W » A large number of patients who develop the condition have an associated prior infection, classically with *Campylobacter jejuni*.

P » Several subtypes and associations exist:
- Miller–Fisher syndrome
  - Anti-GQ1b antibodies detected in a large number
  - Usually **descending** paralysis
  - Ophthalmoplegia, arreflexia, ataxia
- Acute (or chronic) immune demyelinating polyneuropathy (AIDP/CIDP)
- Acute motor/sensory axonal neuropathy (AMSAN/AMAN).

Epidemiology:
- AIDP is the most common form
- Affects men more than women, usually at age 40
- Miller–Fisher syndrome is more common in Asia

Clinical features:
- **Weakness**
  - **Symmetrical, bilateral, ascending** weakness and paralysis
  - Generally does not progress after 4 weeks
- **Sensory disturbances**
  - Paraesthesia in distal extremities
  - Reduced or absent reflexes
- **Pain**
  - Back pain, limb pain or neuropathic pain
- **Autonomic dysfunction** (e.g. sweating, urinary retention)
- **Respiratory muscle paralysis**

Investigations
- Diagnosis is made **clinically**
- **Pulmonary function tests** may be utilised
- If the diagnosis is unclear, further testing with LP, or antibody testing with anti-ganglioside antibodies or GQ1B to help diagnose Miller–Fisher syndrome may be utilised

Management
Patients may require airway support, and referral to ITU is indicated if the patient has an FV <1.5L.

Stepwise management of Guillain–Barré syndrome

1 **Arrange intravenous immunoglobulin/plasma exchange**
- IVIG more likely to be completed than plasma exchange
- IVIG after plasma exchange has no additional benefit

2 **Symptom control should also be offered**

E ≫ Corticosteroids do not improve symptoms, and may in fact delay recovery from the condition. Prognosis is generally excellent if the patient makes a full recovery. Up to 10% may die from respiratory complications.

5.14.2 Charcot-Marie-Tooth disease

Charcot–Marie–Tooth disease (CMT) refers to a group of hereditary sensory and motor neuropathies (HSMN). It affects 1 in 2500 people. Multiple modes of inheritance have been documented, but the most common is autosomal dominant. Clinical presentation may vary but the classic features include:
- Lower limb muscle weakness and wasting
- Classic 'champagne-bottle' legs
- Foot drop
- Small-muscle wasting of the hand, causing finger curling or 'claw hand'
- Pes cavus (see *Fig. 5.24*)
- Neuropathic pain

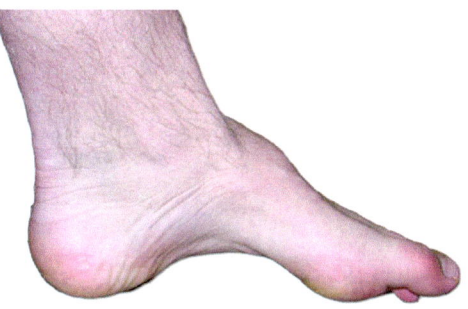

Fig. 5.24 *Pes cavus.*

W ≫ The pathogenesis of most cases of CMT involves duplication of a genetic segment on the short arm of chromosome 17. Some of these mutations affect eventual coding of mitochondrial proteins, which are required in axons and Schwann cells for optimal nerve functioning.

The diagnosis is clinical, but can be confirmed with nerve conduction studies or genetic testing.

Management involves appropriate mild exercise, foot and ankle braces to help stability and surgical correction of deformities.

P ≫ Drugs that cause peripheral neuropathy (e.g. isoniazid, vincristine) are contraindicated in all patients with CMT.

5.15 Diseases of the neuromuscular junction

5.15.1 Myasthenia gravis

Definition: Myasthenia gravis is an autoimmune condition that affects the neuromuscular junction, with auto-antibodies against the acetylcholine receptor in the vast majority of cases. The aetiology is unclear.

Epidemiology:
- Affects women more than men
- Women affected earlier (at approximately 30–40)
- Men typically affected around age 60

E ≫ Myasthenia gravis is associated with other autoimmune conditions, **thymomas (10–15%)** and **thymic hyperplasia (50%)**.

W ≫ Antibodies against the acetylcholine receptor at the neuromuscular junction cause autoimmune destruction, reducing the number of available binding sites for acetylcholine and thus decreasing the regularity of action potential generation. This manifests as muscle weakness, particularly over time.

Clinical features:
- **Easy fatigability**
  - Characteristically better in the morning and worse in the evening
  - Worsens with exercise, activity or use
  - May be limited or generalised
  - Typically affects **eyes** initially (Class I or initial myasthenia gravis), causing bilateral **ptosis or diplopia**
  - Limb weakness or general weakness
  - Patients may develop a characteristic 'myasthenic snarl' on smiling
  - Voice may become softer on counting to 50

E ≫ Note that muscle tone and reflexes are intact. There is unlikely to be obvious muscle wasting or sensory deficits in myasthenia gravis.

- Patients with emotional distress, pregnancy, certain medications or intercurrent illness are likely to experience worsening of symptoms
- Progression of the disease may lead to **dysphagia** or **respiratory compromise** that requires ventilation

P ≫ Lambert–Eaton myasthenic syndrome is another differential diagnosis when considering the symptoms presented in these patients. The condition is thought to arise as a result of auto-antibodies against **voltage-gated calcium channels**. The condition is rare, and is associated with malignancy, particularly small cell lung cancer. Differentiating it from myasthenia gravis may be achieved in smaller cases clinically (reflexes may be depressed in Lambert–Eaton myasthenic syndrome) but more reliably on detection of antibodies to voltage-gated calcium channels. Treatment is with 3,4-diaminopyridine or IVIG.

Investigations

W ≫ A simple test in the early consideration of myasthenia gravis, particularly in the emergency department, is the **ice test**. The physician presses ice held in a latex glove against the patient's eyes for a few minutes. If the patient has myasthenia gravis, this will improve the ptosis seen. This is because the cold reduces acetylcholinesterase-mediated breakdown of acetylcholine at the neuromuscular junction. This test is highly sensitive and specific.

Stepwise plan:

1 **Carry out auto-antibody testing**
- 85% of patients have auto-antibodies to the acetylcholine receptor
- Edrophonium (Tensilon) testing is rarely performed, as it may result in life-threatening bradycardia

2 **Arrange pulmonary function tests**

3 **Provide CT scan of thorax**
- To exclude associated thymomas

Management

Stepwise management of myasthenia gravis

1 **Prescribe anticholinesterase inhibitors**
- Pyridostigmine
- Improves muscle weakness

2 **Provide immunosuppression**
- For generalised disease
- Steroids help in the short term and for relapses
- Treatment may include IVIG, cyclosporin, methotrexate or azathioprine

3 **Consider thymectomy**

5.16 Muscular dystrophies

Muscular dystrophies refer to a collection of genetic disorders characterised by progressive muscle weakness, degeneration and wasting.

5.16.1 Duchenne muscular dystrophy

Duchenne muscular dystrophy is the most common form of muscular dystrophy. Features include:
- X-linked recessive inheritance

- Mutation in the dystrophin gene, coding for dystrophin, a protein observed in muscle cells

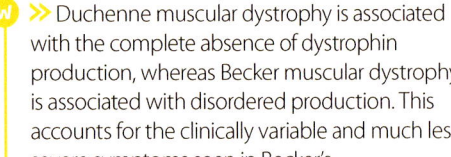

W ≫ Duchenne muscular dystrophy is associated with the complete absence of dystrophin production, whereas Becker muscular dystrophy is associated with disordered production. This accounts for the clinically variable and much less severe symptoms seen in Becker's.

- Patients are generally symptomatic before the age of 4
  - Delayed motor milestones (occasionally speech and language delay)
  - Gait abnormalities
  - Proximal myopathy and wasting
  - Calf pseudohypertrophy

> **E** ≫ The Gower sign, in which the patient has to use their hands and arms to arrive at a standing position, is a classic feature of Duchenne muscular dystrophy (see *Fig. 5.25*).

Patients may be diagnosed clinically, and an initially grossly elevated creatine kinase (CK) is seen in the condition. Parents should undergo genetic testing and counselling and be given emotional support.

Patients require orthopaedic support and monitoring for cardiorespiratory complications. The prognosis is poor, with few patients surviving past young adulthood.

5.16.2 Becker muscular dystrophy

Becker muscular dystrophy is also an X-linked recessive disease that presents with similar progressive proximal muscle wasting and weakness. The symptoms are far less severe, and patients are generally diagnosed in adolescence.

CK may be moderately elevated, and patients should be offered physiotherapy, be advised to exercise regularly and optimise nutrition.

> **P** ≫ Dilated cardiomyopathy is a common complication associated with Becker, and cardiovascular function should be monitored as soon as the diagnosis is made.

5.16.3 Facioscapulohumeral muscular dystrophy

Facioscapulohumeral muscular dystrophy (also known as Landouzy–Dejerine muscular dystrophy) is an autosomal dominant inherited muscle disorder, characterised primarily by **facial and shoulder girdle muscle weakness**. Patients are also likely to present with foot drop and winging of the scapula, and may be at risk of eye dryness, as they are unable to shut their eyes during sleep. Diagnosis is usually made in adolescence, and investigations may show an elevated CK.

5.16.4 Myotonic dystrophy

Myotonic dystrophy refers to an inherited autosomal disorder that causes progressive muscle wasting and weakness. Two major variants exist: type 1 (which has a more severe, congenital form); and type 2, which presents with milder symptoms.

While the presentation may vary (even between types 1 and 2), some features include:
- Prolonged muscle contractions; impairment of muscle relaxation

5

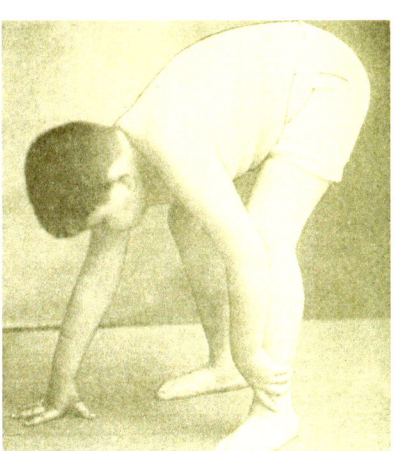
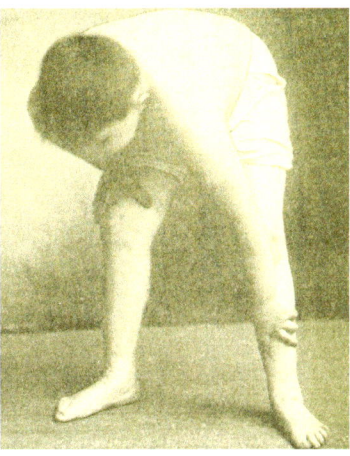

Fig. 5.25 *The Gower sign.*

5

- Muscle wasting and weakness, particularly of the head (temporal) and neck (see *Fig. 5.26*)
- Type 2 myotonic dystrophy is associated with proximal muscle weakness
- Endocrine abnormalities: frontotemporal male pattern baldness, insulin resistance
- Cataracts
- Heart block or cardiomyopathy

There is unfortunately no cure for the condition, and management at present involves treating symptoms and preventing complications.

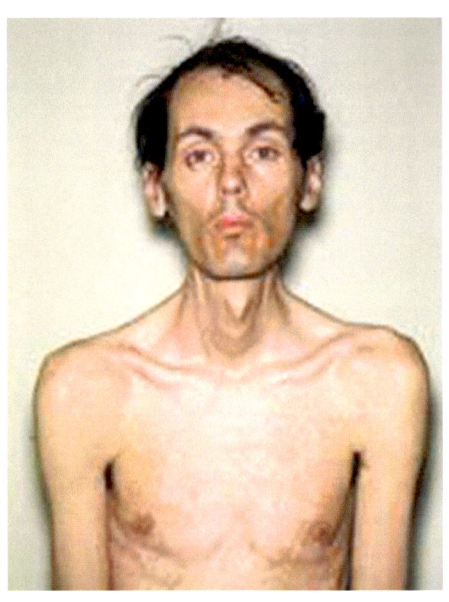

Fig. 5.26 *A patient with myotonic dystrophy. Note the extensive generalised muscle wasting.*

5.17 Neuro-cutaneous disorders

5.17.1 Neurofibromatosis

Neurofibromatosis refers to a group of autosomal dominant conditions that produce cutaneous and neuromuscular symptoms. Two major variations exist:
- Neurofibromatosis Type I (von Recklinghausen disease)
  - More common variant; cutaneous features predominate
  - Cutaneous neurofibromas (see *Fig. 5.27*)
  - At least 6 café-au-lait spots ≥5mm in diameter in children under 10; or ≥15mm in adults (see *Fig. 5.28*)
  - Inguinal/axillary freckling
  - Optic glioma
  - Lisch nodules (iritic hamartoma) visualised on slit-lamp (see *Fig. 5.29*)
  - Musculoskeletal deformities

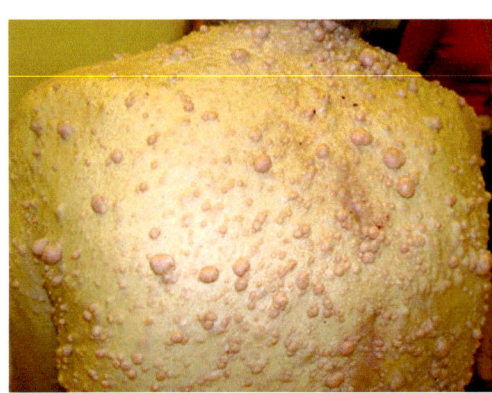

Fig. 5.27 *Neurofibromas over a patient's back.*

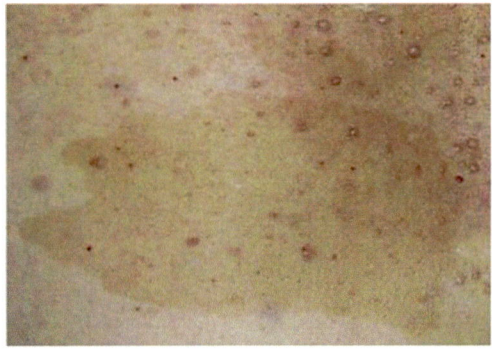

Fig. 5.28 *Café-au-lait spot.*

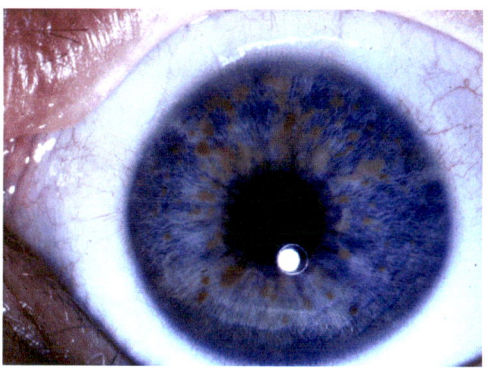

Fig. 5.29 *Lisch nodules (greyish spots in iris).*

- Neurofibromatosis Type II
  - CNS lesions predominate
  - Classically presents with bilateral Schwannomas (vestibular neuromas), visible on MRI
  - Meningiomas, ependymomas or gliomas may be observed

5.17.2 Tuberous sclerosis

Tuberous sclerosis refers to an autosomal dominant condition that presents with both systemic and neuro-cutaneous abnormalities.

- Neurological abnormalities
  - Variable degree of learning difficulty
  - Behavioural disturbances and autism may also be present
  - Intracranial lesions (classically, astrocytomas that obstruct the flow of CSF)
- Skin abnormalities
  - Adenoma sebaceum – reddish lesions that appear in a butterfly distribution over cheeks and nose (see *Fig. 5.30*)
  - Periungual fibromas – fleshy growths under fingernails and toenails
  - Hypomelanotic macules ('ash-leaf' spots); may require UV light to demonstrate in patients with fair skin (see *Fig. 5.31*)
  - Shagreen patches – rough, leathery patches of skin found on the neck and back
- Systemic abnormalities
  - Cystic lesions in the lung
  - Renal angiomyolipomata
  - Cardiac rhabdomyomas
  - Retinal hamartomas (see *Fig. 5.32*)

> **P** ≫ Hamartomas in tuberous sclerosis affect the retina, whilst hamartomas seen in neurofibromatosis affect the iris (Lisch nodules).

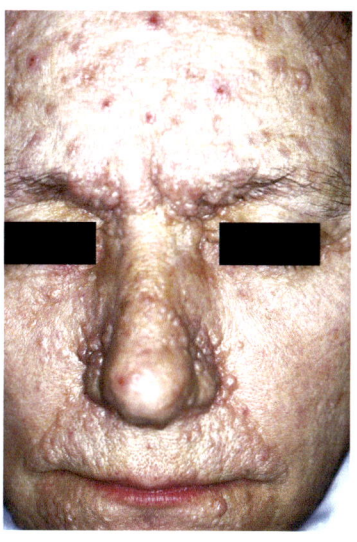

Fig. 5.30 *Adenoma sebaceum.*

5

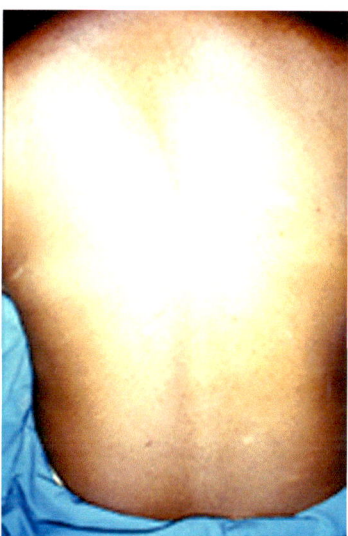

Fig. 5.31 *'Ash-leaf' spots.*

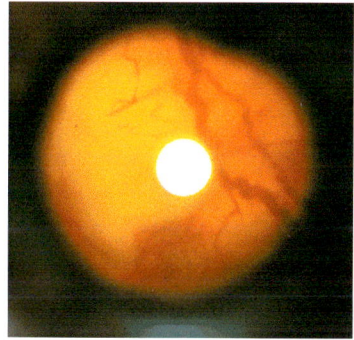

Fig. 5.32 *Retinal hamartomas.*

5

5.18 Delirium

Approach to delirium (NICE 2010, CG103)

Delirium refers to an acute confusional state; NICE defines it as a clinical syndrome, characterised by disturbed consciousness, cognitive function or perception, which has a fluctuating course. Patients rapidly become delirious; and appropriate investigation and treatment should proceed expeditiously, as the condition is associated with poor outcomes. Features include:

- Hyperactive state: arousal, restlessness, agitation
- Hypoactive state: drowsy, quiet
- The elderly, those with intercurrent illness and medical/surgical inpatients are at greater risk for delirium
- Diminished cognition, visual or auditory hallucinations

Table 5.15 Management of delirium – OHIO MED

Orientate	Nurse in a well-lit environment, attempt to re-orientate and calm patient; use clock, familiar objects
Hydrate	Assess hydration status and ensure adequate fluid intake
Infection	Screen for infection, request blood tests and manage accordingly
Oxygen	Correct and address any associated hypoxia
Metabolic	Correct and assess for any metabolic conditions (e.g. diabetes, endocrinopathies)
Electrolytes	Correct any electrolyte abnormalities
Drugs	Review medications (Are they sedative? Do they impair renal function?)

E ≫ Managing delirium ultimately involves finding and treating the underlying cause. Patients who are particularly aggressive and who are not responding to conservative management may be treated with haloperidol.

P ≫ In some cases, finding and stopping a medication-provoked delirium may be difficult. When faced with this possibility, consider stopping non-essential medications in order to assess for signs of improvement. These medications can always be re-titrated and re-introduced at a later date when the patient is stable.

5.19 Dementia

Dementia refers to a collection of symptoms that follow a progressive decline in baseline cognitive ability, characterised largely by impaired memory, loss of independence in daily living and/or behavioural disturbances.

P ≫ Mild cognitive impairment (MCI) is a term used to describe (in theory) a stage between what is thought to be normal ageing and dementia (i.e. pre-dementia). In practice, however, bear in mind that there may be overlaps between the stages, and delineation is not always crystal clear.

The most common aetiology for dementia is a neurodegenerative process, with vascular aetiologies making up about 20%. There are also rarer, potentially treatable causes, such as thyroid disorders, nutritional deficiencies (e.g. pellagra) or syphilis, but these account for a tiny proportion of cases.

E ≫ Vascular neurocognitive disorder is a newer term used to describe a range of pathology from mild cognitive impairment to pure vascular dementia. In practice, there may often be a mixed aetiology but evidence of cerebrovascular disease (either on imaging or clinically), in the context of cognitive impairment, is said to confer the diagnosis. The treatment for dementia caused by vascular disease is not the same as that for dementia related to neurodegenerative processes. Lifestyle modification related to risk factors should be pursued as much as possible, with aggressive lipid-lowering therapy instituted if necessary.

5.19.1 Alzheimer disease

Alzheimer disease is the most common cause of dementia. It is a progressive, neurodegenerative condition, characterised by accumulation of neuronal amyloid plaques (as well as phosphorylated *tau* protein), which form neurofibrillary tangles.

Epidemiology:

- Largely affects older individuals, above the age of 65
- More common in women
- Thought to have an increased risk when cardio-metabolic risk factors are also implicated (e.g. hypertension, hyperlipidaemia and diabetes mellitus)
- Genetics:
  - Apolipoprotein E on chromosome 19 thought to confer increased **risk** for the condition
  - Presenilin 1, presenilin 2 and amyloid precursor protein are thought to herald a **hereditary** cause, which usually has an earlier onset

Diagnosis criteria

The National Institute of Neurological and Communicative Disorders and Stroke and the Alzheimer's Disease and Related Disorder Association (NINCDS-ADRDA, 1984) group the diagnosis of Alzheimer disease into four subgroups (covering eight domains of cognition – memory, attention, language, constructive ability, problem solving, etc.):

- Probable Alzheimer disease
  - Progressive cognitive deficits in 2 or more domains
  - Age of onset between 40 and 90
  - Exclusion of other possible causes, including delirium
- Definite Alzheimer disease
  - Features of probable Alzheimer disease, with histological features on biopsy or at autopsy
- Possible Alzheimer disease
  - Atypical onset
  - Comorbid conditions that may be implicated in aetiology
- Unlikely Alzheimer disease

Other investigations that can aid diagnosis are screening tools (MMSE/MOCA), neuroimaging (particularly MRI) and blood tests used to exclude other aetiologies/types of delirium.

NICE also recommends the use of single photon emission CT (SPECT) when attempting to distinguish Alzheimer disease from vascular/frontotemporal dementia, if necessary.

Management

- Multidisciplinary individualised approach to care with home modification and suitable adjustment of daily activities
- Screening for depression
- Pharmacological therapy
  - Acetylcholinesterase inhibitors
    - Donepezil, rivastigmine, galantamine
    - Contraindicated in severe disease
  - NMDA antagonists
    - Memantine (second-line agent, usually in moderately severe disease)

> **E** » The key takeaway fact about pharmacological intervention in Alzheimer's or neurodegenerative dementia is that these treatments do not cure or halt progression. They merely provide symptomatic benefit and some improvement in the patient's activities of daily living.

5.19.2 Dementia with Lewy bodies

Dementia with Lewy bodies is another type of neurocognitive dementia that presents similarly to Alzheimer disease, with several key distinguishing features:

- Pathophysiological process involves aggregation of alpha-synuclein (Lewy bodies) in the brain (note that a similar process occurs in Parkinson disease and Parkinson plus syndromes)
- Patients present with classic features of dementia (also seen in Alzheimer's) but may also have:
  - Fluctuating levels of cognitive impairment and/or attention
  - Visual hallucinations

Patients who have dementia with Lewy bodies may also have symptoms of parkinsonism on examination. Distinguishing between the two may aid in treatment, as acetylcholinesterase inhibitors may improve dementia with Lewy bodies, whilst drugs used to treat parkinsonism may yield more benefit in a primarily Parkinsonian diagnosis.

- If symptoms of dementia develop before or concomitantly with parkinsonism, dementia with Lewy bodies is the more likely diagnosis
- If symptoms of dementia develop at least a year after motor parkinsonism, Parkinson's is the more likely diagnosis

5

5.19.3 Frontotemporal dementia

Frontotemporal dementia is characterised by atrophy of the frontal and temporal lobes (as the name suggests) – unlike the more diffuse atrophy seen in conditions such as Alzheimer disease.

- It has variable presentations (behavioural variant, forms of primary progressive aphasia)
- There are symptomatic overlaps with Parkinson plus syndromes (particularly progressive supranuclear palsy and corticobasilar degeneration)
- The presenting hallmark is changes in personality and behaviour, which may range from apathy to frank disinhibition (behavioural variant)
- Younger age of onset, usually between 30 and 60 years of age
- Pathophysiology includes involvement and neuronal accumulation of the following proteins:
  - *Tau* protein
  - Transactivating-response DNA binding protein 43 (TDP-43)
  - Fused-in sarcoma gene protein (FUS)
- There is, at present, no treatment for frontotemporal dementia
- Management is largely supportive and directed at symptom alleviation

5.20 Von Hippel–Lindau disease

Von Hippel–Lindau disease is an autosomal dominant disorder caused by a mutation in the von Hippel–Lindau tumour suppressor gene on chromosome 3. There are various subtypes of the disease, and classification depends on presenting features.

The diagnostic criteria include:
- A positive family history and the presence of:
  - A hemangioblastoma (either in the retina or CNS, but most often in the cerebellum) or a renal cell carcinoma **or**
- No positive family history, but the presence of:
  - Hemangioblastomas, renal cell carcinomas **and** the presence of phaeochromocytomas or other tumours of the pancreas

Screening for these characteristic features, particularly in the light of a positive family history, is essential, as it improves the prognosis. Management of the condition is undertaken in a multidisciplinary setting.

Chapter 6
Haematology, oncology and palliative medicine

Hwan Juet Khaw, Kelsey Wai Jan Wong, Ian Wu and *Tan Chuen Wen*

Bridge to clinical medicine

Blood is a type of connective tissue, consisting of a cellular component and an extracellular matrix (known as plasma). What makes blood unique is its fluidity, which allows it to be circulated throughout the body. The cellular component of blood (see *Fig. 6.1*) is primarily made up of:

- Red blood cells (erythrocytes), which play a key role in transporting oxygen
- White blood cells (leucocytes), which play a key role in the body's defence system
- Platelets (thrombocytes), which play a key role in haemostasis

Plasma, a straw-yellow fluid, makes up about 55% of blood. It is 92% water, with the rest consisting of plasma proteins (i.e. albumin, globulins, etc.) and coagulation factors. Serum is the name given to plasma without its clotting factors.

Haematopoiesis

Haematopoiesis refers to the production of blood cells. This primarily occurs in the bone marrow, but extramedullary haematopoiesis may also occur in the liver and spleen (in the case of bone marrow failure). All blood cells are derived from pluripotent haematopoietic stem cells. These cells have the unique ability to differentiate into two main hierarchies of stem cell lineages, namely (see *Fig. 6.2*):

- Myeloid stem progenitor stem cells
  - Proerythroblasts → erythrocytes
  - Megakaryoblasts → platelets

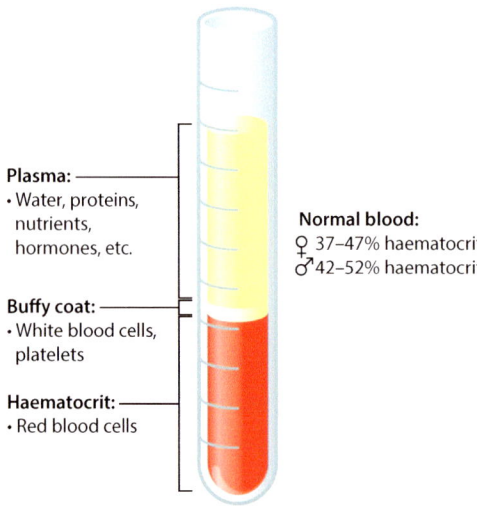

Plasma:
- Water, proteins, nutrients, hormones, etc.

Normal blood:
♀ 37–47% haematocrit
♂ 42–52% haematocrit

Buffy coat:
- White blood cells, platelets

Haematocrit:
- Red blood cells

Fig. 6.1 *Components of blood.*

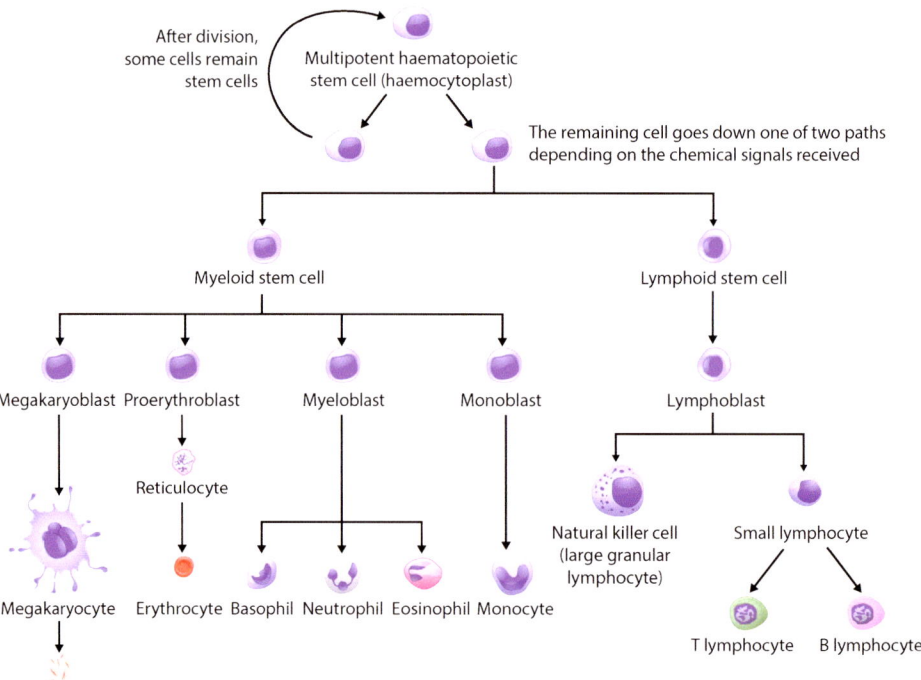

After division, some cells remain stem cells

Multipotent haematopoietic stem cell (haemocytoplast)

The remaining cell goes down one of two paths depending on the chemical signals received

Myeloid stem cell

Lymphoid stem cell

Megakaryoblast Proerythroblast Myeloblast Monoblast

Lymphoblast

Reticulocyte

Natural killer cell (large granular lymphocyte)

Small lymphocyte

Megakaryocyte Erythrocyte Basophil Neutrophil Eosinophil Monocyte

T lymphocyte B lymphocyte

Platelets

Fig. 6.2 *Haematopoiesis.*

- Myeloblasts → neutrophils, eosinophils, basophils
- Monoblasts → monocyte
- Lymphoid progenitor stem cells
  - Natural killer (NK) cell
  - Lymphocytes → T cell, B cell

Subsequent cell production and differentiation is regulated by chemicals known as haematopoietic growth factors. For example, erythropoietin (EPO), produced in the liver and kidneys, is responsible for red cell differentiation and proliferation.

Haemostasis

Haemostasis refers to the body's innate ability to respond to vascular injury and prevent extensive blood loss. This involves a complex interplay of systems between the vessel wall, platelets, coagulation factors and fibrinolytic enzymes. Disruption of these mechanisms gives rise to bleeding and thrombotic (clotting) disorders. Haemostasis can be divided into four distinct stages:

1. **Vessel wall response and platelet adhesion**
   - When the vascular endothelium is breached, endothelin is released, initiating vasoconstriction (vasospasm); this leads to a reduction in blood flow and thus, extensive blood loss
   - Exposure of the subendothelial collagen results in platelet-binding (via GP1a receptors) as well as the release of tissue factor (TF) – activating factor of the coagulation cascade
2. **Platelet plug formation**
   - Subendothelial-bound von Willebrand factor (vWF) interacts with platelets (via GP1b receptors), causing further adhesion
   - Bound platelets subsequently release activation factors (COX-induced prostaglandins, thromboxane A2 and ADP), stimulating further platelet aggregation

E ≫ Antiplatelet drugs work by inhibiting these activation factors, e.g. aspirin (COX-inhibitor) and clopidogrel (ADP-inhibitor). Newer antiplatelet agents, prasugrel and ticagrelor, are variants of ADP-inhibitors.

3. **Coagulation**
   - The coagulation cascade is traditionally divided into extrinsic and intrinsic pathways; both cascades eventually converge at the activation of factor X that leads to a final common pathway (see *Fig. 6.3*)

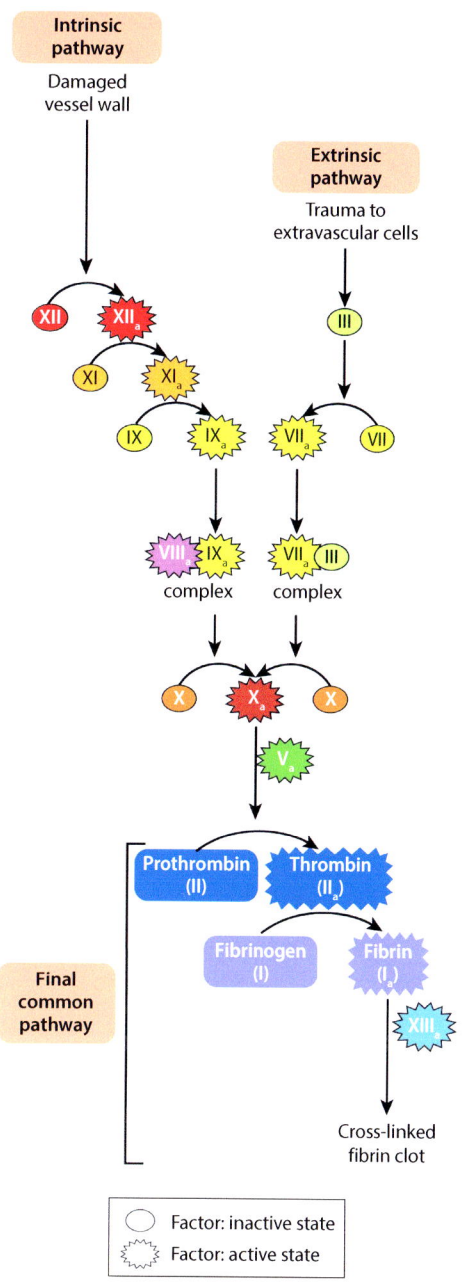

Fig. 6.3 *Coagulation cascade.*

- Coagulation is typically initiated by the extrinsic pathway, triggered when TF binds to factor VII; this occurs over seconds and is further amplified by the intrinsic pathway
- The intrinsic pathway involves a stepwise activation of factors XII, XI, IX and VIII, usually completed after minutes

- Activated factor X, catalysed by activated factor V, converts prothrombin (factor II) into its active form, thrombin
- Thrombin is responsible for converting insoluble fibrinogen (factor I) into its soluble form, fibrin
- Fibrin strands then bind with platelets (via its GPIIb/IIIa receptors); in the presence of factor XIII, fibrin cross-links are formed, stabilising the clot
- Coagulation is regulated by the presence of physiological anticoagulant enzymes
- These enzymes include antithrombin (which cleaves and inactivates factors X and II) and activated protein C (with co-factor protein S), a vitamin K-dependent enzyme that inactivates factors V and VIII as well as inducing fibrinolysis

4. **Fibrinolysis**
   - This refers to the reversal of clotting, restoring normal blood flow after vascular injury
   - The conversion of plasminogen (inactive form) into plasmin is induced by tissue plasminogen activator (t-PA), released from the subendothelial layer
   - Plasmin breaks down fibrin cross-links into fibrin degradation products (FDPs) and D-dimer

E ›› Anticoagulation agents are commonly used in clinical practice. They are frequently used in the treatment and prophylaxis of venous thromboembolisms and prevention of stroke in atrial fibrillation. These agents act at various points of the coagulation cascade.

Table 6.1 *Mechanism of action of common oral anticoagulants*

Anticoagulant	Action	Clotting factors
Heparin	Potentiates antithrombin	Mainly Xa, II
Warfarin	Vitamin-K antagonist (reduces hepatic production of clotting factors)	II, VII, IX and X
Fondaparinux	Pentasaccharide, synthetic factor Xa inhibitor	Xa
Apixaban, rivaroxaban	Direct Xa antagonist	Xa
Dabigatran	Direct thrombin inhibitor	IIa

Blood typing

The discovery of the major blood group types in the early 1900s revolutionised clinical medicine and the way we deliver blood product transfusions. The two most common blood typing systems, used almost universally, are the **ABO system** and the **Rhesus (Rh) system**.

The ABO system is characterised by the presence of specific erythrocyte surface antigens and serum antibodies. *Table 6.2* illustrates the antigens and antibodies that are present in the different blood groups. It is important to note that there is a co-dominant inheritance between groups A and B.

Table 6.2 *Blood groups*

Group	Surface antigen	Serum antibodies	Compatibility
A	A	Anti-B	A and O
B	B	Anti-A	B and O
AB	A and B	None	A, B and O
O	None	Anti-A and anti-B	O

ABO incompatibility occurs when an incompatible blood group is transfused, resulting in intravascular agglutination and subsequently haemolysis.

The Rh system refers to the presence or absence of the Rh antigens on the erythrocyte surface membrane. Although multiple Rh antigens have been identified (e.g. C, E, K, etc.), the D antigen remains the most clinically significant. Therefore, patients with D Rh antigens are described as RhD-positive.

P ›› Problems associated with RhD status occur most commonly during pregnancy. This is particularly prevalent in second pregnancies, when a RhD-negative mother has been sensitised to her first-born's RhD-positive red blood cells, and thus produces anti-RhD antibodies. These antibodies will then react with her second child's (if RhD-positive) red blood cells, resulting in haemolytic disease of the newborn.

Transfusion reactions

Since the introduction of vigorous and strict safeguards in transfusion protocols, transfusion complication rates have fallen substantially.

Table 6.3 *Transfusion reactions and their management*

Reaction	Timing	Features	Management
Mild allergy	Immediate	Rash, itch, urticaria	**Slow** transfusion, antihistamine
Severe allergy	Immediate	Bronchospasm, angioedema, ↓BP	**Stop** transfusion, antihistamine, steroid, salbutamol nebs
Haemolysis (ABO incompatibility)	Within minutes	Rigors, fever, dyspnoea, ↓BP, DIC, haemoglobulinuria	**Stop** transfusion, inform labs, IV fluids, treat DIC
Febrile non-haemolytic	Hours	Fever (isolated T ≥38°C), rigors	**Slow** transfusion, paracetamol
Bacterial contamination	Within 24 hours	High fevers, ↓BP, shock	**Stop** transfusion, antibiotics, Sepsis 6 Protocol, return blood to labs
Transfusion-related acute lung injury (TRALI)	6–24 hours	ARDS, acute SOB and cough, **normal** CVP/JVP	**Stop** transfusion, oxygen, treat ARDS
Fluid overload	6–24 hours	Acute SOB, **raised** CVP/JVP	**Slow** transfusion, oxygen, IV furosemide

Adverse transfusion reactions still occur in around 3% of patients. These are usually mild reactions, but it is important to be aware of severe complications that may occur. These reactions and their treatment are shown in *Table 6.3*.

Haematopoietic stem cell transplantation

Haematopoietic stem cell transplantation (HSCT), also known as bone marrow transplant (BMT), is increasingly used in the treatment of various haematological conditions – mainly haematological malignancies. There are two main types of HSCT: allogeneic HSCT and autologous HSCT.

Allogeneic HSCT involves transfusing donor haematopoietic stem cells, preferably HLA-matched, into a recipient who has been conditioned for transplant. The conditioning process often requires high-dose chemotherapy (with or without radiotherapy), which has the dual function of destroying malignant cells and inducing temporary immunosuppression.

E ≫ Graft versus host disease (GVHD) is a complication related to alloimmunity, caused by the cytotoxic effects of the donor's T-lymphocytes ('the graft') towards the host cells. This may occur in up to one-third of patients and can be traditionally classified as acute (within the first 100 days) or chronic (≥100 days from transplant). Immunosuppressive agents (e.g. methotrexate, cyclosporin) are given to reduce the chance of developing GVHD.

P ≫ GVHD should not be confused with 'graft versus disease' effect, which refers to a beneficial mechanism of allogeneic HSCT. This effect occurs as a result of the donor's immune system recognising and eliminating the host's residual malignant cells.

Autologous HSCT differs, in that 'self' haematopoietic stem cells are harvested prior to conditioning therapy. These harvested cells are then re-infused post-chemotherapy.

6.1 Anaemia

Approach to anaemia

Anaemia is defined as a decrease in the number of red blood cells or a decrease in the oxygen-carrying capacity of blood cells.

E ≫ The World Health Organization broadly categorises anaemia as a haemoglobin level that is below 13g/dl in men and below 12g/dl in women.

As anaemia is more of a symptom than a disease in itself, one approach is to consider three mechanisms that can potentially lead to anaemia – **decreased red blood cell** (RBC) **production**, **increased RBC lysis** and **loss of blood**. Looking at the morphology of blood cells also offers a clue to the type of anaemia, i.e. **microcytic**, **normocytic** or **macrocytic**.

A normal **mean corpuscular volume** (MCV), which is a measurement of the average volume of RBCs, is 80–100 femtolitres (fl). A microcytic anaemia is characterised by an MCV <80fl, and a macrocytic anaemia is characterised by an MCV >100fl.

The most common causes of a microcytic anaemia are iron-deficiency anaemia and thalassaemia. Sideroblastic anaemia (see *Section 6.1.3*) is generally microcytic, but may present with a normocytic anaemia.

Common causes of macrocytic anaemias include excess alcohol, folate and/or vitamin B12 deficiency (from pernicious anaemia or inadequate dietary intake), various medications and myelodysplasia. Patients with anaemia may suffer from fatigue, dyspnoea and headaches, but other systemic features (particularly weight loss, night sweats and fevers) should prompt a more thorough evaluation, and an attempt to elicit an underlying cause.

6.1.1 Microcytic anaemias

Iron-deficiency anaemia

Definition: iron-deficiency anaemia (IDA) refers to a condition caused by inadequate iron intake, which leads to decreased RBC production.

Epidemiology:
- Most common cause of anaemia globally
- Premenopausal women are most at risk of IDA, due to blood loss during menstruation

> **E** ≫ GI bleeding is the most common cause of anaemia in men and postmenopausal women.

Aetiology/pathophysiology:
- Three major causes of IDA exist:
  - Insufficient dietary intake of iron or malabsorption of iron (e.g. in coeliac disease)
  - Increased loss of iron (e.g. GI bleeding, cancer, ulcerative colitis or endemic infectious diseases such as hookworm infections or schistosomiasis)
  - Increased demand for iron (e.g. during pregnancy)

- Iron is an essential component in the formation of the haem group in haemoglobin; a decreased level of iron, relative to bodily requirements, will eventually result in impaired haemoglobin synthesis.

Clinical features:
- Patients with IDA may be **asymptomatic**
- Presenting symptoms include fatigue, dyspnoea and headaches
- More alarming symptoms, such as chest pain and severe dyspnoea, do not occur until the haemoglobin level drops significantly
- Examination findings may include koilonychia (spoon-shaped nails; see *Fig. 6.4*) and angular chelitis (see *Fig. 6.5*)

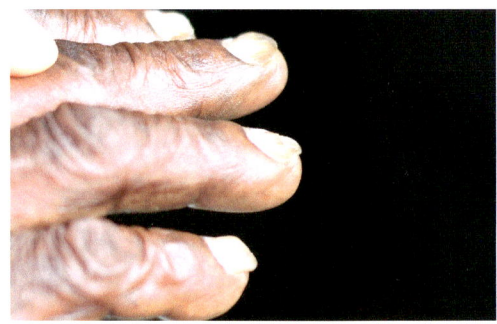

Fig. 6.4 *Koilonychia.*

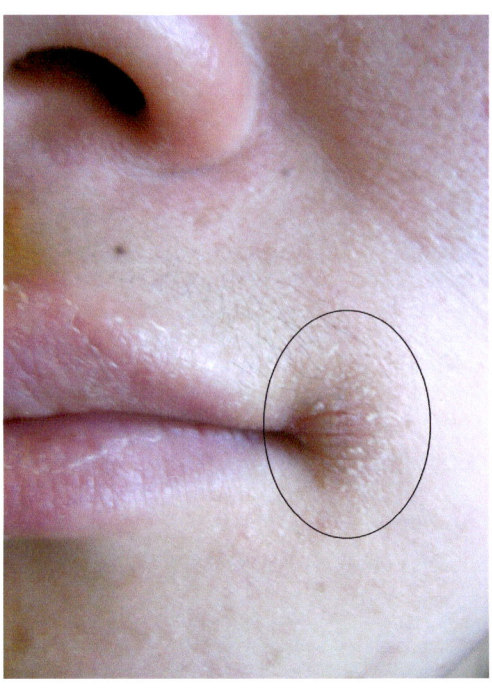

Fig. 6.5 *Angular chelitis.*

P ≫ Plummer–Vinson syndrome (also known as Paterson–Kelly–Brown syndrome) is characterised by a triad of symptoms: **iron-deficiency anaemia, oesophageal webs** and **dysphagia**. It may also present with glossitis. The exact aetiology is unclear. Treatment involves iron replacement and endoscopic dilatation of the oesophagus. A careful assessment is warranted, as patients with this syndrome are also at higher risk of developing oesophageal carcinomas.

Investigations

Stepwise plan:

1 **Arrange initial tests, including a full blood count, peripheral smear and iron studies**
- Will indicate a hypochromic (central pallor of RBC), microcytic anaemia
- Low iron levels, but **increased** total iron binding capacity (TIBC)
- **Serum ferritin <12ng/ml is diagnostic**

W ≫ One important consideration when evaluating ferritin is that ferritin (much like transcobalamin) is an acute phase reactant, and levels may be falsely elevated in acute inflammatory illnesses. The gold standard test in determining IDA is Prussian blue staining of bone marrow biopsy, but, as one might imagine, this is rarely carried out to elicit the diagnosis.

2 **If patients are asymptomatic or have GI symptoms, further investigation with endoscopy is warranted**

3 **Patients should also be tested for coeliac disease serology if indicated clinically**

Management

Stepwise management of iron-deficiency anaemia

1 **Oral iron replacement is the first-line treatment**
- Oral ferrous sulphate/fumarate
- May take up to 2 months for haemoglobin levels to normalise

2 **Patients who do not respond to oral iron, or are intolerant, may be considered for IV iron replacement**

E ≫ It is important to warn patients about side effects pertaining to treatment with iron supplementation, namely black stools, constipation and nausea.

Thalassaemia

The word thalassaemia is originally derived from the Greek word *thalassa*, meaning 'from the sea', highlighting the fact that people of Mediterranean heritage tend to inherit this condition.

Two important forms exist – alpha thalassaemia and beta thalassaemia. The disease process is typically associated with gene deletions and point mutations respectively, leading to improper synthesis of adult haemoglobin, which is composed of two alpha globin chains and two beta globin chains.

E ≫ Haemoglobin possesses a haem subunit that interfaces with paired globin chains. These may be variations of alpha, beta, gamma or delta globin chains, producing various types of haemoglobin. Some of the more common variants include:
- Haemoglobin A (HbA): two alpha chains, two beta chains (96–98% of Hb)
- Haemoglobin A2 (HbA2): two alpha chains, two delta chains (2–3% of Hb)
- Haemoglobin F (HbF): two alpha chains, two gamma chains (1–2% of Hb), primarily produced by the foetus

The effect of these mutations on symptoms may vary, depending on the type and extent of involvement, and thalassaemia may at times be classified as minor, major or intermedia.

Beta thalassaemia is more likely to affect people of Mediterranean origin, whilst alpha thalassaemia is more likely to affect Asians. Up to 2% of individuals are carriers of beta thalassaemia worldwide. Around 5% of people are estimated to be carriers of alpha thalassaemia.

6

Alpha thalassaemia

Table 6.4 *Pathophysiology of alpha thalassaemia*

Pathophysiology	Features	Outcome/management
One gene deletion α,-/α,α	Alpha thalassaemia trait; Hb levels usually normal; may have slight anaemia	Usually asymptomatic
Two gene deletions α,-/α,- or -,-/α,α	Alpha thalassaemia trait; microcytic, hypochromic anaemia; Hb levels usually normal	Usually asymptomatic
Three gene deletions α,-/-,- (HbH disease)	Significantly anaemic; significantly low MCV, Hb Hepatosplenomegaly, jaundice	Clinically significant anaemia; may require blood transfusions
Four gene deletions -,-/-,- (Bart's Hb)	Death *in utero*; incompatible with life	Hydrops fetalis

Beta thalassaemia

The majority of beta thalassaemias are caused by point mutations in the beta globin gene, resulting in dysfunctional haemoglobin synthesis. These produce three clinically significant forms of beta thalassaemia – beta thalassaemia minor, beta thalassaemia intermedia and beta thalassaemia major (see *Table 6.5*).

P ≫ In some cases, bony abnormalities, such as frontal bossing, expansion of the maxilla in beta thalassaemia major ('chipmunk facies') and the 'hair on end' appearance on X-ray, are described as key distinguishing features. In practice, however, these generally develop much later in the disease process, and are more prominent in patients who have yet to receive treatment.

E ≫ Regular blood transfusions are not without complications. The body does not have a natural means of excreting excess iron, and so iron overload from frequent blood transfusions may occur in the long term. This excess iron is deposited in various organs and may cause fibrosis, organ failure and endocrinopathies if endocrine organs are affected.

Iron chelation helps reduce the risk of this, to some degree. Desferrioxamine, an iron chelator, is one of the more traditional agents, mostly because it is given subcutaneously. Oral iron chelators (such as **deferasirox** and **deferiprone**) are also available, and the use of these agents is proving more popular because of their route of administration.

6.1.2 Anaemia of chronic disease

The anaemia of chronic disease is incompletely understood, but is thought to occur as a result of cytokine-mediated iron retention and suppression of erythropoiesis.

6.1.3 Sideroblastic anaemia

Sideroblastic anaemia is a congenital or acquired form of anaemia that occurs as a result of dysfunctional erythropoiesis, leading to excess iron deposition in RBC precursors and the formation of ringed sideroblasts in the bone marrow (see *Fig. 6.6*).

Table 6.5 *Classification of beta thalassaemia*

Classification	Features	Outcome/management
Beta thalassaemia minor	Hypochromic, microcytic anaemia; elevated levels of **HbA2**	Usually asymptomatic
Beta thalassaemia major	Severe anaemia begins to develop early on in infancy, when HbF levels begin to fall; presents with jaundice, sleepiness and failure to thrive; may have bony abnormalities; elevated levels of HbF and HbA2	Patients require lifelong blood transfusions and iron chelation
Beta thalassaemia intermedia	Patients typically present with anaemia, but may vary in presentation with regard to jaundice, bony abnormalities and other symptoms	In these patients, the need for transfusions depends on the severity of their disease

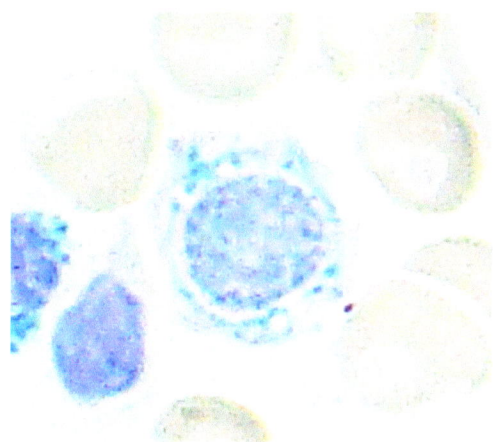

> >> Dietary folate is converted to methyl-tetrahydrofolate (MTHF) in the plasma and cells. The metabolism of homocysteine to methionine is essential to produce tetrahydrofolate (THF) from MTHF. Vitamin B12 is an important co-factor that functions to catalyse this reaction. THF is then incorporated into the DNA cycle and ultimately metabolised into DNA. Impaired nuclear maturation ensues, resulting in nucleocytoplasmic dysynchrony. The resultant cells (megaloblasts) are larger in size, with disproportionately enlarged nuclei.

Fig. 6.6 *Sideroblast – iron accumulation in the mitochondria surrounding the nucleus (blue specks).*

Acquired forms of the disease may occur as a result of chronic infections, systemic lupus erythematosus (SLE), drug therapy or lead poisoning. This disease is clinically indistinguishable from other forms of anaemia, but iron studies will demonstrate high iron levels. A definitive diagnosis is made on demonstrating ringed sideroblasts on bone marrow studies. Treatment is generally supportive and involves removing the underlying cause. Pyridoxine (vitamin B6) may be useful in treating congenital forms of this disease.

6.1.4 Macrocytic anaemia

As discussed previously, macrocytic anaemias are characterised by an MCV of >100fl. They can be categorised into megaloblastic anaemias or non-megaloblastic anaemias.

Megaloblastic anaemia

This form of anaemia is caused by deficiencies in either vitamin B12 or folic acid. These micronutrients are essential in DNA synthesis, and reduced levels will result in impaired haematopoiesis. The biochemical mechanism of folate and vitamin B12 in megaloblastic anaemia is shown in *Fig. 6.7*.

Vitamin B12 deficiency

As discussed in *Chapter 3*, dietary vitamin B12 binds to intrinsic factor produced by gastric parietal cells and this complex is subsequently absorbed in the terminal ileum. Hence, the causes of vitamin B12 deficiency can be divided, based on these factors:

- **Insufficient dietary vitamin B12 intake** – e.g. vegans and vegetarians
- **Gastric pathology** – pernicious anaemia (*see below*), gastrectomy
- **Small bowel pathology** – ileal resection, inflammatory bowel disease (IBD), malabsorption disorders (e.g. SIBO, tropical sprue; *see Chapter 3*)

Folate deficiency

Dietary folate is found in leafy vegetables (e.g. broccoli, spinach) and animal protein (e.g. liver). It is present as polyglutamates which are subsequently converted into the monoglutamate form in the proximal small bowel (mainly the jejunum) and actively absorbed into the plasma. Folate deficiency can be caused by:

- **Reduced dietary intake** – alcohol excess, malnutrition
- **Increased metabolic demand** – pregnancy (most common cause), proliferative diseases, malignancy
- **Malabsorption disorders** – IBD, small intestinal bacterial overgrowth (SIBO), tropical sprue
- **Antifolate drugs** – e.g. phenytoin, methotrexate, trimethoprim

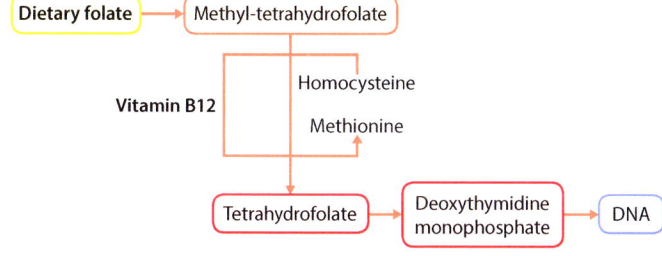

Fig. 6.7 *The role of vitamin B12 and folate in megaloblastic anaemia.*

Patients with folate deficiency are often asymptomatic but may sometimes present with glossitis.

Pernicious anaemia

Pernicious anaemia is an autoimmune condition characterised by atrophic gastritis and destruction of parietal cells. It is commonly found in the elderly population, with an average age of onset of 60. Auto-antibodies towards parietal cells are found in up to 90% of patients. These auto-antibodies are responsible for the atrophic cellular destruction and subsequent loss of intrinsic factor production. The use of the Schilling test has fallen out of favour, due to its limited availability.

> **E** ≫ Other autoimmune associations include Addison disease, vitiligo, Hashimoto thyroiditis and Graves disease. Hence, patients should be screened for these conditions. Patients with pernicious anaemia should have endoscopic upper GI evaluation performed at diagnosis due to their susceptibility to all types of gastric tumours.

Non-megaloblastic anaemia

Macrocytosis can also occur in conditions without megaloblastic changes. These include:

- Physiological changes, e.g. pregnancy
- Alcohol excess

> **P** ≫ Chronic alcohol excess has myriad effects on haematopoiesis. It primarily causes bone marrow suppression, leading to a reduction in blood cell precursor. Apart from microcytosis, alcohol may also cause sideroblastic, megaloblastic and haemolytic anaemias.

- Liver disease
- Other haematological conditions, e.g. aplastic anaemia, reticulocytosis, myelodysplasia
- Hypothyroidism

Investigations

Stepwise plan:

1   **Perform a full blood count, reticulocyte count and a peripheral blood film**
- Reticulocyte – may be low
- Blood film – megaloblasts (vit B12 and folate deficiencies) or target cells (alcohol; see *Fig. 6.9*)

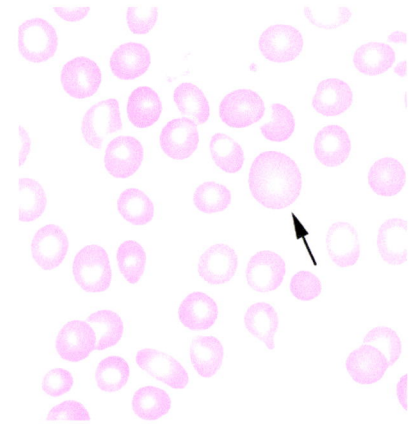

Fig. 6.8 *Macrocytosis.*

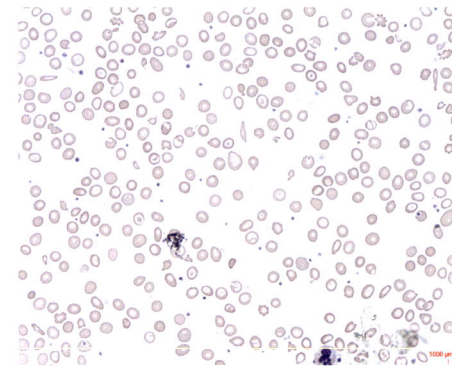

Fig. 6.9 *Target cells (Mexican hat) with their characteristic bull's eye-like appearance.*

2   **Check vitamin B12 and folate levels**

3   **Arrange other blood tests – LFTs, TFTs**

Management

The treatment of macrocytic anaemia depends on its underlying cause.

Stepwise management of macrocytic anaemia

1   **Vitamin B12 deficiency can be treated with an initial loading regime of 6 doses**
- 1mg (IM injections) over a period of 2 weeks, followed by 1mg every 3 months

2   **Oral preparations of vitamin B12 have since been shown to have similar efficacy**
- These may be used as an alternative if PA is absent

3   **Folate is usually replaced daily – 5mg for the first 3 weeks**
- This is followed by a once-weekly maintenance dose

In a patient with both deficiencies, it is important to replace vitamin B12 in the first instance, to prevent exacerbation of neurological symptoms.

6.1.5 Sickle cell anaemia

Definition: sickle cell diseases are a spectrum of haemoglobinopathies in which sickle cell haemoglobin (HbS) is present, due to an autosomal recessive gene mutation. Sickle cell traits (carrier) are the result of inheriting a sickle gene from one carrier parent, while sickle cell anaemia occurs when both parents are carriers. This section focuses on sickle cell anaemia.

Epidemiology:
- 30–40% prevalence of carriers in sub-Saharan Africa
- Sickle cell anaemia is the most common severe genetic disease in the UK
- Sickle cell traits are protective against malaria

Aetiology/pathophysiology:
- The major adult haemoglobin (HbA) comprises two alpha and two beta globin chains (α2β2)
- In sickle cell diseases, an autosomal recessive mutation of the beta globin gene substitutes glutamic acid for valine at the sixth amino acid, resulting in the formation of HbS

Major genotypes of sickle haemoglobinopathies:
- Sickle cell carriers – 40% HbS and 60% HbA
- Sickle cell anaemia – 100% HbS
- Sickle beta thalassaemia:
  - Beta-0 – 100% HbS
  - Beta-+ – 60% HbS and 40% HbA
- Haemoglobin SC – 50% HbS, 50% HbC

Red cells containing HbS are reversibly deformed into sickle (crescent) shapes when deoxygenated; in this state their membranes are 'stickier'. They adhere to vascular endothelium and occlude small vessels, leading to microinfarctions and ischaemic pains, known as vaso-occlusive crises. The red cells are also recognised as abnormally shaped by the spleen, resulting in haemolytic anaemia.

>> Hypoxia, acidosis, dehydration, infection, cold, strenuous exercise, anxiety and fever are precipitants of sickle cell crises.

Clinical features:

>> Sickle cell anaemia is usually diagnosed before or at birth. However, in undiagnosed infants, presentation tends to occur in the first few months of life – corresponding to the falling concentrations of HbF.

There is great clinical variability between patients; some remain asymptomatic until adulthood, whilst others suffer multiple 'attacks' that vary in severity. Patients may present with the following:
- Anaemia, jaundice, lethargy, pallor, weakness, growth restriction
- Recurrent infections, splenomegaly
- Delayed puberty

Some patients may also present initially with sickle cell crises (see *Table 6.6* for further details and management).

Investigations

Stepwise plan:

1 Arrange antenatal diagnosis
- In both parents who are sickle cell carriers, there is a 25% risk of sickle cell anaemia in their offspring
- Chorionic villus sampling or amniocentesis are options for antenatal diagnosis

2 Provide neonatal screening
- Heel-prick test in the first few days of birth

3 Obtain bloods
- Full blood count with peripheral blood smear shows Hb of 6–8g/dl with increased reticulocytes (10–20%) and sickled red cells on peripheral blood film (see *Fig. 6.10*), iron studies

4 Sickle solubility test
- Normal haemoglobin appears clear, whilst HbS precipitates and is turbid

5 Haemoglobin electrophoresis
- This is diagnostic; 80–95% HbS with no HbA, with 2–20% HbF

6 Arrange other investigations, including bloods (U&Es, LFTs, PFTs)
- For monitoring of disease and screening for complications, as outlined in *Table 6.6*

6

Table 6.6 *Sickle cell crises and their management*

Sickle cell crises/presentations	Management
Vaso-occlusive crisis: presents as skeletal (bone marrow) pain due to bone infarction or avascular necrosis. In children, dactylitis is very common, whilst in adults, bone pain is usually confined to the axial skeleton **Almost any other vessel may be involved:** bowel ischaemia, renal papillary necrosis, retinal haemorrhage and detachment, cerebral infarction (especially in children)	1. Adequate analgesia 2. Supplemental oxygen 3. Aggressive hydration 4. Investigation and correction of underlying causes (infection, acidosis) 5. Transfusions are only indicated in symptomatic anaemia
Sequestration crisis: presents in infants and young children with acute splenomegaly, pallor, haemodynamic instability, acute drop in haemoglobin levels secondary to the trapping of red cells in the spleen	1. Transfusions 2. Splenectomy in recurrent cases of sequestration
Acute chest syndrome: vaso-occlusive crisis in the lungs, presents with chest pain, fever, dyspnoea; seen on chest X-ray as a new pulmonary infiltrate. Difficult to distinguish from other differentials of chest pain	1. Oxygen therapy is priority; analgesia 2. Caution with hydration to prevent pulmonary oedema
Aplastic crisis: associated with parvovirus B19 infection, causing severe anaemia from transient cessation of erythropoiesis. Clinical picture may be similar to heart failure	Usually requires transfusion, occasionally spontaneously resolves

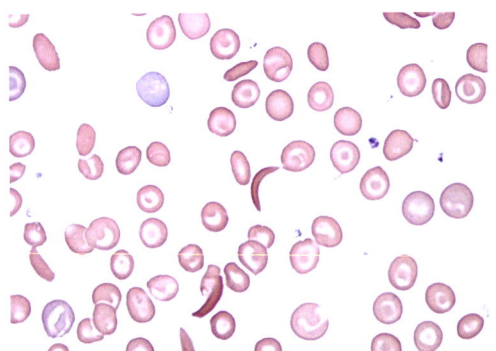

Fig. 6.10 *Sickle cell on blood film.*

Complications

> » Sickle cells are more rigid and more prone to clumping. Increased blood viscosity occurs as a result, eventually leading to vascular occlusion. Interrupted oxygenation may lead to end-organ infarction.

Ongoing management of chronic disease:

- Monitoring and managing complications: anaemia, cholelithiasis, cardiomegaly and congestive heart failure, leg ulcers, pulmonary hypertension, priapism, proliferative retinopathy, renal failure, developmental delay, subacute central nervous system damage
- Supportive care, including pain management
- Hydroxyurea: increases concentration of HbF

- Blood transfusions: especially pre-surgically
- Bone marrow transplantation: consider in children with severe recurrent complications
- Patient education about complications and recognition of signs and symptoms, genetic counselling
- Post-splenectomy vaccinations

6.1.6 Aplastic anaemia

Aplastic anaemia is a rare haematological condition, characterised by pancytopenia and bone marrow hypocellularity. It has an annual incidence of 2 per million cases. These can be divided into primary and secondary causes.

- Primary
  - Idiopathic
  - Congenital
    - Fanconi anaemia
    - Shwachman–Diamond syndrome
- Secondary
  - Drugs
    - Antibiotics – sulphonamides, linezolid
    - Cytotoxic drugs – penicillamine, gold
    - Anti-inflammatory – NSAIDs, naproxen
    - Anti-epileptics – phenytoin, carbamazepine
  - Chemicals – benzene, organophosphates
  - Paroxysmal nocturnal haemoglobinuria
  - Viral hepatitis – EBV
  - Pregnancy

Patients present with symptoms of bone marrow failure – anaemia, recurrent infections and bleeding.

E >> Diagnosis depends on the presence of:
- Hypocellular bone marrow and at least 2 of the following:
  - Hb <10g/dl
  - Neutrophil count $<1.5 \times 10^9$/L
  - Platelet count $<50 \times 10^9$/L

Patients with aplastic anaemia usually require regular FBC monitoring and infection surveillance.

Management
Management involves supportive treatment, with blood product transfusion and aggressive antibiotic therapy as well as immunotherapy.
- Younger patients (<50 years old)
  - Allogeneic stem cell transplant – offers a curative option
- Elderly patients (>50 years old)
  - Immunotherapy (typically with cyclosporin and antithymocyte globulin (ATG) regime) – improves 5-year survival

6.1.7 Haemolytic anaemia
Haemolytic anaemias are a group of conditions characterised by premature death or destruction of red cells. They can occur either within the vessel (intravascular) or outside it (extravascular).

Physiologically, red cells are broken down by the reticulo-endothelial system in the liver or spleen and the majority of these haemolytic anaemias develop extravascularly. *Figure 6.11* illustrates the different causes of haemolytic anaemia.

Inherited haemolytic anaemias
Red cell membrane defects: hereditary spherocytosis
This is an autosomal dominant condition caused by defects in structural proteins of red cell membranes. It is the most common inherited haemolytic anaemia, affecting around 1 in 5000 people annually.

The proteins affected are spectrin (both alpha and beta subtypes), ankyrin, band 3 protein and protein 42. These proteins function primarily to maintain RBC deformability. Defects in these structural proteins result in increased RBC fragility, particularly when passing through the spleen. Extravascular haemolysis develops as a consequence of this.

Patients are typically jaundiced since birth and may often have splenomegaly. They also often experience:
- Haemolytic crisis – rare but can occur with severe infections
- Megaloblastic crisis – folate deficiency
- Aplastic crisis – associated with parvovirus B19 infection in children

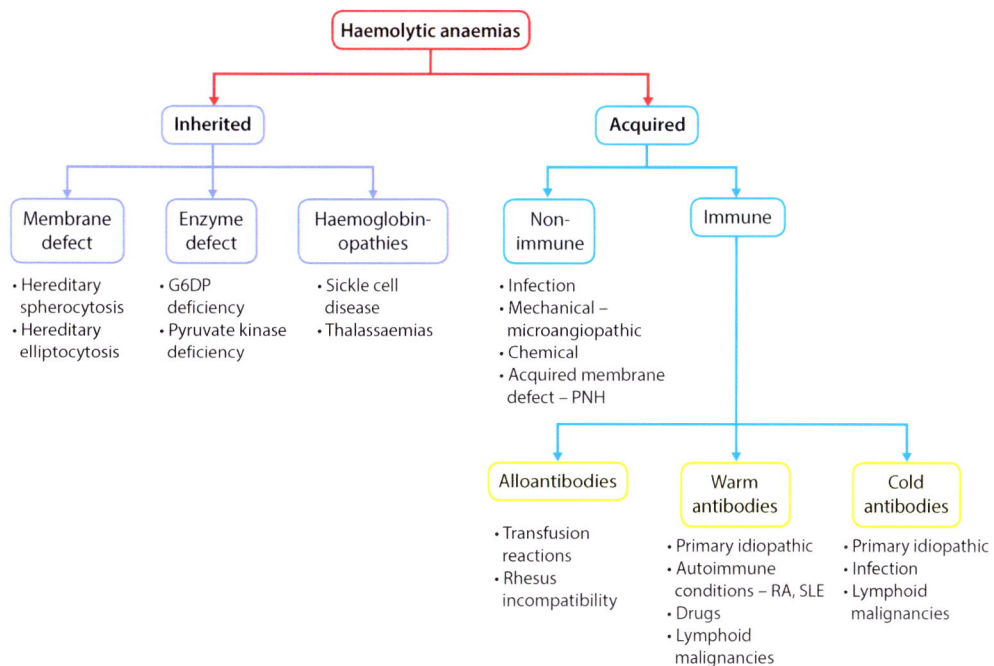

Fig. 6.11 *Causes of haemolytic anaemia.*

≫ One of the major associations of hereditary spherocytosis is the development of gallstones. This is due to red cell lysis and subsequent accumulation of unconjugated bilirubin in the gall bladder, promoting pigmented gallstone formation.

Investigations

Stepwise plan:

1 **Peripheral blood film**
- Spherocytes are diagnostic (see *Fig. 6.12*)
- Reticulocytes may also be present

2 **Osmotic fragility test (OFT)**
- This is rarely performed in clinical practice due to its lack of sensitivity and specificity. However, it may be useful if blood film results are inconclusive

3 **EMA binding test by flow cytometry**

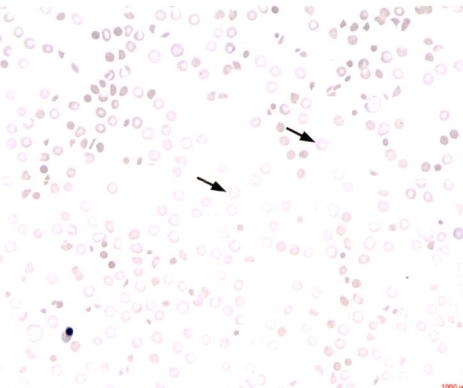

Fig. 6.12 *Spherocytes seen on a peripheral blood film. Note that they lack the classic biconcave disc shape.*

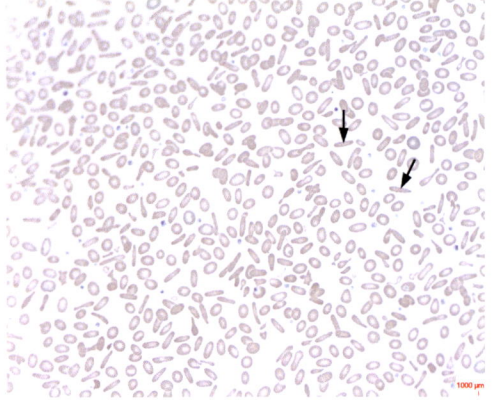

Fig. 6.13 *Elliptocytes seen on a peripheral blood film.*

Stepwise management of hereditary spherocytosis

1 **Folate replacement and splenectomy are the mainstay treatments for hereditary spherocytosis**

2 **Splenectomies are usually held off until after the age of 6 to prevent the risk of sepsis**

3 **Post-splenectomy management should be commenced**

Hereditary elliptocytosis

This is a cell membrane disorder characterised by defects in the structural proteins alpha-spectrin and protein 4.1. These defects result in production of elliptocytes (see *Fig. 6.13*). Like hereditary spherocytosis, this condition has an autosomal dominant inheritance. However, hereditary elliptocytosis is much less common, with an annual incidence of only 1 in 10,000. Most patients are asymptomatic and rarely require active treatment.

Red cell enzyme defects

The red blood cell, just like any other cell, requires energy (in the form of ATP) to maintain its function and protect itself from oxidative stress. Two main enzyme pathways (namely, the hexose monophosphate and Embden–Meyerhof glycolytic pathways) exist to facilitate glucose metabolism in RBC. *Figure 6.14* is a simplified representation of these processes.

 ≫ Enzyme defects in the hexose monophosphate pathway (e.g. glucose-6-phosphate dehydrogenase (**G6PD**)) result in decreased glutathione production. This makes the RBC more susceptible to oxidative stress and intermittent haemolysis. On the other hand, defects in the Embden–Meyerhof pathway (e.g. **pyruvate kinase**) affect ATP production and therefore cause premature RBC haemolysis.

Glucose-6-phosphate dehydrogenase (G6PD) deficiency

G6PD deficiency is an X-linked condition affecting the hexose monophosphate pathway of glucose metabolism, resulting in intolerance of oxidative stress and subsequently haemolysis. It affects about 10% of the population and, being an X-linked condition, it is considerably more common in men. Rarely, heterozygous females can be affected in the early stages of life. There are almost 400 variants of this condition.

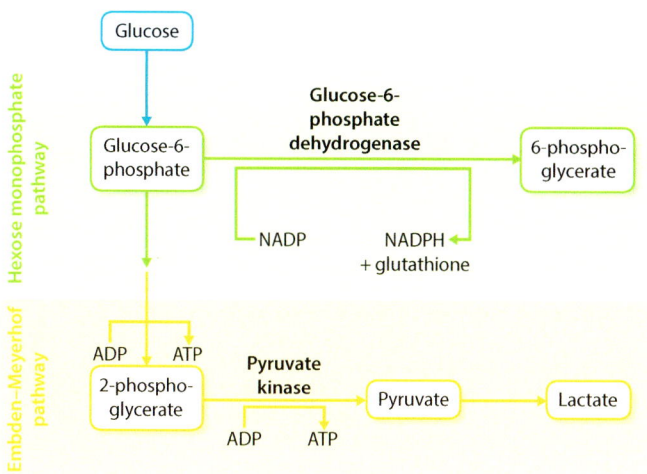

Fig. 6.14 *Glucose metabolism in RBC.*

E ≫ Haemolysis in G6PD deficiency is usually associated with a trigger, most commonly a drug or infective cause. Triggers include:
- Drugs – antimalarials, aspirin, antibiotics (sulphonamides, ciprofloxacin), quinidine, vitamin K
- Acute infection
- Exposure – fava or broad beans, mothballs (naphthalene)

W ≫ Fava beans are rich in vicine and divicine, which are reducing agents that reduce oxygen to hydrogen peroxide. This, in turn, increases oxidative stress.

Patients tend to present acutely with symptoms of haemolysis (jaundice and anaemia).

Investigations

Stepwise plan:

1 **Carry out a full blood count with a peripheral blood film**
- **Blister (or bite) cells** and **Heinz bodies** may be seen during an acute attack
- Elevated reticulocyte count as a result of haemolysis may also be present

2 **Obtain G6PD levels**
- These can be indirectly measured but caution should be exercised, as an acute episode may produce a false normal result

Management
Management of an acute haemolytic event primarily involves:
- Treating the underlying cause
- Stopping and avoiding any precipitating triggers

Acute transfusions may be necessary in life-threatening cases.

Pyruvate kinase deficiency

An RBC enzymopathy of autosomal recessive inheritance that affects the Embden–Meyerhof glycolytic pathway of glucose metabolism. It is much less common than G6PD deficiency. Reduced ATP production results in rigid red cells that become spiculated when passing through the spleen. **'Prickle' cells** are typically seen on blood film. Presentation is variable with anaemia and splenomegaly. Transfusions may be necessary and splenectomy is reserved for patients requiring frequent transfusions.

Acquired haemolytic anaemias
Autoimmune haemolytic anaemia (AIHA)

AIHAs are a group of disorders characterised by RBC destruction as a result of auto-antibodies. These are classically divided into **warm** and **cold** subtypes, depending on the optimum temperature at which the antibodies are most active. The differences between these subtypes are shown in *Table 6.8*. AIHAs are typically direct Coombs test-positive, which indicates the presence of auto-antibodies towards RBCs.

6

E ≫ The Coombs (antiglobulin) test is a qualitative test used to detect the presence of antibodies. The Coombs test consists of two different tests, namely direct (DAT) and indirect (IAT). Antihuman antibodies IgG (Coombs reagent, CR) are used to detect the presence of antibodies.

Table 6.7 Comparison between direct Coombs and indirect Coombs test

Test	Direct Coombs (DAT)	Indirect Coombs (IAT)
Indication	• Haemolytic anaemia • Transfusion reactions	• Prenatal rhesus testing • Cross-matching
Function	Detects antibodies **bonded to the RBC**	Detects antibodies in the **plasma**
Mechanism	Coombs reagent binds directly to auto-antibodies attached to RBC and causes agglutination	Plasma antibodies are first exposed to the donor's blood. Recipient antibodies will interact with the donor's RBC antigens in the event of incompatibility. CR is added, resulting in agglutination

Patients usually present with intermittent episodes of haemolysis (jaundice and anaemia) as well as splenomegaly. This is often an underlying trigger (i.e. infection, folate deficiency) or associated condition (e.g. SLE, lymphoproliferative disorder).

P ≫ Chronic cold agglutinin disease (CHAD) is a condition commonly associated with B-cell lymphoma causing *acrocyanosis*, a condition that is similar to the Raynaud phenomenon, in which intravascular haemolysis results in painful and blue extremities.

Investigations

Stepwise plan:

1 **Obtain FBC and peripheral blood film**
- **↓Hb, ↑reticulocyte, ↑MCV, ↑LDH**
- Spherocytosis is commonly seen as a result of RBC damage

2 **Direct Coombs test**
- Positive result

Management

- Principles involve treating the underlying cause and stopping any offending agents
- Corticosteroids are often used and are effective in inducing remission in warm AIHA; however, this treatment can take up to 3 weeks to take effect
- Splenectomy may be considered in patients who fail to respond to corticosteroids

Non-immune haemolytic anaemia

Acquired haemolytic anaemias not attributable to an immune cause may be due to mechanical trauma, infections (e.g. malaria, *Clostridium perfringens*) or acquired membrane defect (i.e. paroxysmal nocturnal haemoglobinuria).

Mechanical traumas causing intravascular haemolysis include:
- Mechanical heart valves – high velocity resulting in shear stress
- Microangiopathic haemolytic anaemia (MAHA) – caused by fibrin deposition in capillary beds. This is associated with:
  – Haemolytic uraemic syndrome (HUS)

Table 6.8 Comparison between warm AIHA and cold agglutinin disease

	Warm AIHA	Cold agglutinin disease
Temperature	Ideally 37°C	Best at 4°C
Epidemiology	Affects both sexes, all ages; most common in middle-aged females	Usually occurs in the elderly population
Antibody	IgG	IgM
Causes	• Primary idiopathic • Rheumatic conditions (e.g. SLE, RA) • Drugs (e.g. interferon, NSAIDs, penicillin, etc.) • Lymphoid malignancy	• Primary idiopathic • Infections (i.e. EBV, CMV, mycoplasma) • Lymphoid malignancy • Paroxysmal nocturnal haemoglobinuria (PNH)

– Thrombotic thrombocytopenia purpura (TTP)
– Disseminated intravascular coagulation (DIC)
- Burns causing thermal injury and fragmentation of RBC

Paroxysmal nocturnal haemoglobinuria (PNH)

PNH is a rare, acquired form of haemolytic anaemia, in which there is non-malignant clonal expression of haematopoietic stem cells with absent GPI-anchor proteins. These proteins act as attachment sites for complement defence proteins (e.g. CD55 and 59). Uncontrolled complement activation results in haemolysis and pro-thrombosis.

 ≫ PNH can present with:
- Intravascular haemolysis, resulting in haemoglobinuria
- Thrombosis – both arterial and venous
- Deficient haematopoiesis – ranging from mild anaemia to severe pancytopenia or aplastic anaemia

The recommended management for PNH is supportive care, such as intermittent blood transfusions and long-term anticoagulation. Eculizumab, an anticomplement C5 monoclonal antibody, has revolutionised PNH treatment.

6.2 Bleeding disorders

Approach to bleeding

Haemostasis is the body's complex mechanism that maintains the balance between bleeding and clotting. As described in earlier sections, this exact mechanism can be divided into three distinct processes, namely:
1. Vessel wall TF activation
2. Platelet plug formation
3. Activation of the coagulation cascade

Defects or disorders in any of these processes will result in abnormal clotting or coagulation. Congenital (inherited) causes will be present at birth and are usually associated with a strong family history of bleeding disorders; whereas acquired conditions tend to be related to an underlying disease or concurrent drug use. *Figure 6.15* illustrates the various aetiologies of bleeding disorders.

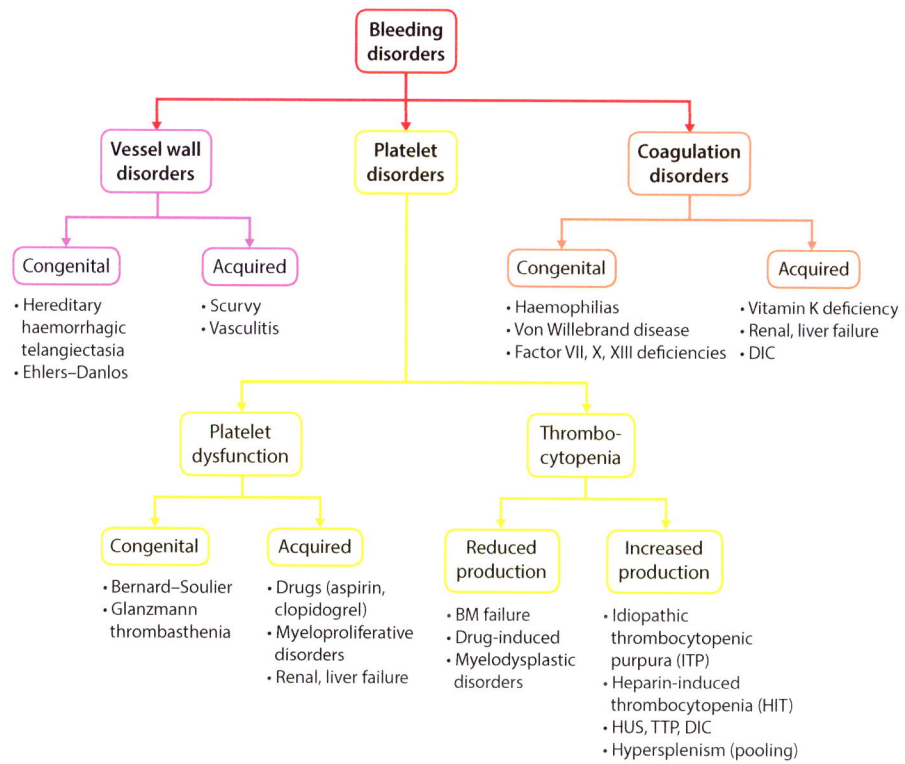

Fig. 6.15 *Bleeding disorders.*

It is important to distinguish vessel wall and platelet (clotting) disorders from a coagulation defect. This distinction can usually be elicited by the clinical presentation or laboratory findings (see *Table 6.9*).

Table 6.9 *Comparison between clotting and coagulation disorder*

	Clotting disorder	Coagulation disorder
Site	Bleeding within skin (bruising, purpura) or mucosal membranes (GI, uterine)	Bleeding tends to involve joints (haemarthroses) or muscles (haematoma)
Timing	Occurs spontaneously	Occurs within hours to days

Coagulation screen

Coagulation tests (see *Table 6.10*) are important in determining the cause of a bleeding disorder. They are also often used to monitor anticoagulation therapy.

Table 6.10 *Coagulation screen*

Test	Assessment	Clinical utility
Platelet count	Platelets	Thrombocytopenia
Bleeding time	Platelets	Platelet dysfunction, von Willebrand disease
Activated partial thromboplastin time (APTT)	Intrinsic pathway (factors II, V, VIII, IX, X and XI)	Monitor heparin therapy, haemophilia, DIC
Prothrombin time (PT), INR	Extrinsic pathway (factors II, V, VII, X)	Liver disease, monitor warfarin therapy, DIC
Fibrinogen levels	Final common pathway	Liver failure, DIC

6.2.1 Vessel wall disorders

Vascular abnormalities can be divided into congenital and acquired causes:
- Congenital – HHT and Ehlers–Danlos
- Acquired
  - Scurvy – vitamin C deficiency results in abnormal collagen formation, predisposing to bleeding and bruising
  - Vasculitis – Henoch–Schönlein purpura
  - Infection – meningococcal rash

Hereditary haemorrhagic telangiectasia (HHT)

HHT is a rare, autosomal dominant condition characterised by mutations in genes responsible for blood vessel development. These mutations give rise to abnormal expression of vascular TGF-ß receptors, resulting in:
- **Telangiectasia** – tortuous dilatation of end-capillaries, particularly in the fingers, toes, lungs, GI tract and nose (see *Fig. 6.16*)
- **Arteriovenous malformations** (AVM) – predisposing to right–left shunting, leading to hypoxaemia and paradoxical embolisms

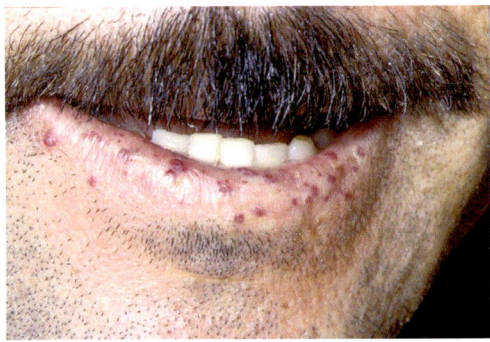

Fig. 6.16 *Telangiectasia of the lip, commonly seen in HHT.*

Patients typically present with recurrent epistaxis or GI bleeds, resulting in iron-deficiency anaemia. If suspected, patients should be screened for AVMs and these should be ablated if detected.

6.2.2 Platelet disorders

Bleeding can occur as a result of a reduced platelet count (thrombocytopenia) or platelet dysfunction (thrombocytopathy).

Platelet dysfunction

Disorders of platelet dysfunction can be either be acquired or congenital (see *Table 6.11*). Clinically, drug-induced thrombocytopathy is the most common cause.

Table 6.11 *Acquired and congenital causes of platelet dysfunction*

Acquired	Congenital
• Drugs – antiplatelet agents (e.g. aspirin, clopidogrel, glycoprotein IIb/IIIa inhibitors) • Renal and liver disease • Myeloproliferative disorders	• Glanzmann thrombasthenia • Bernard–Soulier syndrome • Storage pool disorder

>> Platelet dysfunction, secondary to renal disease, is multifactorial. Uraemia induces vascular synthesis of platelet-inhibitory prostaglandins and nitric oxide. This is in addition to intrinsic inhibition of thromboxane A2 production, resulting in uraemic thrombocytopathy.

P >> Glanzmann thrombasthenia and Bernard–Soulier syndrome are rare congenital abnormalities of platelet membrane glycoprotein deficiency. Deficient glycoprotein Ib (in Bernard–Soulier syndrome) results in failure of platelet adhesion, whereas absent glycoprotein IIb/IIIa complex (in Glanzmann's) results in ineffective fibrin activation and platelet aggregation.

Thrombocytopenia

Thrombocytopenia is defined as a reduced platelet count of $<150 \times 10^9$/L. However, severe spontaneous bleeding is unusual with counts above 20×10^9/L. The causes of thrombocytopenia can be broadly categorised into disorders affecting platelet production or platelet consumption.

- Reduced platelet production
  - Bone marrow failure
    - Aplastic anaemia
    - Megaloblastic anaemia
    - Infiltration secondary to malignancy
    - Cytotoxic drug and alcohol
  - Inherited thrombocytopathies
    - Bernard–Soulier syndrome
    - Alport syndrome
    - Wiskott–Aldrich syndrome
- Increased platelet consumption
  - Immune
    - Immune thrombocytopenic purpura (ITP)
    - Heparin-induced thrombocytopenia (HIT)
  - Non-immune
    - DIC, HUS, TTP
    - Sepsis
    - Drug-induced – penicillin, quinine, thiazides
  - Splenic pooling
    - Hypersplenism

Immune thrombocytopenic purpura (ITP)

Definition: ITP refers to an autoimmune condition characterised by a low platelet count, in the absence of other causes or associated underlying disorders.

Like most autoimmune conditions, ITP is more common in females.

 >> Auto-antibodies directed towards platelets results in premature platelet splenic clearance. Recent evidence has also suggested antibody-mediated suppression of megakaryocyte development in the bone marrow.

Clinical features:
- Presents more acutely, often triggered by an infection and has a self-limiting course in children
- Insidious onset and has a chronic course in adults
- There is often an associated autoimmune condition (e.g. SLE, CLL, CTDs, HIV)
- Mild bleeding (epistaxis, menorrhagia) and easy bruising

Investigations
- Initial investigations should include FBC and peripheral blood film to exclude other causes of thrombocytopenia
- In ITP, these results will essentially be normal – apart from a low platelet count
- Bone marrow biopsy is recommended in patients over the age of 60

Management
- Acute attacks should be treated with short courses of corticosteroids
- IV Ig may be considered as an adjunct in severe cases
- Second-line therapies include splenectomy, thrombopoietin mimetics, danazol and other immunosuppressive agents (e.g. rituximab, azathioprine, cyclosporin, etc.)

Heparin-induced thrombocytopenia (HIT)

HIT is an uncommon but dangerous complication of heparin therapy, typically occurring 5–10 days after commencement. It is a severe pro-thrombotic disorder with paradoxical thrombocytopenia. Antibodies towards platelet factor 4 (pf4) and heparin complexes on platelet surfaces result in platelet activation and a subsequent coagulation cascade. The 4T score can indicate the likelihood of HIT in a patient with thrombocytopenia. Anti-pf4 ELISA may be used in cases with moderate to high clinical likelihood to aid the diagnosis. Heparin should be stopped immediately, and alternative anticoagulation should be started.

6

E ≫ HIT is far more common with unfractionated heparin (UFH), compared to low molecular weight heparin (LMWH). This is due to the formation of ultra-large complexes (ULCs) with the relatively larger-sized UFH molecules. Thus, the difference in developing HIT can be attributed to the effective molecular weight.

6.2.3 Congenital coagulation (bleeding) disorders

Haemophilia A

Definition: an X-linked recessive coagulation disorder characterised by a deficiency in clotting factor VIII.

E ≫ Haemophilia is almost exclusively a male disorder. Rarely, females with abnormal lyonisation, Turner syndrome and mosaicism may be affected.

Epidemiology:
- Affects 1 in 5000 of the male population

Pathophysiology:
- Mutations of the factor VIII gene on chromosome X result in reduced expression and circulating volume of factor VIII
- Factor VIII is crucial in the formation of thrombin via the intrinsic pathway
- Reduced levels of factor VIII result in abnormal coagulation and this prolongs activated partial thromboplastin time (aPTT)

Clinical features:
The severity and presentation depend heavily on the residual level of factor VIII. Haemophilia can be categorised as shown in *Table 6.12*.

Table 6.12 *Classification of severity of haemophilia A*

Severity	Levels (%)	Presentation
Mild	>5	Only bleed after major trauma or surgery
Moderate	1–5	Occasional spontaneous bleeding or after minor surgery
Severe	<1	Severe spontaneous bleeding, most commonly into joints and haematomas

P ≫ Psoas and calf haematomas can be complicated by femoral nerve complication and compartment syndrome, respectively. Recurrent haemarthroses lead to cartilage destruction and joint deformities.

Investigations
Coagulation screen should be performed in all patients. This will reveal:
- Normal PT, bleeding time and VWF levels
- Prolonged APTT
- Significantly ↓ factor VIII

Management
Treatment strategy depends on the severity of the bleed.

Stepwise management of haemophilia A

1 **For acute major bleeds, offer IV plasma-derived or recombinant factor VIII**
- Complications include development of factor VIII inhibitor

2 **For minor bleeds and in patients with residual levels >0.1, consider IV or intra-nasal desmopressin (DDAVP)**

W ≫ DDAVP has an indirect effect on factor VIII, as factor VIII is stored with VWF as complexes in vascular endothelial cells. Stimulation of the release of VWF by DDAVP will also increase the levels of factor VIII.

3 **Offer lifestyle advice**
- Avoid contact sports, NSAIDs and IM injections

Haemophilia B (Christmas disease)
Haemophilia B, much like haemophilia A, is an X-linked recessive bleeding disorder which causes a deficiency in factor IX. It is less common than its counterpart, but they have almost identical presentations. Treatment of haemophilia B is with plasma-derived or recombinant factor IX. Desmopressin has no effect on the release of factor IX and is therefore ineffective.

Von Willebrand disease
Von Willebrand disease (VWD) is a relatively common inherited coagulation disorder caused by defective or deficient VWF. VWF binds factor VIII in circulation, and unbound factor VIII degrades rapidly. Mutations of the VWF gene on chromosome 12 are responsible for the development of this condition. There are

many variants of this condition. However, VWD can be broadly divided into the three types shown in *Table 6.13*.

Table 6.13 *Von Willebrand disease subtypes*

Type	Inheritance	Abnormalities
1	A. dominant	Partial quantitative deficiency
2	A. dominant	Defective protein structure (qualitative)
3	A. recessive	Severe quantitative deficiency (almost absent)

Presentation can be variable and type-dependent. In general,

- Types 1 and 2 have milder symptoms and tend to exhibit symptoms that are more consistent with a clotting defect (e.g. epistaxis, menorrhagia or bleeding post-surgery)
- Type 3 patients may experience more severe and spontaneous bleeding but haemarthroses are uncommon

> **E** ≫ Patients with VWD have coagulation test findings that are consistent with a mixed defect, with **both prolonged bleeding time and APTT**. This is because abnormal VWF delays platelet activation and the coagulation cascade is also affected, due to reduced factor VIII levels.

DDAVP is used to promote the release of VWF in mild and moderate cases. Intermediate purity factor VIII concentrate (plasma-derived, containing intact VWF) may be used in more severe cases.

6.2.4 Acquired coagulation (bleeding) disorders

Vitamin K deficiency

Vitamin K is an essential co-factor in the coagulation cascade, imperative for the carboxylation of glutamic acid of factors II, VII, IX and X. This primes the coagulation factors for calcium binding and subsequent activation.

Vitamin K deficiency can be caused by:

- Drugs – excess anticoagulation (e.g. coumarins, warfarin)
- Malnutrition – poor dietary intake (↓ green leafy vegetables intake, alcoholism)
- Malabsorption – CD, IBD, cholestatic disease, tropical sprue

Both APTT and PT will be prolonged as both the intrinsic and extrinsic pathways are involved. Replacement with IV vitamin K (5–10mg) is the mainstay of treatment. For warfarin reversal management, see *Appendix 3*.

Liver disease

As discussed in *Chapter 3*, the liver is responsible for the synthesis of important coagulation factors, namely factors V, VII, VIII, IX, X, XI, prothrombin and fibrinogen. In patients with liver disease (e.g. cirrhosis), the production of these factors is significantly impaired, resulting in abnormal coagulation.

Thrombocytopenia, secondary to hypersplenism and consumptive DIC in acute liver failure, is also a potential mechanism of hepatic coagulopathy.

6

6.3 Thrombophilia

Thrombophilia refers primarily to both inherited and acquired conditions or hypercoagulable states, predisposing to clot formation (thrombosis). Thrombus formation is a complex process and has been extensively described in the *Bridge to Medicine* section. Thrombosis can develop in an artery or a vein.

Arterial thrombi are usually a result of localised atherosclerosis, commonly occurring at sites of turbulent flow (e.g. coronary arteries and carotid bifurcation). Venous thrombi, on the other hand, often arise due to the presence of one or more risk factors seen in the Virchow triad.

> **E** ≫ The Virchow triad broadly describes the three main risk factors for thrombosis:
> - **Hypercoagulability** – alteration of blood components (e.g. increased levels of clotting factors)
> - **Vessel wall injury** – trauma (shear stress) to the endothelium
> - **Changes to blood flow** – both turbulent and static flow predisposes to clot formation

6.3.1 Inherited thrombophilia

Factor V Leiden (FVL)

A hypercoagulable state caused by a single-base mutation, resulting in abnormal factor V expression. The result is a defective factor V protein with increased resistance to breakdown by activated protein C. FVL affects 3–5% of the healthy Caucasian population and is very rare in the Far East. The risk of thrombosis is significantly elevated by the concurrent use of COCP.

Antithrombin (AT) deficiency

AT deficiency is commonly inherited in an autosomal dominant fashion. AT is a protease inhibitor, responsible for inactivating various activated clotting factors. For this reason, it is the site of target of heparin therapy – potentiating its activity. Hence, decreased levels of AT will result in unregulated coagulation, predisposing to thrombosis. Recurrent clots are common in childhood and VTE risk is significantly raised during pregnancy.

Protein C and S deficiency

Similar to AT deficiency, both these deficiencies have an autosomal dominant inheritance. Both function to inactivate factors Va and VIIa. Risk of thrombosis is increased five-fold and homozygous forms of this condition present with life-threatening neonatal purpura fulminans.

6.3.2 Acquired coagulation (thrombotic) disorders

Antiphospholipid syndrome (APS)

APS is an autoimmune clinicopathological condition characterised by recurrent thrombosis, obstetric complications and the presence of antiphospholipid antibodies (APAbs). The underlying mechanism is unclear. However, auto-antibody activation of complement, platelets and coagulation factors has been observed in animal models.

> **E** >> APS is associated with other autoimmune conditions, particularly HLA DR7 and DR4-related conditions. This includes SLE (APAbs present in up to 30% of patients), RA, sero-negative arthropathies, vasculitides, etc.

Diagnostic criteria

The diagnosis of APS is based on clinical and biochemical findings. According to the International Consensus Statement, a patient with APS must fulfil a least one clinical and one laboratory criterion.

- Clinical criteria
  - >1 episode of vascular thrombosis
  - Obstetric morbidity – >3 spontaneous miscarriages (<10 weeks) or >1 unexplained foetal death (>10 weeks)
- Laboratory criteria – presence of any of the following auto-antibodies on ≥2 separate occasions, >12 weeks apart:
  - Lupus anticoagulant
  - Anticardiolipin antibodies
  - Anti-b2 glycoprotein I antibodies

> **P** >> Other systemic presentations include livedo reticularis (caused by capillary thrombosis), valvular heart disease and thrombocytopenia.

Patients with a confirmed diagnosis of APS should be started on lifelong anticoagulation therapy; warfarin is the agent of choice. Aspirin and low molecular weight heparin may be used during pregnancy.

Thrombotic thrombocytopenia purpura (TTP)

TTP is a rare, but serious autoimmune condition characterised by severe thrombosis and paradoxical consumptive thrombocytopenia.

> **W** >> Auto-antibodies directed towards the ADAMTS-13 enzyme are responsible for this condition. In normal circumstances, this enzyme functions to cleave large VWF multimers to smaller functional units. However, in TTP, VWF remains in its larger form, causing microvascular occlusion.

> **E** >> TTP is associated with a clinical pentad. However, only a few patients present with all five of the following symptoms:
> - Thrombocytopenia
> - MAHA
> - Neurological symptoms
> - Fever
> - Acute kidney injury

Plasmapheresis should be initiated as soon as the diagnosis is made. Corticosteroid therapy (with or without rituximab) is used to treat the underlying autoimmune process.

Disseminated intravascular coagulation (DIC)

DIC is a severe, life-threatening acquired coagulopathy, usually occurring in the context of an underlying acute illness. These conditions include:

- Severe septicaemia – meningococcal, *E. coli* O157 infections
- Paraneoplastic – haematological malignancies and solid tumours
- Severe trauma and burns
- Obstetric complications – HELLP syndrome, placental abruption

Underlying causes of DIC should be managed promptly, and correction of coagulopathy is only indicated in the context of active bleeding. Antifibrinolytic agents may cause further micro-deposition of fibrin and should be avoided in DIC.

W ≫ In DIC, there is systemic activation of both the clotting and coagulation pathway, usually as a result of cytokine-mediated processes and monocyte-induced TF expression. Consequently, there is significant platelet and coagulation factor consumption as well as subsequent production of FDPs.

E ≫ Patients with DIC present with paradoxical symptoms of both bleeding and thrombosis. Consumptive thrombocytopenia causes severe haemorrhage, whereas thrombotic symptoms are caused by platelet and fibrin aggregation. Therefore, coagulation testing often reveals global haemostasis failure, indicated by prolonged bleeding time, PT and APTT.

6

6.4 Haematological malignancies

Malignant disorders of the haematological system may affect the blood, bone marrow or the lymphatic system. These include leukaemias, lymphomas and plasma cell dyscrasia.

6.4.1 Leukaemias

Leukaemias are malignancies of haematopoietic stem cells, characterised by the abnormal proliferation of leucocytes and their precursors in the bone marrow and peripheral blood. They can be classified according to their germ line type (i.e. myeloid or lymphoid) or the extent of cell differentiation (i.e. acute or chronic). They can be divided into:

- Acute myeloid leukaemia (AML)
- Acute lymphoblastic leukaemia (ALL)
- Chronic myeloid leukaemia (CML)
- Chronic lymphocytic leukaemia (CLL)

P ≫ It is a common misconception that the words 'acute' or 'chronic' refer to the duration of the disease in the leukaemia subtype. However, these descriptions in fact refer to the maturity of the cells. In acute leukaemias, there is abnormal proliferation of undifferentiated and immature blast cells (>20% of peripheral and bone marrow cells). In contrast, in chronic leukaemias, malignant cells are able to differentiate and partly mature.

The exact aetiology of leukaemia is unknown in most patients. However, it is thought that interactions between several genetic and environmental risk factors underpin the pathogenesis of many of these subtypes (see *Table 6.14*).

Table 6.14 *Risk factors associated with leukaemia*

Genetics	• High concordance in identical twins • Chromosomal abnormalities (Philadelphia (Ph)) • Associated with trisomy 21, Fanconi anaemia and Li–Fraumeni syndrome
Viruses	• Human T-cell lymphotropic type 1 retrovirus
Radiation exposure	• Increased incidence of leukaemia seen after the atomic bomb explosions in Hiroshima and Nagasaki • Radiotherapy for spinal cancer or X-ray exposure during pregnancy
Drugs and toxins	• Benzene exposure (smoking) • Alkylating agents (e.g. melphalan)

Acute myeloid leukaemia

Definition: a malignant disorder of the bone marrow that involves abnormal clonal proliferation of cells of the myeloid lineage.

Epidemiology:
- Prevalence of 6 per 100,000 of the population
- Median age of onset of 65
- Equal age distribution in the younger population but men are more frequently affected after the age of 60 (3:2 ratio)

Classification
The FAB (French–American–British) classification of AML is now outdated and the newer WHO classification (revised 2008) is regarded to be more clinically relevant, providing better prognostic information. The WHO classification subdivides AML on the basis of its potential aetiology.
- AML with recurrent genetic abnormalities
  - Cytogenetic abnormalities involving t(8;21), inv(16) and t(15;17) are associated with the best prognosis

> **P** ≫ The chromosomal translocation t(15;17) is the characteristic feature of a subtype of AML known as acute promyelocytic leukaemia (APML). The translocation down-regulates the expression of the RAR-alpha (PML-RARA) gene, resulting in abnormal proliferation of immature granulocytes known as promyelocytes.

> **W** ≫ DIC is a life-threatening and common complication of APML, with up to 85% of patients eventually developing it. This is a result of increased tissue factor (TF) production by the promyelocytes, a key component in the initiation of the coagulation cascade.

- AML with myelodysplastic-related changes
  - Patients with a pre-existing myelodysplastic or myeloproliferative disease (e.g. CML, myelofibrosis) that have undergone acute malignant transformation
- Therapy-related AML – associated with previous chemotherapy
- AML not otherwise specified

Clinical features:
- As there is immature myeloid proliferation, the presentation of AML is reflective of bone marrow failure:
  - Anaemia – usually presenting as fatigue and breathlessness
  - Neutropenia – recurrent infections
  - Thrombocytopenia – bleeding, bruising, petechiae

> **E** ≫ The total WCC is significantly elevated, but this represents the overproduction of non-functional, immature blast cells.

- End-organ infiltration – common sites include:
  - Liver and spleen – hepatosplenomegaly
  - Gums – gingivitis and bleeding
  - Skin – leukaemia cutis is an uncommon sign

Investigations

Stepwise plan:

1 **Arrange blood test and film**
- ↓Hb, ↑WCC, ↓plts
- Blast cells and Auer rods may be seen on peripheral blood smear

2 **Arrange BM aspirate**
- >20% blast cells and Auer rods are diagnostic (see *Fig. 6.17*)

3 **Carry out cytogenetic analysis**
- This is performed to guide treatment

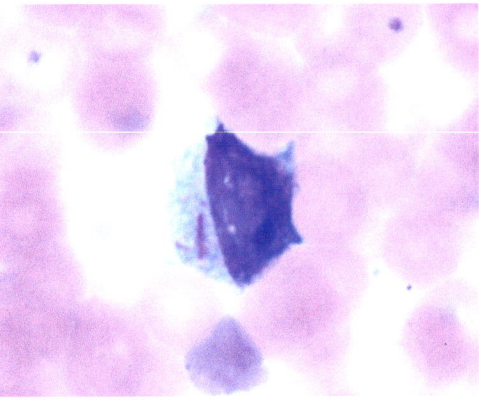

Fig. 6.17 *Auer rods (purple) seen in the cytoplasm of the blast cell.*

Management
The treatment of AML involves supportive therapy, chemotherapy and bone marrow transplantation.

Stepwise management of acute myeloid leukaemia

1 **Arrange supportive therapy**
- **Transfusion** – RCC and platelets may be required
- **Prophylactic antibiotics, antivirals** and **antifungals** may be indicated
- Treatment of neutropenic sepsis (see *Chapter 12*) should be commenced promptly

- Adequate **hydration** and **allopurinol** or **rasburicase** should be commenced to control hyperuricaemia (usually secondary to tumour lysis syndrome)

> **E** >> Tumour lysis syndrome refers to a group of metabolic disturbances which commonly occur as a result of chemotherapy. The death (lysis) of abnormal cells releases high cellular material into the bloodstream. This usually results in hyperuricaemia, hyperkalaemia, hyperphosphataemia and hypocalcaemia, followed by acute renal failure.

- **Leucopheresis** may be considered, prior to chemotherapy, to reduce the number of circulating white cells
- This may prevent sequelae of hyperviscosity and improve outcomes

2 Provide chemotherapy
- Three distinct stages exist in the treatment of acute leukaemias:
  - Remission induction
  - Remission consolidation
  - Maintenance therapy
- Treatment regimes are tailored to the patient's AML subtype and should be performed at specialist centres
- Cytarabine, an antimetabolic agent that interferes with DNA synthesis is commonly used in AML
- Intra-thecal therapy may be required in CNS disease or high-risk subgroups
- All-trans retinoic acid (ATRA; e.g. tretinoin) in combination with other agents may be used in patients with APML
- Palliative chemotherapy may be considered in advanced cases

> **W** >> ATRAs are especially effective in APML because of their agonistic properties on RAR-alpha receptors, restoring the differentiation of promyelocytes (usually arrested in APML). A common complication of this is differentiation syndrome, which patients should be monitored for. Effectively, this makes APML one of the most curable subtypes of AML.

3 Consider stem cell transplantation (SCT)
- Allogeneic SCT may be considered in high-risk patients, and those who have relapsed or fail to response to initial chemotherapy

Acute lymphoblastic leukaemia (ALL)

Definition: a malignant disorder of the bone marrow that involves abnormal clonal proliferation of cells of the lymphoid lineage. ALL developing from precursor B cell lineage (80%) is more common than the T-cell lineage.

Epidemiology:
- Annual incidence of 3 per 100,000
- Mainly affects children with a peak age of 2–4 years
- 75% of cases occur in patients under 6 years

Risk factors:
- Strong association between trisomy 21 and ALL (10–20x risk)
- Multiple recurring cytogenetic abnormalities (most often chromosomal translocations) have been identified, e.g. the BCR-ABL fusion gene as a result of the Philadelphia chromosome t(9:22) (more common in adults; see *CML section* below)
- Environmental – radiation, organophosphate exposure

Clinical features:
- Generalised fatigue and malaise are common first symptoms
- BM failure symptoms – anaemia, recurrent infections, bleeding
- Infiltrative signs and symptoms
  - Thymic mass (more common in T-cell ALL)
  - Lymphadenopathy, splenomegaly (with or without LUQ pain)
  - Purpura and gingival hypertrophy
  - Testicular enlargement
  - Meningeal (CNS) involvement – headache, neck stiffness, cranial nerve palsies

> **W** >> CNS involvement is more common in ALL, compared to AML, as lymphocytes pass more readily through the blood–brain barrier. T-cell phenotyping and elevated lymphoblasts in the CSF are risk factors for developing CNS recurrence (50–70% in the absence of prophylaxis) 1 year post-remission. Note that <10% of patients have CNS involvement at the time of diagnosis.

Investigations

> **Stepwise plan:**

1 Obtain FBC, peripheral blood film and BM aspirate
- ↑WCC, ↓Hb, ↓platelets
- >20% lymphoblasts seen on blood film or BM aspirate is diagnostic of ALL

6

  2 Arrange immunophenotyping and cytogenetics analysis of BM aspirate

  3 Carry out other tests
- CXR may be useful in identifying mediastinal masses
- LP for CSF cytology and flow cytometry to assess for CNS involvement

Management
As with AML, the management of ALL involves supportive therapy, chemotherapy and bone marrow transplantation.

> **Stepwise management of acute lymphoblastic leukaemia**

  1 Arrange supportive therapy

  2 Provide chemotherapy
- The three phases of chemotherapy approach is also utilised in ALL
- However, the chemotherapy agents used in ALL vary from those used in AML

  3 Consider bone marrow transplantation

E ≫ Prophylactic intra-thecal therapy is often given to reduce the rate of CNS recurrence.

Chronic myeloid leukaemia (CML)

Definition: CML is a myeloproliferative disorder of the bone marrow haematopoietic stem cells, resulting in clonal expansion of the myeloid lineage.

Epidemiology:
- Accounts for about 15% of all leukaemias
- Almost exclusively a condition of the elderly population, with a median diagnosis age of 55 years
- Annual incidence of 1 per 100,000

Pathophysiology:
- Radiating exposure is the main risk factor identified
- This fusion gene encodes a BCR-ABL protein which amplifies tyrosine kinase activity and thus increases cell proliferation and differentiation
- CML usually develops and progresses in three distinct phases (see *Fig. 6.18*)
- Most cases (80–90%) are diagnosed in the chronic phase.

E ≫ CML is characterised by the presence of the Philadelphia chromosomal (Ph) abnormality, the result of reciprocal translocations of the ABL gene on chr9 with the BCR gene on chr22 (see *Fig. 6.19*).

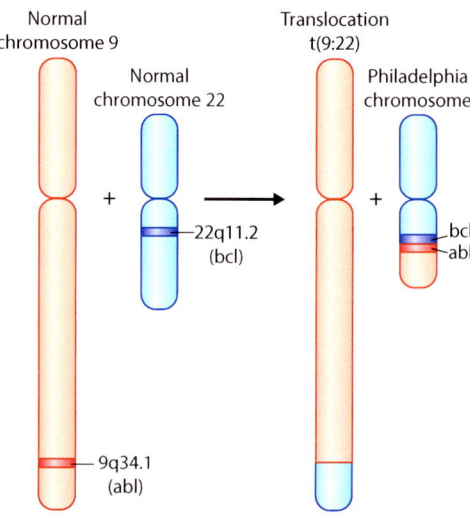

Fig. 6.19 *Philadelphia chromosomal abnormality.*

Clinical features:
- Presentation is insidious, with generalised and vague symptoms of fatigue, malaise, night sweats and weight loss
- Significant hepatosplenomegaly may occasionally cause unspecific abdominal discomfort

Investigations
Like most other leukaemias, investigations of CML include

> **Stepwise plan:**

  1 Arrange FBC, peripheral blood film and BM aspirate/biopsy
- ↑WCC and ↑↑platelets (may be present in up to 30% of patients)
- Elevated neutrophil count and its precursors are seen on blood film and BM aspirate
- Increased myeloblasts is indicative of the accelerated (10–19%) or blastic (>20%) phase.

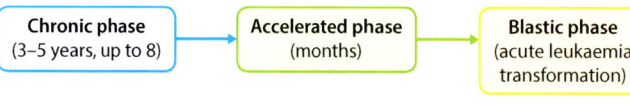

Fig. 6.18 *Phases of CML.*

2 **Cytogenetic analysis – should reveal t(9:22) Ph chromosome**

Management

The treatment of CML has been revolutionised since the advent of tyrosine kinase inhibitors (e.g. imatinib, nilotinib).

Chronic lymphocytic leukaemia (CLL)

Definition: a malignant disorder of the bone marrow, causing clonal expansion of B-cell lymphocytes.

Epidemiology:

- Most common leukaemia in the West, accounting for 30% of all cases
- Annual incidence of 4 per 100,000
- Male preponderance of 2:1 and has a median age of onset of 70

Clinical features:

- CLL often develops insidiously, with 90% of patients being asymptomatic on presentation
- Diagnosis is usually made incidentally on routine blood tests but symptoms may arise during the later stages of disease
- 'B' symptoms include fatigue, fever, night sweats and weight loss
- Infiltration – hepatosplenomegaly (sometimes massive), lymphadenopathy (often symmetrical and painless)
- Anaemia – due to BM infiltration or AIHA

> **W** >> AIHA and ITP are common complications of CLL. When these conditions occur simultaneously, due to autoimmune mechanisms, they are collectively known as Evans syndrome.

Staging

The Binet classification is most commonly used in Europe, whereas the Rai classification is used in the USA. These classification systems aim to guide treatment and provide disease prognostic indicators. *Table 6.15* shows the Binet staging.

Investigations

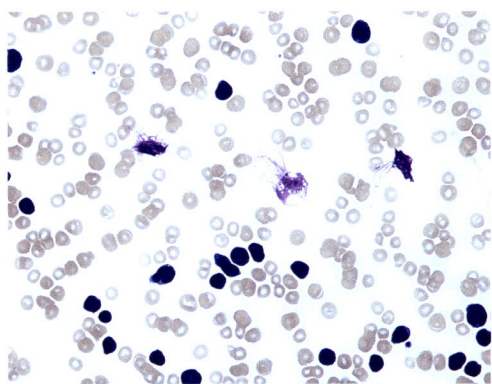

Fig. 6.20 *Smudge cell.*

> **Stepwise plan:**

1 **Arrange FBC, peripheral blood film**
- ↑WCC (lymphocytosis) ± ↓Hb, ↓platelets

2 **Smudge/smear cells may be seen on blood film (see *Fig. 6.20*)**
- These are caused by smearing of abnormally fragile lymphocytes during preparation

3 **Lymph node biopsy and immunophenotyping are required**

> **E** >> Unlike other leukaemias, BM aspirate/biopsy is not always necessary in CLL. Nevertheless, it may occasionally be useful in establishing a diagnosis.

Management

The treatment of CLL depends on the stage of disease. In general, no treatment is necessary for stage A CLL. Patients with stage B and C should be offered supportive care, chemotherapy or BMT as appropriate.

> **P** >> The Richter transformation, the lymphomatous conversion of CLL to large B-cell lymphoma, may occur in 5–10% of all cases.

Table 6.15 *Binet classification of CLL*

Stage	Lymphadenopathy	Anaemia	Low platelets	Survival (years)
A	<3	No	No	>10
B	>3	No	No	~7
C	Any	Yes	Yes	~5

6.4.2 Lymphomas

Lymphomas are malignancies of the lymphoid tissue, most commonly occurring in the lymph nodes. They usually originate from the B-cell lineage. Lymphomas are divided based on the histopathological findings and they can be primarily categorised into either:

- Hodgkin lymphoma (HL)
- Non-Hodgkin lymphoma (NHL), which accounts for 90% of all lymphomas
  - B-cell lymphomas
    - High grade (70%)
      - Diffuse large B-cell lymphoma (30–50%)
      - Mantle-cell lymphoma
      - Burkitt lymphoma
    - Low grade (30%)
      - Follicular lymphoma (FL, 20–25%)
      - MALT-omas
  - T-cell lymphomas

Hodgkin lymphoma (HL)

Definition: a malignant disorder of the lymphatic system, characterised histologically by the presence of Reed–Sternberg cells.

Epidemiology:

- Annual incidence of 2 per 100,000
- Bimodal distribution – first peak at age 25 and a further peak at 60

> **E** ≫ Infective mononucleosis (EBV infection) and immunosuppression are strong risk factors for HL. Elevated EBV titres seen in up to 40% of patients. It has been hypothesised that viral proteins trigger abnormal B cells to undergo uncontrolled proliferation and evade apoptosis.

Classification

Classical HL can be further categorised into four subtypes, based on distinct histological appearance:

- Nodular sclerosing (70%)
- Mixed cellularity (20%)
- Lymphocyte-rich (<5%)
- Lymphocyte-depleted (<1%)

> **P** ≫ Nodular lymphocyte-predominant HL (NLPHL) is an HL variant, distinguished by the presence of 'popcorn cells'. It represents 5% of all HL cases.

Clinical features:

- Painless, asymmetrical lymphadenopathy (commonly cervical) is often the first presenting complaint
- Chest symptoms (discomfort, SOB) may be present, secondary to mediastinal lymphadenopathy in younger patients
- Constitutional 'B' symptoms – fever, night sweats and weight loss

Investigations

All patients with suspected lymphoma should be investigated as follows.

> **Stepwise plan:**

1. **Obtain baseline bloods and peripheral blood film**
   - FBC may be normal or reveal mild lymphopenia
   - ↑ESR and LDH are poor prognostic markers
   - Baseline LFTs and U&Es are required prior to treatment
   - Blood film may reveal Reed–Sternberg cells (see *Fig. 6.21*)

2. **Obtain radiological imaging**
   - Pan-CT (neck, C/A/P) ± PET scan is useful in detecting lymphadenopathy and aids staging of disease (see *Fig. 6.22*)

3. **Arrange lymph node biopsy**
   - Performed either surgically or under radiological guidance

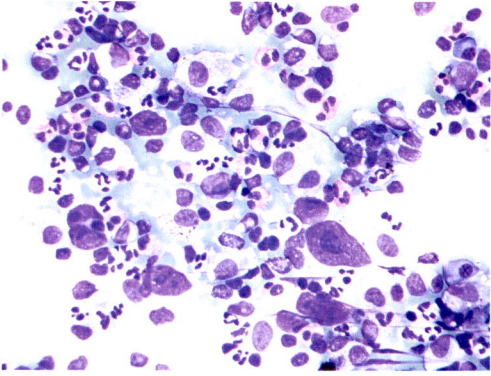

Fig. 6.21 *Reed–Sternberg cells with their characteristic nucleosis.*

Staging

HL has been traditionally staged using the Ann Arbor classification. However, Cotswold modification of the conventional system is now more common and is widely used in clinical practice (see *Table 6.16*).

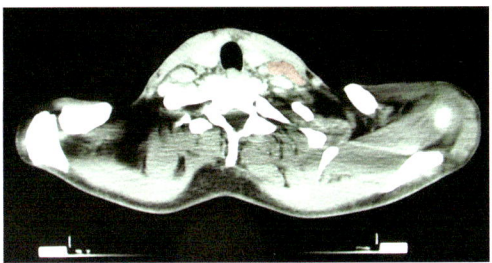

Fig. 6.22 *CT neck showing an enlarged lymph node on the left side of the neck (red area).*

Table 6.16 *Ann Arbor with Cotswold modification Hodgkin lymphoma staging system*

Stage	Description (lymphatic involvement)
I	Single-LN region or lymphoid structure (e.g. spleen, thymus)
II	>2 LN regions on the same side of the diaphragm
III	Involves LN regions on both sides of the diaphragm
IV	Extra-lymphatic metastasis (e.g. BM, liver)

The following suffixes may be added to denote the presence of other features: A (no B symptoms), B (B symptoms present), X (bulky disease, LN >10cm) or E (extra-lymphatic involvement).

Management

Chemotherapy and radiotherapy are the mainstay treatment modalities used in patients with HL. Treatment choice is stage-dependent. Follow-up PET scanning is used to evaluate disease response.

Stepwise management of Hodgkin lymphoma

1 In early disease (stages I and II)
- Radiotherapy monotherapy was used historically; however, the advent of chemotherapy has significantly limited the need for irradiation and may be avoided entirely in selected cases
- Chemo-radiotherapy is now the therapy of choice, and is curative in up to 90% of patients.

2 In advanced disease (stages III and IV, or I and II with unfavourable features)
- Combination chemotherapy with the **ABVD regime** (doxorubicin, bleomycin, vincristine and dacarbazine) is one of the most commonly used treatments
- A curative effect can be achieved in 50–60% of patients

E ≫ The main side effects of the ABVD regime are myelosuppression, mucositis, cardiac and pulmonary toxicity.

Non-Hodgkin lymphoma (NHL)

Definition: NHL primarily refers to a heterogeneous group of lymphoproliferative malignancies. There are over 60 variants of this condition, but they can be broadly divided into B-cell NHL or T-cell NHL as per the WHO classification.

Epidemiology:
- Sixth most common cancer in the UK
- Annual incidence of 5–10 per 100,000
- Male preponderance
- Peak incidence at the age of 65–75

Aetiology/risk factors:
NHL is associated with a number of conditions and infections such as the ones listed below.
- Familial – Wiskott–Aldrich syndrome, ataxia telangiectasia
- Viral infections
  - EBV – Burkitt lymphoma, T-cell lymphoma
  - HSV-8 – AIDS-related lymphoma
  - Human T-cell lymphocytic virus 1 – T-cell lymphoma
  - *Helicobacter pylori* – gastric MALToma
- Autoimmune diseases – SLE, coeliac disease, RA
- Immunosuppression – drugs, HIV, post-transplantation

P ≫ Burkitt lymphoma (BL) is an aggressive, rapid-growing, high-grade B-cell NHL. It is more common in children. BL has a very strong association with EBV, chronic malaria and AIDS. As it is a fast-growing lymphoma, it is very chemotherapy-sensitive, with survival rates of >90% in low-risk patients.

Clinical features:
- The clinical presentation of NHL is dependent on its grade and subtype (see *Table 6.17*)
- The most common initial finding is painless lymphadenopathy, but unlike HL, these lymphomas tend to be disseminated across multiple sites
- Symptoms vary and are classically related to the site of extra-nodal involvement
- Hepatosplenomegaly is also a relatively common finding

6

Table 6.17 *Comparison of clinical features in high-grade and low-grade NHL*

	High-grade NHL	Low-grade NHL
Onset	Rapid-growing, bulky tumours	Slow-growing and insidious
B symptoms	Common	Uncommon
Extra-nodal involvement	Common, affecting GI, GU, CNS, thyroid	Uncommon, unless in advanced disease
BM infiltration	Uncommon	Common

Investigations

These are similar to those carried out for HL.

> **Stepwise plan (NICE 2016, NG52):**

1 Obtain baseline bloods and peripheral blood film
- FBC may reveal cytopenias (BM involvement), ↑LDH (associated with poor prognosis)
- Blood film typically shows normal lymphocytes

2 Arrange LN biopsy, which is regarded as the gold standard diagnostic procedure
- Can be done either surgically or percutaneously under radiological guidance
- Immunocytochemistry and FISH analysis should be performed to allow accurate disease subclassification

3 Carry out PET-CT staging
- This allows appropriate staging of the disease
- The Ann Arbor classification is used to stage NHL

4 Carry out bone marrow aspirate/biopsy
- To assess for BM involvement if the diagnosis is confirmed

Management

> **Stepwise management of non-Hodgkin lymphoma (NICE 2016, NG52):**

1 In low-grade NHL (e.g. follicular lymphoma)
- Watchful waiting in asymptomatic patients
- Localised disease can be treated with radiotherapy with curative intent
- Chemotherapy regimens (e.g. CVP, CHOP, MCP) in combination with rituximab (for B-cell lymphoma) are recommended as options in symptomatic patients with stages III and IV disease

- Maintenance rituximab monotherapy may be used in patients with advanced disease (stages III and IV), who have relapsed
- Autologous BMT may be considered in cases of transformational disease (low-grade → high-grade lymphoma)

2 In high-grade NHL (e.g. DLCBL)
- Chemotherapy regime – commonly CHOP (cyclophosphamide, doxorubicin, vincristine and prednisolone), in combination with rituximab (for B-cell lymphoma), are first-line agents
- CNS prophylaxis with intrathecal chemotherapy should be offered to patients with testis, breast, adrenal or renal involvement
- Salvage therapy – combination high-dose chemotherapy regimens and allogeneic/autologous BMT may be considered in patients with refractory disease

> **W** ➤ Rituximab is a monoclonal antibody, targeting the CD20 protein found on B-cell membranes. It increases the elimination of B cells, promoting the development of healthy B-cell colonies. This makes it particularly effective in lymphoproliferative disorders, involving the B-cell lineage.

Waldenström macroglobulinaemia (WG)

WG, also sometimes known as lympho-plasmacytoid lymphoma, refers to a rare, **IgM** paraprotein-related haematological malignancy. It is primarily a disease of the elderly, with a median age of onset of 70 years. Patients usually present with hyperviscosity symptoms (i.e. headache, epistaxis), lymphadenopathy and occasionally splenomegaly.

Acute hyperviscosity episodes should be treated with plasmapheresis. Chemotherapy and rituximab have been shown to be effective in inducing remission in up to 50% of patients and may be used if clinically appropriate.

Cryoglobulinaemia

Cryoglobulinaemia is a condition in which cryoglobulins, immune complexes that precipitate below resting body temperature (<37°C), are present in the plasma. In simple cryoglobulinaemia (type 1), monoclonal IgM are produced by malignant B cells.

E ≫ Cryoglobulinaemia is associated with the classic Meltzer triad of symptoms:
- Purpura (due to end-capillary haemorrhage)
- Weakness
- Arthralgia

P ≫ Strictly speaking, type 2 and 3 (mixed) cryoglobulinaemia are not paraproteinaemias, as they tend to be polyclonal, most commonly forming complexes with rheumatoid factor (RF) in up to 75% of cases. Hepatitis C infection has been identified as the main cause in most cases of mixed cryoglobulinaemia.

6.4.3 Plasma cell dyscrasia

Plasma cell dyscrasia refers to a constellation of disorders associated with abnormal proliferation of plasma cells and monoclonal gammopathy.

Table 6.18 Causes of monoclonal and polyclonal gammopathy

Monoclonal gammopathy	Polyclonal gammopathy
• Monoclonal gammopathy of uncertain significance (MGUS) • Multiple myeloma • Lymphomas • Amyloidosis, CTDs	• Acute infection • Chronic inflammatory disorders – sarcoidosis, autoimmune conditions

E ≫ Monoclonal gammopathies are usually caused by clonal expansion of plasma cell, releasing abnormally high amounts of immunoglobulins or monoclonal proteins (also known as paraproteins or M-proteins).

Monoclonal gammopathy of uncertain significance (MGUS)

MGUS is a relatively common, benign paraproteinaemia affecting up to 2% of the population. Its prevalence increases with age and peaks at 70 years. The paraprotein can be derived from IgG, IgM or IgA. Patients are asymptomatic, and diagnosis is often made incidentally on biochemical testing. No treatment is required for MGUS. However, there is a 25% risk of malignant (myeloma) transformation after 20 years.

Multiple myeloma (MM)

Definition: MM is a paraproteinaemia, a disorder of plasma cell origin, which can be preceded by MGUS (*see above*). The disease is characterised by monoclonal antibody production and bone marrow infiltration by plasma cells.

Epidemiology:
- Second most common haematological malignancy
- 15–20% mortality from haematological cancers and 2% of all cancers
- Affects males more than females
- More common in Afro-Caribbeans than in Caucasians, with a median age of 63–70 at diagnosis

Aetiology/pathophysiology:
- Genetically, abnormalities are most common on chromosome 14, where translocation results in an oncogene placed with an immunoglobulin (Ig) heavy chain gene; other chromosomes (e.g. 13) may also be involved.
- This leads to the proliferation of malignant plasma cells (also known as MM cells), which secrete a single (monoclonal) type of Ig or fragments of Ig in serum and urine
- Normal Ig production is impaired, increasing risk of infections
- MM cells infiltrate bone marrow, increase osteoclast activity (osteoclastic activating factors produced by MM cells) and inhibit osteoblast function, leading to lytic bony lesions and subsequently, hypercalcaemia
- Marrow is replaced by tumour cells, leading to anaemia
- Free light chains produced by MM cells are excreted in the urine (known as Bence Jones proteins)
- In excess, these are deposited in the distal tubules, causing acute kidney injury

W ≫ The frequency of myelomas correlates roughly with the serum concentration of heavy chain classes; thus IgG myelomas are the most common subtype.

Clinical features:

E ≫ 80% of patients present with lethargy secondary to anaemia and bony pain, most commonly back pain (secondary to bony lesions). MM can also present as a medical emergency, with sepsis, hypercalcaemia, hyperviscosity symptoms or spinal cord compression secondary to vertebral lesions.

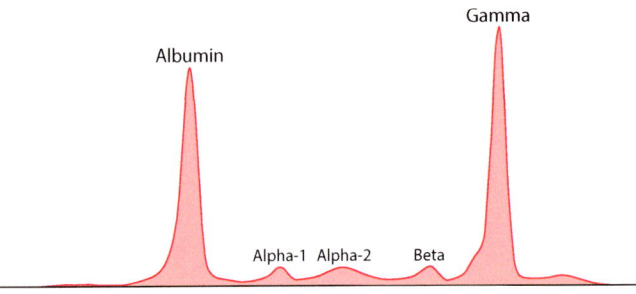

Fig. 6.23 *A serum protein electrophoresis showing two peaks – first peak is represented by albumin (control) and second peak shows the presence of elevated paraproteins (gammopathy).*

Other clinical features include:
- Pathologic fractures as a result of lytic bony lesions
- Hypercalcaemia
- Recurrent bacterial infections
- Proteinuria or dehydration secondary to renal impairment

Investigations

The diagnosis of MM involves laboratory and imaging investigations.

Stepwise plan:

1   Arrange blood testing
- FBC – normocytic, normochromic anaemia ± pancytopenia
- U&Es – $\uparrow Ca^{2+}$, $\uparrow ALP$, $\uparrow ESR$
- Peripheral blood film – rouleaux formation as a result of increased paraproteins and plasma cell

2   Carry out serum protein electrophoresis and immunofixation
- To confirm the presence of paraproteins (see *Fig. 6.23*)

3   Arrange bone marrow aspirate or biopsy
- To allow plasma cell percentage and phenotyping (see *Fig. 6.24*)
- FISH cytogenetic analysis and immuno-phenotyping to allow assessment of prognosis

4   Obtain imaging
- Skeletal survey to look for lytic lesions (see *Fig. 6.25*)
- Full body MRI and PET-CT can sometimes be considered

Management

The treatment of MM mainly involves supportive therapy, immuno-/chemotherapy and bone marrow transplantation.

Stepwise management of multiple myeloma

1   Offer supportive therapy
- Renal disease – provide adequate IV fluid rehydration

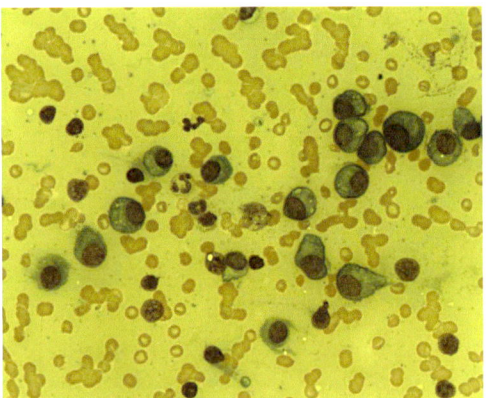

Fig. 6.24 *Plasma cell infiltrate on a BM aspirate.*

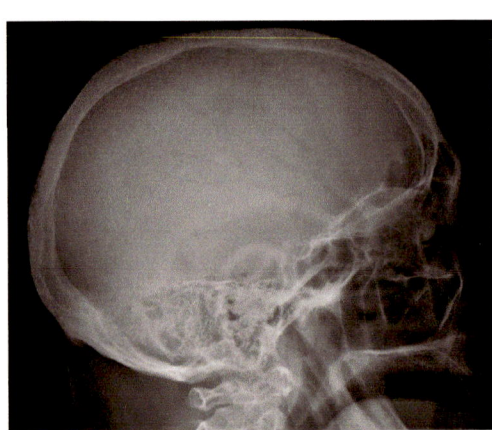

Fig. 6.25 *Plain skull X-ray showing multiple lytic lesions indicative of MM.*

- Bone disease (pain) – this is most effectively treated by radiotherapy or dexamethasone; bisphosphonates may also be used to reduce osteoclast activity and prevent hypercalcaemia
- Infection prophylaxis – offer seasonal influenza and pneumococcal vaccinations and prophylactic antiviral post-chemotherapy
- Thromboprophylaxis (LMWH or aspirin) should be considered

2 Provide immuno-/chemotherapy
- Combination of proteasome inhibitor (e.g. bortezomib)/immunomodulatory agents with steroids, with/without chemotherapy should be offered. The most common combination is VCD (bortezomib + cyclophosphamide + dexamethasone).
- Consider autologous SCT for transplant-eligible patients post-induction therapy

6.4.4 Myeloproliferative disorders

These represent a group of chronic conditions, characterised by abnormal clonal proliferation of one or more cell lines of myeloid lineage. They usually arise as a result of Janus kinase 2 (JAK2) mutations. Chronic myeloid leukaemia (see *Section 6.4.1*) is also classified as a myeloproliferative disorder.

> **W** >> JAK2 is a tyrosine kinase protein, responsible for cell signalling in bone marrow haematopoietic stem cells. Genetic mutations, most commonly V617F, up-regulate the sensitivity towards haematopoietic growth factors such as erythropoietin and thrombopoietin.

Polycythaemia vera (PV)

PV, traditionally known as polycythaemia rubra vera, is a trilineage myeloproliferative disorder affecting the mainly erythroid but also myeloid and megakaryocyte cell lines. PV often affects the elderly population, with an average age of onset of 60 years. Around 90% of patients are JAK2-positive and the presence of JAK2 is diagnostic in PV.

Presentation is often insidious, with:
- Hyperviscosity syndrome (30%)
- Pruritus (30–40%) and splenomegaly (70%)
- Occasionally (<5%), patients complain of acute burning and erythema of the hands and feet; this is known as erythromelalgia

> **E** >> Hyperviscosity syndrome is a constellation of symptoms, caused by high cell counts resulting in high serum viscosity, producing symptoms of:
> - End-organ congestion – visual disturbances, neurological symptoms (headache, dizziness, tinnitus), cardiac (angina, SOB)
> - Reduced blood flow (stasis) – recurrent thrombosis, bleeding (due to high shear force through the capillaries)

In PV, there is usually elevated Hb/Hct, JAK2 mutation, hypercellular marrow and reduced erythropoietin level.

The aim of management is to keep the Hct <0.45ml/L. This is usually achieved by weekly venesections, long-term aspirin or hydroxycarbamide (in higher-risk patients). There is a 30% risk of MF transformation.

Essential thrombocythaemia (ET)

This is a chronic myeloproliferative disorder characterised by abnormal proliferation of megakaryocytes. Patients have an elevated platelet count (typically >600 × 10^6/L) but normal RBC and WBC levels. Bleeding and thrombosis are common presentations, due to platelet dysfunction.

Diagnosis depends on excluding other causes of thrombocytosis. Unlike in PV, the presence of the JAK2 mutation (~50%) is supportive rather than diagnostic. Treatment involves hydroxycarbamide or anagrelide (megakaryocyte maturation inhibitor) to reduce platelet levels, and long-term aspirin.

Myelofibrosis (MF)

Definition: primary MF is a rare condition, characterised by multi-lineage clonal proliferation (in particular, abnormal megakaryocytes), resulting in PDGF-induced reactive fibrosis of the bone marrow. MF may also be secondary, progressing from PV, ET or other chronic conditions.

Clinical features:
- Initially, patients present with constitutional 'B' symptoms and often massive splenomegaly
- Bone marrow failure symptoms may become apparent in later stages

Investigations

In MF, there is evidence of BM fibrosis on biopsy and JAK2 or MPL mutation, in combination with clinical findings and the presence of leucoerythroblastosis and poikilocytes on peripheral blood film.

Management
- Treatment is supportive, with transfusions and hydroxycarbamide
- Splenectomy may be considered for symptomatic control
- Allogeneic BMT may be curative in younger patients
- Ruxolitinib, a JAK2 inhibitor, can be considered in some patients

6

6.4.5 Myelodysplastic syndrome (MDS)

MDS is a heterogeneous group of malignant disorders characterised by dysplastic haematopoiesis, affecting one or more lineages with varying risk of developing AML. They can occur primarily (usually as a result of cytogenetic abnormalities) or secondary to previous chemo-/radiotherapy (10%). The annual incidence of MDS is 4 per 100,000 and it is more common in the elderly. Presentation is variable, with consequences of bone marrow failure.

Patients with MDS have peripheral blood film showing dysplastic blood cells, often revealing dysmorphic RBC and hypogranular ± hyper-/hypo-segmented WBCs. BM aspirate or biopsy is often hypercellular, with

the presence of blast cells (<20%). MDS is classified according to the World Health Organization (WHO) Revised Classification 2008.

Risk stratification of MDS can be calculated using different means, but these scoring systems generally include analysis of peripheral cytopenias, BM blast percentages, and cytogenetic characteristics.

Management is based on the risk stratification of the disease and includes:
- Supportive care (including transfusion support, erythropoietin-stimulating agents (ESA), growth factor support and antibiotics for infections)
- Hypomethylating agents (e.g. azacitidine)
- Allogeneic SCT – the only curative modality in suitable candidates

6.5 Oncology

Oncology is a branch of medicine that relates to the understanding of the development, progression and treatment of neoplastic conditions. The prevalence of these conditions has steadily risen and has considerable impact on the global burden of disease.

6.5.1 Breast cancer

Definition: breast cancer is a malignancy most commonly originating from epithelial cells lining the ducts or lobules of the breast. Breast cancer may also occur secondary to sarcomas/lymphomas.

Epidemiology:
- 1 of 10 newly diagnosed cancers annually
- Females: 1 in 8 lifetime risk in the UK
- Incidence in females compared to males is 150:1
- Benign masses are 15x more common than malignant masses

Aetiology/pathophysiology:
- **Hereditary:** genetics (inherited mutations) accounts for only 2–5% of all breast cancers. However, carriers of the BRCA1 or BRCA2 mutations have an 87% lifetime incidence of breast cancer. Others include the Li–Fraumeni syndrome (inherited mutation of p53 tumour-suppressor gene) and PTEN gene.
- **Sporadic:** major risk factors (relative risk >4.0) include age, family history, past history of cancer, atypical ductal hyperplasia. Other important risk factors involve exposure to oestrogen and progesterone (nulliparity, long-term HRT, first

child >35 years, early menarche, late menopause). Acquired mutations p53, PTEN and oncogene are observed in non-hereditary breast cancer.
- **Secondary metastases:** not discussed in this section.

> W >> Hormone-dependent nature of breast cancer – role of endogenous and exogenous oestrogen in stimulation of mammary tumours.

- Breast carcinomas arise from the epithelium of ducts or terminal ducts of the lobule, and may be non-invasive (ductal carcinoma *in situ*, lobular carcinoma *in situ*) or invasive.
- Less commonly, other invasive subtypes include mucinous, tubular, medullary and papillary subtypes. Paget disease of the breast is a carcinoma of the nipple epithelium.

Clinical features:

> E >> Firm, painless, irregular mass commonly in the upper outer quadrant, may increase in size non-cyclically (compare fluctuating size of fibrocystic disease). Pain, if present, is non-cyclical in nature.

- Skin changes: puckering/tethering (peau d'orange), rash, ulceration, thickening, discoloration
- Nipple discharge (typically blood-stained)
- Axillary lymphadenopathy

Investigations

- Women aged between 50 and 70 are invited for screening mammography every 3 years in England and Wales

E >> Diagnosis of breast cancer is made by a triple assessment of clinical examination + imaging + cytology. Further investigations are warranted if results are inconsistent with the clinical presentation.

- Clinical examination
- Mammography and/or ultrasound (see *Figs 6.26* and *6.27*)
- Core biopsy and/or fine needle aspiration cytology: to establish receptor status (oestrogen receptor & human epidermal growth factor receptor 2 (HER2))

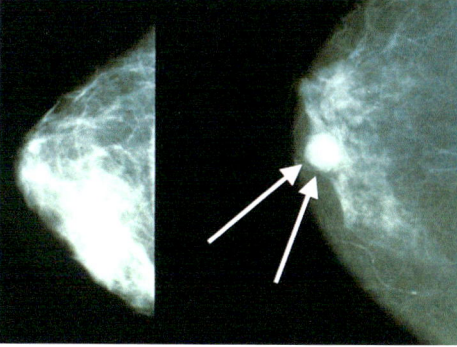

Fig. 6.26 *Mammography showing a calcified breast mass suspicious of a tumour.*

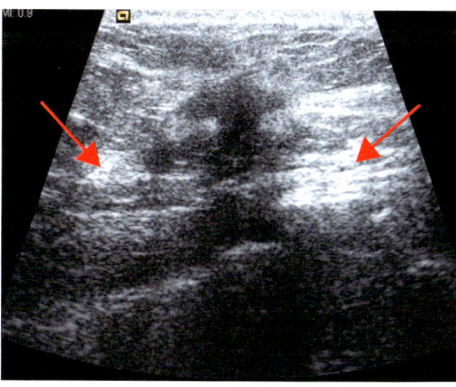

Fig. 6.27 *Breast ultrasound showing an invasive ductal cancer.*

P >> Mammography features suspicious for malignancy include irregular spiculated mass, clustered micro-calcifications, linear branching calcifications.

W >> In younger women, ultrasound is a better modality for evaluating breast masses due to breast tissue density. Sensitivity of mammography versus ultrasound is based on age.

P >> Most malignant cells maintain their expression of steroidal hormone receptors (and therefore hormonal dependence), allowing hormonal manipulation to be used as a therapeutic strategy.

Stepwise management of breast cancer

1 Staging of breast cancer
- TNM (tumour/node/metastasis)

2 Surgery
- Breast-conserving surgery (preferred where possible) or mastectomy
- Delayed or immediate reconstruction options are discussed, depending on planned adjuvant therapies

3 Further investigations
- These include pre-surgical axillary staging with ultrasound and sentinel lymph node biopsy (SLNB) – to determine whether axillary lymph node dissection is warranted

4 If suspicions are present, patients undergo investigations for metastatic disease
- These investigations include X-rays, CT scans, bone scans (hot spots indicate increased metabolic uptake), PET scans, MRI

Adjuvants

Local therapy
- Radiotherapy is used post-DCIS, and in early invasive cancer with high risk of local recurrence and if axillary clearance is not possible following positive SLNB

Systemic therapy
- Chemotherapy is indicated in sentinel node/systemic involvement (≥TNM Stage 2), and is a combination of adriamycin, cyclophosphamide, methotrexate and 5-fluorouracil
- Endocrine therapy is indicated in receptor-positive tumours
  - HER2+: trastuzumab (Herceptin) monoclonal antibody
  - ER+: non-selective anti-oestrogen (tamoxifen), selective oestrogen receptor modulators

6

(raloxifene), aromatase inhibitors (block conversion of androgens to oestrogen), GnRH analogues (decrease endogenous oestrogens)

Table 6.19 *Management strategy based on extent of disease*

Disease extent	Summary of treatment options/principles
Localised disease (DCIS)	Surgery (breast-conserving) + radiotherapy; SLNB not routine
Early invasive	Surgery + axillary staging + systemic therapy
Locally advanced	Surgery + radiotherapy + systemic therapy
Metastatic	Systemic therapy, supportive care

Prognostic factors include tumour size, type, grade, receptor status, lymph node status, vascular/lymphatic invasion.

Complications include lymphoedema.

HRT is not offered in women with menopausal symptoms and a history of breast cancer.

6.5.2 Ovarian cancer

Definition: ovarian cancer refers to a group of malignancies resulting from malignant transformation of ovarian cells, or secondary metastases from other parts of the body.

Epidemiology:
- Lifetime risk 2%, more common in Caucasians
- Incidence increases with age
- Highest mortality rate amongst gynaecological cancers due to its vague symptoms and late presentation

Aetiology/pathophysiology:
- **Hormonal:** nulliparity, early menarche, late menopause, IUCDs, infertility, endometriosis, obesity
- **Genetics:** BRCA1 and BRCA2 (44% lifetime incidence in carriers), family history of ovarian/breast cancer, Lynch syndrome
- Ovarian cancer spreads by direct implantation on adjacent structures (commonly right liver edge, omentum, diaphragm peritoneum), or lymphatic drainage

Subtypes
- **Epithelial tumours (85–90%)** arise from the epithelial surface of the ovary, occur primarily

in older women; subtypes include serous (most common), mucinous, endometroid, clear cell, undifferentiated tumours
- **Germ cell tumours (2–10%)** are most prevalent in women <35 years. These tumours are derived from primitive germ cells of embryonic gonads. Types include dysgerminoma (most common), endodermal sinus (yolk sac), teratoma, choriocarcinoma, sarcomas. These are most prognostically favourable.
- **Sex cord-stromal tumours (<5%)** originate from connective tissue cells and include granulosa cell, Sertoli–Leydig, fibrosarcoma and fibroma
- **Secondary to other tumours** include gastrointestinal, breast, haematopoietic, uterus and cervix

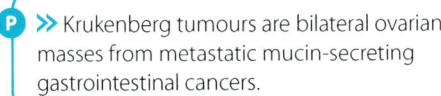
P ➤➤ Krukenberg tumours are bilateral ovarian masses from metastatic mucin-secreting gastrointestinal cancers.

Clinical features:
- Initially asymptomatic or vague symptoms, including persistent abdominal bloating, early satiety, nausea and vomiting
- Constitutional symptoms of fatigue, weight loss, anorexia
- Other late symptoms include persistent pelvic pain or pressure, changes in bowel habits, urinary urgency and/or frequency, abnormal uterine bleeding, ascites and pleural effusion

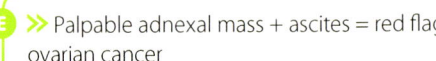
E ➤➤ Palpable adnexal mass + ascites = red flag ovarian cancer

Investigations

Stepwise plan (NICE 2011, CG122):

1 **Measure serum CA 125**
- Include α-fetoprotein and β-hCG in women <40 years to detect non-epithelial ovarian cancer, and ultrasound of abdomen and pelvis

2 **Calculate risk malignancy index (RMI)**
- Score of ≥250 warrants referral to a specialist multi-disciplinary team

3 **Carry out further investigations to determine the extent of disease**
- Include CT abdomen/pelvis (and thorax if clinically indicated)

P ≫ RMI: ultrasound features × menopausal status × serum CA 125
- Ultrasound features (0–1 features = 1 point, ≥2 = 3 points): solid areas, multilocular cyst, bilateral involvement, ascites, intra-abdominal metastases
- Menopausal status (pre = 1 point, post = 3 points)
- Serum CA 125 levels are measured in IU/ml

Fédération Internationale de Gynécologie et d'Obstétrique (FIGO) staging
- I: tumour confined to ovaries
- II: tumour extends to pelvic tissues
- III: spread to peritoneum outside pelvis and/or retroperitoneal lymph nodes
- IV: distant metastasis (liver, lung)

Stepwise management of ovarian cancer (NICE 2011, CG122):

1 Stage I
- Surgery for staging and optimal debulking: total abdominal hysterectomy with bilateral salpingo-oophorectomy and infracolic omentectomy, including peritoneal biopsies and retroperitoneal lymph node assessment (but not dissection)
- Adjuvant chemotherapy is offered to high-risk stage I and consists of six-cycle carboplatin

2 Stages II–IV
- Surgery may be performed before or after neoadjuvant chemotherapy, aiming for complete resection of all macroscopic disease
- If surgery has not been performed, tissue diagnosis is usually obtained before commencing cytotoxic chemotherapy, via percutaneous image-guided biopsy, laparoscopic biopsy or laparotomy
- Chemotherapy agents include cisplatin/carboplatin (platinum-based therapy), as single agents or in combination with paclitaxel and/or bevacizumab

6.5.3 Prostate cancer

Definition: a malignancy arising from the prostate gland, with 75–80% of cancers developing in the peripheral zone of the prostate.

Epidemiology:
- Most common cancer in men
- 26% of all male cancer diagnoses in the UK
- Lifetime risk is 1 in 9 men in the UK
- Median age of diagnosis is 68 years

W ≫ Due to the insidious onset and slow growth of most prostate cancers, screening is unlikely to be beneficial in men with a life expectancy of 10–15 years.

Aetiology/pathophysiology:
- Risk factors: age >50 years, family history, African-Caribbean ethnicity; also high animal fat diet, chronic inflammation, UV radiation
- The most likely precursor is high-grade prostate intra-epithelial neoplasia (PIN), which displays intermediate histology between normal and malignant cells
- Prostate cancer initially spreads locally, progressing to periprostatic tissue, seminal vesicles and bladder neck; then metastasises via haematogenous route, most frequently involving bone, then lung and liver

Clinical features:
- Local disease: lower urinary tract symptoms of hesitancy, frequency, urgency, weak stream, incomplete emptying, incontinence; may also present with urinary tract infection
- Locally invasive disease: haematuria, perineal/suprapubic pain, obstructive symptoms (anuria, loin pain, kidney disease), impotence, tenesmus
- Metastatic disease: bone pain, spinal cord compression (paraplegia), lymphadenopathy, weight loss

Investigations

Stepwise plan:

1 Clinical: digital rectal examination (DRE)
- Findings include firm palpable nodules or indurations, gland asymmetry, lack of mobility of prostate (from adhesions), palpable seminal vesicles

2 Biochemistry: total prostate-specific antigen (PSA) levels
- Free PSA levels, PSA doubling time and PSA velocity are other parameters used in predicting response to treatment or in monitoring disease

E ≫ PSA levels normally increase with age – the relative annual increase rather than absolute levels suggest cancer. Prostate cancer cannot be diagnosed on biochemistry alone.

6

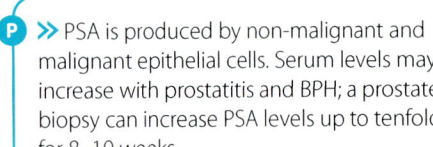

P ≫ PSA is produced by non-malignant and malignant epithelial cells. Serum levels may increase with prostatitis and BPH; a prostate biopsy can increase PSA levels up to tenfold for 8–10 weeks.

P ≫ Androgen deprivation therapy is effective in castrate-sensitive prostate cancer, by lowering testosterone levels. This may be achieved surgically via bilateral orchidectomy or chemically with luteinising hormone-releasing hormone (LHRH) antagonists/agonists.

3 Biopsy: transrectal ultrasound-guided (TRUS) biopsy
- Findings are graded histologically via Gleason score
- Decision to biopsy should take into account DRE findings and other risk factors, rather than be solely based on the PSA

4 Consider MRI to evaluate if a re-biopsy is warranted, in a negative TRUS biopsy

P ≫ The Gleason score is derived from the sum of the two most prominent tissue types on biopsy. Grade 1 indicates the most well architecturally differentiated tumour, while grade 5 indicates the most poorly differentiated. The score is prognostic (75% ten-year risk of local progression if score >7).

5 Investigate for metastases
- Bone scan, X-rays, pelvic CT/MRI

Management (NICE 2014, CG175)

W ≫ Brachytherapy is the transperineal implantation of radioactive seeds directly into the prostate. Its goal is to minimise radiation to surrounding tissues, and it is associated with fewer side effects than external beam radiotherapy.

Adverse effects of radical treatment and management:
- Sexual dysfunction – phosphodiesterase-5 inhibitors, vacuum devices, intraurethral inserts, penile injections, penile prostheses
- Urinary incontinence – continence clinic, pelvic floor exercises, bladder retraining, pharmacotherapy, artificial urinary sphincter
- Radiation-induced enteropathy – involve gastroenterologists
- Specific to hormone therapy
  - Hot flushes: medroxyprogesterone, cyproterone acetate
  - Osteoporosis: assess fracture risk, consider bisphosphonates or denosumab
  - Gynaecomastia: prophylactic radiotherapy, tamoxifen
  - Fatigue: aerobic exercise
- Relapse: reassess and consider options as per *Table 6.20*

6.5.4 Testicular cancer

Definition: testicular cancer is a malignancy of germ cell origin, and usually affects a younger population, with excellent curability.

Epidemiology:
- 1% of all male cancer diagnoses
- Peak incidence in men aged 20–40 years
- More common in white males

Table 6.20 *Management of prostate cancer*

Risk stratification: PSA + Gleason score + clinical stage (TNM)	Treatment options
1. Low-risk or intermediate-risk localised cancer 2. Post-treatment monitoring	Active surveillance Monitoring of PSA levels, DRE, prostate re-biopsy; men with disease progression may be offered individualised radical treatment
1. Low-risk or Intermediate-risk localised cancer 2. High-risk localised 3. Locally advanced	Radical prostatectomy: removal of prostate gland and seminal vesicles; may include pelvic lymph node dissection Radiotherapy (brachytherapy and/or external beam radiation) Androgen deprivation therapy
1. Metastatic cancer	Curative intent: bilateral orchidectomy Symptomatic therapy should be targeted towards sites of metastases • Sexual function: androgen deprivation therapy • Painful bone metastases: bisphosphonates, strontium • Urinary tract obstruction: percutaneous nephrostomy, JJ stent insertion

Aetiology/pathophysiology:

- Risk factors – history of malignancy in contralateral testis, cryptorchidism, testicular maldescent, Klinefelter syndrome, male infertility, infantile hernia
- Genetics: chromosome 12 abnormality is present in almost all testicular cancers
- Testicular cancer is classified based on its pathological origin (see *Table 6.21*), with 90–95% of cases being germ cell tumours.

Clinical features:

- Painless testicular lump
- Testicular discomfort, swelling, abdominal pain
- Usually no inguinal lymphadenopathy
- Gynaecomastia
- Features of seminomatous and non-seminomatous germ cell tumours (GCTs) are described in *Table 6.22*

Table 6.21 *Pathological classification of testicular cancer*

Germ cell tumours (GCTs)	Seminoma
	Non-seminoma
Sex cord/stromal tumours	Leydig, Sertoli, granulosa
Other stromal tumours	

Table 6.22 *Features of seminomatous and non-seminomatous GCTs*

Seminomatous GCTs	Non-seminomatous GCTs
50% of all GCTs, median age of presentation – fourth decade	Most frequent in third decade of life
	Histological subtypes: embryonal carcinoma, teratoma, choriocarcinoma, endodermal sinus (yolk sac) tumour
More indolent, rarely metastasises, better prognosis	More aggressive, early metastasis to retroperitoneal lymph nodes, lung parenchyma
Can present with raised hCG/LDH	AFP is specific to non-seminoma

Investigations and management (BAUS 2015)

Initial investigations:

- Clinical examination
- Blood tests for tumour markers: human chorionic gonadotrophin (hCG), alpha feto-protein (AFP), lactate dehydrogenase (LDH)
- Imaging: bilateral testis ultrasound, CT chest, abdomen, pelvis

- Further investigations (bone scan, brain CT/MRI) are indicated in symptomatic patients, depending on initial findings

> **Stepwise management of testicular cancer**

1 Inguinal exploration and orchidectomy is performed
- To obtain tissue histology for TNM staging
- In life-threatening situations (due to extensive metastasis), chemotherapy is given before surgery

2 If the diagnosis is unclear, a testicular biopsy may be taken
- Consider biopsy of the contralateral testis in high-risk patients

3 Organ-preserving surgery may be considered in special cases

4 Chemotherapy
- Agents used include carboplatin-based (used as single agent, usually only for stage I seminoma) and bleomycin, etoposide, cisplatin as combination agents (BEP)

W ➤➤ Tumour markers must be repeated 5–7 days after orchidectomy to ensure predicted decline of serum levels, as this points to recurrence or persistence of the tumour (the half-lives of hCG and AFP are 24–36 hours and 5–7 days, respectively).

Management according to subtype

Table 6.23 *Management of testicular cancer*

	Seminomatous GCTs	Non-seminomatous GCTs
Stage I	Surveillance, carboplatin chemotherapy	Surveillance or single course of chemotherapy
Stages IIA/B (metastatic)	Radiotherapy or 3–4 courses of chemotherapy	3–4 courses of chemotherapy or retroperitoneal lymph node dissection with surgical resection of residual masses if indicated
Stage IIC	3–4 courses of chemotherapy	

E ➤➤ When tumours present as mixed seminoma and non-seminoma, they are treated as the more aggressive non-seminoma subtype.

Other considerations:

- Fertility and sperm storage are pre-surgical considerations, as semen quality is reduced after orchidectomy
- Patients should be offered testicular prostheses

- Post-chemotherapy complications include peripheral neuropathy, hearing loss, Raynaud phenomenon
- Increased risk of cardiac events

6.6 Palliative medicine

From the Latin word *palliare* (meaning 'to cloak or disguise'), this specialty focuses on symptom relief without curative intent. Palliative care is broad and complex and encompasses a multi-disciplinary approach aimed at maintaining the best possible quality of life in the context of a person's disease, regardless of the stage they are at.

In the course of incurable disease, palliative care extends from diagnosis to transition from curative to palliative intent, to ongoing deterioration, terminal stage and bereavement. The palliative care role is influenced by factors such as cultural perceptions of death and dying, desire for cure, age of the patient and their familial responsibilities. The essence of palliative care is well-summarised by the '7 Cs' (communication, coordination, control of symptoms, continuity, continued learning, carer support, and care of the dying), developed by the Gold Standards Framework (GSF), a UK-based training primary care initiative to improve end-of-life care.

> **W** ›› Palliative care aims neither to hasten nor prolong the dying process and is unambiguously distinct from euthanasia. The principle of double effect focuses on the intent of relieving suffering, but acknowledges that, in terminal phases, abatement of futile life-sustaining treatment may foreseeably but unintentionally alter the time of death.

6.6.1 Common symptoms and management

Pain

Around 70% of patients with advanced cancer suffer from some form of pain. The choice of analgesia depends on several factors, including the mechanism of pain, its severity, and the patient's analgesia naivety. The WHO analgesia ladder offers a guide to the use of analgesics (see www.who.int).

- **Somatic**: well localised, may be due to bony and capsulated organ (liver) metastases, post-op, may be exacerbated by activity (incident/episodic

pain). Use NSAIDs and opioids, and pre-emptively use breakthrough doses (e.g. before shower or dressing).
- **Visceral**: vague and poorly localised pain, may present with autonomic features (sweating, tachycardia, hypotension). Common causes include bowel and biliary obstruction. Opioids are analgesia of choice, spasmolytics such as hyoscine (Buscopan) may be beneficial in colicky pain.
- **Neuropathic**: shooting or burning pain, may be accompanied by numbness, tingling. Neuralgia, peripheral neuropathy, plexus involvement, spinal cord compression. Tricyclic antidepressants, mood stabilisers, NMDA, GABA agonists.
- **Psychosocial**: psychotherapy, counselling.

Guidelines for opioid prescribing

- Oral medications are preferable where tolerated; titrate required dose with sustained-release preparation, and include PRN immediate-release doses for breakthrough pain, for instance
  - a total maximum of 30mg morphine a day =
    - 10mg sustained-release morphine 12-hourly +
    - 5mg immediate-release morphine 4-hourly PRN
- Increase/decrease doses based on previous day's use of PRNs, aiming to prevent pain rather than relieve it; to obtain 'breakthrough'/PRN doses, divide the total daily dose by 6
- Parenteral medications may be used if indicated (e.g. nausea, bowel obstruction, dysphagia) and are usually administered via a subcutaneous needle or continuous infusion with a syringe driver

Nausea and vomiting (N&V)

Multiple pathways, involving the higher cerebral centres, chemoreceptor trigger zone (CTZ), vestibular input, GIT and vagus, feed back to the vomiting centre (VC) (see *Table 6.25*).

Non-pharmacological antinausea strategies include avoiding the smell of cooking food, frequent and smaller meal portions, anxiety management techniques and acupuncture.

Table 6.24 *Opioid conversion chart*

PO:PO ratio	Oral (PO)	Oral (PO)	Parenteral (SC)	PO:SC ratio
–	–	30mg morphine	10mg SC morphine	3:1
1:10	10mg morphine	100mg codeine	–	–
1:10	12mg morphine	120mg tramadol	100mg tramadol	1.2:1
3:2	15mg morphine	10mg oxycodone	5mg SC oxycodone	2:1
5–7.5:1	15mg morphine	3mg hydromorphone	1mg SC hydromorphone	3:1
Variable 3–20:1	morphine	20mg methadone	10mg methadone	2:1

Table 6.25 *Mechanism of action of common anti-emetics*

Medications	Mechanism of action and indications
Metoclopramide (peripheral and central) **Domperidone** (peripheral only)	• Dopamine receptor antagonists; prokinetic agents which relax the pylorus and duodenum and increase lower oesophageal sphincter tone • Used in gastric stasis, gastric irritation, reflux (GORD), ileus; exercise caution in small bowel obstruction
Haloperidol	• Central D_2 receptor antagonist (acts on CTZ) • Effective in opioid-induced N&V, chemical and metabolic causes such as uraemia and hypercalcaemia
Ondansetron **Dolasetron** **Tropisetron**	• $5HT_3$ antagonist at central (CTZ, VC) and peripheral (enterochromaffin cells in upper GI, vagal afferents) sites • Effective in post-operative, chemo-/radio-induced N&V
Cyclizine **Promethazine**	• H_{1-2} and ACh (muscarinic) receptor antagonist at the vestibular system and VC • Used for N&V due to motion sickness, vertigo, bowel obstruction, raised intracranial pressure
Prochlorperazine	• Central dopamine and noradrenergic receptor antagonist, broadly acts on CTZ, VC, vestibular system and gut
Dexamethasone	• Mechanism of action unclear, but appears effective at reducing oedema and inflammation around tumours • Used in raised intracranial pressure, hepatomegaly
Lorazepam	• Acts on GABA and higher cerebral centres • Effective for anxiety-related nausea and pre-medication

Respiratory symptoms

- **Dyspnoea:** manage correctable causes such as pneumonia, asthma, COPD, anaemia, heart failure, pleural effusion. Strategies include upright posture, loose clothing, controlled expiration, relaxation, chest physiotherapy, airy environment. Trial of benzodiazepines and/or opioids if anxiety-related.
- **'Death rattle':** noisy breathing caused by increased upper airway secretions in the terminal phases. This is usually distressing to family rather than the patient. Anticholinergics (such as hyoscine, atropine and glycopyrrolate) reduce the secretions and gurgling.

Fatigue

Fatigue is usually multidimensional and may be due to correctable causes (anaemia, infection, respiratory illness, endocrine cause) or subjectively related to terminal illness and deconditioning. Strategies such as exercise, activity planning, sleep hygiene, vitamin and biochemical correction, glucocorticoids may be trialled.

Terminal restlessness

This is multifactorial (secondary to pain, discomfort, opiate toxicity, psychological distress). Practise good sleep hygiene; drugs of choice are diazepam, levomepromazine and midazolam.

6

Delirium and depression

Look for reversible causes.

The first-line drug treatment is haloperidol. Second-line treatments include: benzodiazepines (lorazepam, midazolam, temazepam).

It may be challenging to differentiate appropriate responses to illness and major depression but it is important, as depression is treatable. Apart from supportive psychotherapy, there should be a low threshold for initiating pharmacologic measures.

Other important considerations

- **Anticipatory prescribing** is a hallmark of palliative care and should be instituted for the above and other symptoms not discussed (e.g. anxiety, constipation, diarrhoea, loss of appetite, dysphagia, xerostomia, hiccups, insomnia, itch). Correctable causes should be identified and treated, apart from implementing various adjunct strategies.
- Legal issues may include discussions surrounding resuscitation status, appointing a power of attorney and guardianship. Documentation of a will should occur sooner rather than later. Seek local guidelines for specific requirements.
- Spiritual and psychosocial support.
- Prognostication is challenging but models are used to estimate disease trajectories of cancer, organ failure and dementia.
- Catastrophic haemorrhage/emergencies include GI bleeding, fatal haemoptysis, status epilepticus. Stay with patient, use dark towels, palliative sedation.
- Clinician self-care includes debriefing with other team members, identifying emotions, self-awareness, and personal life outside work, which can all affect one's outlook and ability to care for patients.

Chapter 7
Nephrology

Amar Vaswani, Hwan Juet Khaw and *Samantha Jingyun Koh*

Basic principles

Nephrology is a branch of clinical medicine that deals with diagnosing and managing disorders of the body's filtering and excreting system, known as the renal system. Conditions affecting the renal system typically involve electrolyte disturbances. This chapter describes these conditions as well as providing a systematic approach to electrolyte abnormalities.

Bridge to clinical medicine

- The kidneys are paired, bean-shaped organs that lie in the retroperitoneum at the level of about T12 to L3

> E >> The right kidney sits slightly lower than the left as it is displaced downwards by the liver.

- They are encapsulated by a fibrous capsule and further protected by a thick fat pad, allowing for shock absorption
- Nephrons are the main functional unit of the renal system, responsible for the kidney's filtration, excretion and fluid balance maintenance functions; the nephrons have three distinct components:
  - **The glomerulus**, which carries out ultrafiltration of the blood
  - **Renal tubules**, including the **loop of Henle**, which carry out excretion and reabsorption of electrolytes
  - **Collecting duct**, which carries out reabsorption of water

The glomerulus

- Around 25–30% of cardiac output goes directly to the kidneys via the renal arteries. The renal arteries divide into interlobular arteries and eventually form afferent arterioles.

- These arterioles supply a specialised, tightly packed capillary bed, known as the glomerulus, and emerge as efferent arterioles. The pressure (hydrostatic and osmotic) gradient between the capillaries and the Bowman capsule influences the glomerular filtration rate (GFR).
- Specialised cells, known as **podocytes** (see *Fig. 7.1*), wrap around the glomerular capillaries, forming filtration slits, acting as the first line of filtration in the glomerulus.
- The **basement membrane** forms the second line of filtration, situated between the capillary lumen and the lumen of the Bowman capsule. The resultant filtrate is then funnelled down into the proximal convoluted tubule.

Renal tubules and the collecting system

- Filtrate from the Bowman capsule moves into the proximal convoluted tubule (PCT). The majority of electrolytes (e.g. Na, K, Ca, Mg and glucose) are reabsorbed here, facilitated by microvilli on the lumen (see *Fig. 7.2*).
- Active secretion of waste products (e.g. urea, drugs, toxins, etc.) also occurs at the renal tubules.

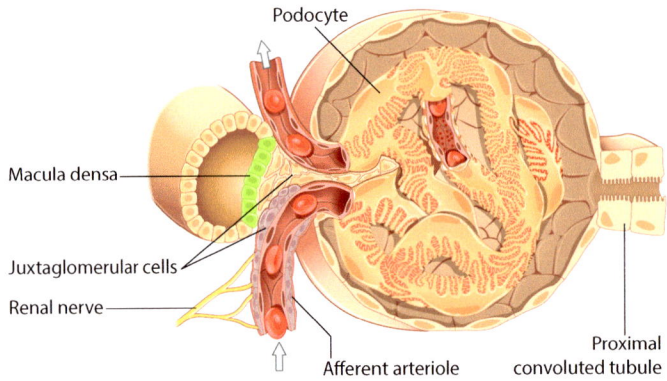

Podocyte

Macula densa

Juxtaglomerular cells

Renal nerve

Afferent arteriole

Proximal convoluted tubule

Fig. 7.1 The glomerulus; note the position of the juxtaglomerular cells in relation to the macula densa (distal collecting tubules) and arterioles.

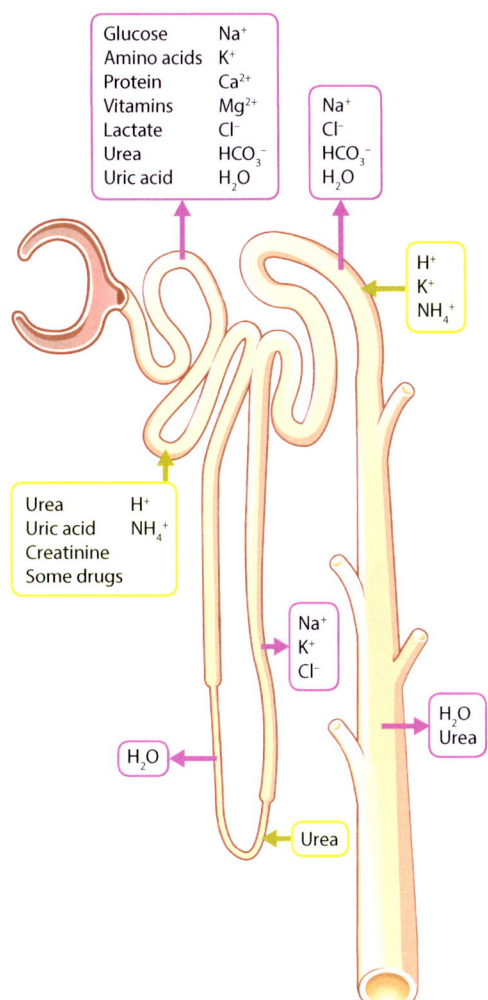

Fig. 7.2 *Sites of reabsorption and secretion in a nephron.*

- The loop of Henle consists of a thin descending portion and a thick ascending portion. This unique system allows a phenomenon (known as the **counter-current multiplier system**) to occur.
- Na/K ATPase actively pumps Na ions from the lumen of the ascending loop into the interstitial space between the loops. This creates a hyperosmolar area and provides an osmotic gradient for the reabsorption of water via the descending loop.
- Further reabsorption and secretion occurs in the distal convoluted tubules (DCT).
- Specialised cells (known as **macula densa cells**) are responsible for detecting any changes in the Na concentration and filtrate osmolality. They regulate the **release of renin** by the **juxtaglomerular cells**, situated adjacent to the Bowman capsule and afferent arterioles (the effects of renin are discussed in the section below).

- The function of the collecting ducts is mainly to regulate urine osmolality and in turn serum osmolality. They do this via **aquaporin channels**. When stimulated by **ADH** released from the posterior pituitary gland (see *Chapter 4*), aquaporin channels insert themselves onto the apical side of the collecting ducts. This allows water to move via osmosis into the interstitial spaces, resulting in more **concentrated urine**.

The renin-angiotensin-aldosterone system (RAAS)

- Renin, also known as angiotensinogenase, is a renally produced hormone that functions to break down angiotensinogen (produced by the liver) into angiotensin I (see *Fig. 7.3*)
- Angiotensin I is then converted into its active metabolite, angiotensin II, by an angiotensin-converting enzyme (ACE) released by the lungs

E ≫ This ACE enzyme is the pharmacological target of ACE inhibitors, used in blood pressure regulation.

- Angiotensin II is a potent vasoconstrictor, which increases systemic blood pressure by:
  - Direct arteriole vasoconstriction, which increases intracellular calcium
  - Sympathetic activation, which increases noradrenaline release at postganglionic receptors
  - Aldosterone secretion by the adrenal cortex, which results in sodium reabsorption and potassium secretion at the DCT and collecting ducts
  - ADH release, which increases water reabsorption at the collecting ducts

Evaluation of kidney function

- Measuring GFR allows for an assessment of functional impairment of the kidneys (this is not an exact correlation)
- Creatinine, a substance produced by muscle metabolism and from consumption of meat, is filtered through the glomerulus without reabsorption; it is therefore most commonly used as a marker of GFR, but it is also not an exact measure of GFR
- Variations in the amount of muscle mass can also affect creatinine levels, with no change in GFR
- Isotopes that are not secreted and filtered by the kidneys (and thus provide an accurate measure of GFR) are not readily available and are expensive

7

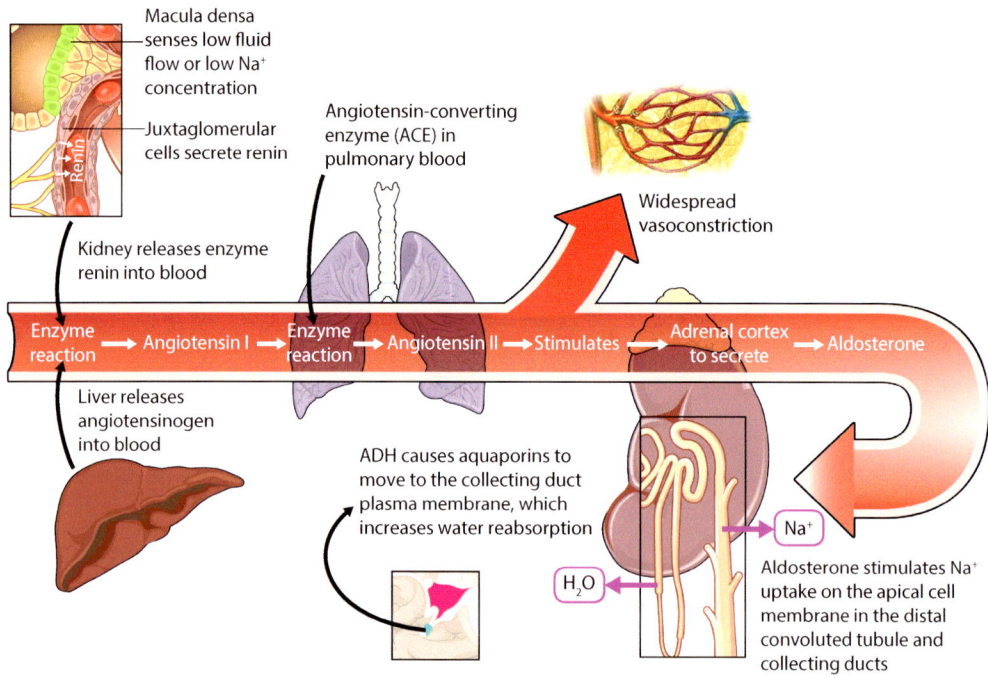

Fig. 7.3 *The renin–angiotensin–aldosterone system (RAAS).*

- Instead, equations – such as the Cockcroft–Gault equation, the modification of diet in renal disease (MDRD) equation and the chronic kidney disease epidemiology collaboration (CKD-EPI) – are used to estimate GFR
- However, these equations are limited in their usefulness because each was developed in a different study population and measures a different domain
- Of the equations listed above, the MDRD is most often employed, but underestimates the GFR at levels above 60ml/min/1.73m^2
- Conversely, the CKD-EPI equation estimates GFR more accurately at higher levels

- The Cockcroft–Gault equation has been used for a far longer period of time, and provides the basis for guidelines on drug dosing, but is less accurate than the MDRD and CKD-EPI when estimating GFR

> **E** ≫ Note that eGFR is only validated in patients with chronic kidney disease and should not be used when assessing or monitoring a patient in the acute phase. Serum creatinine levels should be used instead.

7.1 Acute kidney injury (AKI)

Definition: AKI refers to an abrupt decline in renal function from the baseline. NICE (2013, CG169) advises that acute kidney injury, previously known as acute renal failure, encompasses a wide spectrum of injury to the kidneys, not just kidney failure. The definition of acute kidney injury has changed in recent years, and detection is now mostly based on monitoring creatinine levels, with or without urine output.

Epidemiology:
- Commoner in the elderly
- Determining prevalence is complex, as different criteria are used to define the condition across various healthcare systems
- Associated with up to 5% of hospital admissions, and up to 30% of ICU admissions

Aetiology/pathophysiology:

Aetiology can be helpfully classified into three major groups: pre-renal factors, renal factors and post-renal factors.

- **Pre-renal causes:**
  - These generally encompass reduced renal perfusion with no structural damage to the kidney
  - May include haemorrhage, hypovolaemia, **sepsis**, heart failure, nephrotoxics
  - Renovascular disease (e.g. renal artery stenosis)

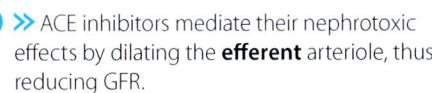 ACE inhibitors mediate their nephrotoxic effects by dilating the **efferent** arteriole, thus reducing GFR.

- **Renal causes**
  - These generally refer to **intrinsic** renal disease
  - They may include glomerulonephritis, vasculitis and acute tubular necrosis (ATN)
    - **ATN is the most common cause of AKI (implicated in 50–70% of cases)**
    - Tubular cell death – either **ischaemic ATN** or **nephrotoxic ATN**
    - Ischaemic ATN – hypoperfusion of kidneys, emboli
    - Nephrotoxic ATN – nephrotoxic medications (e.g. aminoglycosides, cisplatin)

W >> Tubular cells are highly susceptible to ischaemic injury because of their high metabolic activity and regular cell renewal. This is also why patients who develop ATN are likely to recover once the underlying cause is treated.

  - Acute interstitial nephritis (AIN):
    - Implicated in approximately 10% of AKI
    - **Almost always occurs secondary to medication side effects**
    - Beta lactams, NSAID use (nephrotic syndrome, gradual onset) most implicated
    - Only one-third (or less) of patients present with the classic triad of fever, eosinophilia and a rash
    - Withdraw causative agent, prescribe steroids
  - Chronic tubulointerstitial nephritis
- **Post-renal causes**
  - Obstruction to urinary outflow tract
  - Caused by tumours, clots, calculi, strictures, etc.

W >> Obstruction causes a build-up of renal pressure and causes atrophy on a cellular level. Leucocyte infiltration and cytokine release are also implicated in the development of AKI if it is due to an obstructive, post-renal cause.

Clinical features

Presentations are often related to the complications of renal failure. These include:

- Uraemia – general malaise, lethargy, pruritus, paraesthesia, altered mental state, pericardial rub, pale skin
- Hyperkalaemia – palpitations, chest pain
- Acidosis – Kussmaul breathing, confusion
- Fluid overload – peripheral oedema, breathlessness, raised JVP

E >> Patients with underlying illness, kidney disease or diabetes, or those who are undergoing surgery or being given contrast agents, are at much higher risk of developing AKI. For patients who require unavoidable contrast agents, aggressive hydration prior to the administration of contrast is said to decrease the incidence of contrast-induced nephropathy. The evidence also does not support the use of routine acetylcysteine.

Investigations (NICE 2013; CG169)

The development of criteria for the diagnosis of AKI has been carried out with RIFLE (Risk, Injury, Failure, Loss and End-stage disease) and has been improved upon by AKIN (Acute Kidney Injury Network) and consolidated by KDIGO (Kidney Disease: Improving Global Outcomes).

Stepwise plan (NICE 2013, CG169):

1. **Detect acute kidney injury, in line with the RIFLE, AKIN or KDIGO definitions, by using any of the following criteria**
- A rise in serum creatinine of ≥26.5 micromol/L within 48 hours
- A ≥50% rise in serum creatinine known or presumed to have occurred within the past 7 days/an increase of 1.5-fold from baseline
- A fall in urine output to <0.5ml/kg/hour for >6 hours in adults and >8 hours in children and young people

7

- A ≥25% fall in eGFR in children and young people within the past 7 days

2 Monitor serum creatinine regularly in all adults, children and young people with or at risk of acute kidney injury

3 Investigate the underlying cause, as treatment of the underlying cause will improve symptoms. Investigations include the following
- Medication review
- Urinalysis
- Blood tests – FBC, U&Es, LFTs, glucose, coagulation screen, glomerulonephritis/vasculitis screen (serology)
- ECG – look for signs of hyperkalaemia
- Fractional excretion of sodium (FE_{Na})
  - FE_{Na} <1% likely pre-renal cause
  - FE_{Na} >2% likely ATN
- Urgent renal ultrasound to exclude any post-renal causes
- Relevant radiology (e.g. CT KUB, CXR)

Management

Treatment is generally supportive, with rehydration therapy being the mainstay. Treatment mainly involves treating the underlying cause.

Stepwise management of acute kidney injury (NICE 2013, CG169):

1 Ensure accurate fluid balance monitoring
- Fluid balance (intake and output) chart with **daily weights** and urinary catheterisation if necessary
- Encourage oral hydration and supplement with IV fluid therapy as appropriate

2 Review medications
- Consider withholding and avoiding nephrotoxic medications (e.g. NSAIDs, ACE inhibitors, metformin, etc.)

3 Identify and treat underlying cause

4 Provide supportive therapy
- Offer supplementary oxygen if patient is breathless, and transfuse if they are anaemic

5 Arrange urgent urology referral if severe obstructive conditions predominate
- Or refer to a nephrologist if patient is unresponsive to medical therapy or requires renal replacement therapy (NICE)

6 Monitor renal function daily
- Or even arrange twice-daily U&Es

7 NICE also advises against routinely offering loop diuretics to treat acute kidney injury

> **P** ≫ When to refer for renal replacement therapy (RRT)
>
> A helpful mnemonic (based on the guidelines) is '**POPAC**':
> **P**ulmonary oedema
> **O**edema (general)
> **P**otassium (hyperkalaemia)
> **A**cidosis
> **C**omplications of uraemia (e.g. pericarditis, encephalopathy)

7.1.1 Rhabdomyolysis

Definition: rhabdomyolysis refers to a clinical condition characterised by skeletal muscle breakdown and release of cellular contents, causing acute kidney injury and electrolyte abnormalities.

> **W** ≫ Myocyte cellular metabolism is interrupted when damage or trauma occurs, disrupting homeostasis and causing cellular necrosis and release of substances extracellularly. One of these substances is myoglobin, which, when filtered by the kidneys, predisposes to AKI because of its toxic nature outside myocytes. This causes myoglobinuria, which results in darker, brown urine. Electrolyte abnormalities (such as hyperkalaemia, hyperphosphataemia and hypercalcaemia) also occur as a result of cellular necrosis.

Aetiology:
- There are a number of possible causes, as any type of muscle necrosis or myoglobinuria can increase the risk of developing rhabdomyolysis
- Some of these include alcoholism, DKA, infections, ischaemia, trauma (particularly crush injuries and burns), falls, long lies, compartment syndrome and seizures

Clinical features:
- Reddish-brown 'tea-coloured' urine (see *Fig. 7.4*)
- Muscle swelling, pain or limb paraesthesia
- Fever, nausea, vomiting
- Hyperkalaemia
- Hypocalcaemia (myoglobin binds calcium to it)

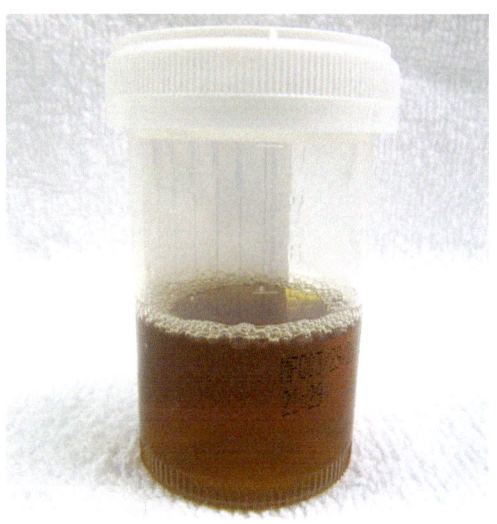

Fig. 7.4 *Reddish-brown urine of a patient with rhabdomyolysis.*

Approach to rhabdomyolysis

The diagnosis is usually made on clinical grounds. Symptoms include:

- Haematuria on urinalysis
- Hyperkalaemia, hypocalcaemia and hyperphosphataemia
- CK is significantly elevated, up to 5 times baseline

Treatment involves aggressive fluid therapy and correction of electrolyte abnormalities, particularly if hyperkalaemia or hypocalcaemia are life-threatening.

> **P** ≫ Statins carry a very small risk of rhabdomyolysis (<1%).

7.2 Chronic kidney disease

7

Definition: chronic kidney disease refers to kidney damage for 3 or more months, secondary to structural or functional disorders or disease that presents with an estimated glomerular filtration rate (eGFR) <60ml/min/1.73m^2 on two separate occasions.

Chronic kidney disease in adults: assessment and management (NICE 2014, CG182)

Table 7.1 *Classification of CKD according to eGFR*

Stage	Severity	eGFR
1	Normal/high	≥90
2	Mild reduction	60–89
3a	Mild/moderate	45–59
3b	Moderate/severe	30–44
4	Severe	15–29
5	Kidney failure	≤15

NICE advises that an increased ACR and a decreased GFR are associated with an increased risk of poorer outcomes, and this risk is multiplied if increased ACR and decreased GFR occur together.

Bear in mind that the KDIGO guidelines also include the degree of albuminuria (which also reflects kidney disease and mortality) in their stratification of CKD.

Classifying persistent albuminuria:

- Mild <30mg/g
- Moderate 30–300mg/g
- Severe >300mg/g

> **E** ≫ Note that in patients with extreme amounts of muscle mass (e.g. bodybuilders) eGFR results should be interpreted with caution.

Epidemiology:

- Incidence has increased
- Affects almost 10% of adults worldwide
- Commonly seen in older patients with long-standing DM or hypertension
- Afro-Caribbean and Asian populations are at greater risk

Aetiology/pathophysiology:

Table 7.2 *Causes of CKD*

Common causes	Other causes
• Diabetes mellitus • Hypertension	• Renovascular disease • GN, SLE • Interstitial disease (often drug-induced) • Polycystic kidney disease

P ≫ Patients are said to have accelerated progression of disease if there is a change in GFR category or a sustained decrease in GFR of ≥25% within 12 months or <15ml/min/1.73m^2 per year.

Clinical features:
- Patients may be asymptomatic until a late stage
- Symptoms classically associated with CKD (such as pruritus, polyuria, oedema, fatigue and muscle weakness) largely occur in severe CKD
- Patients with CKD typically have other comorbid conditions as well, e.g. coronary artery disease, hypertension, dyslipidaemia, and mineral and bone disorders

Investigations

Stepwise plan (NICE 2014, CG182):

1 Assess kidney function
- Measure eGFR
- Advise patients to abstain from eating meat 12 hours before eGFR measurement
- Urine ACR >3mg/mmol

2 Arrange blood tests and urine dipstick
- Normochromic normocytic anaemia
- Auto-antibody testing if underlying disease is suspected

3 Obtain renal ultrasound
- Offer if patients have:
  - Symptoms of obstruction
  - Accelerated progression of disease
  - Family history of polycystic kidney disease
  - Visible or persistent microscopic haematuria

Management
Educate patients about their condition, and encourage them to stop smoking and adjust their calorie, potassium, phosphate and salt intake. Low-protein diets are not recommended, as there is insufficient evidence to recommend their use at present. Nephrotoxic medications should be withheld.

Stepwise management of chronic kidney disease (NICE 2014, CG182)

1 Manage blood pressure
- Target: <140/90
- Target: <130/80 if ACR >70mg/mmol
- Offer ACE inhibitors first line; stop anti-hypertensives if hyperkalaemia develops

2 Manage cardiovascular disease
- Optimise risk factors, prescribe statins and antiplatelet agents as appropriate
- Consider the use of apixaban instead of warfarin, if patients have AF and Stage 3b CKD or if they have a history of DM, heart failure, or previous cerebrovascular events

3 Check for renal bone disease and electrolyte abnormalities
- Measure calcium, phosphate, PTH and Vit D levels if eGFR <30ml/min/1.73m^2
- Attempt to normalise calcium and phosphate levels
- Offer bisphosphonates, as appropriate, for prevention and treatment of osteoporosis
- KDIGO guidelines recommend alkali supplementation (e.g. sodium bicarbonate) to keep serum bicarbonate in the normal range, as lower levels of bicarbonate have been associated with poorer outcomes

4 Manage anaemia
- Screen and correct for iron deficiency
- Offer erythropoietic-stimulating agent as appropriate

5 Manage oedema
- Offer loop diuretic (e.g. furosemide 40mg) as appropriate

6 Provide renal replacement therapy
- This is recommended for end-stage disease

W ≫ Renal osteodystrophy refers to a disorder in bone mineralisation secondary to chronic kidney disease. This occurs because a reduced ability to excrete phosphate develops as CKD progresses, leading to hyperphosphataemia and secondary hyperparathyroidism. As 1-Alpha hydroxylation of vitamin D is carried out by the kidneys, there is an impaired conversion of vitamin D to its active form, leading to decreased uptake of calcium in the small intestine.

E ≫ Elevated PTH levels cause osteoclastic breakdown of bone and predisposition to osteoporosis or osteomalacia. Treatment of renal osteodystrophy involves phosphate binders, e.g. sevelamer or Calcichew (calcium carbonate and vit. D$_3$), calcium and vitamin D supplementation and/or cinacalcet (a calcimimetic used to reduce PTH levels in secondary hyperparathyroidism).

7.3 Glomerulonephritis

Glomerulonephritis is an umbrella term encompassing various disease manifestations and presentations with regard to renal disease. These may be largely **nephrotic** or **nephritic** in nature, or may present as a combination of the two, and the variability of symptoms (nephrotic or nephritic) is based on the disease process observed.

It is therefore helpful to classify these diseases (for learning purposes) as **largely nephrotic, largely nephritic** and **mixed nephrotic and nephritic**. Note that actual presentations may vary in clinical practice, but learning the disease processes this way helps solidify understanding and diagnostic approach.

7.3.1 Nephrotic syndrome

E » Very broadly, **nephrotic disease**, specifically **nephrotic syndrome,** is characterised by:
- **Proteinuria**
  - >3g/24 hours **or** urine protein:creatinine ratio >300mg/mol
- **Hypoalbuminaemia**
  - <25g/L
  - Associated with hyperlipidaemia
- **Oedema**
- **Hyperlipidaemia**.

Minimal change nephropathy
- Most common cause of nephrotic syndrome in children (90%) and <20% in adults
- Exact aetiology and pathophysiology unknown
- Fatigue, peripheral or general oedema with features of nephrotic syndrome
- **Normal** light microscopy, but demonstrates **podocyte (foot processes) fusion on electron microscopy**
- Treat with **prednisolone** – most patients recover within 6 to 8 weeks, but may experience frequent **recurrences**
- Prognosis is excellent, with very few patients progressing to end-stage disease

Focal segmental glomerulosclerosis (FSGS)
- 'Focal' – particular glomeruli involved
- 'Segmental' – involves only a part of the glomerulus, as opposed to the whole of it
- Accounts for 15% of nephrotic syndrome approximately
- May be idiopathic
- Associated with Afro-Caribbean populations, **HIV**, drug abuse (heroin in particular)

- Biopsy may indicate **IgM deposition** (see *Fig. 7.5*)
- Treatment with steroids or immunosuppressive agents in patients who are unresponsive to steroids
- 50% progress, up to 50% experience remission

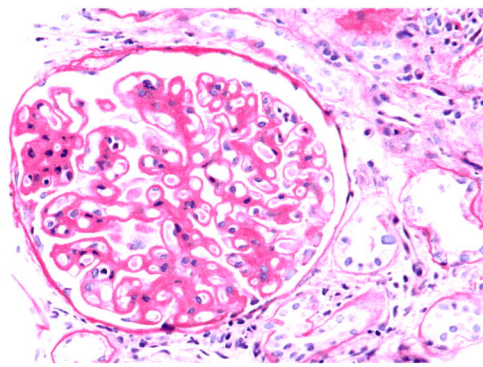

Fig. 7.5 *Histology of FSGS.*

Membranous nephropathy
- Usually affects adults, most common cause of nephrotic syndrome in **adults**
- Vast majority are **idiopathic**
- Secondary causes include malignancy (lung and colon), other autoimmune diseases, penicillamine use, gold
- Characterised by granular IgG deposits enveloped by basement membrane in a **'spike and dome'** pattern (see *Fig. 7.6*)
- Treatment is with steroids and immunosuppressive drugs
- Prognosis is based on the **rule of thirds**: one-third undergo spontaneous remission; one-third respond to treatment; and one-third progress to end-stage disease

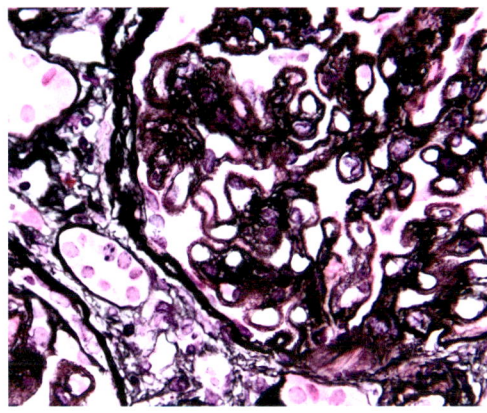

Fig. 7.6 *Silver staining histology showing basement membrane spike formation.*

7

7.3.2 Nephritic syndrome

Very broadly, **nephritic syndrome** is characterised by:
- Haematuria (microscopic/macroscopic)
- Hypertension
- Associated proteinuria with oedema (particularly periorbital/pulmonary)

Thin basement membrane disease
- Common cause of glomerulonephritis
- Autosomal dominant
- Usually presents incidentally with **asymptomatic** benign microscopic haematuria
- Excellent prognosis, reassure patient

IgA nephropathy (Berger disease)
- Most common cause of glomerulonephritis worldwide
- Classically associated with visible frank haematuria in a younger adult a few days post-URTI
- Urinalysis may demonstrate proteinuria and albuminuria along with haematuria
- Renal biopsy showing **mesangial deposition of IgA** is required to confirm the diagnosis (see *Fig. 7.7*)
- **No specific therapy**; steroids may be beneficial in some cases
- 25% progress to end-stage disease

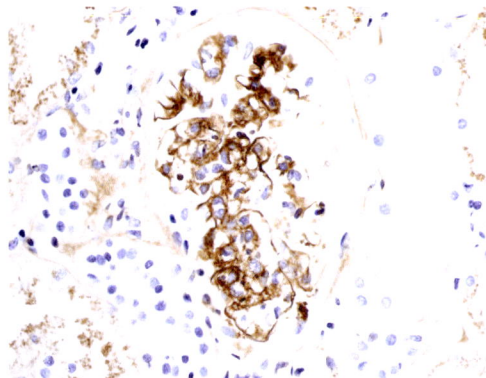

Fig. 7.7 *Immunostaining revealing mesangial IgA deposition.*

> P >> Henoch–Schönlein purpura is said to exist as a variant of IgA nephropathy, as there is some relationship between the two.

Post-streptococcal glomerulonephritis (PSGN)
- Patients usually present **1–2 weeks** after initial infection
- Features include myalgia, headache, haematuria and proteinuria
- Associated with **increased anti-streptolysin O titre (ASOT)** and a **decreased C3 level**
- Supportive management, excellent prognosis

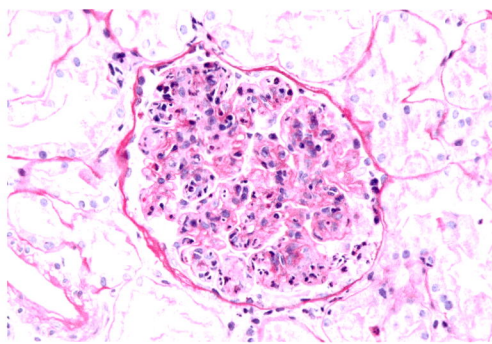

Fig. 7.8 *Micrograph of PSGN.*

Rapidly progressive glomerulonephritis (RPGN) aka Crescentic GN
- Aggressive decline in renal function, may occur as a sequela of other glomerulonephritides
- Will progress to end-stage renal failure if left untreated
- **Type I – Goodpasture syndrome**
  - Auto-antibody-mediated damage via anti-glomerular basement membrane (anti-GBM) antibodies to **type IV collagen**
  - Twice as common in men, bimodal distribution
  - Causes **haematuria** and **haemoptysis** (**RPGN** and **pulmonary haemorrhage)**
  - Approximately 70% have both lung and kidney involvement
  - Diagnosis made based on linear IgG deposits on biopsy; treatment is with plasmapheresis, steroids and immunosuppression

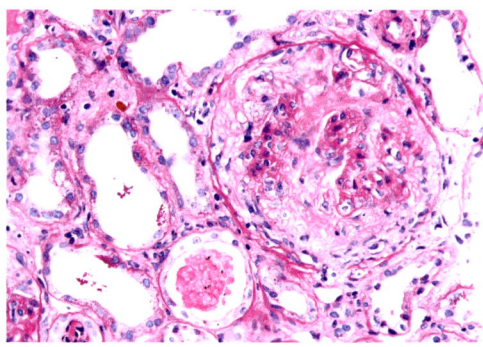

Fig. 7.9 *Micrograph of RPGN caused by Goodpasture syndrome.*

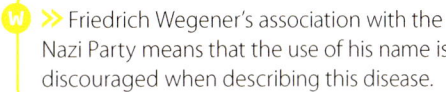

E » IgG puts the G in Goodpasture. Note that DL_{CO} may also be elevated because of possible pulmonary haemorrhage.

- **Type II – Immune complex mediated disease**
  - Sequelae of any immune complex deposition, e.g. SLE, PSGN, etc.
- **Type III – Pauci immune**
  - Associated with vasculitis, including ANCA-positive vasculitides
  - pANCA: microscopic polyangiitis, Churg–Strauss syndrome
  - cANCA: **granulomatosis with polyangiitis (GPA) (aka Wegener granulomatosis)**

Granulomatosis with polyangiitis

This condition is characterised (and classified) according to **ELK** involvement, namely, **E**NT, **l**ungs and **k**idney involvement. Features include:
- cANCA-positive RPGN
- Haemoptysis
- Otitis, epistaxis, sinusitis, rashes
- Saddle-shaped nose deformity
- Conjunctivitis
- Episcleritis

Approach to granulomatosis with polyangiitis

- Asymptomatic patients or those with no organ damage may be given methotrexate
- Immunosuppression with cyclophosphamide (and adjunctive prednisolone) for symptomatic severe disease
- NICE recommends rituximab as an alternative to cyclophosphamide, particularly if it is poorly tolerated or the patient is fairly unresponsive to therapy
- Steroids are given as adjuvant therapy for 1 year, after which they can be titrated down, provided improvement occurs

- Patients in remission can be switched from cyclophosphamide to methotrexate or azathioprine
- Surgical treatment can be offered for correction of nasal deformity

W » Friedrich Wegener's association with the Nazi Party means that the use of his name is discouraged when describing this disease.

7.3.3 Mixed nephrotic and nephritic

Membranoproliferative glomerulonephritis
- Also known as mesangiocapillary glomerulonephritis
- Proliferation of mesangial cells and basement membrane thickening
- Uncommon, associated with **SLE** and **cryoglobulinaemia**
- Half of all patients progress to end-stage disease within 10 years

Alport syndrome
- >80% of all cases have an X-linked dominant inheritance
- Type IV collagen defect, which affects the eyes, ears and kidney basement membrane
- Presents with haematuria and progressive proteinuria, sensorineural deafness and lens abnormalities (e.g. cataracts and lenticonus – a spherical projection of the lens anteriorly or posteriorly)
- No specific therapy, but ACE inhibitors control hypertension and can slow disease progression

 » Sensorineural deafness in Alport's is rarely congenital – it usually presents in childhood, prior to the onset of renal disease.

7.4 Renal vascular disease

Renovascular disease is an umbrella term used to describe causes of hypoperfusion in the kidneys. The vast majority (about 80% of cases) occur secondary to atherosclerotic disease, but there are other causes, such as renal vein thrombosis, fibromuscular dysplasia (particularly in younger women), embolism and post-transplant renal artery stenosis.

 » **Features:**
- Renovascular disease, via RAAS activation, is an important cause of secondary hypertension, and this is generally resistant to medical therapy
- Decrease in renal function with risk factors or ACE inhibitor/ARB treatment
- Recurrent pulmonary oedema in the absence of systolic impairment (aka 'flash' pulmonary oedema).

7

Approach to renovascular disease

Renal ultrasound, while helpful (may show asymmetrical, different-sized kidneys), cannot confirm the diagnosis. **Angiography** is the gold standard investigation. MR angiography may also be used in proximal disease.

> **P** ≫ Fibromuscular dysplasia associated with medial fibroplasia may have a 'beads on a string' appearance on angiography (see *Fig. 7.10*).

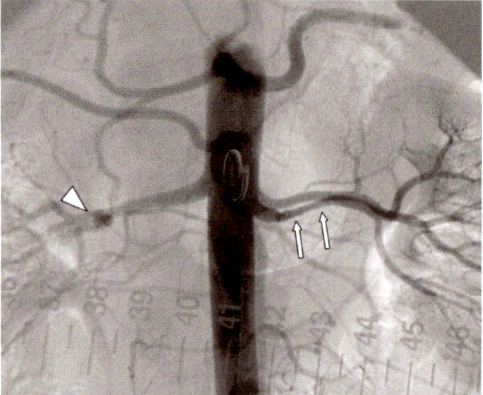

Fig. 7.10 *Renal artery angiography showing a right renal artery aneurysm (triangle) and 'beads on a string' sign (arrows) of an accessory left renal artery seen in a patient with fibromuscular dysplasia.*

Treatment involves optimising risk factors, avoiding nephrotoxic agents and managing hypertension. Whilst medical management without angioplasty is preferable if the patient is clinically stable, angioplasty should be offered if:

- Flash pulmonary oedema is present
- Hypertension is refractory to medical therapy

7.4.1 Haemolytic uraemic syndrome (HUS)

Haemolytic uraemic syndrome (HUS) is a microvascular renal disorder characterised by thrombotic angiopathy resulting in endothelial dysfunction. HUS primarily affects children (90% of cases), often related to a gastroenteritis outbreak of *E. coli* O157:H7 strain. A sporadic, less common form of HUS exists which tends to affect adults.

- Enterohaemorrhagic *E. coli* O157:H7 produces verotoxins (i.e. Shiga-like toxins) that bind to receptors on the surface of endothelial cells of the microvasculature
- This causes endothelial cells to break down, resulting in platelet activation (via tissue factor, TF) exposure, and ultimately leading to intravascular thrombosis
- Endothelial dysfunction also results in erythrocyte fragmentation and haemolysis
- This, in combination with glomerular microvascular thrombosis, leads to renal impairment

Patients with HUS often present with bloody diarrhoea and abdominal pain in the initial stages, which may progress with thrombocytopenia, jaundice and renal failure. A blood film may reveal schistocytes (erythrocyte fragmentation as a result of intravascular damage). The condition usually resolves spontaneously with conservative management. However, dialysis and plasma exchange may be required in some patients.

7.5 Cancers of the kidneys and urinary tract

Carcinomas of the kidney and bladder are discussed below. For prostate and testicular cancers, see *Chapter 5*.

7.5.1 Renal cell carcinoma

Renal cell carcinoma is the most common tumour of the kidney presenting in the adult population.

- It is more likely to present in older individuals; a small number have hereditary associations, e.g. **von Hippel–Lindau** disease
- Patients who smoke, have hypertension and have undergone long-term renal replacement therapy are at greater risk

- A significant proportion are detected incidentally, but the disease is said to present with a classic triad of symptoms:
  - Haematuria
  - Loin pain
  - Flank mass

> **E** ≫ Compression caused by renal cell carcinomas may lead to the development of varicoceles, and while this is frequently tested in exams (e.g. an asymptomatic patient with polycythaemia and a varicocele), the vast majority of tumours are picked up on imaging, and this presentation is relatively rare in practice.

- Increased red cell production (due to increased erythropoietin production)
- Renal cell carcinomas are also classically associated with **cannonball** metastases to the lung
- Treatment of renal cell carcinoma involves staging the tumour, surgical resection and adjunct chemoradiotherapy

7.5.2 Bladder cancer

Definition: bladder cancer refers to neoplastic transformation of cells or the bladder urothelium.

Epidemiology:
- Squamous cell carcinoma (SCC) is the most common type worldwide
- Transitional cell carcinoma (TCC) is the most common type in developed nations

> **E** >> Frank haematuria in an older patient is bladder cancer until proven otherwise. All individuals above the age of 45 with visible haematuria and no UTI should be referred urgently.

Aetiology/pathology:
- Patients may present with macroscopic haematuria and microscopic haematuria in about 20% of cases

- Some patients also experience dysuria and increased frequency, or bone pain/breathlessness if metastasis has occurred
- Risk factors include
  - Smoking (both SCC and TCC)
  - Schistosomiasis (SCC)
  - Aromatic amines in dyes and paints (TCC)

Investigations

> **Stepwise plan:**
>
> 1 **Attempt to rule out infective aetiologies with appropriate blood tests**
>
> 2 **Diagnosis is made on cystoscopy and biopsy**
>
> 3 **TNM staging of the disease with CT or MRI should be carried out before initiating therapy**

Management
- T1 or carcinoma *in situ* (80% of patients): transurethral resection of bladder tumour (TURBT) plus intravesical chemotherapy
- T2 or T3: radical cystectomy with ileal conduit + adjunct chemoradiotherapy
- T4: palliative chemoradiotherapy; may require long-term catheter

7.6 Infections of the urinary tract

7.6.1 Urinary tract infection (UTI)

Definition: A urinary tract infection refers to an infection of the urethra, bladder or kidneys. Of these, a bacterial infection of the bladder (cystitis) is the most common form.

Epidemiology:
- Very common – UTIs make up 2% of GP consultations
- Vast majority of UTIs are experienced by women, due to shorter urethra length
- UTIs in men should always warrant added clinical suspicion, although UTIs do typically affect older men

Aetiology/pathophysiology:

> **E** >> The most common organism causing a UTI is *E. coli*.

- Apart from infection, UTIs may also be iatrogenic
- May be caused by sexual activity or a new partner (classically described as 'honeymoon cystitis')
- Risk factors include immunosuppression, diabetes, and underlying renal tract abnormalities

> **P** >> UTIs may be classified as:
> - **Uncomplicated**
>   - Normal underlying genitourinary anatomy and physiology
> - **Complicated**
>   - Underlying anatomical or physiological abnormality predisposes to UTI (e.g. outflow obstruction, response to medications)
> - **Recurrent**
>   - Repeat infection with a new organism
> - **Relapsing**
>   - Repeat infection with the same organism

Clinical features:
- Patients typically present with:
  - Dysuria (pain or discomfort on passing urine)
  - Increased urinary frequency or urgency
  - Foul-smelling urine
- Patients with upper urinary tract infections are more likely to present with:
  - Fever, systemically unwell
  - Loin pain
  - Back pain

Investigations
NICE (CKS 2015) recommends that we:
Make a working diagnosis of UTI, given the presence of:
- Typical symptoms
- Leucocyte esterase and nitrites on urinary dipstick
  - If both are negative, UTI is unlikely
  - If leucocyte esterase is positive only, there is an intermediate chance of a UTI
  - If nitrites are positive, UTI is very likely (irrespective of leucocyte esterase level)

Management
Patients should drink more fluids, and women should be advised to wipe from front to back after urination.

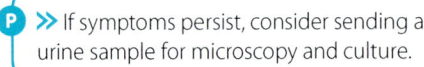

Stepwise management of UTI (NICE CKS 2015)

1 **In men:**
- Offer symptomatic relief with paracetamol and treat lower UTI without associated indwelling catheters with a course of trimethoprim 200mg BD for 7 days

2 **In women:**
- Offer symptomatic treatment with paracetamol or NSAIDs
- Uncomplicated UTI:
  - Trimethoprim 200mg BD for 3 days **or**
  - Nitrofurantoin 50mg QDS for 3 days
- Complicated UTI:
  - Consider prolonging antibiotic therapy for up to 10 days

P ≫ If symptoms persist, consider sending a urine sample for microscopy and culture.

E ≫ All pregnant patients with asymptomatic bacteriuria should have urine sent for culture and be treated with antibiotics (nitrofurantoin) for 7 days.

W ≫ The evidence base for the use of cranberry juice remains poor at the moment.

7.6.2 Pyelonephritis
Definition: pyelonephritis refers to an infection of the renal pelvis and parenchyma, and may be acute or chronic.

Clinical features:
- Pyelonephritis is most commonly a sequela of ascending UTI, likely to be caused by *E. coli*, *Proteus* or *Klebsiella*
- Acute pyelonephritis affects mostly women and the elderly
- Structural and functional urinary tract abnormalities, as well as diabetes mellitus, are risk factors for the development of pyelonephritis
- Classically characterised by a triad of fevers/rigors, loin pain and costovertebral angle tenderness, with or without nausea and vomiting
- Patients with a history of vesicoureteric reflux are more likely to develop chronic pyelonephritis

Investigations
- Urinalysis may demonstrate haematuria, proteinuria and nitrites
- Blood inflammatory markers are likely to be elevated
- **Ultrasound** is the first-line investigation
- A CT scan may be required to confirm the diagnosis in certain cases

Management
- In the acute setting, patients should be managed with analgesia, fluids and anti-emetics
- Patients should be started on **empirical antibiotic therapy**
- **Ciprofloxacin** or **co-amoxiclav** are recommended first-line therapies for 7 days

7.6.3 Prostatitis
Definition: prostatitis refers to inflammation of the prostate gland. Patients may present with systemic upset, pyrexia, dysuria, urgency or back, abdominal or pelvic pain. Patients often complain of **pain on ejaculation**. The condition has two major subtypes:
- **Bacterial prostatitis**
  - Most common form in younger men; largely caused by Gram-negative organisms
  - May also be due to sexually transmitted infections
  - May be acute or chronic

- Patients with acute prostatitis present as very systemically unwell; and the diagnosis is made on blood and urine culture
- Chronic bacterial prostatitis is likely to present with recurrent UTI
- Treat patients with antibiotics, urgently in acute prostatitis and over a prolonged period (up to 8 weeks) to allow antibiotics to reach the prostate (e.g. fluoroquinolones)

- **Non-bacterial prostatitis/chronic prostate pain syndrome**
  - Chronic prostate-related pain with no discernible cause
  - Pelvic, perineal or genital pain longer than 3 months
  - Pain on ejaculation is a commonly reported symptom

7.7 Polycystic kidney disease

Two types exist – autosomal dominant polycystic kidney disease (ADPKD) and autosomal recessive polycystic kidney disease (ARPKD).

ADPKD
- Most common inherited renal disease, affects 1:1000 individuals
- Genetic abnormalities are classified as PKD1 (most common, chromosome 16), PKD2 or PKD3
- Patients may present with:
  - Loin pain
  - Hypertension
  - Enlargement of the kidneys
  - Haematuria, kidney stones or infection

P >> Other forms of congenital kidney disease, such as horseshoe kidney (fusion of both kidneys secondary to embryological malformation) or medullary sponge kidney (cystic dilatation of ducts within the kidney) also put the patient at greater risk for stones or infection.

E >> Berry aneurysms are an important association in patients with PKD, but deciding when to intervene (and how best to) requires careful consideration, particularly if picked up incidentally.

Investigations
- Urinalysis: haematuria
- Blood tests: polycythaemia secondary to increased erythropoietin
- **Ultrasound** is the **investigation of choice** in demonstrating polycystic kidneys, and for screening relatives, particularly if there are two unilateral cysts or one cyst in each kidney in patients at risk under the age of 30
- A **CT scan** may be considered (see *Fig. 7.11*)

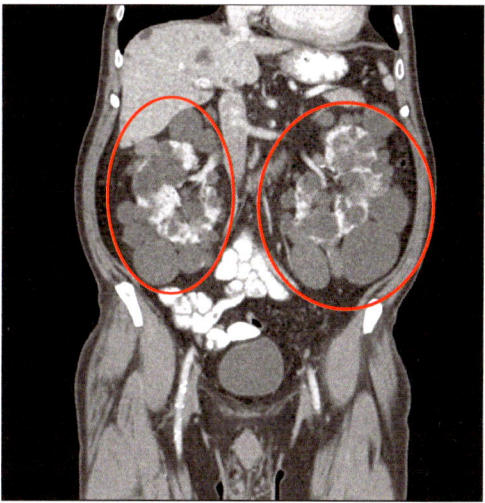

Fig. 7.11 *Coronal view of an abdominal CT showing extensive cyst formation over both kidneys and liver in a patient with ADPKD.*

Management
- Avoid contact sports
- Reduce salt intake
- Treat associated hypertension (target 130/80 with an **ACE** inhibitor)

P >> Almost half of all patients with ADPKD will develop end-stage renal disease by the age of 70.

- Manage concomitant infections (e.g. UTI, pyelonephritis)
- Pain related to cyst formation may be treated with NSAIDs or cysts may be removed surgically (drainage or laparoscopically)
- Patients will likely require a transplant or dialysis as the disease progresses

ARPKD
- Far more likely to present in infancy or childhood
- Infants are usually several months old, and may present with organomegaly, kidney disease that reaches end-stage in their teenage years and hepatic fibrosis
- Patients who present in childhood are more likely to develop liver abnormalities and have a variable degree of renal impairment

- Ultrasound is the investigation of choice in infants; CT may be used in children
- Infants require monitoring in intensive care; and liver/renal transplants may be required in the long term

7.8 Nephrolithiasis/urolithiasis

Definition: kidney stones refer to the presence of calculi within the urinary tract (from kidneys to bladder)

Epidemiology:
- Lifetime risk between 5 and 12%
- Typically affects more men than women
- More common in hot, dry or tropical regions, probably because dehydration is an important risk factor for stone formation

Aetiology/pathophysiology:
- Kidney stones are more likely to develop in urine supersaturated by compounds and minerals
- Stones may be:
  - Non-infective
    - Calcium oxalate (most common)
    - Calcium phosphate
    - Urate

> **W** >> One theory postulates that calcium oxalate stones develop due to the adherence of hydroxyapatite (calcium phosphate) crystals to the urothelial lining, creating a scaffolding called a Randall plaque. This serves as a nidus for calcium oxalate deposition and the formation of stones.

  - Infective
    - Magnesium ammonium phosphate (struvite), which may cause characteristic 'staghorn' calculi, caused by urease-producing bacteria
  - Hereditary
    - **Cystinuria** (not cystinosis!)
    - Lesch–Nyhan syndrome (see *Chapter 10*)
- Risk factors include inadequate fluid, hypercalciuria, hyperparathyroidism and disturbed oxalate metabolism

> **P** >> Cystinosis is an AR disorder causing cysteine accumulation in the renal tubules, leading to Fanconi syndrome, hypothyroidism, failure to thrive, renal disease and visual problems. Cystinuria, on the other hand, refers to an AR condition characterised by impaired amino acid absorption, saturating urine with hexagonal cysteine crystals and predisposing to stones.

Clinical features:
- Patients are likely to present with:
  - Sudden loin to groin pain (renal colic)
  - Pain radiating to the labia or scrotum
  - Haematuria, dysuria or urinary retention

Investigations

> **Stepwise plan (European Urology Association 2015):**
>
> 1 **Arrange non-contrast CT KUB (see *Fig. 7.12*)**
> - More sensitive and specific than X-ray KUB
> - Demonstrates 99% of stones on CT and allows for visualisation of anatomy
>
> 2 **Obtain blood tests, screening and urine dipstick**
> - Urine dip may demonstrate haematuria
> - Consider other aetiologies, e.g. hyperparathyroidism, congenital disorders, etc.

Management

> **Stepwise management of kidney stones**
>
> 1 **Provide analgesia and IV fluids**
> - NSAIDs recommended as first-line treatment (ibuprofen 400mg, diclofenac 75mg IM/PR)
> - Morphine may be used in severe cases

2 Definitive management
- Intervention depends on the size of the stone (see *Table 7.3*)

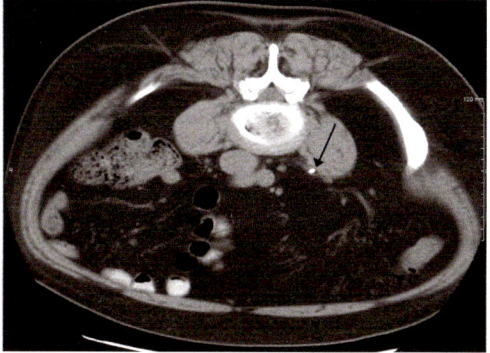

Fig. 7.12 *Non-contrast CT KUB showing a 3mm left ureteric stone.*

Table 7.3 *Management of stones in relation to their diameter*

Stone diameter	Resolution
<0.5cm	Usually resolve spontaneously
<0.5–1cm	Resolve spontaneously in 50% of cases; may require alpha blockers (tamsulosin)
>1cm	Requires intervention; consider extra-corporeal shockwave lithotripsy (avoid in pregnancy)
>2cm	Requires percutaneous nephrolithotomy

E ≫ Pregnant patients should be offered utero-scopy (passing a ureteric scope into the urinary and renal tracts to alleviate the condition) should stones occur.

7.9 Renal tubular disease

7.9.1 Renal tubular acidosis

Renal tubular acidosis (RTA) occurs as a result of **acid accumulation** due to impaired kidney excretion. Patients with RTA generally have poor acidification of the urine, and are predisposed to develop a **hyperchloraemic metabolic acidosis** with a **normal anion gap**. Note that there are several types of RTA and the condition may have a variable presentation.

W ≫ Type 3 RTA is now thought to be a combination of type 1 and 2 RTA, and is rarely discussed in modern classification.

- Type 1 (**distal**) RTA
  - Acid accumulation results from inability to acidify urine at the distal tubule
  - May develop as a primary disorder, or associated with inherited (e.g. Marfan, Ehlers–Danlos syndrome) or autoimmune disorders (e.g. SLE, Sjögren syndrome)
  - Presents with **high urinary pH, hypokalaemia, renal stones and progressive renal failure** if left untreated
  - Ensure electrolyte abnormalities are corrected; chronic disease is treated with oral bicarbonate
- Type 2 (**proximal**) RTA
  - Acid accumulation results from impaired bicarbonate resorption at the proximal tubule
  - May present with hypokalaemia, polyuria, osteomalacia or rickets

P ≫ Fanconi syndrome refers to a defect in tubular transport at the **proximal convoluted tubule**. The condition may be idiopathic, inherited (possibly alongside other conditions such as Wilson disease) or acquired (e.g. from tubular damage or nephrotoxic drugs such as cisplatin or aminoglycosides). Fanconi renal syndrome causes impaired absorption of potassium, amino acids, bicarbonate and glucose.

- Usually co-presents with **Fanconi** syndrome
- Treat with bicarbonate, correct hypokalaemia and vitamin D supplementation
- Manage Fanconi syndrome by replacing lost substances and correcting other underlying abnormalities
- Type 4 (**hyperkalaemic**) RTA
  - Associated with conditions or medications causing lowered **aldosterone**, e.g. Addison's, amyloidosis, diabetes, ACE inhibitors
  - Treat underlying cause and replace mineralo-corticoid loss with fludrocortisone if necessary

7.9.2 Hereditary tubulopathies

Bartter syndrome
This is a rare inherited renal tubulopathy characterised by mutations affecting the Na-K-Cl

co-transporter at the ascending loop of Henle. This results in impaired sodium reabsorption, leading to chronic salt wasting. The clinical biochemical picture of Bartter syndrome is similar to a patient taking a loop diuretic (e.g. furosemide) – hyponatraemia, hypokalaemia and alkalosis.

Gitelman syndrome

Gitelman syndrome is an autosomal recessive condition, characterised by NCC (Na-Cl symporter) dysfunction at the DCT. This leads to reduced Na-Cl reabsorption and chronic salt wasting. The syndrome is similar to a patient treated with a thiazide diuretic. Biochemical analysis will reveal hypokalaemia, hypomagnesaemia, alkalosis and hypocalciuria.

7.10 Renal replacement therapy

Renal replacement therapy is an important treatment modality in the management of chronic kidney disease and acute kidney injury.

Four main options are available:
- Conservative therapy
- Dialysis
- Haemofiltration
- Renal transplant

Conservative therapy
- Usually in patients with end-stage disease
- Dialysis confers no further benefit
- Symptomatic control is the goal of therapy (e.g. with dietary modification, erythropoietin, vitamin D analogues)
- Allows for better quality of life

Dialysis
- Patients are usually started on dialysis when their GFR reaches 10ml/min
- Early referral (GFR levels around 30ml/min) helps reduce morbidity
- There are two types – haemodialysis and peritoneal dialysis

Haemodialysis
- Blood is pumped past a semi-permeable membrane that acts as a substitute for the damaged kidney
- An electrolyte-rich fluid, called the dialysate, runs counter-current to the blood; and the concentration of electrolytes can be varied specifically
- Diffusion along each solute's osmotic gradient takes place, effectively removing waste products
- Ultrafiltration is used to maintain water balance
- Advantages: conducted by healthcare professionals, more emotional support available, three times a week at minimum

W >> Adequate vascular access is needed for haemodialysis, which usually involves the creation of an arteriovenous fistula between a peripheral artery and vein. This should be carried out 3–6 months prior to haemodialysis. Patients opting for haemolysis may do so daily, but a more common regimen is three times a week for 4 hours at a time.

Peritoneal dialysis
- The peritoneum acts as the 'kidney substitute'
- A Tenckhoff catheter allows infusion of fluid into the peritoneal cavity, allowing diffusion between peritoneal capillaries and the solution
- This method is more flexible, with multiple regimens
- Patients can perform continuous ambulatory peritoneal dialysis (CAPD), for four 20-minute episodes distributed throughout the day
- Advantages: flexibility, able to conduct it during sleep

E >> **Complications**
Both types of dialysis can lead to complications. Haemodialysis can be complicated by site infections, thrombosis or aneurysm formation, anaphylaxis and muscle cramps.

Peritoneal dialysis may lead to peritonitis (often complicated by *S. epidermidis*), blockage or leaking of the catheter or the development of hernias.

Despite the various complications associated with dialysis and renal replacement therapy in general, most patients on dialysis are still more likely to die from cardiovascular disease.

Haemofiltration

- Used to treat unwell patients with acute kidney injury or multi-organ dysfunction or sepsis
- Does not use diffusion as a principle
- Instead, uses convection to remove waste products steadily through a permeable membrane
- Less useful for patients who require frequent dialysis

Renal transplant

- Cadaveric (85%) or live donor (better outcomes)
- Provides best long-term outcomes
- Requires long-term immunosuppression, induction with basiliximab, followed by maintenance with triple therapy of a calcineurin inhibitor (tacrolimus or cyclosporin), mycophenolate mofetil and prednisolone

 Complications of renal transplant

- Immunosuppressive complications: increased incidence of cancers and opportunistic pathogens
- Build-up of toxic metabolites
- Recurrence of initial disease in transplanted kidney

 Rejection of the graft may also occur; this may present in various ways:

- Hyperacute rejection
  - Occurs within minutes
  - Rare, because of better HLA matching
  - Requires removal of the transplanted kidney
- Acute graft failure
  - <6 months
  - T-cell mediated or CMV-related
- Chronic graft failure
  - >6 months
  - Slow decline in renal function (rise in creatinine)
  - Vascular changes, fibrosis of kidney

Both acute and chronic graft rejection may be treated with intensification of immunosuppression and steroids, but acute rejection is more likely to respond to treatment.

7

Chapter 8
Metabolic medicine and toxicology

Samantha Jingyun Koh and *Kimberly Shuyi Loh*

Basic principles

Regulation of fluids, electrolytes and pH in the body is key in maintaining homeostasis. The kidneys, along with hormonal and neural influences, accomplish this by controlling the composition and volume of urine.

Bridge to clinical medicine

Fluids composition and compartments

Water makes up 45–75% of our total body weight. Solutes present in our body include electrolytes (such as inorganic salts, acids and base) and non-electrolytes (such as glucose, lipids and urea).

Fluids are distributed in the body in compartments: within the cells and outside the cells. Two-thirds of fluids are inside cells (intracellular), and the remaining one-third are outside cells (extracellular).

Approximately 80% of extracellular fluids are interstitial, while 20% are within the plasma (a component of blood). The transcellular compartment makes up a small percentage of the extracellular compartment, where fluid is generally not significant.

Examples include cerebrospinal fluid, synovial fluid, peritoneal fluid and pleural fluid. Osmotic and hydrostatic pressures regulate exchange of fluids between the compartments (see *Fig. 8.1*).

> **E** ≫ 'Third spacing' refers to the abnormal collection of fluids in a non-functional area that is not usually supposed to contain fluids. Fluids 'leak out' of the intravascular compartments, causing hypotension and tachycardia. At the same time, the accumulation of fluid in the abnormal space can compress nearby structures, resulting in organ dysfunction or obstruction. Conditions in which third spacing occurs include burns, pancreatitis, ascites and angioedema.

Water intake and output

Water is mostly ingested as liquids or in food, and it is absorbed via the gastrointestinal tract. A minimal portion of water comes from metabolic water produced during aerobic cellular respiration.

Regulatory hormones

These hormones regulate fluid and electrolyte balance.

- **Antidiuretic hormone**, also known as vasopressin, is produced in the posterior pituitary; it functions by:
  - Promoting water reabsorption in the distal convoluted tubules and collecting ducts of the nephron
  - Acting on the hypothalamic thirst centre to increase water consumption
- **Aldosterone** is produced by the adrenal cortex; it is released in response to low sodium levels, and angiotensin II released from the renin–angiotensin system, and acts by:
  - Increasing sodium reabsorption in the distal convoluted tubules and collecting ducts of the nephrons. This subsequently increases water reabsorption via osmosis
- **Atrial natriuretic peptide** is released from the atria in response to elevated blood pressure and volume – this results in:
  - A decrease in aldosterone release, thereby increasing sodium and water excretion in the urine
  - A decrease in ADH release, therefore reducing water reabsorption
  - A decrease in thirst, lowering water consumption

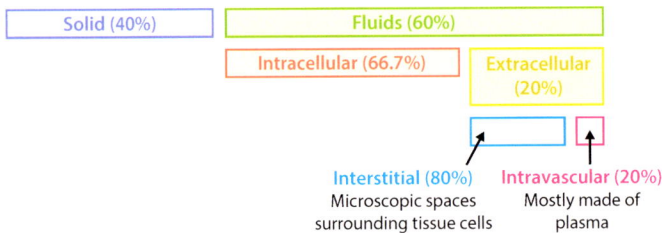

Fig. 8.1 *Fluid compartments.*

Fluid balance assessment

It is important to be able to perform a proper fluid balance assessment. A number of clinical parameters are often used to determine a patient's fluid status (see *Table 8.1*).

Table 8.1 *Clinical features of a patient's fluid status*

Parameter	Hypovolaemia	Hypervolaemia
Vital signs	↑HR, ↓BP	↑RR, ↓SpO$_2$
JVP	Not visible	↑
Urine output	↓	=/↑
Clinical signs	• Cool peripheries • ↓ skin turgor, dry mucous membranes • ↓ cap. refill time	• Pitting oedema • Crackles in lung bases, pulmonary oedema on CXR

E ≫ Performing daily weights is a good and accurate way of monitoring a hypervolaemic patient's fluid status. It is often used as a measure and a guide to diuresis therapy.

Fluid prescribing (NICE 2017, CG174)

Intravenous fluid therapy is indicated when fluid and electrolyte needs cannot be met via oral or enteral routes.

Fluid resuscitation

Stepwise management of fluid resuscitation

1 **Assess haemodynamic status**
- Indications of hypovolaemia include low blood pressure, tachycardia, increased capillary refill time, and reduced skin turgor

2 **Identify cause of deficit**

3 **If patient is haemodynamically unstable, administer immediate fluid bolus of 500ml crystalloid over 15 minutes**
- e.g. 0.9% saline, Hartmann's or Plasmalyte

4 **Reassess fluid status and repeat fluid resuscitation, up to 2000ml if needed**

5 **Seek expert help if >2000ml given and signs of shock present**

Fluid maintenance

In well and haemodynamically stable patients, fluid intake should be maximised via the oral route. The aim of maintenance fluids is to meet daily fluid and electrolyte requirements when oral/enteral intake is insufficient, and to ensure insensible losses (500–1000ml) are accounted for.

P ≫ **Daily requirements:**
- Water 25–30ml/kg/day
- Sodium, potassium and chloride 1mmol/kg/day
- Glucose 50–100g/day.

In the elderly, the malnourished, or in patients with renal or cardiac comorbidities, fluids should be given at a lower rate so as to prevent overload. Intravenous fluids that may be chosen for maintenance include: isotonic saline with/without potassium, dextrose 5% solution and dextrose saline.

Fluid replacement

In some cases, fluid maintenance is insufficient to rectify existing or ongoing fluid and electrolyte imbalances.

Stepwise management of fluid replacement

1 **Check any existing fluid or electrolyte imbalances**
- Such as dehydration, fluid overload, hypokalaemia or hyperkalaemia

2 **Check any ongoing fluid and electrolyte losses**
- Such as vomiting, diarrhoea or high biliary drain output

3 **Check any issues with fluid distribution between the fluid compartments**
- In the case of sepsis, organ failure or post-operative fluid retention

4 **Adjust the fluid prescription**
- By adding or subtracting from maintenance needs to account for the existing imbalances, ongoing losses and abnormal distribution

8

8.1 Acid–base balance

The pH of body fluids is kept within narrow limits (between 7.35 and 7.45) to allow normal cellular function to occur. Acids are generated by the metabolism of protein, fat and sugar. These are then removed via pulmonary exchange (as CO_2) or via the kidneys (through HCO_3^-). The lungs and kidneys operate jointly to maintain the pH range, with buffers playing a crucial role in minimising drastic changes in H^+ concentration. Bicarbonate (HCO_3^-) is the main extracellular fluid buffer. It combines with H^+ to form H_2CO_3, thus reducing the amount of H^+ in the blood.

$$HCO_3^- + H^+ \leftrightarrow H_2CO_3 \leftrightarrow CO_2 + H_2O$$

Acid–base disturbances may be caused by:
1. Disruptions in the regulation of CO_2 in the lungs: respiratory acidosis/alkalosis
2. Disruptions in the regulation of bicarbonate and other buffers in the blood: metabolic acidosis/alkalosis

Approach to acid–base disturbances

A stepwise approach to interpreting an ABG has been discussed (see *Chapter 2*). *Table 8.2* demonstrates the various biochemical patterns of these disturbances.

Table 8.2 *Patterns of acid–base disturbances*

		PaCO₂	HCO₃⁻
Acidosis pH <7.35	Metabolic	Normal or ↓	↓↓
	Respiratory	↑↑	Normal or ↑
Alkalosis pH >7.45	Metabolic	↑	↑↑
	Respiratory	↓↓	↓

> **W** ≫ The body attempts to compensate for pH changes by regulating HCO_3^- or CO_2 excretion. For example, metabolic acidosis causes hyperventilation (hence pCO_2 reduction) via stimulation of medullary chemoreceptors. Respiratory acidosis results in increased renal retention of HCO_3^-. This compensatory response acts in a way that allows HCO_3^- concentration and pCO_2 to move in the same direction following a primary abnormality.

8.1.1 Metabolic acidosis

The main mechanisms giving rise to metabolic acidosis are:
- **Increased acid generation** – lactic acidosis, diabetic ketoacidosis, salicylate poisoning
- **Loss of bicarbonate** – severe diarrhoea, type 2 (proximal) renal tubular acidosis
- **Diminished renal acid excretion** – renal failure, type 1 (distal) renal tubular acidosis

> **E** ≫ The serum anion gap is helpful in narrowing the differentials in a patient with metabolic acidosis. It represents the concentration of all the unmeasured anions in the plasma.
>
> **Serum anion gap** = measured cations – measured anions
>
> $$= (Na^+ + K^+) - (Cl^- + HCO_3^-)$$
>
> **Albumin** is the major unmeasured anion and contributes almost the whole of the value of the anion gap. Every 1g decrease in albumin will decrease the anion gap by 2.5 to 3mmols. As a result, the anion gap must be adjusted upwards in patients with hypoalbuminaemia.
>
> Corrected serum anion gap = (Serum anion gap measured) + [2.5 x (4.5 – observed serum albumin)]
>
> **Elevated anion gap:** usually results from increased acid generation
>
> **Normal anion gap:** usually results from a loss of bicarbonate or diminished renal acid excretion, which causes a compensatory rise in plasma chloride concentration.

8.1.2 Metabolic alkalosis

The main mechanisms giving rise to metabolic alkalosis are:
- **Intracellular shift of H^+**: hypokalaemia (causes transcellular shift of K^+ out of the cell in exchange for H^+)
- **Gastrointestinal loss of H^+**: vomiting
- **Excessive renal H^+ loss**: primary mineralocorticoid excess, loop/thiazide diuretics, Bartter and Gitelman syndromes, hypercalcaemia and the milk-alkali syndrome
- **Administration and retention of HCO_3^-**

8.1.3 Respiratory acidosis

Respiratory acidosis occurs as a result of hypercapnia ($PaCO_2$ elevation) from either increased CO_2 production or reduced elimination (alveolar ventilation).

The following give rise to respiratory acidosis:
- COPD or other underlying lung disorders
- Central disorders: stroke, obstructive sleep apnoea, brainstem disease
- Neuromuscular disorders: Guillain–Barré syndrome, myasthenia gravis, chest wall deformities
- Sedative use: benzodiazepines, opioids

8.1.4 Respiratory alkalosis

Respiratory alkalosis usually occurs as a result of alveolar hyperventilation leading to hypocapnia (decrease in $PaCO_2$).

The following give rise to respiratory alkalosis:
- **Stimulated respiratory drive**: cerebrovascular accident, psychogenic
- **Hypermetabolic**: thyrotoxicosis, fever, anxiety, pain, salicylate toxicity
- **Iatrogenic**: mechanical ventilation
- **Hypoxia induced**: pulmonary embolism, heart failure, asthma, altitude acclimatisation

8.2 Electrolyte disorders

8.2.1 Hypernatraemia

Definition: hypernatraemia is defined as a sodium concentration >145mmol. As plasma sodium concentration is dependent on the sodium and water content in the plasma, hypernatraemia can be a result of water loss, resulting in a relative effect of higher sodium content, sodium gain or both.

> E ≫ Hypernatraemia is uncommon outside the hospital setting, and patients who are elderly, young, unwell, or are receiving intravenous fluids are more likely to develop hypernatraemia.

The causes of hypernatraemia can be divided according to a patient's fluid status (see *Fig. 8.2*).

Clinical features:
- Patients with hypernatraemia tend to have CNS symptoms, such as fatigue, weakness and seizures and cerebral oedema at dangerous levels
- High sodium levels are usually diagnosed incidentally
- Diabetes insipidus, if suspected, should also be investigated

Management

Management involves treating the underlying cause, drinking plenty of water and correcting the abnormality slowly.

8.2.2 Hyponatraemia

Definition: hyponatraemia is defined as serum sodium <135mmol/L. As with hypernatraemia, the causes of hyponatraemia can be classified according to a patient's fluid status (see *Fig. 8.3*).

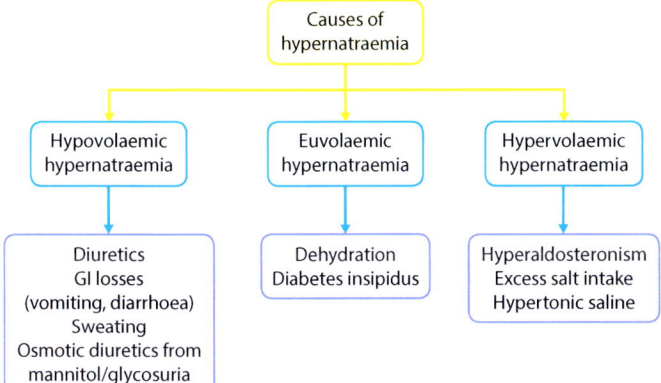

Fig. 8.2 *Hypernatraemia causes according to fluid status.*

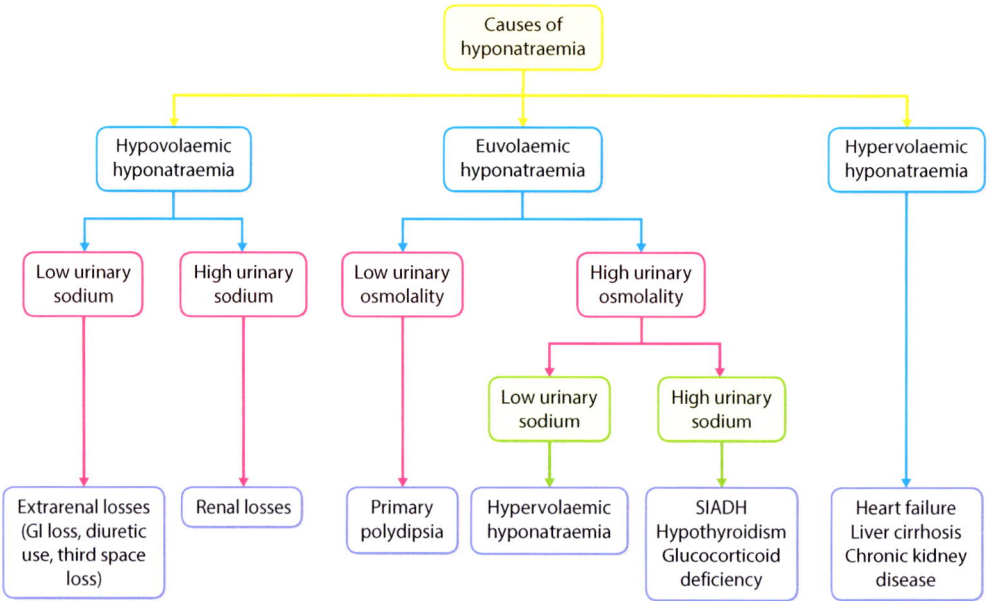

Fig. 8.3 *Causes of hyponatraemia.*

E ≫ Common drugs causing hyponatraemia are diuretics, tricyclic antidepressants, SSRIs and proton pump inhibitors.

P ≫ Sodium levels can be erroneously low due to:
1. Improper blood sampling (obtaining blood from the drip arm)
2. Hyperglycaemia
   - Presence of glucose in the plasma causes osmotic shifts of water from intracellular to extracellular space, reducing serum sodium concentration
3. Pseudo-hyponatraemia
   - Pseudo-hyponatraemia refers to low plasma sodium concentration being measured, when, in actual fact, the plasma sodium concentration is normal
   - Water makes up 93% of blood plasma volume, and 7% solids (largely lipids and proteins). Hyperlipidaemia and hyperproteinaemia result in a decrease in the ratio of water to solids. As sodium is present only in the water fraction of the plasma, this leads to an abnormally low sodium measurement
   - A direct ion-sensitive electrode (which measures only the water component), can be used in order to avoid spuriously low sodium measurements.

Clinical features:
- Symptoms include lethargy, fatigue, confusion, headache, nausea and muscle cramps
- Serum sodium levels below 115mmol/L put the patient at severe risk of developing seizures, respiratory arrest and coma
- Acute hyponatraemia (<48 hours onset), where there is a rapid drop in sodium levels, is often more dangerous than chronic hyponatraemia (>48 hours), due to lack of neuronal adaptation to the rapid alteration in serum osmolarity, causing cerebral oedema
- Acute hyponatraemia is commonly seen during the post-operative period
- In contrast, chronic hyponatraemia (>48 hours) is mostly asymptomatic or presents with mild symptoms such as impaired gait and reduced congnitive ability

Investigations

Stepwise plan:

1. **Arrange blood tests (including U&Es and TFTs)**
- To exclude hypothyroidism

2. **Perform Synacthen test**
- To exclude Addison disease (see *Chapter 4*)

3. **Obtain urinary and serum osmolality as well as urinary sodium levels**
- To guide identification of underlying cause

Management

Stepwise management of hyponatraemia

1   **Is the hyponatraemia acute or chronic?**

2   **Are the symptoms mild, moderate or severe?**

3   **Check the patient's fluid status:**
- If hypervolaemic, treat the underlying cause and fluid restrict
- If hypovolaemic, rehydrate with normal saline
- If euvolaemic, identify and treat underlying cause
- Refer to *Fig. 8.4* for details of management

W ≫ Rapid correction of sodium in non-emergency situations may lead to osmotic demyelination, and a condition known as cerebral pontine myelinolysis, leading to quadriplegia, paralysis and pseudo-bulbar palsy secondary to large osmotic shifts.

8.2.3 Hyperkalaemia

Hyperkalaemia refers to an elevation in serum potassium levels above 5.5mmol/L.

Classification of hyperkalaemia (ERC 2015)
- Mild 5.5–5.9
- Moderate 6.0–6.4
- Severe >6.5

Causes of hyperkalaemia
- Renal disease (AKI/CKD)
- Medications, e.g. ACE inhibitors, NSAIDs, cyclosporin, some antifungals
- Rhabdomyolysis, crush injuries, burns
- Acidosis, e.g. DKA

- Addison disease
- Excess administration

P ≫ Pseudo-hyperkalaemia refers to a false elevation in serum potassium level based on laboratory findings as a result of improper due process, e.g. obtaining a blood sample from a limb receiving IV potassium.

Patients may present non-specifically or with muscle weakness, palpitations or chest pain. Very severe hyperkalaemia can precipitate cardiac arrhythmias.

Apart from investigating serum urea and electrolytes, obtain an ECG.

E ≫ Features of **hyperkalaemia** on ECG (see *Fig. 8.5*):
- Flattened or absent P waves
- PR prolongation
- Broadening of the QRS
- Tall tented T waves.

Management
For emergency management of hyperkalaemia, see *Chapter* 12.

Stepwise management of hyperkalaemia

1   **Stabilise cardiac membrane, using calcium gluconate**

2   **Shift potassium intracellularly**
- Insulin/dextrose infusion, salbutamol nebs

3   **Carry out elimination**
- Binders (e.g. calcium resonium), haemofiltration/dialysis

4   **Treat underlying cause**

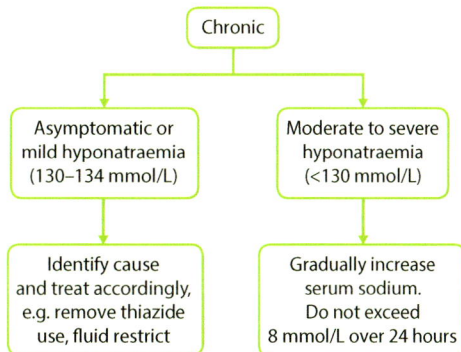

Fig. 8.4 Management of hyponatraemia.

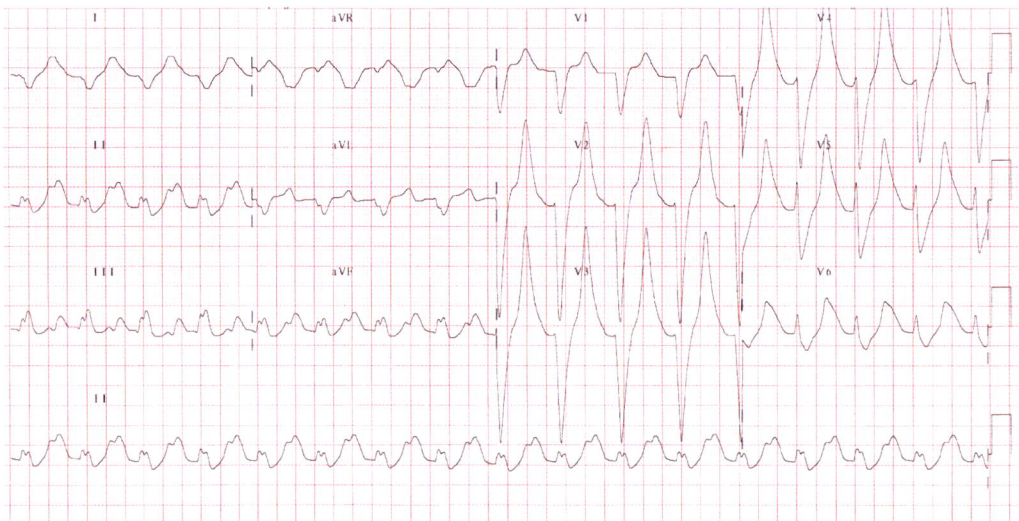

Fig. 8.5 *ECG showing tall peaked T waves, prolonged PR intervals and widening of the QRS complexes in a hyperkalaemic patient.*

8.2.4 Hypokalaemia

Definition: hypokalaemia refers to serum potassium that is <3.5mmol/L.

Aetiology:
- Reduced oral intake or GI losses
- Medication-related – diuretics, insulin
- Endocrine – Conn or Cushing syndrome
- Renal losses – hereditary tubulopathies (see *Chapter 7*)

> **W** ≫ Refeeding syndrome is a complication that occurs when a previously malnourished patient receives adequate nutrition. Reintroduction of nutrition, particularly carbohydrates, causes insulin release and increased cellular uptake of phosphate, potassium and magnesium. In this context, hypokalaemia and hypophosphataemia can provoke life-threatening arrhythmias. Careful reintroduction of feeds is therefore very important, with approximate intake at 10 kcal/kg/day, titrated up to full support by the end of the week.

Clinical features:
- Patients with hypokalaemia tend to present with muscle weakness
- They may also have cramps that may progress to paralysis and respiratory failure at dangerously low levels (<2.5mmol/L)

> **P** ≫ Check the patient's magnesium levels, as hypomagnesaemia can impair potassium retention by the kidneys, causing hypokalaemia!

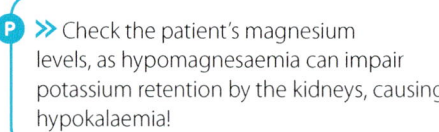
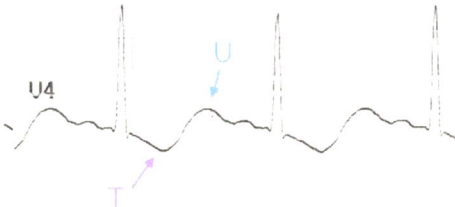

Fig. 8.6 *ECG segment showing T-wave inversion and a U wave seen in hypokalaemia.*

> **E** ≫ Features of **hypokalaemia** on ECG include (see *Fig. 8.6*):
> - Flattened T waves
> - U waves
> - ST depression.

Management

Generally, oral replacement is preferred, particularly if the hypokalaemia is not severe. If potassium is less than 2.5mmol/L, consider IV KCl (not exceeding 20mmol/h).

E » Higher rates of infusion require senior assistance, central infusion and continuous cardiac monitoring. Boluses of IV KCl should never be given under any circumstances.

8.2.5 Hypercalcaemia

Definition: hypercalcaemia refers to an elevation in serum calcium level.

Aetiology:
- Hypercalcaemia is most commonly caused by **malignancy** or as a result of **primary hyperparathyroidism**
- Other causes include exogenous administration of vitamin D, myeloma, dehydration and sarcoidosis

Clinical features:

E » **Table 8.3** *Presentations of hypercalcaemia*

Bones	Bone pain
Stones	Kidney or ureteric stones
Groans	Abdominal pain, pancreatitis
Moans	Behavioural disturbances, depression

Investigations
- Urea and electrolytes
- Calcium, phosphate, albumin
- PTH
- Vitamin D
- ECG
- CXR
- Myeloma screen
- TFTs
- ALP

P » Calcium levels need to be corrected in the setting of hypoalbuminaemia, using the formula:

Corrected calcium = Measured calcium + (0.8 × (4 – serum albumin))

Management

Stepwise management of hypercalcaemia

1 **Treat underlying cause**

2 **Provide urgent rehydration with IV fluids**

3 **Use calcitonin to lower calcium levels**
- This acts by increasing renal excretion of calcium and reducing bone resorption
- Note that calcitonin has a much weaker effect than bisphosphonate

4 **Administer bisphosphonates (pamidronate or zoledronic acid)**
- These act by preventing bone resorption

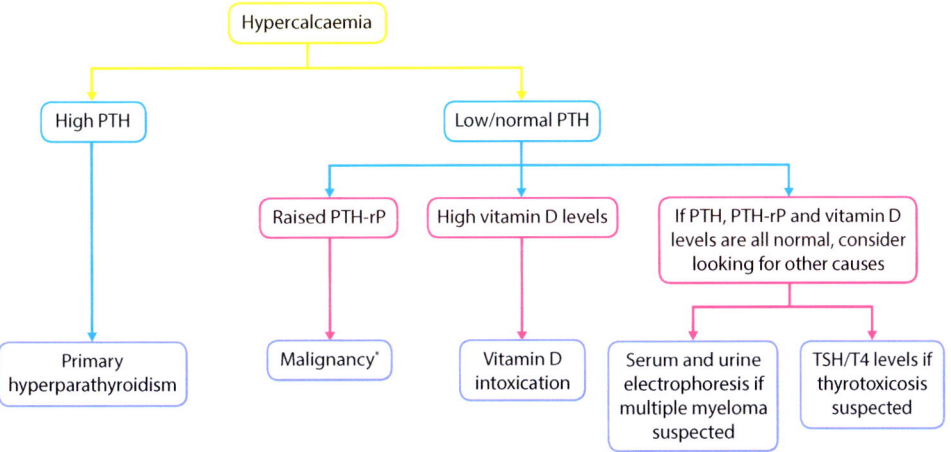

Fig. 8.7 *Diagnostic approach to hypercalcaemia.*
*PTH-rP levels are generally not needed for diagnosis as hypercalcaemia of malignancy tends to present quite obviously with symptoms and recent onset.

8.2.6 Hypocalcaemia

Definition: hypocalcaemia refers to a reduction in serum calcium level.

Aetiology:
Common
- Post-surgery (thyroid, parathyroid surgery)
- Vitamin D deficiency
- Hypomagnesaemia
- Hypoalbuminaemia

Uncommon
- Hypoparathyroidism
- Pseudo-hypoparathyroidism
- Chronic kidney disease
- Pancreatitis
- Hypermagnesaemia
- Rhabdomyolysis

Clinical features:
- Clinical features correlate with the severity of the hypocalcaemia
- Patients can present with paraesthesia of the fingers and toes, perioral paraesthesia, muscle cramps and carpopedal spasm
- In severe cases, there may be laryngospasm causing airway obstruction

> **E** »» Hypocalcaemia is associated with two eponymous signs – the Trousseau sign (carpal spasm elicited by inflating a BP cuff) and the Chvostek sign (facial spasm elicited by tapping the facial nerve).

Investigations
- U&Es, calcium, phosphate, and PTH and vitamin D. The biochemical pattern of various aetiologies varies (see *Table 8.4*)
- Check CK levels if rhabdomyolysis is suspected, and amylase if acute pancreatitis is suspected.
- ECG may show a prolonged QT interval

Table 8.4 Biochemical patterns of hypocalcaemia aetiologies

	Ca	PO$_4$	PTH
Hypoparathyroidism	↓	↑	↓
Pseudo-hypoparathyroidism	↓	↑	↑
Vitamin D deficiency	↓	↓	↑
Chronic kidney disease	↓	↑	↑

Management
- IV calcium gluconate/chloride is given in acute severe symptomatic hypocalcaemia
- Oral calcium tablets may be necessary for maintenance of calcium levels in persistent hypocalcaemia
- Patients with hypoparathyroidism generally require both calcium and vitamin D supplementation for their lifetime
- Treat any associated hypomagnesaemia to ensure effective treatment of hypocalcaemia
- Nutritional vitamin D deficiency is treated with ergocalciferol or cholecalciferol

> **W** »» PTH is required for renal conversion of inactive 25-hydroxyvitamin D to active 1-25 dihydroxyvitamin D. Therefore, patients with hypothyroidism and kidney disease will require the active forms of vitamin D supplements such as alfacalcidol and calcitriol.

8.2.7 Magnesium disorders

Hypermagnesaemia
- This condition almost always develops in individuals with renal failure who are unable to excrete magnesium, especially if additional magnesium-containing products are taken (e.g. antacids)
- May cause non-specific weakness
- Clinical levels >7 may predispose to **bradyarrhythmias** and **heart block**

> **W** »» Magnesium antagonises the cardiac effects of calcium, producing bradyarrhythmias.

- Severe disease is treated with IV calcium gluconate
- Diuretics may also be used to increase magnesium excretion, but the best therapy is to prevent excess ingestion

Hypomagnesaemia
- May be caused by nutritional deficiency, excess alcohol, severe vomiting and diarrhoea, and diuretic use
- Causes weakness, muscle cramps, arrhythmia and tetany
- Treatment with oral or IV magnesium salts, depending on severity

8.2.8 Phosphate disorders

Hyperphosphataemia
- Most commonly due to chronic kidney disease, but can also be caused by tumour lysis syndrome, rhabdomyolysis, or phosphate-containing laxatives
- The mainstay of hyperphosphataemia treatment in chronic kidney disease patients is the use of phosphate binders such as calcium carbonate, calcium acetate and sevelamer

Hypophosphataemia
- Causes include vitamin D deficiency, primary hyperparathyroidism, alcohol withdrawal and refeeding syndrome
- Treatment is with oral or IV phosphate supplementation
- IV phosphate should be used with caution as it can precipitate hypocalcaemia, renal failure and arrhythmias

8.2.9 Hyperuricaemia

Hyperuricaemia refers to an abnormally high level of uric acid in the blood. Homeostasis of serum urate levels largely depends on intake (typified by purine-rich food) and urinary excretion. Patients with hyperuricaemia may be symptomatic, presenting with gout or kidney stones, or may remain asymptomatic. Symptomatic patients should be treated (see *Chapter 10*), whilst treatment is generally not recommended for patients with asymptomatic hyperuricaemia.

> **E** >> Alcohol intake (not purine intake) is primarily implicated in the pathogenesis of hyperuricaemia. If patients with gout or asymptomatic hyperuricaemia are to make a single lifestyle modification, reducing their alcohol intake would therefore be the modification of choice.

8.3 Metabolic bone disease

8.3.1 Paget disease of bone

Definition: Paget disease of bone refers to a skeletal disorder characterised by increased breakdown of bone and haphazard remodelling, leading to bones that are both structurally and functionally weaker.

Epidemiology:
- The axial skeleton and long bones are most commonly affected
- The disease has a slightly greater predilection for males

Clinical features:
- The disease may be picked up incidentally
- If the patient is symptomatic, they are likely to describe bone pain, skeletal deformities (often hats that don't fit) or experience pathological fractures

> **W** >> Patients may also describe hearing loss as an associated symptom if the skull is affected, particularly if there is compression of the facial nerve or bony deformities of the ossicles.

- Patients with Paget disease usually have normal levels of calcium, phosphate and PTH, but have a significantly elevated bone-specific alkaline phosphatase

Management
- Alkaline phosphatase activity is also used to monitor response to treatment
- There is no specific therapy available for Paget disease
- Bisphosphonates are currently the treatment of choice, although surgical correction of deformities may be considered if medical therapy proves ineffective
- Bone healing after surgery is delayed, and it may take a significant length of time for full improvement to take place

8.3.2 Achondroplasia

Definition: achondroplasia is a common cause of dwarfism secondary to a mutation in fibroblast growth factor receptor 3 (FGFR3). This mutation may occur sporadically, or be inherited in an autosomal dominant fashion. Sporadic mutations, however, are associated with an increased paternal age. The condition may be diagnosed using prenatal ultrasound, or clinically and radiologically using skeletal surveys and X-rays.

8

Clinical features:

- Patients with the condition are likely to present with an enlarged cranium, abnormally shortened limbs and increased laxity of joints
- Other features include frontal bossing of the forehead, a flattened nose, kyphosis or lordosis, short digits and recurrent otitis

Management

- At present, the condition has no specific treatment; some centres advocate the use of growth hormone therapy, but results are not particularly encouraging
- Surgical lengthening of bones is an alternative, albeit controversial, treatment modality
- Patients should also be followed up for dental abnormalities or the presence of sleep apnoea

8.3.3 Osteomalacia

Definition: osteomalacia is a disorder of mineralisation of bone matrix (osteoid). Rickets is a disorder of mineralisation of cartilage in the epiphyseal growth plates of children.

Aetiology:

- The most common cause of osteomalacia is vitamin D deficiency (defined as serum 25-hydroxyvitamin D (25OHD) concentrations of <30nmol/L)
- Osteomalacia is associated with 25OHD levels of <20nmol/L
- This can be secondary to poor dietary intake, conditions leading to malabsorption, inadequate sun exposure, renal disease, anticonvulsant use and liver disease
- Other causes include hereditary or acquired disorders of phosphate wasting, type 2 renal tubular acidosis, or excessive use of mineralisation inhibitors (bisphosphonates)

Clinical features:

- Bone pain and tenderness (especially in the long bones and pelvis)
- Muscle weakness (usually proximal)
- Fractures with little or no trauma (ribs, vertebrae, long bones)
- Poor mobility and impaired gait
- Signs of hypocalcaemia: muscle spasms, cramps, tetany
- May also be asymptomatic and present radiologically as osteopenia

Investigations

- Calcium ($\downarrow$ or normal)
- Phosphate ($\downarrow$ or normal)
- Alkaline phosphatase ($\uparrow$)
- Serum 25OHD ($\downarrow$)
- PTH ($\uparrow$)
- U&Es (to check for underlying CKD)
- X-ray
  - Diffuse demineralisation
  - Pseudofractures (Looser zones)
  - Coarsened trabeculae
  - Insufficiency fractures

Management

> **Stepwise management of osteomalacia**

1   Treat vitamin D deficiency
- Commence a loading regimen to provide a total of approximately 300,000IU vitamin D, given either as separate weekly or daily doses over 6–10 weeks
- Follow with maintenance therapy of 800–2000IU daily (occasionally up to 4,000IU daily), given either daily or intermittently at higher doses

2   Monitor serum calcium concentration
- Following initiation of treatment, after 1 month and 3 months
- Then less frequently (every 6 to 12 months)

8.3.4 Osteoporosis

Definition: osteoporosis is a disease characterised by decreased bone mass and structural deterioration of bone tissue, with a consequent increase in bone fragility and susceptibility to fracture.

The World Health Organization (WHO, 2008) has defined osteoporosis in postmenopausal women or men as existing when axial bone density T-score (measured by dual-energy X-ray absorptiometry (DXA)) at the femoral neck falls 2.5 standard deviations or more below the average value in young healthy women (T-score $\leq$−2.5SD).

Severe osteoporosis is said to exist when there is bone mineral density (BMD) that is 2.5SD (T-score) or more below the young female adult mean, in the presence of one or more fragility fractures.

Fragility fractures are caused by mechanical forces that would not ordinarily result in fracture, known as low-level trauma. These forces are quantified as being equivalent to a fall from a standing height or less.

Epidemiology:

- Has been estimated to contribute to nearly 9 million fractures annually worldwide
- Over 300,000 patients present with fragility fractures to hospitals in the UK each year as a result of osteoporosis
- The prevalence of osteoporosis increases markedly with age, from 2% at 50 years to more than 25% at 80 years in women

Aetiology

- An imbalance between rate of bone formation and resorption results in accelerated bone loss
- BMD changes with age – the maximum BMD (peaked bone mass) is achieved around age 30–40; thereafter there is age-related bone mass, with an accelerated loss in women following menopause
- The following are associated with increased bone loss:
  - Family history
  - Lifestyle: reduced exercise, poor diet, alcohol excess, smoking
  - Drugs: steroids, cytotoxics, heparin
  - Endocrine causes: Cushing's, osteomalacia, hyperthyroidism
  - Malabsorption: coeliac disease
  - Liver disease
  - Renal disease

Clinical features:

- Usually asymptomatic, until the patient presents with a fracture, with resulting pain and deformity
- Fragility fractures
  - Most commonly in the vertebrae, proximal femur and distal radius
  - May also occur in the humerus, pelvis, ribs and other bones

Investigations

- Dual-energy X-ray absorptiometry (DXA) scan at the femoral neck (gold standard) (see *Fig. 8.8*)
- FBC, ESR
- U&E, LFTs, TFTs, serum calcium
- Testosterone/gonadotrophins in men
- Serum immunoglobulins and paraproteins, urinary Bence Jones proteins

Management

Stepwise management of osteoporosis

1 Alleviate symptoms

2 Reduce risks with lifestyle advice and education

- Stop smoking
- Carry out weight-bearing exercise
- Follow a diet that includes adequate calcium and vitamin D

8

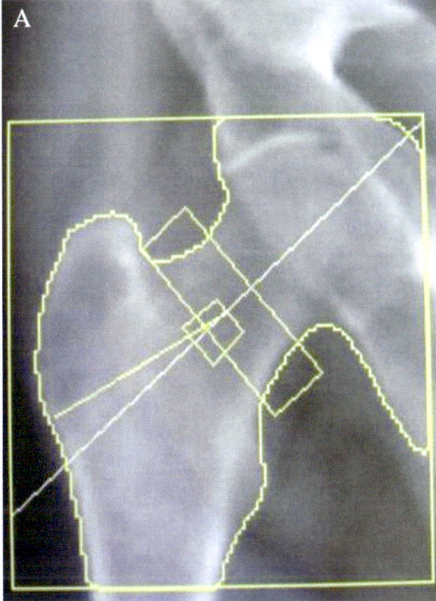
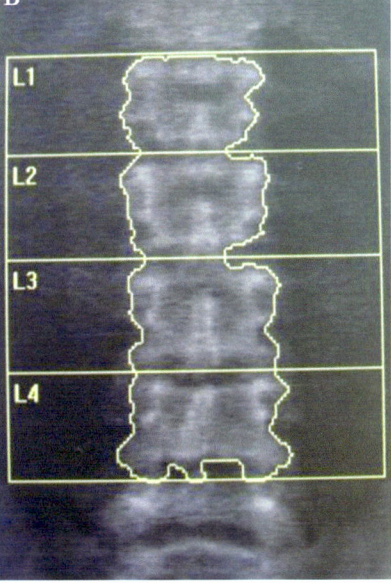

Fig. 8.8 *DXA scan of the femoral neck and lumbar spine.*

3 Use pharmacological treatment to deal with underlying causes
- Bisphosphonates (e.g. alendronate, risedronate, zoledronate), which work via osteoclast inhibition
- Selective oestrogen receptor modulators (raloxifene)
- Denosumab, which reduces osteoclastogenesis
- Strontium, which is restricted to individuals with severe osteoporosis for whom treatment with other approved drugs is not possible

 P ≫ **FRAX** calculates the 10-year probability of a major osteoporotic fracture in people aged 40–90 (with or without BMD result)

QFracture score calculates the 10-year probability of developing an osteoporotic fracture in people aged 30–99 (without BMD result)

8.4 Vitamin deficiencies

Table 8.5 *Vitamin deficiencies*

Vitamin/mineral	Clinical features
A (Retinol, retinal)	Night blindness, hyperkeratosis
B1 (Thiamine)	Beriberi, Wernicke–Korsakoff syndrome
B2 (Riboflavin)	Cheilitis, angular stomatitis
B3 (Niacin)	Pellagra – dermatitis, dementia and diarrhoea (3 Ds)
B5 (Pantothenic acid)	Paraesthesia
B6 (Pyridoxine)	Peripheral neuropathy
B7 (Biotin)	Dermatitis, GI upset
B9 (Folic acid)	Megaloblastic anaemia, neural tube defects in pregnancy
B12 (Cobalamin)	Megaloblastic anaemia, SCDC
C (Ascorbic acid)	Scurvy
D (Cholecalciferol)	Osteomalacia, rickets in children
E (Tocopherol)	Spinocerebellar ataxia (very rare deficiency)
K (Phylloquinone)	Bleeding diathesis, haemorrhagic disease of the newborn

 P ≫ Vitamin K is synthesised by gut bacteria. All newborns are at risk of Vitamin K deficiency, as vitamin K development and production are associated with adequate proliferation of gut bacteria.

 W ≫ Scurvy is a complication of vitamin C deficiency, characterised by bleeding gums, poor dentition, mottled skin and fatigue. Vitamin C is a necessary factor in the production of collagen. Patients may die from this disease, as a result of bleeding. Therapy includes introducing vitamin C-rich foods into the diet (e.g. citrus fruits and cruciferous vegetables). The disease was historically associated with sailors probably because a diet of foods rich in vitamin C (specifically oranges and lemons) was found to cure the sailors of this ailment. Scurvy was thought to be a gastrointestinal disorder in the 18th century.

 E ≫ Vitamins A, D, E and K are fat-soluble vitamins. Patients with diseases related to fat malabsorption (e.g. cystic fibrosis) are at risk for conditions linked to deficiencies in these vitamins.

8.5 Glycogen storage diseases

Glycogen storage diseases are a group of inherited or acquired defects in glycogen storage, synthesis or breakdown. There are various types, and some of the more prominent forms are listed here:

- **Type 1**: glucose-6-phosphatase deficiency (von Gierke disease) is the most common glycogen storage disorder caused by autosomal recessive impairment of liver gluconeogenesis, leading to hypoglycaemia, lactic acidosis and hyperuricaemia

- **Type 2:** acid alpha-glucosidase deficiency (Pompe disease) is an autosomal recessive disorder characterised by glycogen accumulation in the lysosomes, leading to widespread indiscriminate muscle weakness, resulting in impairment of skeletal muscle and cardiomyopathy

- **Type 3**: glycogen debranching enzyme deficiency (Cori disease) is an autosomal recessive disorder

8.6 Porphyria

Porphyria refers to a group of inherited metabolic conditions involving enzyme deficiencies in haem synthesis. The overproduction and accumulation of haem precursors (porphyrins) is responsible for the various clinical presentations of the disease. They are usually caused by inherited genetic mutations with both autosomal dominant and recessive inheritance. Porphyrias are classified by their different enzyme deficiencies. However, they can be broadly categorised as acute, cutaneous and mixed (see *Table 8.6*).

Table 8.6 *Types of porphyria*

Acute	• Acute intermittent porphyria (AIP) • Aminolaevulinic acid dehydratase porphyria
Cutaneous	• Porphyria cutanea tarda (PCT) • Erythropoietic protoporphyria • Congenital erythropoietic porphyria
Mixed	• Hereditary coproporphyria • Variegate porphyria

8.6.1 Acute intermittent porphyria (AIP)

This condition affects twice as many women as men.

Aetiology:
- Attacks may be precipitated by certain medications (e.g. barbiturates, anti-epileptics, COCP)
- Other possible triggers include alcohol, dehydration and infection as well as physical and emotional stress

Clinical features:
- Symptoms occur intermittently, and patients may be asymptomatic between attacks

- Symptoms may include reddish, dark urine (see *Fig. 8.9*) and fever, episodic abdominal pain, nausea and vomiting
- Sympathetic activation – ↑BP, HR, sweating
- Neuropsychiatric symptoms – seizures, psychosis, neuropathy

> **E** ≫ AIP is an important differential diagnosis of an acute surgical abdomen. It should be excluded prior to surgery, as certain anaesthetic agents may trigger or worsen acute porphyria.

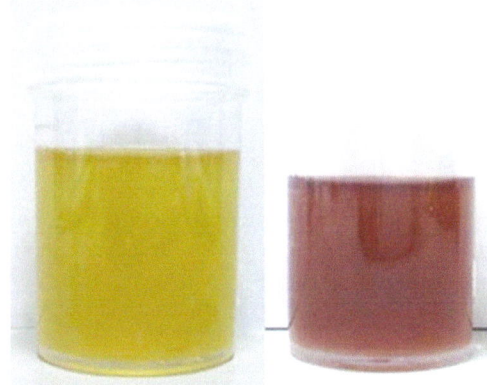

Fig. 8.9 *Normal-coloured urine on the left, compared to reddish urine seen in a patient with acute porphyria.*

Management
- Diagnosis is made based on the presence of increased urinary porphobilinogen (PBG) and total porphyrins

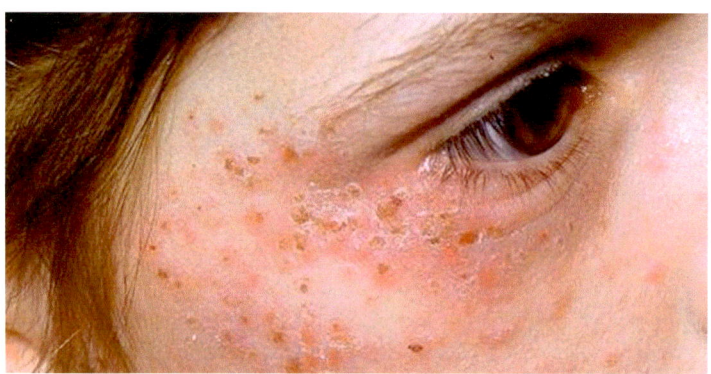

Fig. 8.10 Cutaneous manifestation of porphyria.

- Management remains largely supportive – precipitants and underlying causes should be avoided and treated
- IV haemin may be used in more severe acute attacks

8.6.2 Porphyria cutanea tarda

This is the commonest form of porphyria, affecting 2–5 per million of the UK population.

Aetiology:
- Occurs as a result of deficiency in hepatic uroporphyrinogen decarboxylase enzyme (UROD)
- Unmetabolised substrates accumulate and are deposited at cutaneous tissues

Clinical features:
- Presents **with blistering, photosensitive skin lesions** (see *Fig. 8.10*)
- Other signs include skin hyperpigmentation and reddish, dark urine
- Liver failure may develop as a result of ferritin accumulation

Management
- Treatment involves sunlight avoidance and regular phlebotomy to reduce serum ferritin
- Chloroquines may be used alternatively, when phlebotomy is contraindicated

8.7 Toxicology

Toxicology is the study of the adverse effects of chemical or physical agents on living organisms. Suspected poisoning, which may include accidental exposures, deliberate self-poisoning, drug misuse and therapeutic errors, is a common reason for presentation to health services.

About 140,000 people with suspected poisoning are admitted to hospitals across the UK each year. Many more are seen in emergency departments and discharged, or managed in primary care, frequently using NHS advice lines such as NHS 111, NHS Direct (Wales) and NHS 24 (Scotland). The National Poisons Information Service (NPIS) provides information and advice to support the management of these patients, using information from the poisons information database TOXBASE.

8.7.1 Paracetamol overdose

Paracetamol (acetaminophen in the USA) overdose is the most common toxicological emergency and the most common cause of liver transplant and death due to poisoning.

Pathophysiology:
- In a normal individual, 90% of paracetamol is conjugated in the liver with glucuronide and sulphate conjugates and then excreted in the urine
- About 2% is eliminated by the kidneys, and the remaining 8% is metabolised oxidatively by the cytochrome P450 system in the liver – during this process, a hepatotoxic compound N-acetyl-p-benzoquinone imine (NAPQI) is created which rapidly binds to glutathione and is cleared
- However, once glutathione levels are depleted, NAPQI accumulates and is free to bind to hepatocellular membranes, resulting in cell death and ultimately, liver failure
- Toxicity has been demonstrated at single paracetamol ingestion doses of >150mg/kg taken in less than 1 hour, or 12g in adults
- However, the threshold is lowered in patients with an induced P450 system (hence increased rate of NAPQI formation) or with low glutathione stores (such as HIV, or cystic fibrosis, or anorexic patients)

Clinical features:

- Patients usually look well initially, with minimal or no symptoms; therefore, despite a lack of significant early symptoms, patients who have taken an overdose of paracetamol should be transferred to hospital urgently
- A decrease in GCS should prompt the search for ingestion of other drugs
- **Phase 1** (up to 24 hours): anorexia, nausea and vomiting
- **Phase 2** (24–72 hours): right subcostal pain and tenderness
- **Phase 3** (72–96 hours): jaundice, encephalopathy, cerebral oedema, hypoglycaemia coagulopathy, acute renal failure, death
- **Phase 4** (4–14 days): recovery

Investigations

- Full blood count, U&Es, liver function tests, prothrombin time, clotting, INR, glucose
- Serum paracetamol levels (ideally 4 hours post-ingestion)

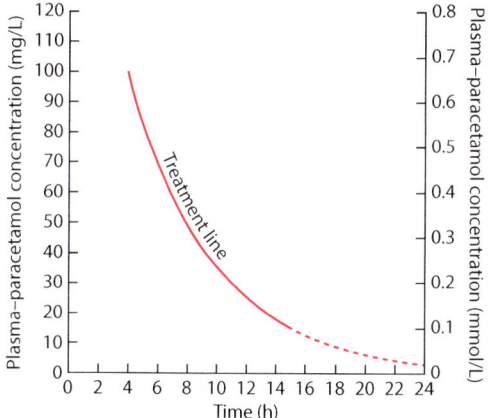

Fig. 8.11 *Paracetamol overdose treatment nomogram.*

Management (BNF/TOXBASE)

Stepwise management of paracetamol overdose

1 For acute overdose

- Administration of activated charcoal if ≥150mg/kg paracetamol ingested in ≤1 hour
- Commence acetylcysteine immediately in patients:

  – Whose plasma–paracetamol concentration falls on or above the treatment line on the paracetamol treatment graph (see *Fig. 8.11*)
  – Who present 8–24 hours after taking an acute overdose of more than 150mg/kg of paracetamol, even if the plasma–paracetamol concentration is not yet available

2 For staggered overdose, uncertain time of overdose, or therapeutic excess

- Commence acetylcysteine immediately, unless >24 hours since the last ingestion, the patient is asymptomatic, the plasma–paracetamol concentration is undetectable, and liver function tests, serum creatinine and INR are normal

3 When treating with acetylcysteine

- This protects the liver if infused up to, and possibly beyond, 24 hours of ingesting paracetamol
- Most effective if given within 8 hours of ingestion, after which effectiveness declines
- Administer via three consecutive intravenous infusions over 21 hours:
  1. 150mg/kg, in 200ml 5% dextrose, over 1 hour
  2. 50mg/kg, in 500ml 5% dextrose, over 4 hours
  3. 100mg/kg, in 1000ml 5% dextrose, over 16 hours
- Common side effects: flushing, urticaria, pruritus – treat with antihistamines

8.7.2 Salicylate overdose

Salicylates are used as analgesic agents and are found in numerous over-the-counter medications, the most common being aspirin. While not as common as paracetamol ingestion, salicylate overdose still accounts for a significant number of poisoning incidents.

Pathophysiology:

- Inhibition of cyclo-oxygenase contributes to platelet dysfunction and gastric mucosal injury
- Stimulation of the chemoreceptor trigger zone in the medulla causes nausea and vomiting
- Activation of the respiratory centre in the medulla results in hyperventilation and respiratory alkalosis
- Alterations in cellular metabolism lead to metabolic acidosis

8

Clinical features:

- Unlike paracetamol overdose, the onset of symptoms begins relatively early following salicylate overdose (1–2 hours; peaking at 12–24 hours)
- Fatal aspirin intoxication can occur after the ingestion of 10–30g by adults and as little as 3g by children

> E ≫ Patients present with an initial respiratory alkalosis and subsequently a metabolic acidosis.

- Plasma concentrations 6 hours after an overdose roughly correlate with degree of toxicity
  - **Mild** toxicity (300–500mg/L): ototoxicity (especially tinnitus), hyperpnoea with respiratory alkalosis, sweating
  - **Moderate** toxicity (500–700mg/L): vomiting, severe hyperpnoea, hyperthermia, dehydration, abdominal pain
  - **Severe** toxicity (>750mg/L): CNS depression, seizures, coma, metabolic acidosis, pulmonary oedema, acute renal failure, death due to cardiovascular collapse/respiratory failure/CNS failure

Investigations

- Initial and serial (every 2 hours) salicylate levels until levels fall
- U&Es, liver function tests, INR, glucose
- ABG, serum bicarbonate and pH
- Urinalysis, urine output

Management

> **Stepwise management of salicylate overdose (TOXBASE)**
>
> 1 **Administer activated charcoal**
>   - If ≥125mg/kg salicylate ingested in ≤1 hour
>
> 2 **Replace fluid losses**
>
> 3 **For urine alkalinisation and correction of metabolic acidosis**
>   - Administer intravenous sodium bicarbonate to enhance urinary salicylate excretion (optimum urinary pH 7.5–8.5)
>
> 4 **Correct plasma–potassium concentration before giving sodium bicarbonate**
>   - As hypokalaemia may complicate alkalinisation of the urine

> 5 **Consider haemodialysis**
>   - This is the treatment of choice for severe salicylate poisoning, when the plasma–salicylate concentration >700mg/L or in the presence of severe metabolic acidosis

8.7.3 Organophosphate poisoning

Organophosphorus is one of the commonest insecticides, used in several products.

Pathophysiology:

- Organophosphorus is absorbed through the bronchi and intact skin, as well as through the gut
- Toxicity occurs through the inhibition of cholinesterase activity via the active agent parathion
- This prolongs and intensifies the effects of acetylcholine

Clinical features:

- The clinical features of organophosphate poisoning are the result of muscarinic and nicotinic effects of excess acetylcholine
- They include anxiety, restlessness, dizziness, headache, miosis, nausea, hypersalivation, vomiting, abdominal colic, diarrhoea, bradycardia and sweating
- Muscle weakness and fasciculation may develop and progress to generalised flaccid paralysis, including the ocular and respiratory muscles
- Convulsions, coma, pulmonary oedema with copious bronchial secretions, hypoxia, and arrhythmias occur in severe cases

Management

- Avoid further absorption
- Implement airway protection, optimisation of breathing and adequate ventilation and oxygenation
- Gastric lavage may be considered, provided the airway is protected
- Intravenous injection – atropine 2mg (20micrograms/kg) every 5 to 10 minutes until the skin becomes flushed and dry, the pupils dilate, and bradycardia is abolished
- **Pralidoxime chloride** (cholinesterase reactivator) can be used as an adjunct to atropine in moderate or severe poisoning, and continued until the patient has not required atropine for 12 hours

8.7.4 Opiate/opioid overdose

Opioids are psychoactive substances which act on opioid receptors in the body when administered, resulting in reduced perception of pain. They include both prescription analgesics (e.g. morphine, codeine, tramadol, fentanyl) and illegal drugs (e.g. heroin). Worldwide, opioids are responsible for a high proportion of drug-related deaths from overdose, due to their effects on the nervous system.

Clinical features:
- Respiratory depression
- Pinpoint pupils
- Hypotension
- Bradycardia
- Coma

Investigations

Stepwise plan:

1 Obtain FBC, U&Es, creatine kinase, ABG

2 Measure ± blood paracetamol levels

3 Arrange ECG

4 Establish and maintain a clear airway, adequate ventilation and oxygenation

Management

Stepwise management of opiate/opioid overdose

1 Administer intravenous naloxone
   - 0.4–2.0mg (adult), and 0.01mg/kg (child), if coma or respiratory depression is present
   - Repeat at 2- to 3-minute intervals, if necessary, until the patient is breathing adequately

2 If no intravenous access, administer intramuscular naloxone

3 Carry out frequent measurements of observations (especially respiratory rate) and mental status

4 Observe for at least 6 hours after the last administration of naloxone

P ≫ Naloxone is an opioid antagonist with a much shorter half-life than most opioids. In opioid-dependent users, naloxone may precipitate a withdrawal syndrome (agitation, abdominal pain, nausea).

8.7.5 Carbon monoxide poisoning

Despite public awareness campaigns, carbon monoxide poisoning continues to be an important preventable cause of morbidity and mortality, with most exposures occurring in the home.

Pathophysiology:
- The lethality of carbon monoxide stems from its ability to bind preferentially to haemoglobin and myoglobin, reducing the oxygen-carrying capacity of the blood
- This leads to reduced oxygen delivery and utilisation, and oxidant stress injury in various tissues, including diffuse brain demyelination
- Organs with higher metabolic demands are more sensitive to the effects of CO exposure

Clinical features:
- **CNS:** headache, altered mental state, cerebral oedema, memory impairment, ataxia, coma, delayed neuropsychiatric effects
- **Cardiovascular:** tachycardia, hypotension, ST changes, angina, myocardial infarct, cardiac arrest
- **Respiratory:** tachypnoea, dyspnoea, pulmonary oedema
- **Others:** oliguria, tissue hypoxia, rhabdomyolysis

Investigations
- FBC, capillary glucose, U&Es
- ABG with COHb
- 12-lead ECG

Management
Immediate treatment is essential.

Stepwise management of carbon monoxide poisoning

1 Orotracheal intubation if ventilation/ oxygenation is compromised

2 100% oxygen via a tight-fitting mask with an inflated face seal

3 Intravenous infusion of mannitol for cerebral oedema

4 Intravenous infusion of sodium bicarbonate for significant metabolic acidosis

5 Referral for hyperbaric oxygen treatment
   - Discuss with the National Poisons Information Service (NPIS)

8

8.7.6 Snake bites and bee stings

Snake bites

These are relatively uncommon in the UK.

Clinical features:

- A snake bite may cause local and systemic effects
- Local effects: pain, swelling, bruising and tender lymphadenopathy
- Systemic effects: early anaphylactic symptoms (transient hypotension with syncope, angioedema, urticaria, abdominal colic, diarrhoea, and vomiting), with later persistent or recurrent hypotension, ECG abnormalities, spontaneous systemic bleeding, coagulopathy, adult respiratory distress syndrome, and acute renal failure

Management

Stepwise management of snake bites

1. **Adrenaline (for anaphylactic symptoms)**

2. **10ml anti-venom (if systemic envenoming)**
   - By intravenous injection over 10–15 minutes
   - Or by intravenous infusion on 0.9% NaCl over 30 minutes
   - Repeat after 1–2 hours if symptoms persist

Bee stings

Bee stings cause local pain and swelling but seldom cause severe direct toxicity unless multiple stings are inflicted at the same time. If the sting is in the mouth or on the tongue, local swelling may threaten the upper airway.

Management

Stepwise management of bee stings

1. **Remove the sting and clean the area with a topical antiseptic**

2. **Use an intramuscular adrenaline (EpiPen) for anaphylactic reactions**

3. **Use an inhaled bronchodilator for asthmatic reactions**

4. **Antihistamines or topical corticosteroids may help reduce inflammation and relieve itching**

8

Chapter 9
Infectious diseases

Amar Vaswani and *Hwan Juet Khaw*

Basic principles

Infectious diseases, a group of disorders largely caused by microscopic organisms, are some of the leading causes of death worldwide. In low-income countries, they make up the leading cause of death – in the form of respiratory infections.

Bridge to clinical medicine

Bear in mind that the list of pathogenic organisms and antibiotics that follows is by no means exhaustive. In this chapter, we have focused on the more commonly tested/encountered organisms and their key associations/antibiotic choices.

Bacteria

Being prokaryotic organisms invisible to the naked eye and on light microscopy, bacteria require staining in order to be adequately visualised. Chief amongst these stains is the Gram stain, which helps differentiate bacteria by largely subdividing them into two groups – Gram-positive (blue) and Gram-negative (red). *Figs 9.1, 9.3* and *9.4* provide a broad overview of some of these common bacteria.

> **W** ≫ This difference is accounted for by the difference in the composition of the cell walls of these organisms. Gram-positive bacteria have a thick cell wall, composed of peptidoglycan. The blue dye used in Gram staining is therefore taken up and intermeshed within the wall. Gram-negative organisms have thinner walls and a lipid-rich outer membrane (see *Fig. 9.1*). This prevents the Gram stain from being taken up, whilst allowing these organisms to absorb the red safranin counter-stain applied thereafter. Variations in structure and cellular composition also explain why specific antibiotics work against particular groups of bacteria, targeting certain structures or enzymes within them.

- The outer membrane of Gram-negative organisms contains lipopolysaccharide (LPS). A major component of LPS is **lipid A**, also known as **endotoxin**

> **P** ≫ *Listeria* spp. is the only Gram-positive group of bacteria that contains endotoxin.

- Bacteria may be classified by shape:
  - Bacillus (rod)
  - Coccus (circular)
  - Spirochaetes
  - Curved rods
- Bacteria also have various structures that function as **virulence factors** (e.g. pili, toxins, spores and capsules)
- Spores are inactive forms of bacteria that are extremely durable; they can withstand extremes of temperature and various chemicals, and are therefore far more difficult to eradicate
- There are six main types of bacterial genus that are Gram-positive

> **E** ≫ Mycobacteria (which cause tuberculosis and leprosy) are partially Gram-positive. The preferred stain of choice is the acid-fast (Ziehl–Neelsen) stain to visualise these bacteria.

- Spirochaetes are Gram-negative organisms but cannot be identified on Gram stain with light microscopy; these spiral-moving bacteria can thus be visualised using **dark field microscopy** (see *Fig. 9.2*)

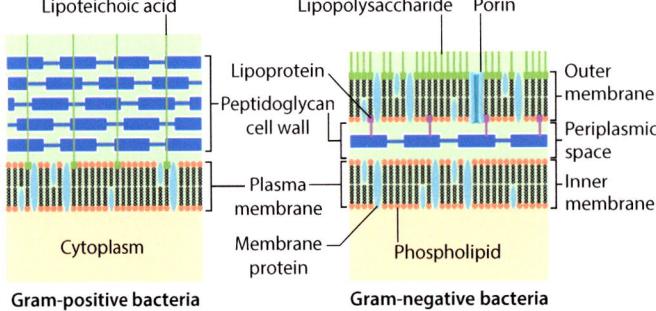

Fig. 9.1 *Comparison of cell wall structure between Gram-positive and Gram-negative bacteria.*

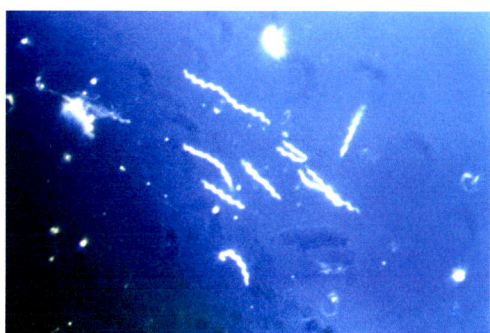

Fig. 9.2 Borrelia burgdorferi, *a spirochaete bacteria, visualised as 'corkscrews' under dark field microscopy.*

Antimicrobials

Penicillins

- Initially 'discovered' by Alexander Fleming, this original version is known as Penicillin G (usually given IM or IV)
- It binds to transpeptidase on the bacterial cell walls and inhibits further synthesis
- Over time, resistance developed, leading to production of beta-lactamases by various bacteria (most notably *Staph. aureus*)
- Further modification of penicillin structure led to the development of beta-lactamase resistant penicillins – namely, methicillin, nafcillin, cloxacillin and dicloxacillin, which are effective against *Staph. aureus*

Gram-positive bacteria

Streptococci (cocci in strips)

Group A Strep
- Beta haemolytic
- URTI with purulent tonsillar exudate
- Cellulitis
- Scarlet fever
- Rheumatic fever
- Glomerulonephritis

Group B Strep
- Beta haemolytic
- May be part of vaginal flora
- Neonatal meningitis/sepsis

S. pneumoniae
- Encapsulated organism
- Pneumonia
- Meningitis

S. viridans
- Alpha haemolytic
- Subacute bacterial endocarditis

Staphylococcus (cocci in clusters)

Staphylococcus aureus
- Various forms of infection/sepsis

Staphylococcus epidermis
- Normal skin commensal
- Hospital-acquired infections
- Prosthetic infections

Gram-positive bacteria

Clostridium (spore forming rod)

C. tetani
- Tetanus

C. botulinum
- Botulism
- Botox

C. difficile
- Pseudomembranous colitis

C. perfringens
- Gas gangrene

Bacillus (spore forming rod)

Bacillus cereus
- Food poisoning

Bacillus anthraces
- Cutaneous and systemic anthrax

Listeria (non-spore forming rod)

Listeria monocytogenes
- Neonatal meningitis
- Immunocompromised individuals

Corynebacterium (non-spore forming rod)

Corynebacterium diphtheriae
- Diphtheria

9

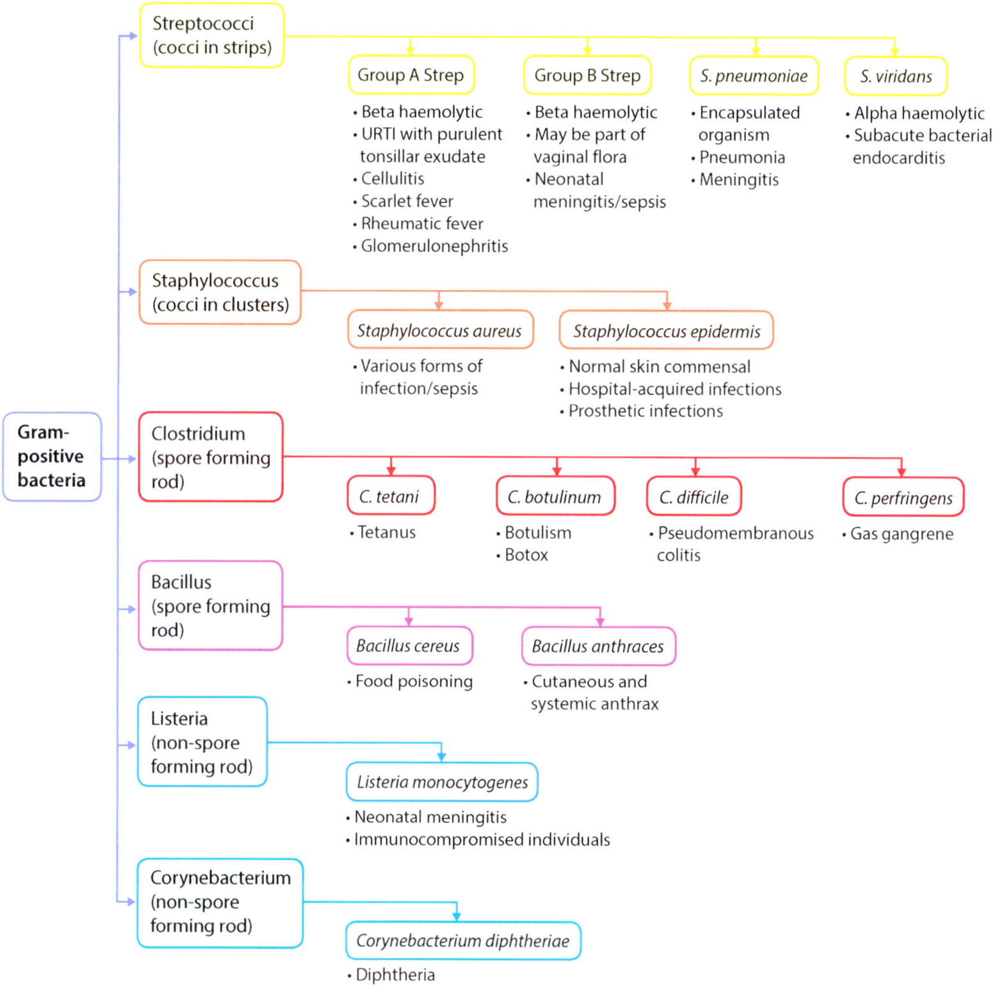

Fig. 9.3 *Schematic diagram showing the different types of Gram-positive bacteria.*

Gram-negative bacteria

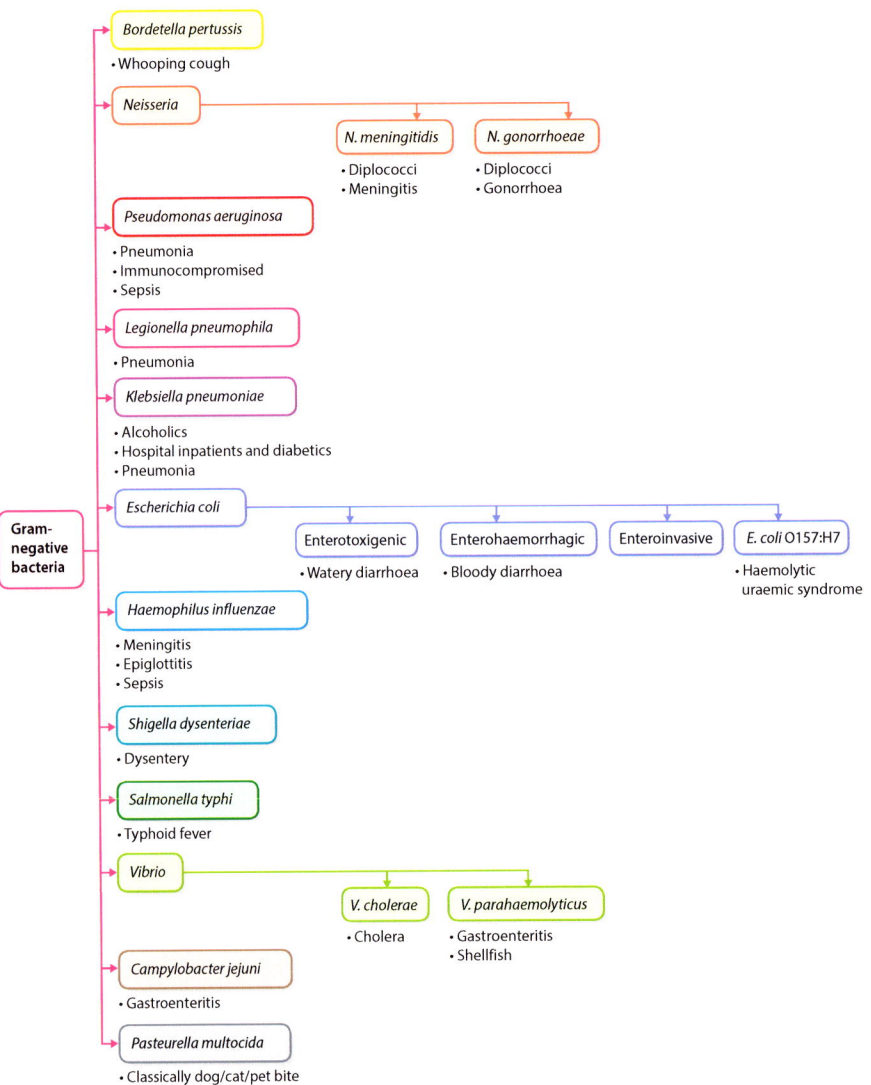

Fig. 9.4 *Schematic diagram showing the different types of Gram-negative bacteria.*

- *Pseudomonas* spp. are notoriously difficult to eradicate, but can be dealt with using anti-pseudomonal penicillins, such as piperacillin (frequently given with tazobactam as Tazocin) or ticarcillin
- Penicillins may also be used in combination with beta-lactamase inhibitors to increase their potency (e.g. amoxicillin can be given together with clavulanic acid as co-amoxiclav) and cover a broad range of bacteria

Cephalosporins

- There are several generations of cephalosporins available, each of which has a distinct effect
- As a general rule, the spectrum for coverage of Gram-positive organisms decreases from first generation to third generation

E >> The most common side effects noted in patients taking cephalosporins are gastrointestinal in nature.

- First generation
  - Examples include **cephalexin** and **cefazolin**
  - Gram-positive activity, weak efficacy against Gram-negatives
  - Not effective against MRSA
- Second generation
  - Examples include **cefoxitin, cefuroxime** and **cefotetan**
  - Greater Gram-negative activity than first-generation cephalosporins
- Third generation
  - Third-generation cephalosporins have broad-spectrum activity and excellent efficacy against Gram-negative organisms
  - First-line treatment for meningitis
  - Examples include **ceftriaxone** and **cefotaxime**
- Fourth generation
  - Better efficacy against both Gram-positive and Gram-negative agents than third-generation cephalosporins
  - Examples include **cefepime** and **cefpirome**
  - Effective against *Pseudomonas* spp.
- Fifth generation (novel)
  - **Ceftaroline**, a fifth-generation cephalosporin, is a broad-spectrum antibiotic, which acts against Gram-positive and Gram-negative organisms

P >> Ceftaroline is also the only cephalosporin that has activity against MRSA.

Carbapenems

- These are broad-spectrum agents generally used in individuals who have hospital-acquired infections, or organisms with multi-drug resistance
- These are common treatment modalities in cases of neutropenic sepsis

E >> Carbapenems are also beta-lactam antibiotics, much like the penicillins and cephalosporins.

Aminoglycosides

- Aminoglycosides are antibiotics with anti-ribosomal properties, inhibiting organism protein synthesis

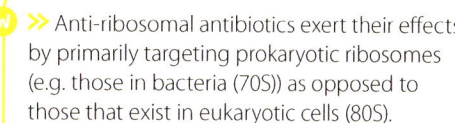

W >> Anti-ribosomal antibiotics exert their effects by primarily targeting prokaryotic ribosomes (e.g. those in bacteria (70S)) as opposed to those that exist in eukaryotic cells (80S).

- Examples include **gentamicin, tobramycin** and **amikacin**
- Doses need to be titrated carefully and by weight, as the drug has a narrow therapeutic window

E >> Aminoglycosides are **ototoxic** and **nephrotoxic**.

Tetracyclines (includes doxycycline, demeclocycline and minocycline)

- These disrupt prokaryotic bacterial synthesis by targeting the small ribosomal subunit

E >> Side effects of doxycycline include tooth discoloration in children, photosensitivity and type II renal tubular acidosis.

Macrolides

- Examples include **clarithromycin, erythromycin** and **azithromycin**
- Antifungals, such as amphotericin B and nystatin, are macrolide derivatives
- They primarily target Gram-positive organisms, with some Gram-negative activity

P >> Macrolides may sometimes interact negatively with statins, particularly clarithromycin and erythromycin, by inhibiting the cytochrome P450 system, and may cause muscle pain and damage. Macrolide antibiotics may also prolong the QT interval and, rarely, lead to polymorphic ventricular tachycardia. They may also cause GI upset and should not be co-administered with colchicine.

Clindamycin

- Despite having similar nomenclature and a similar mechanism of action (anti-ribosomal activity), clindamycin is not a macrolide

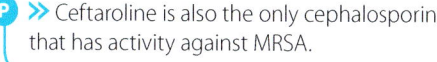

9

Chloramphenicol

- This is an anti-ribosomal antibiotic
- Side effects include **grey baby syndrome**, and **bone marrow suppression**

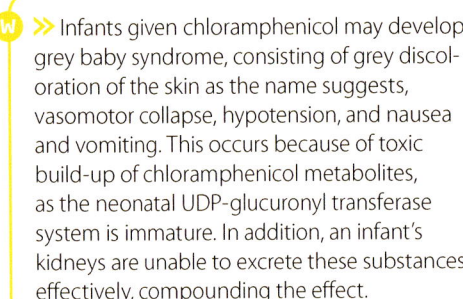 **W** ≫ Infants given chloramphenicol may develop grey baby syndrome, consisting of grey discoloration of the skin as the name suggests, vasomotor collapse, hypotension, and nausea and vomiting. This occurs because of toxic build-up of chloramphenicol metabolites, as the neonatal UDP-glucuronyl transferase system is immature. In addition, an infant's kidneys are unable to excrete these substances effectively, compounding the effect.

Fluoroquinolones

- These broad-spectrum antibiotics work by inhibiting DNA gyrase
- Examples include **ciprofloxacin, levofloxacin, moxifloxacin**
- They are contraindicated in pregnancy and patients with neurological disease

Trimethoprim-sulfamethoxazole (co-trimoxazole)

- Mechanism of action involves folate antagonism
- Commonly used to treat bladder infections, and first line for *Pneumocystis* pneumonia
- Contraindicated in pregnancy, may cause photosensitivity, rash and GI upset

Vancomycin

- Recommended as a first-line treatment for MRSA infections, skin and bone infections, and orally for the treatment of *C. difficile* infections
- Vancomycin is generally infused slowly, to prevent the occurrence of thrombophlebitis and **red man syndrome**, in which flushing and redness occur soon after the infusion, secondary to mast cell degranulation

Fungi

- Fungi are eukaryotic organisms that are unable to photosynthesise
- The fungal cell wall contains sterols, most specifically ergosterol, which is a prime target for various antifungal medications, either by competitive inhibition (e.g. amphotericin) or inhibiting synthesis (e.g. ketoconazole)

- Fungi are generally considered opportunistic infections, and are most likely to pose a serious threat to immunocompromised individuals, but may affect immunocompetent hosts as well
- Specific fungal infections are discussed separately in other chapters (e.g. *Aspergillus* spp. in *Chapter 2*, and superficial *Tinea* infections in *Chapter 11*)

Viruses

- Viruses are organisms containing genetic material enclosed within a **capsid** or membrane
- They do not have organelles, and require host machinery to replicate
- They may be classified as DNA or RNA viruses, and further classified into **single-stranded** or **double-stranded** (see *Table 9.1*)

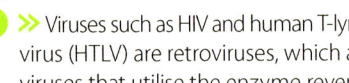 **E** ≫ Viruses such as HIV and human T-lymphotropic virus (HTLV) are retroviruses, which are RNA viruses that utilise the enzyme reverse transcriptase to produce DNA.

Table 9.1 *Classification of viruses*

	DNA viruses	RNA viruses
Single-stranded	Parvovirus	Coronavirus Picornavirus Togavirus Paramyxovirus Orthomyxovirus Rhabdovirus Bunyavirus
Double-stranded	Hepatitis B virus Poxvirus Human herpes viruses (HHV) Papovavirus Adenovirus	Reovirus

P ≫ Streptococci may be distinguished on blood agar by their degree of haemolysis. For example, beta haemolytic streptococci leave hollow zones behind, indicating that complete haemolysis has taken place. On the other hand, alpha haemolytic organisms are unable to completely metabolise haemoglobin, and leave behind a green pigment, indicating that partial haemolysis has taken place.

9.1 Sexually transmitted diseases (STDs)

9.1.1 Syphilis

Definition: syphilis refers to a sexually transmitted infection caused by *Treponema pallidum*.

Epidemiology:

- Common, global condition, 10.6 million new cases from 2005 to 2008
- Approximately 60% attributed to men who have sex with men (MSM)
- Co-infection with HIV merits a high index of suspicion

Aetiology:

- Syphilis may be:
  - Acquired: subdivided into primary, secondary, latent and tertiary syphilis
  - Congenital (transplacental infection)

Clinical features:

- Primary:
  - Development of an indurated, **usually painless** syphilitic ulcer with **non-tender** lymphadenopathy at the site of infection (oral, anal or genital; note that the lesion may be in the cervix in women)
- Secondary:
  - Occurs, on average, 6 weeks after primary infection
  - Presentation is variable, with features such as fever, myalgia and lymphadenopathy predominating
  - A generalised maculopapular rash also may affect the palms, soles, trunk and face (see *Fig. 9.5*)

> **E** >> Secondary syphilis may also be characterised by buccal 'snail-track' ulcers and warty genital lesions known as **condylomata lata**.

- Latent syphilis is defined as positive serology without clinical features of syphilis, with the infection being acquired less than 2 years prior (WHO); this form may relapse to secondary syphilis
- Tertiary:
  - Affects one-third of untreated patients
  - **Syphilitic gummas:** very rare infiltrative, granulomatous lesions that present as firm, necrotic nodules in organs, bone and skin
  - **Cardiovascular sequelae:** commonly include aortitis affecting the aortic root, which may lead to aortic regurgitation or aortic aneurysm

- **Neurological sequelae:** characterised by Argyll–Robertson pupils, tabes dorsalis, ataxia, behavioural disturbances, paralysis and seizures

> **P** >> An Argyll–Robertson pupil (sometimes termed 'prostitute's pupil'), refers to small pupils that accommodate but **do not constrict or react** to a light stimulus.

> **E** >> Tabes dorsalis refers to a demyelinating disorder of the dorsal columns related to syphilis. This condition is characterised by loss of proprioception and vibration, weakness, ataxia and a positive Romberg sign, although these changes may not be present until years after the initial infection.

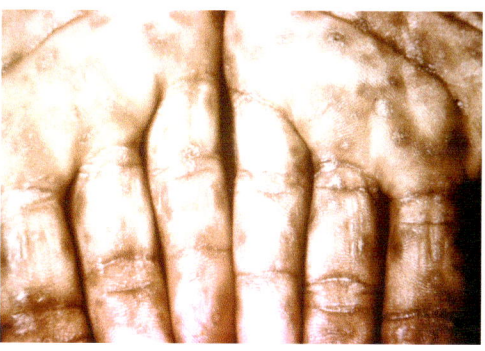

Fig. 9.5 *Secondary syphilitic rash on the palm of the hands.*

Investigations (UK National Guidelines on Syphilis 2008)

Screen for other sexually transmitted infections. Tests for *T. pallidum* can be divided into specific treponemal tests and non-treponemal tests.

> **Stepwise plan:**

1 Arrange treponemal tests
- **Treponemal Enzyme Immunoassay (EIA)** is recommended for screening purposes in national guidelines (IgM acutely and IgG after 4–5 weeks)
- Other treponemal tests, such as the fluorescent treponemal antibody absorbed test (FTA-abs), or TPPA may also be used

9

2 Arrange non-treponemal or cardiolipin tests
- Venereal disease research laboratory (VDRL) or rapid plasma reagin (RPR) test **should be performed when treponemal tests indicate syphilis**
- These are indicators of disease activity but may be false negative

3 Obtain dark field microscopy
- This is the most sensitive and specific test for demonstrating treponemes

4 Arrange other investigations
- These should be relevant neurological or cardiovascular investigations, depending on symptoms

Management

Treatment should be carried out in a genitourinary medicine sexual health clinic.

Stepwise management of syphilis

1 Prescribe penicillin
- IM benzathine penicillin is the first-line treatment for primary, secondary and latent syphilis
- Neurosyphilis may be treated with a 28-day course of doxycycline

2 Treat with azithromycin
- This is used as the second-line treatment

> ≫ The Jarisch–Herxheimer reaction, classically associated with the treatment of syphilis (although it may occur secondary to treatment of any bacterial infection with antibiotics), is characterised by clinical features of shock, fever and rigors within a few hours of antibiotic administration as a result of toxins produced by rapid bacterial death. Treatment with prednisolone and antipyretic agents will help prevent progression of the reaction.

9.1.2 Gonorrhoea

Definition: gonorrhoea refers to a sexually transmitted infection caused by *Neisseria gonorrhoeae*.

Epidemiology:
- Common, global condition
- 10.6 million new cases from 2005 to 2008

- Risk factors include young age, social deprivation, men who have sex with men (MSM) and multiple sexual partners
- Co-infection with HIV and chlamydia are common

> ≫ Neonates may be at risk of developing sepsis and conjunctivitis that progresses to blindness if left untreated (known as **ophthalmia neonatorum**), if they are infected with *Chlamydia trachomatis* or *Neisseria gonorrhoeae* from infected cervical secretions.

Aetiology/pathophysiology:
- *N. gonorrhoeae* has a predisposition for mucosal tissue

Clinical features:
- Men:
  - Urethral discharge, dysuria, epididymo-orchitis (see *Fig. 9.6*)
  - Rectal pain and discharge more common in MSM
- Women:
  - Generally asymptomatic
  - If symptomatic, dysuria, cervicitis or cervical discharge

> ≫ Pelvic inflammatory disease (PID) refers to an infection of the female reproductive tract, secondary to chronic, untreated chlamydia or gonorrhoea infection. This may lead to complications such as scarring of the reproductive system, ectopic pregnancies, dyspareunia, pelvic pain and infertility. Cervical motion tenderness and adnexal pain may be noted on examination. Treatment with antibiotics (IV in severe cases) is recommended.

> ≫ Patients with right upper quadrant pain who suffer from PID are also at risk of developing perihepatitis which may progress to liver capsule inflammation and the formation of adhesions. This is known as Fitz–Hugh–Curtis syndrome.

Investigations
Screen for other sexually transmitted infections.

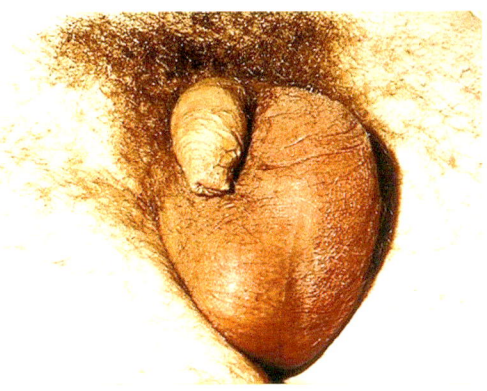

Fig. 9.6 *Epididymo-orchitis.*

1 Carry out nucleic acid amplification test (NAAT)
- NAAT of urine or genital specimens is first-line treatment

2 Grow a culture
- Growing a culture of the organism may help identify and isolate organism

Management
Treatment should be carried out in a genitourinary medicine sexual health clinic.

Stepwise management of gonorrhoea

1 Prescribe antibiotics
- Ceftriaxone 500mg IM and azithromycin 1g PO stat

2 Perform NAAT 2 weeks after treatment
- To confirm eradication

9.1.3 Chancroid

Chancroid is characterised by a typically **painful** tender genital ulcer (see *Fig. 9.7*), caused by infection with *Haemophilus ducreyi* that may also co-present with tender lymphadenopathy or dysuria. Treat with azithromycin.

> E » Chancroid is painful, most people 'du creyi'.

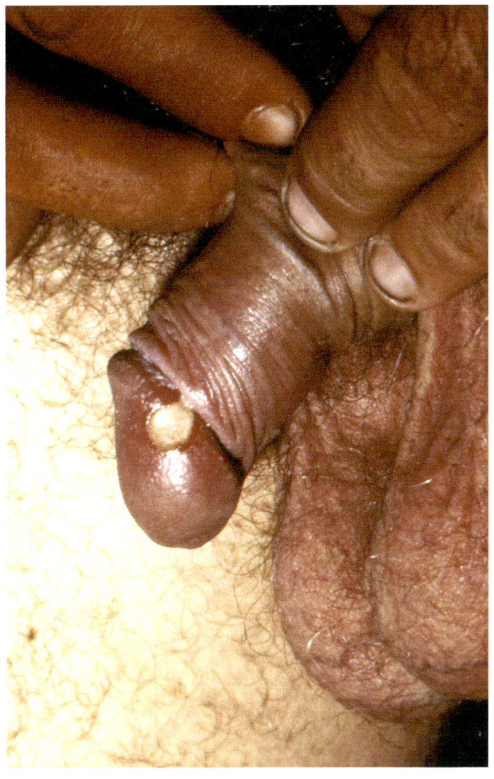

Fig. 9.7 *Penile chancroid lesion.*

9.1.4 Granuloma inguinale (donovanosis)

9

Granuloma inguinale is an infection caused by *Klebsiella granulomatis* that typically presents with an ulcerated genital lesion. The ulcer is usually red and painless (see *Fig. 9.8*) but may be differentiated from syphilis by a relatively decreased incidence of lymphadenopathy and Donovan bodies in tissue samples (characteristically shaped moieties). Treatment is with azithromycin.

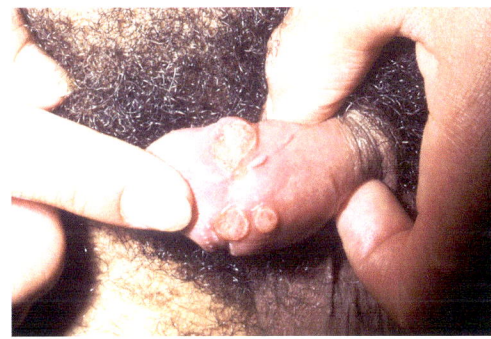

Fig. 9.8 *Granuloma inguinale.*

9.1.5 Chlamydia

Definition: chlamydia infection may refer to several subtypes caused by *Chlamydia trachomatis*:

- Trachoma, an infective conjunctival disease and second most common cause of blindness worldwide, caused by **serotypes A–C**
- Urogenital chlamydia, a common sexually transmitted infection caused by serotypes D–K
- Lymphogranuloma venereum, caused by **L1, L2 or L3 serovars of *C. trachomatis***

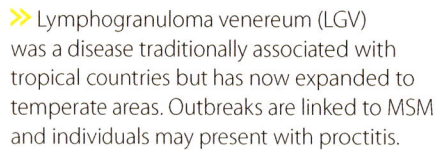

>> Lymphogranuloma venereum (LGV) was a disease traditionally associated with tropical countries but has now expanded to temperate areas. Outbreaks are linked to MSM and individuals may present with proctitis.

Primary LGV:
- Painless ulcer develops (particularly in men; women may be asymptomatic)

Secondary LGV:
- Develops within a month of initial infection
- Characterised by tender inguinal lymphadenopathy, erythema and rash

Tertiary LGV:
- Late sequela, may present years or decades after infection
- May be associated with proctitis, tenesmus, discharge and enlarged rectal nodules
- Elephantiasis of the genitals may occur

Epidemiology:
- Urogenital chlamydia accounted for up to half of all new STDs in England in 2014
- Approximately 100 million new cases a year
- Co-infection with HIV and chlamydia is common

Clinical features:
- Men:
  - Urethral discharge, dysuria
  - May present with testicular pain or epididymo-orchitis

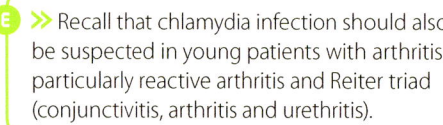

>> Recall that chlamydia infection should also be suspected in young patients with arthritis, particularly reactive arthritis and Reiter triad (conjunctivitis, arthritis and urethritis).

- Women:
  - Generally asymptomatic
  - If symptomatic, dysuria, cervicitis or cervical discharge (see *Fig. 9.9*)

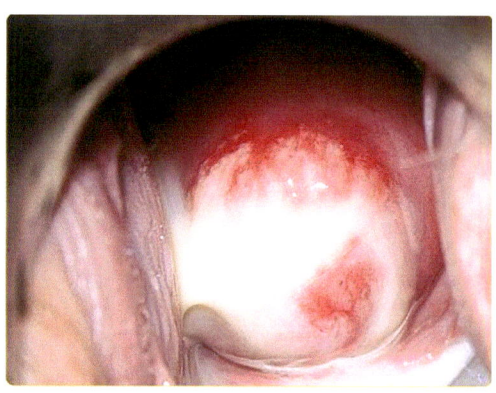

Fig. 9.9 *Chlamydia infection of the cervix.*

Investigations
Screen for other sexually transmitted infections.

Stepwise plan:

1 **Carry out nucleic acid amplification test (NAAT)**
- NAAT of urine or genital specimens is first-line treatment

2 **Grow a culture**
- Growing a culture of the organism may help identify and isolate organism

Management
Treatment should be carried out in a genitourinary medicine sexual health clinic; and testing of young people who are sexually active should be offered at primary care level.

Stepwise management of chlamydia

1 **Prescribe antibiotics**
- Azithromycin 1g PO stat
- Alternatively, doxycycline 100mg BD for 7 days

9.1.6 Human papillomavirus (HPV) infection

Anogenital warts
HPV, particularly **types 6 and 11**, are responsible for the development of anogenital warts in the majority of individuals. They affect both men and women, but they are more likely to affect homosexual men. Screen for other infections. Offer topical podophyllum or cryotherapy first line. Other treatments include topical imiquimod, electrocautery or surgical excision. The disease may sometimes be difficult to treat, and recurrences may be common.

E ≫ HPV types 16 and 18 are linked with the development of cervical cancer. Vaccination is encouraged, alongside regular cervical screening. The quadrivalent vaccine is also protective against types 6 and 11 and has dramatically reduced the incidence of anogenital warts.

9.1.7 Trichomoniasis

Trichomoniasis is a sexually transmitted disease caused by a motile, flagellated protozoa known as

Trichomonas vaginalis. Symptoms include an offensive, yellow discharge in about two-thirds of patients, pruritus, dysuria and cervicitis. The cervix is classically described as a **'strawberry cervix'** because of the accompanying cervicitis.

Note that men usually present asymptomatically with this disease. If they are symptomatic, they usually complain of discharge or dysuria.

NAAT testing is currently recommended first line and treatment is with **metronidazole**.

9.2 Herpetic infections

The herpes virus is a DNA virus, of which there are currently eight identifiable types that belong to three groups – alpha, beta and gamma herpes viruses.

9.2.1 Alpha herpes viruses (HSV-1, HSV-2, VZV/HHV-3)

Herpes simplex virus (HSV-1 and HSV-2)
Bear in mind that there is some overlap between infective symptoms produced by HSV-1 and HSV-2. You should also remember that the features described below are the more common features, rather than those that necessarily **always** appear. Viral DNA remains latent in the dorsal root ganglion.

E ≫ Herpes simplex may also affect the eye (herpes simplex keratitis), causing dendritic herpetic ulcers of the eye. Prompt ophthalmology referral and fluorescein staining is indicated. Treat with topical acyclovir. Steroids should **never** be used, as this may worsen the condition.

HSV-1
- This is generally associated with oral lesions ('cold sores'), causing gingivostomatitis, blisters and pain
- Generally symptomatic treatment is recommended for oral herpes; most cases in immunocompetent individuals resolve spontaneously, but topical acyclovir may prove to have some benefit
- The majority of herpes encephalitis is caused by HSV-1

P ≫ Herpetic whitlow is a herpes infection of the finger, typically affecting healthcare workers, nurses and dental staff who come into contact with oral secretions. Painful vesicular pustules develop. The condition is self-limiting. Topical acyclovir has not been proven to have benefit, and surgical removal may exacerbate the condition.

HSV-2
- Genital herpes is more classically associated with HSV-2, although HSV-1 has been shown to cause it to a large degree
- Transmission occurs sexually or via contact with infected sites (e.g. eyes and skin)
- Genital herpes presents with painful blistering vesicular lesions with accompanying flu-like symptoms
- Tender lymphadenopathy is frequently seen bilaterally
- It has a high rate of recurrence
- Investigate genital herpes with **PCR swab** of the affected lesion **first line**
- Manage with warm baths, topical lidocaine and **oral** valacyclovir

Varicella-zoster virus (human herpes virus 3)
Chickenpox is generally a disease of early childhood caused by the varicella-zoster virus (VZV). The virus, which remains latent in neural tissue, may be reactivated later (usually secondary to a decrease in immune function), resulting in zoster (shingles).

9

Chickenpox

- This is very infectious, and the majority are affected before adolescence
- Transmission occurs via droplet spread
- The first presenting symptom is usually a fever, followed by the development of an itchy, cropped vesicular rash that scabs (see *Fig. 9.10*)
- Diagnosis is clinical, and management in immunocompetent children is supportive, with hydration, anti-pyretics and emollients

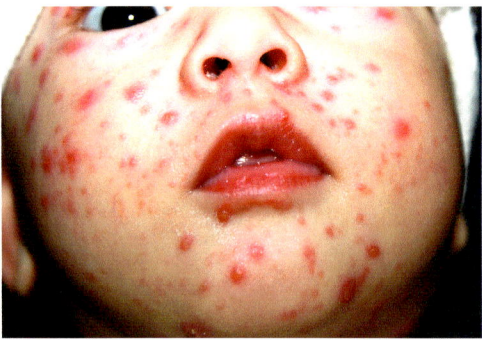

Fig. 9.10 *Classic active VZV (chickenpox) blisters.*

- Acyclovir may be required in high-risk individuals or in the immunocompromised
- Pregnant women who come into contact with a child with chickenpox should be offered varicella antibody testing and varicella-zoster immunoglobulin, to help prevent maternal respiratory infections and foetal varicella syndrome

Zoster

- Zoster, or shingles, is typically caused by reactivation of the latent VZV in the nervous system
- Vesicular eruptions are painful and blistering, and generally occur in a **dermatomal distribution** (see *Fig. 9.11*) as a result of immunosuppression, acute stress or trauma
- Shingles is much more common in older individuals

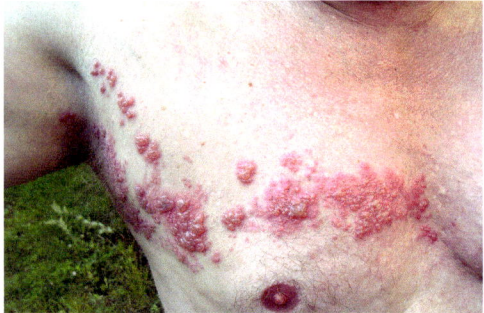

Fig. 9.11 *Typical shingles rash along a T3 dermatomal distribution.*

- The trunk is the site most commonly affected, followed by the ophthalmic division of the trigeminal nerve (**herpes zoster ophthalmicus**) in 10% – referral to ophthalmology is indicated in these cases
- Valacyclovir is the recommended treatment

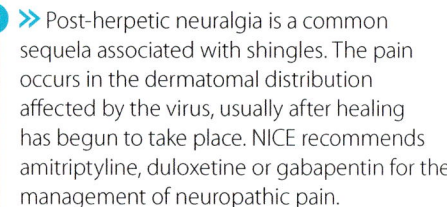 **P** ≫ Post-herpetic neuralgia is a common sequela associated with shingles. The pain occurs in the dermatomal distribution affected by the virus, usually after healing has begun to take place. NICE recommends amitriptyline, duloxetine or gabapentin for the management of neuropathic pain.

9.2.2 Beta herpes viruses (CMV/HHV-5, HHV-6, HHV-7)

HHV-6 and HHV-7

- HH-6 and HH-7 are generally associated with the development of **roseola**, a non-itchy maculo-papular rash that accompanies or follows a fever which spreads from the trunk to the face and limbs
- Treatment is supportive

Cytomegalovirus (CMV or HHV-5)

- Asymptomatic or mild clinical symptoms in immunocompetent hosts; tends to affect the **immunocompromised**
- May affect children transplacentally, causing sensorineural hearing loss, microcephaly and seizures
- Individuals with **transplanted organs** may be at particular risk for CMV as a result of immunosuppression
  - Appropriate screening measures should be taken
- **CMV retinitis** is common in patients with **HIV**
- Investigations include PCR for the virus, and the detection of intranuclear inclusions in tissue samples
- Treatment is with **ganciclovir** or **valganciclovir** first line, or foscarnet second line

9.2.3 Gamma herpes viruses (EBV/HHV-4 and HHV-8)

Epstein–Barr virus (HHV-4)

- Infectivity related to B cells

E ≫ EBV has been linked with the development of Burkitt lymphoma, nasopharyngeal carcinoma (particularly in Asian populations), oral hairy leukoplakia in patients affected by HIV and cases of Hodgkin lymphoma.

P » Infectious mononucleosis, also known as glandular fever, is a self-limiting viral illness caused by EBV (or CMV in a small number of cases) and typically affects young people.

Patients present with a **flu-like illness** with a **sore throat** and **cervical lymphadenopathy and hepatosplenomegaly in some cases**.

Investigation can be carried out using the **Paul–Bunnell** or **monospot** tests. Important management strategies include:

- Avoiding alcohol
- Avoiding contact sports due to risk of splenic rupture
- Supportive therapy; disease is self-limiting

Note that the use of amoxicillin as a means of treatment may precipitate a rash and should be avoided.

Human herpes virus 8 (HHV-8)

- HHV-8 causes **Kaposi sarcoma** (see *Section 9.3.1*).

9.3 HIV/AIDS

Definition: human immunodeficiency virus (HIV) refers to a retrovirus that infects CD4 T cells, eventually decreasing immune function over time. Two forms of the virus exist:
- HIV-1: most common infective form worldwide
- HIV-2: generally endemic in Africa

Acquired immunodeficiency syndrome (AIDS) refers to an immunocompromised condition caused by HIV, usually occurring about a decade after the initial infection if left untreated. It is characterised by opportunistic infections and severely impaired immunity.

E » The progression of HIV to full-blown AIDS has halted to a large degree with the introduction of highly active anti-retroviral therapy (HAART). Some patients on long-term therapy are now able to reach near-normal lifespans.

Epidemiology:
- 35 million people affected worldwide; more than half in Africa
- MSM are particularly at risk, and account for approximately 40% of new cases
- However, in sub-Saharan Africa more heterosexual women are affected than men

Aetiology/pathophysiology:
- Spread of the virus occurs via sexual intercourse, blood and blood products, birth and delivery, breastfeeding and sharing of needles

W » HIV attaches to a glycoprotein (gp120) on CD4 T-lymphocytes, infecting the cell and creating DNA copies of viral RNA via the enzyme **reverse transcriptase**. Mature virions are then formed as viral proteins are synthesized by the human host and cleaved by viral proteases, contributing to an initial spike in viral load early on in the disease process. This eventually subsides as human host immune response takes over, and the efficacy at which immune response occurs and continues is thought to influence the rate of progression of symptoms. This response is thought to be largely genetic.

Clinical features:
Patients infected with HIV at the time of illness are usually asymptomatic. Patients may present at any stage of the illness, encompassing:
- Acute seroconversion
  - 2–6 weeks after infection
  - Symptoms mimic flu-like illness or infectious mononucleosis
  - Presence of risk factors merits a high index of clinical suspicion
- Clinical latent period
  - Generally asymptomatic during this time; may take years
  - Persistent general lymphadenopathy may be present (nodes >1cm in diameter, at least two extra-inguinal sites for more than 3 months)
  - Chronic infection with the virus occurs

9

- AIDS-related complex (ARC)
  - Constitutional symptoms – weight loss, fever, night sweats, heralding the potential early onset of the development of AIDS
  - May have some opportunistic infections, e.g. candidiasis, seborrhoeic dermatitis, oral hairy leukoplakia (see *Fig. 9.12*)
- AIDS
  - Defined in terms of CD4 count <200 cells per microlitre, or presence of characteristic opportunistic infections
  - Increased risk of cancers, particularly those of viral origin, e.g. Kaposi sarcoma (see *Fig. 9.13*), Burkitt lymphoma

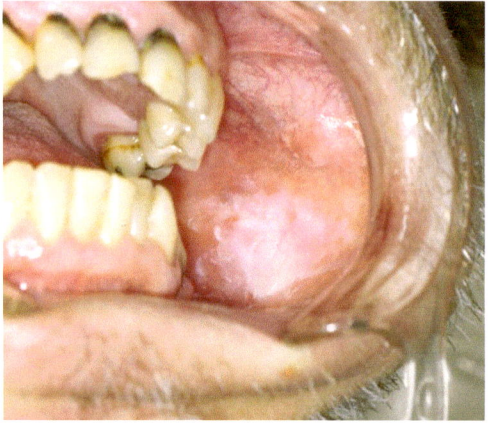

Fig. 9.12 *Buccal leukoplakia.*

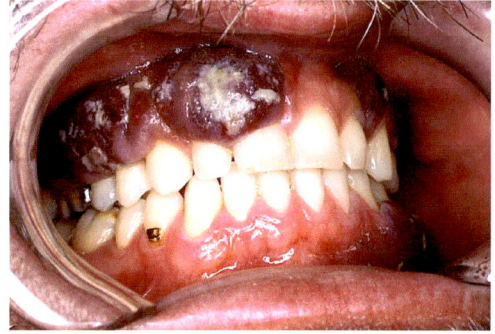

Fig. 9.13 *Peri-oral Kaposi sarcoma with overlying candidiasis.*

Investigations

Stepwise plan:

1   HIV 1/2 antigen–antibody immunoassay
- Initial screening test

2   HIV 1/2 differentiation immunoassay

- Subsequent testing with the differentiation assay is recommended after having a positive antigen–antibody immunoassay
  a. **HIV 1 (+) HIV 2 (–): HIV 1 antibodies present**
  b. **HIV 1 (–) HIV 2 (+): HIV 2 antibodies present**
  c. **HIV 1 (+) HIV 2 (+): HIV antibodies present**
  d. **HIV 1 (–) HIV 2 (–): proceed to Step 3**

3   HIV-1 NAAT
- Only if differentiation sample in step 2 proves negative – a positive NAAT at this stage indicates acute HIV infection

> E ≫ Western blot testing is no longer recommended. If the antigen–antibody immunoassay (Step 1) is negative, but the differentiation immunoassay is positive and/or NAAT – this may indicate a false positive test.

4   Investigate and manage relevant opportunistic infections

9.3.1 Complications of HIV/AIDS infection

The development of HIV/AIDS is associated with superinfections caused by opportunistic pathogens.

Complications include:
- **Pneumonia**
  - Classically associated with *Pneumocystis jirovecii* pneumonia (PCP, organism previously known as *Pneumocystis carinii*)
  - Patients with PCP usually present with fever, a dry cough and dyspnoea on exertion; CXR demonstrates perihilar infiltrates

> E ≫ All patients with a CD4 count below 200, or those who have previously had one infection, should receive prophylaxis against the development of pneumocystis with co-trimoxazole. Acute infection should be treated with IV co-trimoxazole.

  - Pneumonia may also be bacterial in origin (most commonly *S. pneumoniae* and *H. influenzae*)
- **Tuberculosis**
  - Development or reactivation of latent TB
  - Worse in endemic areas

- **Mycobacterium avium complex infections**
  - Associated with CD4 counts <50
  - Prophylaxis with azithromycin
- **CMV infection**
  - Particularly retinitis – decreased visual acuity, eye pain
  - Treat with ganciclovir
- *Cryptosporidium parvum* diarrhoea
  - No specific therapy, manage supportively
- **Candidiasis**
  - Oesophageal, cutaneous or disseminated
- **Cerebral toxoplasmosis**
  - Most common CNS infection, caused by protozoa *Toxoplasma gondii*; animal reservoir is usually cats
  - May present with headache, fevers, encephalitis, focal neurology
  - Investigate with toxoplasma serology and CT scan, which will show **ring-enhancing lesions**
  - Treat with **pyrimethamine and sulfadiazine**
  - Prophylaxis with co-trimoxazole if CD count <100

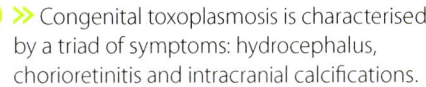

E » Congenital toxoplasmosis is characterised by a triad of symptoms: hydrocephalus, chorioretinitis and intracranial calcifications.

- **Progressive multifocal leukoencephalopathy (PML)**
  - Progressive demyelinating disease caused by the JC virus
  - Presents with focal neurological signs, behavioural changes, paraesthesia, paralysis and dementia
  - Diagnosis based on **PCR** of JC virus
  - **No specific therapy**; course of the disease depends on treatment efficacy of HAART
- **Cryptococcal meningitis**
  - Symptoms may range from mild chronic headaches to meningism to seizures caused by fungus *Cryptococcus neoformans*
  - Definitive diagnosis made on identifying **cryptococcal antigen** in the CSF

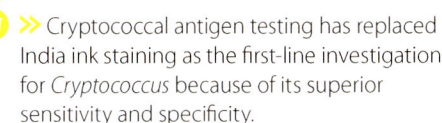

W » Cryptococcal antigen testing has replaced India ink staining as the first-line investigation for *Cryptococcus* because of its superior sensitivity and specificity.

  - Treatment is with amphotericin B and fluconazole first line
- **Kaposi sarcoma**
  - Caused by HHV-8
  - Development of characteristic purple macules or papules that may begin on the face and spread

  - May affect respiratory system and GI tract, causing dyspnoea, haemoptysis and abdominal pain
  - Local lesions are treated with radiotherapy or pegylated intralesional doxorubicin

Management

Baseline blood functions and screening for other investigations should be carried out before instituting HAART. Previous guidelines recommended starting HAART at a particular CD4 count, but the BHIVA 2015 guidelines recommend starting HAART as soon as a diagnosis is reached.

Stepwise management of HIV/AIDS

P » When determining which agent to use in the HAART combination, you should consider comorbidities, particularly with regard to liver function. Note that initiating HAART should not, however, be halted whilst considering drug-mediated liver injury.

1 Decide on drug regimen
- HAART classically consists of a choice between three drugs from a variety of classes, and the associated reduction in viral load is a marker of the efficacy of and adherence to treatment:
- **Nucleoside analogue reverse transcriptase inhibitors (NRTI)**
  - e.g. zidovudine, lamivudine, emtricitabine, tenofovir
  - Side effects: peripheral neuropathy
  - Zidovudine: anaemia, neutropenia, myopathy
- **Protease inhibitors (PI)**
  - e.g. indinavir, darunavir, lopinavir, ritonavir (booster)
  - Side effects: dyslipidaemia, increased risk of diabetes, diarrhoea
  - Indinavir: kidney stones
- **Non-nucleoside analogue reverse transcriptase inhibitors (NNRTI)**
  - e.g. efavirenz, nevirapine
  - Side effects: insomnia, dizziness
- Combination of at least three drugs, usually:
  - **NRTI × 2 + PI**
  - **NRTI × 2 + NNRTI**

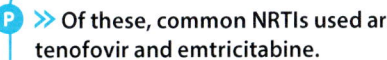

P » Of these, common NRTIs used are tenofovir and emtricitabine.

2 Provide post-exposure prophylaxis
- Post-exposure prophylaxis is an important consideration for healthcare professionals, although the risk of seroconversion post-needlestick injury is <0.5%
- Wash the affected area and attempt to bleed (do not attempt to suck the area)
- Report to occupational health, and follow local procedure guidelines
- Start post-exposure prophylaxis within 72 hours and continue for more than 28 days
- Engage in follow-up testing at 12 and 24 weeks

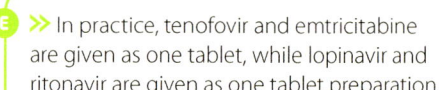 **E** ≫ In practice, tenofovir and emtricitabine are given as one tablet, while lopinavir and ritonavir are given as one tablet preparation.

9.4 Bacterial infections

9.4.1 Respiratory bacterial infections

Pertussis

Pertussis, also known as whooping cough, refers to a respiratory infection characterised by coughing and inspiratory whoops caused by ***Bordetella pertussis***.

The incidence of whooping cough has decreased dramatically since the introduction of the DPT vaccine, but it is important to note that individuals may still contract the disease even after being vaccinated, and some adolescents may also be affected.

P ≫ Whooping cough may be associated with vomiting, and in severe cases, cyanotic episodes after coughing.

E ≫ Pertussis is a **notifiable** disease, and the diagnosis should be confirmed with **nasopharyngeal swabs** (not throat swabs).

Macrolide antibiotics are the first-line treatment, with clarithromycin being used generally and erythromycin in pregnant women. The evidence suggests that the disease course is unlikely to be affected despite treatment; however, it provides symptomatic relief.

Diphtheria

Diphtheria is an infectious disease caused by ***Corynebacterium diphtheriae***, characterised by upper respiratory symptoms, fever and the development of a **greyish-white** pseudomembrane in the throat.

The incidence of the disease has decreased dramatically since the introduction of vaccination, and it is now rare in the developed world. Treatment (particularly if encountered e.g. in developing nations) is with erythromycin.

Scarlet fever

Definition: scarlet fever refers to a **notifiable** condition that presents with fever, rash and upper respiratory symptoms that are caused by reaction to toxins produced by Group A beta haemolytic streptococci.

Epidemiology:
- Typically affects children under the age of 10
- It was associated with serious mortality in earlier centuries, before the development of antibiotics

Clinical features:
- Sudden onset of fever
- Coarse, red rash typically appearing on the neck and chest (face may appear flushed), appearing on the lower extremities later
- Throat examination may demonstrate tonsillitis and a 'strawberry tongue' (see *Fig. 9.14*)

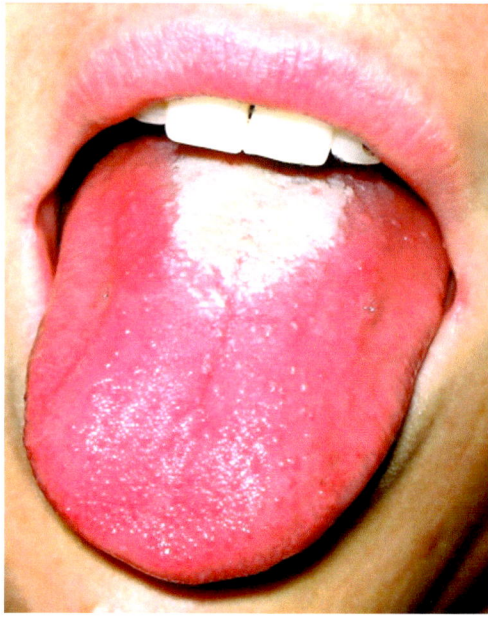

Fig. 9.14 *Strawberry tongue in a patient with scarlet fever.*

9

Management

The diagnosis is largely clinical, although throat swabs and rapid antigen testing may help in uncertain cases. **Penicillin** is the **first-line** antibiotic, with azithromycin being used if patients are allergic.

Complications may include local spread (causing otitis media, peritonsillar abscess, mastoiditis or sinusitis) or systemic spread (causing pneumonia or septicaemia). Uncommon long-term complications include rheumatic fever or post-streptococcal glomerulonephritis (PSGN).

 >> Note that, while penicillin treatment may decrease the risk of developing rheumatic fever, it does not reduce the risk of developing PSGN.

Epiglottitis

Epiglottitis is a severe obstruction of the airway secondary to inflammation of the epiglottis caused by *Haemophilus influenzae*. It usually presents in young children with inspiratory stridor, drooling and pyrexia. Other symptoms include pooling of secretions, odynophagia and a change in voice.

The widespread use of the Hib vaccine has greatly reduced the incidence of this condition. The throat should **not** be examined in suspected epiglottitis. Instead, there should be immediate referral for laryngoscopy, with adequate support for the possibility of eventual intubation and ventilation.

Legionella

Legionnaires' disease is an important differential diagnosis in the assessment of pneumonia, caused by *Legionella pneumophila*. This disease is classically associated with **travel, air conditioning and water tanks**. Culture of the organism from sputum is gold standard, but the urinary *Legionella* antigen test is more commonly used.

In addition to respiratory symptoms, *Legionella* pneumonia is likely to present with deranged LFTs and hyponatraemia. **Erythromycin is the antibiotic of choice**, but alternatives include ciprofloxacin or doxycycline.

9.4.2 Musculoskeletal bacterial infections

Osteomyelitis

Osteomyelitis refers to an infection of the bone and bone marrow. It may be acute or chronic, and spread may be categorised as **haematogenous** (spread from distant focus) or **direct** (e.g. contact between bone and infective agents in trauma or perioperatively).

 >> The first process observed in osteomyelitis is periosteal elevation and thickening, followed by inflammation and necrosis of bone, producing a **sequestrum** (dead bone), which is a nidus for infection. The new bone, or **involucrum**, then begins to undergo remodelling in response.

P >> The most common organism implicated in osteomyelitis is *Staph. aureus*; but do note that *S. typhi* is the most common organism in osteomyelitis developed in the context of sickle cell disease.

- Patients are frequently feverish and have localised pain, immobility and erythema of the affected region
- Swabbing draining sinus tracts is unreliable, as these may be contaminated and may not isolate the causative organism
- **Investigate** with blood cultures, plain films (see *Fig. 9.15*) or **MRI**
- **Acute infections:** IV antibiotics for 4–6 weeks
- **Chronic infections:** IV antibiotics and surgical debridement

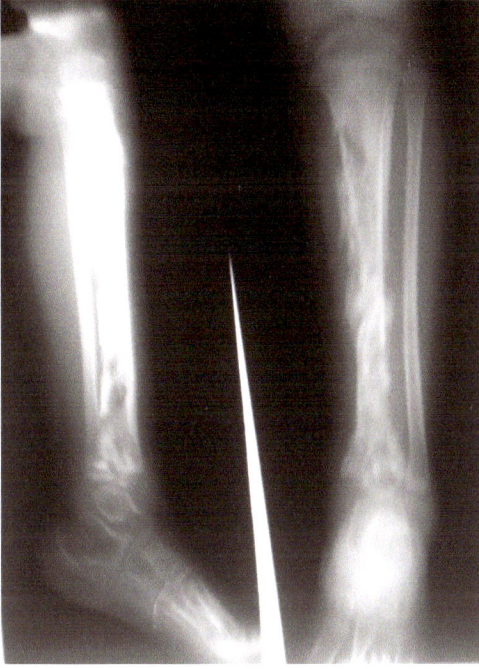

Fig. 9.15 *Left lower leg X-ray showing numerous radiolucencies within the tibia suggestive of bony infiltration and abscess formation.*

Necrotising fasciitis

Necrotising fasciitis is a rare, potentially fatal disease caused by a polymicrobial bacterial infection (type I), or a monomicrobial bacterial infection (type II), classically a **Group A streptococcal** infection.

E ≫ Necrotising fasciitis may masquerade as innocent-seeming cellulitis, but it is important to have a high index of suspicion, especially when considering systemic symptoms that do not quite fit with localised tenderness, as the condition may lead to severe sepsis and shock in a matter of days. Patients with diabetes, liver disease or those who are immunocompromised are at greater risk of developing the condition.

P ≫ Fournier gangrene is a severely progressive form of necrotising fasciitis affecting the groin, genitals or perineal area.

Prompt referral for surgical debridement and empiric, broad-spectrum IV antibiotics are indicated in the treatment of this condition.

9.4.3 Bacterial vaginosis

Bacterial vaginosis, the most common cause of abnormal vaginal discharge in women of reproductive age, is typified by the growth of anaerobic organisms, particularly **Gardnerella vaginalis** (see *Fig. 9.16*).

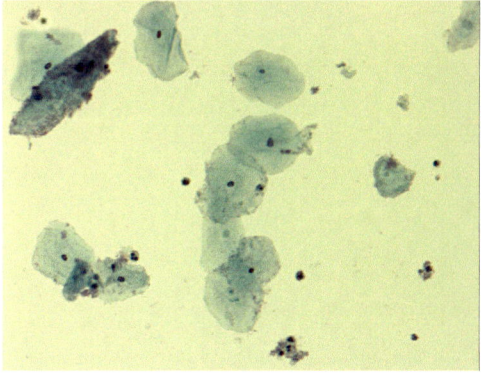

Fig. 9.16 *Micrograph of* Gardnerella vaginalis *(clue cells).*

Clinical features (NICE CKS 2014):
- Approximately 50% of women are asymptomatic
- Characterised by a fishy-smelling, thin, white discharge
- **Not** usually associated with itching or soreness
- Vaginal pH >4.5

Management (NICE CKS 2014)

Treat if symptomatic, even if pregnant. NICE does not recommend screening for bacterial vaginosis.

Stepwise management of bacterial vaginosis

1 Prescribe oral metronidazole
- 400mg twice daily for 5–7 days
- Higher dose may be used, but **not** in pregnant women

2 Prescribe intravaginal antibiotics
- Intravaginal metronidazole or clindamycin gel if patient prefers, or is unable to tolerate oral metronidazole

E ≫ Oral clindamycin or tinidazole are alternatives, but not routinely recommended.

9.4.4 Rickettsial diseases

E ≫ Much of the study of infectious disease (in the exam setting) relies on memorising the various organisms and symptoms. This is not always easy, and so we sometimes use seemingly ridiculous phrases to help us remember them. The phrases below have worked as memory aids for us, and we hope they will work for you too.

Rickettsial diseases are caused by Gram-negative coccobacilli. All the agents, apart from *Coxiella burnetii*, have a vector. Diagnosis is made clinically and confirmed with PCR. Treatment is with **doxycycline**.

Rocky mountain spotted fever
- Caused by *Rickettsia rickettsii*
- Often transmitted by a tick bite
- In addition to flu-like symptoms, the rash is characteristically described as spreading from the palms, soles and trunk to the neck and chest

E ≫ Rocky boxed so hard his hands turned red, it went all the way to his chest.

Endemic typhus
- Caused by *Rickettsia prowazekii*
- With similar flu-like symptoms, the rash travels from the trunk to the extremities and **spares the palms and soles**

E ≫ Endemic disease is so *prowa*ful, it only spares our palms and souls.

Scrub typhus
- Acute febrile illness with **indurated eschar**
- Caused by *Orientia tsustugamushi*

E ≫ She told me she loved using **oriental scrubs** to get rid of her eschar.

Q fever
- Caused by *Coxiella burnetii*
- Linked to animal contact, with sheep, goats and cows being an important risk factor
- This disease may present with a high fever, pneumonia or hepatitis acutely, and may predispose to conditions such as endocarditis if chronic

E ≫ There was no one on the farm when I went looking for Mrs **Burnetii**, so I had to direct some of my Qs to the cattle.

9.4.5 Leprosy (Hansen disease)

Definition: this disease is caused by *Mycobacterium leprae*.

Epidemiology:
- It is endemic in Africa, southeast Asia and South America
- **Two-thirds of all cases occur in India**

Pathophysiology:
- Leprosy may be **tuberculoid leprosy**, characterised by limited growth of *M. leprae* and much less severe disease
- Or it may be **lepromatous leprosy**, characterised by diffuse dermatological involvement and severe bacteraemia

Clinical features:
- 'Leonine' facies associated with lepromatous leprosy (see *Fig. 9.17*)
- Peripheral neuropathy, thickened nerves and neuro-ophthalmic damage
- Hypopigmented plaques with no sensation (see *Fig. 9.18*)

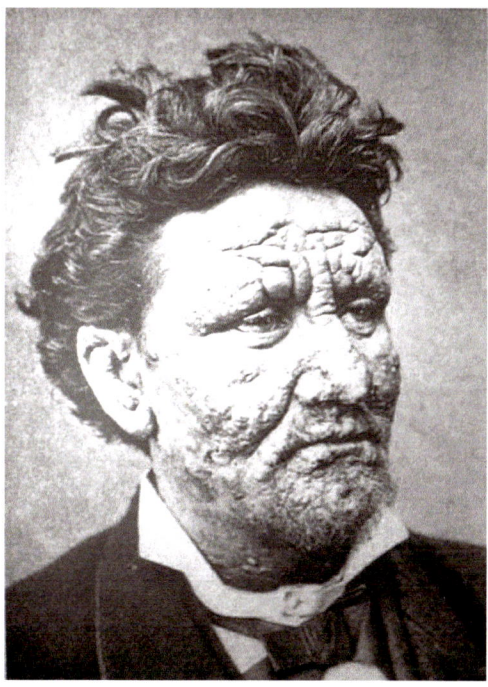

Fig. 9.17 Leonine face.

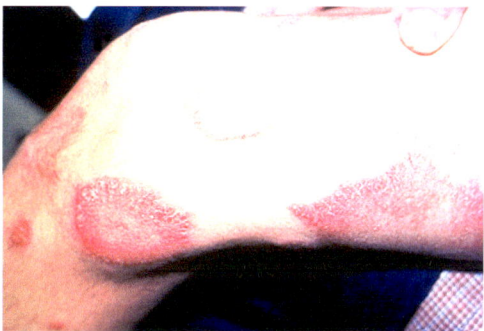

Fig. 9.18 Cutaneous leprosy lesions.

Management
Diagnosis is made upon identifying the agent from biopsy of skin samples, and treatment involves a multi-drug regimen of rifampicin and clofazimine for tuberculoid leprosy for 6 months, with the addition of dapsone to these two agents for two years in lepromatous leprosy.

9.4.6 Tetanus

Definition: tetanus refers to an infection caused by the spore-forming anaerobe, *Clostridium tetani*.

E ≫ Various other strains of clostridium exist, each causing different conditions. *Clostridium difficile* infection leads to pseudomembranous colitis. *Clostridium perfringens* is associated with gas gangrene. *Clostridium botulinum* is associated with botulism.

Tetanus is extremely rare in developed nations following vaccination, but older individuals or people who classically acquire injuries associated with trauma or contamination involving rusty nails or garden soil are at risk.

Clinical features:
- Most common form: generalised tetanus in 80%
  - Descending pattern of disease
  - Flu-like prodrome
- Muscle spasms, which may cause respiratory complications
- Trismus (or lockjaw) and risus sardonicus, an abnormal facial muscle spasm that causes patients to look as if they're smiling – note that this occurs late in the disease process
- Opisthotonus – a hyperextended state in which the patient appears to arch their body (see *Fig. 9.19*)

W ≫ The tetanus toxin produced by the bacteria adversely affects the release of inhibitory neurotransmitters GABA and glycine, causing sustained spasmodic muscle contraction and overactivity.

The diagnosis is made on clinical grounds.

Management
- Consideration of ITU referral (respiratory support may be needed)
- Human tetanus immunoglobulin IV
- Consider the use of metronidazole as an adjunctive therapy

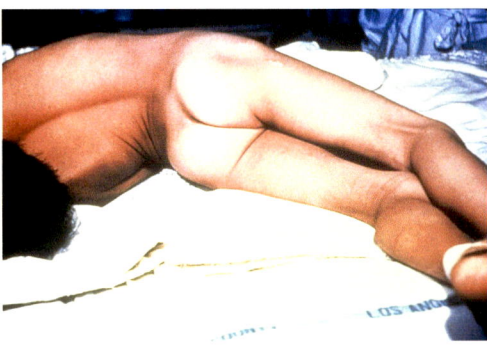

Fig. 9.19 *Opisthotonus secondary to* C. tetani *infection.*

Prevention:
- Patients with high-risk wounds (e.g. fractures) should be given **human tetanus immunoglobulin IV** even if vaccinations have been completed
- If vaccinations are incomplete or the status is unknown, high-risk patients should be given **both** the vaccine and human tetanus immunoglobulin

9.5 Viral infections

9.5.1 Influenza

Definition: influenza infection is characterised by respiratory illness in the context of an influenza infection.

Epidemiology:
- Up to 15% of the population per year
- Newer influenza strains can cause pandemics (exemplified by the H1N1 swine flu pandemic in 2009)

Aetiology/pathophysiology:
- Three serotypes exist, A, B and C, of which A is the most common cause of disease
- Patients with comorbid respiratory disease are at greater risk

- Patients with influenza infection are at risk of developing **staphylococcal pneumonia**
- Transmission is via droplet spread

W ≫ Classification of influenza proceeds via assessment of haemagglutinin (H) and neuraminidase (N) antigens. The virus may undergo minor mutations (**antigenic drift**), causing seasonal outbreaks, or more severely, **antigenic shifts**, which may lead to epidemics.

E ≫ **Shift**ing your car is more sudden and severe than letting it **drift**.

Clinical features:

- Upper respiratory symptoms predominate
- Fever, myalgia and headache

Investigations

Stepwise plan:

1 **The condition may be diagnosed clinically**

2 **Or by using direct viral culture from nasopharyngeal swabs or aspirates**
- Note that this may take up to a week

3 **PCR is much quicker**
- It takes less than 48 hours

Management

Stepwise management of influenza

1 **Uncomplicated disease can be managed relatively easily**
- With home rest, analgesia, anti-pyretics and ensuring adequate fluid intake

2 **For more serious disease, prescribe antiviral medication**
- Oseltamivir or zanamivir may be used, particularly for at-risk individuals, if treatment can begin **less than 48 hours** after symptom onset
- Note that the use of these drugs does not treat the infection; it merely reduces duration of symptoms, and this is especially true in immunocompetent individuals
- These measures do not include treatment during pandemics

P ≫ Annual influenza vaccinations are particularly useful for patients with comorbid heart, liver or renal failure, as well as patients with diabetes or COPD.

9.5.2 Upper respiratory tract infections

Upper respiratory tract infections are mild, self-limiting illnesses usually caused by viruses.
- The **common cold (coryza)** is most often caused by rhinoviruses, coronaviruses or adenoviruses
  - Management is based on symptomatic relief; antibiotics do not alter the course of the disease
- **Sore throat (pharyngitis)**
  - Patients should generally be managed supportively
  - Should be admitted if they present acutely breathless or with stridor

E ≫ NICE recommends the use of the Centor criteria when evaluating a patient with a sore throat. These criteria were developed to predict the likelihood of a Group A beta-haemolytic streptococcal infection (GABHS). The criteria are:
- Presence of tonsillar exudate
- Presence of tender anterior cervical lymphadenopathy
- Pyrexia
- Absence of cough.

The presence of 3 or 4 of the criteria indicates a 40–60% chance that the patient has GABHS and will benefit from antibiotic therapy. Offer phenoxymethylpenicillin first line for 10 days, or a macrolide (erythromycin or clarithromycin) for 5 days if the patient is penicillin-intolerant.

- **Laryngitis**
  - Acute laryngitis (hoarseness) is common, and usually due to viral infection, but may also be caused by bacteria or fungi
  - May also be caused by repeated throat clearing, yelling or voice misuse
  - Acute laryngitis is self-limiting; antibiotics are extremely unlikely to alter the disease course
  - Patients with chronic laryngitis (longer than 3 weeks) should be evaluated for more sinister pathology

9.5.3 Severe acute respiratory syndrome (SARS)/MERS-CoV respiratory virus

- **SARS**
  - Viral disease caused by SARS coronavirus
  - Outbreak occurred in Canada and Asia in 2003–2004
  - Causes acute respiratory distress and pneumonia
  - No specific therapy, treatment is supportive
- **MERS-CoV**
  - Middle East Respiratory Syndrome (MERS) caused by the MERS coronavirus (CoV)
  - Produces a pyrexial pneumonia that may lead to ARDS, which is fatal in 35% of cases
  - Outbreak occurred in South Korea in 2015
  - Diagnosis is made on PCR
  - No specific therapy, treatment is supportive

9

9.5.4 Measles

Definition: measles is an RNA viral infection transmitted by droplet spread. It is highly contagious, but the introduction of the MMR vaccine has greatly reduced its incidence in the population.

Clinical features:
- Patients who develop measles tend to present with a flu-like illness
- They may also present with fever, cough or coryza with a rash

E ≫ The rash observed generally spreads from the face to the neck to the trunk, and then finally to the limbs, and is associated with whitish-blue lesions on the buccal mucosa (known as Koplik spots) in just over two-thirds of patients.

Management
Diagnosis can be made based on measles-specific IgM from a swab or blood sample, and treatment is supportive. Complications can include pneumonia and encephalitis.

P ≫ Subacute sclerosing panencephalitis is a very rare complication of measles, and it only appears 5–10 **years** after the initial infection.

9.5.5 Mumps

Definition: mumps is a viral illness caused by a paramyxovirus and spread by droplet transmission. Like measles, the incidence of this condition has greatly diminished since the introduction of the MMR vaccine.

Clinical features:
- Flu-like illness, high fever
- Parotitis (sometimes described as pain while eating), which may be unilateral or bilateral
- Causes orchitis in males, but generally does not lead to impaired fertility
- May cause pancreatitis, arthritis or a mild viral meningitis

Management
The diagnosis is made on clinical grounds, and treatment is largely supportive.

9.5.6 Rubella

Definition: rubella, also known as German measles, refers to a togavirus-mediated infection spread by droplet transmission. Following the introduction of the MMR vaccine, its incidence has decreased sharply.

Pathophysiology:
- One of the major risks is contracting rubella during pregnancy, as this puts the infant at risk for congenital rubella syndrome
- This may cause sensorineural deafness, microphthalmia, congenital cataracts, and congenital heart disease, among other complications

Clinical features:
- Rubella infection also generally presents with a flu-like prodrome and a non-specific rash

Management
PCR testing for the virus is recommended, and management is supportive.

9.5.7 Other viral haemorrhagic fevers

- **Ebola**
  - *Filoviridae* family
  - Virus transmitted to human beings by the bite of an infected fruit bat, or intermediate hosts
  - Endemic to Africa
  - Symptoms may initially be non-specific, but may rapidly progress to abdominal symptoms such as vomiting
  - Patients who progress with shock, bleeding and neurological manifestations are likely to die (mortality can be anywhere from 20% to 80%)
  - Main confirmatory test is **PCR** for the Ebola virus
  - No specific therapy exists, treatment is supportive
- **Lassa fever**
  - Caused by Lassa virus, mostly endemic to sub-Saharan Africa
  - Begins with non-specific symptoms, and may progress to multi-organ development and death
  - ELISA for antigen and IgM antibodies is diagnosis method of choice
  - Treat with early ribavirin and supportive care
- **Marburg virus**
- **Hantavirus**
  - Viral haemorrhagic fever with pulmonary or renal involvement

9

- **Crimean-Congo haemorrhagic fever**
  - Tick-borne viral disease
  - Asia, Africa and the Middle East, despite the name
  - Flu-like symptoms may progress to shock and disseminated intravascular coagulation
  - Treatment is supportive
- **Zika virus**
  - Zika virus (flavivirus) outbreak occurred in 2016
  - Spread by infected *Aedes* mosquitoes (similar to dengue fever) or by sexual contact and blood transfusions
  - May cause congenital anomalies (e.g. microcephaly) and, rarely, Guillain–Barré syndrome
  - Endemic to South America and the Caribbean
  - The disease is **mostly mild, similar to a milder form of dengue fever**
  - It is particularly dangerous in pregnant women, who are advised to avoid endemic areas
  - Diagnosis is made via **PCR** of viral RNA
  - Treatment is supportive

9.6 Zoonoses

9.6.1 Lyme disease

Definition: Lyme disease is a disease caused by the spirochaete *Borrelia burgdorferi* and is an *Ixodes* tick-mediated infection. Patients tend to acquire the disease after holidays or camping in endemic regions, e.g. forests or countries such as the USA, Germany and France and some parts of Asia.

Clinical features:
- **Early localised disease**
  - Development of a **target rash (erythema migrans)** at the site of tick bite; may have flu-like symptoms
  - This rash is the most common presenting symptom
- **Disseminated disease**
  - Anywhere between a few weeks and a few months after initial infection
  - Unilateral or bilateral **facial palsy**
  - May have meningitis
- **Late disease**
  - Cardiovascular: myocarditis, heart block
  - Neurological: encephalitis
  - Arthritis

Investigations

Stepwise plan:

1 **If classic target rash lesion is present, this is considered sufficient clinical criteria to make the diagnosis**
- Proceed straight to treatment

2 **Carry out ELISA testing**
- If diagnosis is uncertain, but clinical features are present, e.g. facial palsy, etc.

Stepwise management of Lyme disease (NICE CKS 2014)

1 **If the tick is still attached, remove it**
- Use fine-tipped forceps or tweezers, grasping the tick as close to the skin as possible
- Pull away from the skin slowly and firmly, without twisting

2 **Prescribe oral antibiotic of choice**
- Doxycycline 100mg BD for 2 weeks

9.6.2 Leptospirosis

Definition: leptospirosis, also known as Weil disease, is caused by infection with spirochaetes in water or soil, usually secondary to animal (particularly rat) excrement contamination.

Epidemiology:
- The disease is most common in southern Europe and Australasia
- Recreational water sport activities or swimming are a risk factor for the development of the disease

Clinical features:
- Patients may present with a high fever, myalgia, headache and chest pain
- These symptoms may progress to developing jaundice and hepatitis

Management
Diagnosis is made on culture. The use of antibiotics is currently unclear, but if a treatment was to be started, the drug of choice would be doxycycline.

9.6.3 Rabies

Definition: rabies is a viral disease caused by *rhabdovirus* that can present with potentially fatal

9

encephalitis. It is mediated by the bite of an infected animal (classically dogs, bats or monkeys).

Pathophysiology:
- After the initial bite, the RNA virus attacks the nervous tissue, causing pain and tingling at the site of inoculation, before it begins to multiply
- Other early symptoms mimic a flu-like prodrome, with fever, headache and malaise
- The disease then progresses to a neurological phase, characterised by furious rabies or paralytic rabies
    - Furious rabies (60%) – delirium, hyperactivity, muscle spasms, vomiting and hydrophobia
    - Paralytic or 'dumb' rabies (40%) – fever and ascending paralysis without hydrophobia
- The most common cause of death in rabies is respiratory paralysis

Management

> **Stepwise management of rabies**

1 **Carry out wound cleaning, irrigation and post-exposure prophylaxis**
- These measures are almost 100% effective at preventing the onset of the disease
- Without these measures, death is almost certain

2 **Administer vaccine**
- Unimmunised patients should receive 5 doses of the rabies vaccine and the human rabies-specific immunoglobulin

9.6.4 Babesiosis

Babesiosis is a rare, tick-borne parasitic disease caused mainly by *Babesia divergens* in Europe and *Babesia microti* in parts of the USA. Asplenic and immunocompromised patients are particularly susceptible. Patients may be asymptomatic or systemically unwell with jaundice, haemolytic anaemia and renal failure. Diagnosis is made by PCR. Older methods (such as the Giemsa or Wright stain on microscopy) have sensitivities related to parasite load. The disease notably has (Maltese) **cross-shaped** inclusions in erythrocytes. Treat with clindamycin and quinine.

> **E** ≫ That babe is **cross**-eyed.

9.6.5 Cat-scratch disease

Cat-scratch disease, as the name implies, is a disease caused by *Bartonella henselae*, usually transmitted by cat scratches, causing erythematous papular lesions at the site and regional lymphadenopathy. The disease may present with severe systemic features (e.g. pneumonia, encephalitis) in immunocompromised individuals.

Diagnosis is based on indirect fluorescent antibody testing for *Bartonella*, and management is with trimethoprim-sulfamethoxazole, particularly in the immunocompromised.

9.6.6 Plague

Plague is a bacterial disease caused by *Yersinia pestis*, often transmitted by the bite of an infected flea. Virtually all cases today occur in Africa. Patients present as systemically unwell, with characteristic multiplication of the organism in lymph nodes, so-called swollen buboes in **bubonic** plague and pneumonia in pneumonic plague. The diagnosis is made by culturing the organism from infected sites and treatment is with fluoroquinolones.

> **W** ≫ The most famous example of the Plague was the Black Death in the 14th century, with epidemics at that time causing the death of hundreds of millions of people.

9.6.7 Anthrax

Anthrax is a bacterial disease caused by *Bacillus anthracis*, which is generally spread when individuals (e.g. farmers) come into contact with infected animals. The disease may be:
- Cutaneous, in which the patient develops a pruritic papule that ulcerates and **blackens** with oedema
- Inhalational, in which the patient develops respiratory failure
- Gastrointestinal, which is a rare condition, characterised by abdominal pain, nausea and vomiting and bloody diarrhoea

Management
Specimens may be cultured and stained for identification. Prompt administration of ciprofloxacin and clarithromycin is necessary, especially until the organism has been identified.

9.6.8 Other zoonotic diseases

- **Pasteurellosis**
    - Bacterial infection, usually caused by *Pasteurella multocida*
    - Often transmitted from the bite of an infected dog or cat
    - Treat with co-amoxiclav

- **Brucellosis**
  - Rarely fatal
  - Associated with contaminated milk/cheese or animal products
  - Causes non-specific symptoms and undulating fevers

- **Tularaemia**
  - Caused by *Francisella tularensis*, an intracellular organism
  - May cause fever, sepsis and ulcerative, tender lymph nodes
  - Caused by tick bite or contact with an infected animal (particularly rabbits and beavers)
  - Treat with doxycycline

9.7 Tropical infections

9.7.1 Malaria

Definition: malaria is a common, parasitic infection caused by *Plasmodium*.

Epidemiology:
- 207 million cases in 2012, 80% in sub-Saharan Africa
- Tragically, 75% of all deaths were children
- Virtually all cases from non-endemic areas are related to infection via an individual from an endemic area

E ≫ Malaria should be suspected in all individuals who are pyrexial who have returned from an endemic area, regardless of prophylactic treatment taken.

W ≫ The *Anopheles* mosquito injects a number of malarial sporozoites during a blood meal, which travel to the liver, infect hepatocytes and undergo reproduction. At this point, no symptoms occur, which accounts for the incubation period. This is longer in *P. vivax* and *P. ovale*, because of an attributed hypnozoite formation in the liver. Sporozoites in the liver become schizonts, which rupture to release merozoites into the bloodstream. The merozoites invade erythrocytes and cause the red blood cells to rupture – this cycle is variable for each species, accounting for the 'tertian' and 'quartan' nature of malaria. Red blood cell rupture causes cytokine activation by leucocytes, producing characteristic malarial symptoms and fever.

Aetiology/pathophysiology:
- Five main species cause disease in humans, transmitted by *Anopheles* mosquitoes

Table 9.2 Plasmodium *species*

Plasmodium falciparum	• Causes severe disease, associated classically with 'tertian' rhythm, with pyrexia and symptoms every 48 hours • Daily erythrocyte rupture may also be a feature
Plasmodium vivax	• Benign tertian rhythm, fever every third day • Dormant hypnozoites in the liver • Can only be differentiated from *P. ovale* on microscopy
Plasmodium ovale	• Benign tertian rhythm, fever every third day • Dormant hypnozoites in the liver • Can only be differentiated from *P. vivax* on microscopy
Plasmodium malariae	• Classically, a quartan malaria, fever and rupture every fourth day
Plasmodium knowlesi	• Form of parasite found in southeast Asia in primates • Malaria presentation may vary, but severe disease can quickly become fatal, due to rapid multiplication of organisms

P ≫ *P. falciparum* infections are likely to present symptomatically within a month, whereas *P. vivax* and *P. ovale* take up to 6 months to present with symptoms.

Clinical features:
- Fever, chills and rigors
- Symptoms intensify in tandem with erythrocyte rupture
- Hepatosplenomegaly, jaundice
- *Falciparum* infection is more severe, and may lead to thrombocytopenia, acute kidney injury and ARDS

9

Investigations

Stepwise plan:

1 **Carry out thick and thin blood smear with Giemsa stain**
- Gold standard investigation (see *Fig. 9.20*)
- Cheap, high sensitivity and specificity

2 **Perform rapid diagnostic antigen tests (RDTs)**

3 **Arrange blood tests**
- FBC, U&Es, LFTs, blood cultures, ABG
- Check **G6PD status** prior to giving antimalarial medication

Management

The choice of antimalarial depends on the type of parasite isolated. Before travelling to endemic regions, take general preventive measures, e.g. using insect repellent, wearing long-sleeved clothing and taking antimalarial prophylaxis.

Stepwise management of malaria

1 **To treat non-*falciparum* malaria**
- Treat with chloroquine; effective against most non-*falciparum* malaria
- Primaquine is sometimes used to destroy liver hypnozoites

2 **To treat *falciparum* malaria**
- Admit all patients to HDU, with a view to providing step-up care, as patients may deteriorate rapidly
- To treat uncomplicated *falciparum* malaria
  - Artemether with lumefantrine (artemisinin combination therapy is first line)
- To treat severe *falciparum* malaria
  - IV quinine dihydrochloride with ECG monitoring
  - IV artesunate + doxycycline

P » Antimalarial prophylaxis
- *P. falciparum* chloroquine-sensitive or *P. vivax/ovale*:
  - Chloroquine 1 week before, weekly for each week during travel and for 4 weeks after
- *P. falciparum* chloroquine-resistant:
  - Atovaquone + proguanil (Malarone) 2 days before, daily during travel, and for 7 days after
  - Mefloquine 2–3 weeks prior, weekly during travel, and 4 weeks after

E » **Side effects of antimalarial drugs**

Atovaquone + proguanil: headaches, nausea, good side effect profile

Mefloquine: diarrhoea, neuropsychiatric symptoms such as insomnia, dizziness, mental clouding

Chloroquine: blurred vision, abdominal pain, nausea

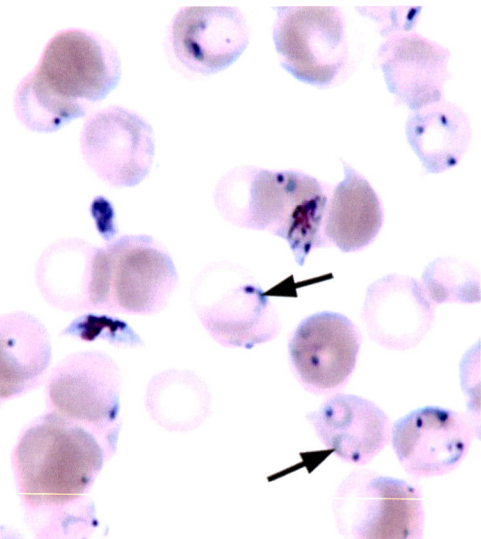

Fig. 9.20 Plasmodium falciparum *gametocytes (ring-like) within erythrocytes.*

9.7.2 Dengue fever

Dengue fever (also colloquially known as break-bone fever) is a vector-borne disease caused by a flavivirus and the mosquito *Aedes aegypti*.

WHO definition of dengue haemorrhagic fever

These features are all required:
- Current or recent fever lasting 2–7 days
- Thrombocytopenia (platelets <100,000mm^3)
- Positive tourniquet test, petechiae, mucosal bleeding
- Evidence of plasma leakage (indicates severity) – increased haematocrit, decreased protein and presence of effusion

The disease is particularly prevalent in South America, southeast Asia and Australia.

E ≫ 95% of dengue haemorrhagic fever occurs in patients below the age of 15. There appears to be some evidence of genetic susceptibility.

P ≫ Chikungunya fever (meaning 'contorted fever') refers to an arbovirus also transmitted by *Aedes aegypti* in warm tropical regions, and may present similarly to dengue fever, but with the addition of disabling polyarthritis. Patients with dengue fever classically tend to describe bone pain and myalgia.

Management
Management of dengue fever is supportive, with prompt administration of fluids, antipyretics and transfusion of blood products as needed.

9.7.3 Yellow fever

Definition: yellow fever is a viral haemorrhagic fever caused by an RNA flavivirus that is spread by several species of mosquito. The disease is particularly endemic in African and Latin American regions.

W ≫ The virus infects leucocytes and hepatocytes, leading to cell breakdown and an enormous release of cytokines, which may predispose the patient to shock.

Clinical features:
- Presents with non-specific fever, malaise
- Rigors in the first few days, before progressing to jaundice, acute kidney injury, bleeding (possibly related to DIC) and shock

Management
Rapid detection methods include ELISA or PCR. There is no specific treatment, and management is supportive. Prevention of the disease is crucial, from using mosquito nets and mosquito control in endemic areas to the use of the **yellow fever vaccine (live vaccine)** before travelling to affected areas.

9.7.4 Cholera

Cholera is a form of acute diarrhoea caused by the organism *Vibrio cholerae*, transmitted by contaminated water or shellfish. It is endemic in parts of Africa, South America, Asia and India. Patients present with severe diarrhoea (classically described

as **rice-water** stools), which leads to major fluid loss and shock. Diagnosis is made based on stool microscopy and culture, and treatment includes vigorous rehydration, electrolyte replacement and ciprofloxacin.

9.7.5 American trypanosomiasis (Chagas disease)

Definition: American trypanosomiasis (also known as Chagas disease) is caused by the parasite *Trypanosoma cruzi*, which is transmitted by an infective reduviid bug. It is particularly endemic in South America and Mexico.

Clinical features:
- Patients may present as acutely systemically unwell
- They may have a **notable conjunctivitis and eye swelling** known as the **Romana sign**
- The disease may lie dormant for many years in its chronic form, leading to enlargement of body organs, causing dilated cardiomyopathy and arrhythmias, megaoesophagus and megacolon

E ≫ The bug that causes Chagas is a **megalo**-maniac.

Management
Diagnosis is made with serological tests, and treatment is with benznidazole or nifurtimox.

9.7.6 African trypanosomiasis

Definition: African trypanosomiasis (also known as **sleeping sickness**) is caused by the parasites *Trypanosoma gambiense* and *rhodesiense*, transmitted by the bite of an infected tsetse fly.

Clinical features:
- The disease presents acutely with systemic illness and an indurated chancre at the site of the bite
- There may also be regional lymphadenopathy in posterior cervical lymphadenopathy, known as the **Winterbottom sign**
- Patients eventually develop CNS symptoms, with increasing daytime somnolence (hence the name), seizures, confusion and coma

Management
Diagnosis is made on Giemsa stain of blood identifying the parasite or the card agglutination test for trypanosomiasis (CATT). The recommended treatment is with **suramin** early in the disease progression, and **nifurtimox-eflornathine** in severe cases.

9

9.7.7 Trematode (fluke) infections

There are several clinically relevant trematode infections. In this section, we will highlight schistosomiasis and *Chlonorchis sinensis* (the Chinese liver fluke), as it is a known risk factor in the development of cholangiocarcinoma. Treatment of this trematode infection involves triclabendazole or praziquantel.

Schistosomiasis

Schistosomiasis is a trematode infection caused by various species of *Schistosoma* and is transmitted by contact with infected water containing contaminated secretions from a particular freshwater snail. The most common endemic region is sub-Saharan Africa.

The disease can present acutely with fever, myalgia and abdominal pain, along with pruritus at the site of infection (colloquially known as a 'swimmer's itch'). The gold standard for diagnosis is microscopic examination of stool or urine, and the condition is treated with **praziquantel**.

 E ≫ *Schistosoma haematobium* is particularly associated with dysuria and haematuria; and it can progress to renal failure if left untreated. It is also a **risk factor for the development of squamous cell carcinoma of the bladder**.

9.7.8 Filariasis

Filariasis is a nematode parasite infection typically caused by *Wuchereria bancrofti* and *Brugia malayi* or *Brugia timori* and spread by the bite of an infected mosquito. There are two major forms – cutaneous and lymphatic.

Lymphatic filariasis classically presents with fever and painful lymphadenopathy acutely, with progression to severe lymphoedema and elephantiasis, with lymphoedema of the limbs and genitals.

Detection of microfilariae in the blood and eosinophilia are helpful in diagnosing the condition. Treatment is with mebendazole.

9.8 Candidiasis

Definition: candidiasis refers to a fungal infection caused by *Candida* spp., which may be a normal commensal, and can cause local or systemic disease. The systemic disease is particularly prevalent in patients who are in immunocompromised states.

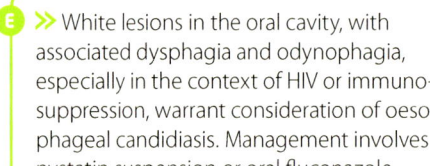 **E** ≫ White lesions in the oral cavity, with associated dysphagia and odynophagia, especially in the context of HIV or immunosuppression, warrant consideration of oesophageal candidiasis. Management involves nystatin suspension or oral fluconazole.

Aetiology/pathophysiology:
- *Candida albicans* is the most common cause

Approach to candidiasis
- Vulvovaginal candidiasis
  - Like most forms of candidiasis, risk factors include immunosuppression, steroid use, antibiotic use and diabetes mellitus

  - Typically presents with pruritus, vulvitis, erythema and a non-offensive 'cottage cheese'-like appearance
  - Treatment includes topical antifungals (e.g. clotrimazole) first line
  - Oral treatments include fluconazole
- Disseminated candidiasis
  - Systemic fungal infection
  - Remove source of infection (if possible) and treat using systemic antifungals or echinocandins

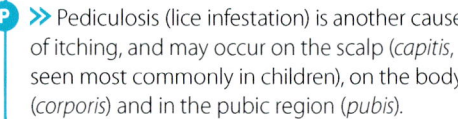 **P** ≫ Pediculosis (lice infestation) is another cause of itching, and may occur on the scalp (*capitis*, seen most commonly in children), on the body (*corporis*) and in the pubic region (*pubis*).

9.9 Prion disease (Creutzfeldt-Jakob disease, CJD)

Prion disease (transmissible spongiform encephalopathy) refers to a rare cluster of neurodegenerative conditions.

 P >> Bovine spongiform encephalopathy (also known as 'mad cow disease') is thought to have arisen from a variant of CJD in cattle.

CJD usually presents with a history (lasting a few weeks) of neuromuscular problems, behavioural problems and memory loss. Neurodegeneration tends to proceed at a rapid rate. Investigations include EEG and CSF biochemical markers. Unfortunately, there is no cure and management is supportive.

9.10 Helminth infections

9.10.1 Nematode (roundworm) infections

Nematodes are a class of helminths (worm) that cause infection.

Types of infection include:
- **Filariasis** (see *Section 9.7.8*)
- **Onchocerciasis (river blindness)**
  - Caused by *Onchocerca volvulus*
  - This parasite is transmitted by the bite of *Simulium* blackflies, which dwell near rivers, giving the disease its name
  - The diagnosis can be made by skin biopsy of lumps where the worm resides
  - Treatment is with **ivermectin**

 E >> (R)iver-mectin for river blindness.

- **Enterobiasis (pinworm infection)**
  - Caused by the pinworm *Enterobius vermicularis*
  - Infection results from ingestion of food or drink containing contaminated eggs
  - The eggs can be demonstrated on microscopy using the **Scotch-tape** test, in which placing transparent tape near the anal area will pick up the eggs
  - Treatment involves copiously disinfecting linen and living spaces, as well as taking albendazole or mebendazole
- **Ascariasis**
  - Caused by the worm *Ascariasis lumbricoides*
  - Transmitted by eating food contaminated by helminth eggs
  - These worms cause diarrhoea, malabsorption, hepatosplenomegaly and can migrate to the lungs to cause breathlessness
  - Treatment is with albendazole or mebendazole

P >> Löffler syndrome refers to an acute respiratory illness characterised by pulmonary eosinophilia secondary to migration of larva in ascariasis or hookworm infection.

- **Trichuriasis (whipworm infection)**
  - Causes abdominal pain, diarrhoea and lethargy
  - Seen mostly in tropical areas with poor sanitation
  - Treatment is with albendazole or mebendazole
- **Hookworm infection**
  - Caused by *Ancylostoma duodenale* or *Necator americanus*
  - Often transmitted via soil
  - These worms are voracious bloodsuckers, and this causes iron-deficiency anaemia and protein deficiency
  - Larval migration can cause **cutaneous larva migrans**, which results in a tunnelling, serpiginous rash in the skin
  - Treatment is with albendazole or mebendazole
- **Dracunculiasis**
  - Caused by the Guinea worm *Dracunculus medinensis* only in Africa
  - 1–2mm wide, and adult females can be up to a metre long!

 W >> The name dracunculiasis refers to infection by 'little dragons' in Latin.

  - Infection occurs after ingesting water contaminated with larvae
  - This is likely to be the first parasitic disease that is successfully eradicated; 3 million cases in 1986 decreased to 22 cases in 2015
  - The worm emerges painfully from the skin at a point during its life cycle

9

- – Treatment is threefold:
  - ○ Submerge the wound in clean water, to reduce cellulitis as the worm attempts to emerge
  - ○ Extract worm by coiling it around a stick as it emerges
  - ○ Offer metronidazole or thiabendazole to help extraction
- **Toxocariasis**
  - – Typically caused by a parasite that affects dogs, *Toxocara canis*
  - – Humans may become affected by touching infected dogs
  - – Causes eosinophilia, blindness (by migration to the eyes), respiratory and abdominal symptoms
  - – Treat with albendazole or mebendazole

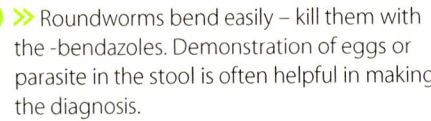 Roundworms bend easily – kill them with the -bendazoles. Demonstration of eggs or parasite in the stool is often helpful in making the diagnosis.

9.10.2 Cestode (tapeworm) infections

Cestode infections typically include:

- **Hydatid disease**
  - – Caused by *Echinococcus granulosus*
  - – Insidious onset – may be asymptomatic for years
  - – Infection occurs when consuming products contaminated with parasite eggs
  - – Causes abdominal pain, jaundice and shortness of breath (cyst rupture produces symptoms)
  - – Investigate with **ultrasound and CT abdomen**
  - – Treatment is **surgical**, but care must be taken to ensure that no cysts rupture during surgery, using albendazole and mebendazole pre- **and** post-operatively
- **Cysticercosis (pork tapeworm)**
  - – Caused by *Taenia solium*, associated with poorly cooked pork
  - – May cause myositis, fever and abdominal pain

 A specific, dangerous complication of *T. solium* infection is **neurocysticercosis**, which presents with hydrocephalus and acute seizures. Once the seizures have been adequately controlled, treat the helminth infection with **albendazole** or **praziquantel**.

- **Taeniasis (beef tapeworm)**
  - – Caused by *Taenia saginata,* associated with poorly cooked beef
  - – Produces abdominal symptoms
  - – Treat with **praziquantel**
- **Diphyllobothriasis (fish tapeworm)**
  - – Caused by *Diphyllobothrium latum*
  - – Common in Japan, because of sushi and sashimi consumption
  - – May be asymptomatic, or cause abdominal discomfort, vomiting or weight loss
  - – Diagnosis based on demonstrating eggs in the stool
  - – Treat with **praziquantel**

9.10.3 Other parasitic infections

- **Loa loa disease**
  - – Filarial eyeworm that causes lymphoedema, swelling, muscle pain and abscesses secondary to granuloma formation
  - – This parasite is called an eyeworm because eye pain may occur as *filariae* migrate across the eyes and bridge of nose
  - – Treat with **diethylcarbamazine**
- **Amoebiasis**
  - – Most common organism implicated is *Entamoeba histolytica*
  - – Associated with abdominal pain, bloody diarrhoea, peritonitis and anaemia due to GI bleeding
  - – Diagnosis may be made on demonstrating cysts in the stool
  - – Treat with **metronidazole**

Chapter 10
Rheumatology and immunology

Amar Vaswani

Basic principles

Rheumatology refers to a branch of internal medicine concerned with the treatment of diseases of the joints and soft tissues. As our understanding of the disease process has evolved, we now know that a significant number of rheumatological diseases originate with immunological dysfunction (e.g. vasculitis, autoimmune disease).

Bridge to clinical medicine

- The musculoskeletal system allows for adequate support and body movement in time and space
- The human body has 206 bones
- The human skeleton may be grossly divided into the **axial** skeleton and the **appendicular** skeleton
- The axial skeleton consists of the skull, the ossicles of the ear, hyoid bone, thoracic cage and vertebral column
- The appendicular skeleton consists of the bones of the upper and lower limbs, as well as the pectoral and pelvic girdles

Joints, articulation and movement

- A joint is a structure in the body at which two skeletal components articulate
- Joints allow for laxity, stability and movement
- Joints may be classified **structurally** and **functionally**

Structural joint classification

- Fibrous – joints articulated with fibrous tissue, with little space in between (three types)
  - Sutures (e.g. in the skull)
  - Syndesmoses (thin fibrous tissue connection present in e.g. tibia/fibula)
  - Gomphoses (e.g. joints holding teeth in place)
- Cartilaginous – joints articulated with cartilage (two types)
  - Synchondroses (epiphyseal plates of children)
  - Symphyses (e.g. pubic symphysis)
- Synovial (see *Fig. 10.1*)
  - Joints articulated with a joint space, cavity and fluid that reduce friction
  - Weakest joint structurally, but most mobile functionally

Functional joint classification

- Synarthroses – virtually no movement at the joint
- Amphiarthroses – little movement at the joint
- Diarthroses – freely movable joint

W ≫ Joints are susceptible to injury and inflammation (arthritis) due to their structure and function. If a single joint is affected, the arthropathy is said to be monoarticular, and if a number of joints are affected, the arthropathy is termed polyarticular. Arthritis has myriad causes, from degeneration of articular cartilage in osteoarthritis and autoimmunity (e.g. rheumatoid arthritis) to crystal deposition (e.g. gout) and infection (septic arthritis).

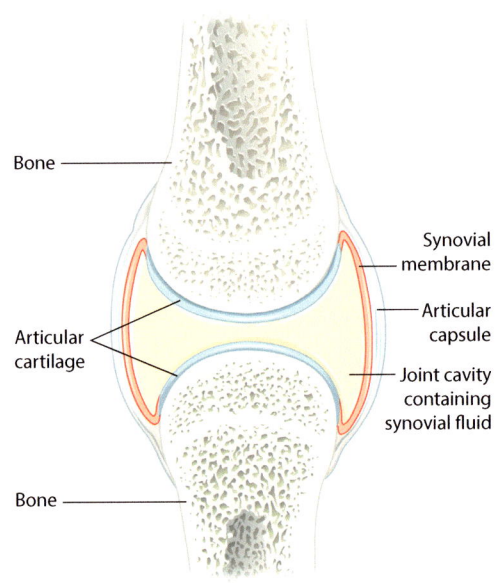

Bone

Synovial membrane

Articular capsule

Articular cartilage

Joint cavity containing synovial fluid

Bone

Fig. 10.1 A synovial joint.

Immunodeficiency and autoimmunity

Immunodeficiency

- Immunodeficiency refers to the intrinsic or extrinsic impairment in the immune system's ability to respond to a potential threat
- Primary immunodeficiencies usually refer to intrinsic impairment, most likely caused by congenital abnormalities
- Secondary immunodeficiencies are more likely to be acquired, and may occur as a result of immunosuppressive medication, infection or malignancy
- Patients may require long-term therapy, possibly involving antibody replacement or recurring antibiotic therapy to keep infections at bay

P ≫ Note that an immunosuppressive state is in itself a risk factor for the development of cancer.

Autoimmunity

- Autoimmunity refers to a form of immunological dysfunction in which an immune response is mounted against the body's own cells and tissues
- Autoimmune diseases occur secondary to impairment, in a phenomenon known as immunological tolerance; this allows the immune system not to react to the body's own cells and structures, whilst remaining active against foreign antigens
- The exact pathogenesis is incompletely understood, but autoimmunity is thought to arise as a result of many factors, including gender (women are more susceptible), environment, pathogens, genetics and molecular mimicry (foreign antigens share similar structural features to host antigens), amongst others

10.1 Osteoarthritis

Definition: osteoarthritis (OA) refers to a clinical state that occurs as a result of a degenerative process involving articular cartilage, extracellular matrix and subchondral bone, causing joint pain and limitation of function.

Epidemiology:

- Typically affects the older population
- More common in men at a younger age; more common in women at an older age
- Knee OA tends to be more common than hip OA

Aetiology/pathophysiology:

E ≫ The development of OA has been attributed to several risk factors, including genetic susceptibility, being female, obesity, intrinsic joint abnormalities or work-related mechanical stress.

- At a biochemical level, osteoarthritis occurs secondary to a disruption in homeostatic mechanisms involving cartilage renewal and breakdown
- A combination of triggers (some of them described above) predispose the joint to inflammation and trauma
- This inflammation and trauma results in matrix metalloproteinases that cause cartilage degradation and a net erosion of articular cartilage

and surrounding structures within the synovium, subsequently producing symptoms

P ≫ OA may be classified as primary or secondary. Primary OA is typically idiopathic, with no discernible underlying cause, whilst secondary OA is more likely to be associated with obesity or an intrinsic joint abnormality.

Clinical features:

- OA typically presents with joint pain, swelling and stiffness that lasts less than 30 minutes in the morning
- The most common joints affected are the knee and hip, followed by the proximal and distal interphalangeal joints (PIP/DIP) and the carpometacarpal joint of the thumb
- The pain of hip OA may present as referred knee or antero-medial groin pain
- The pain of OA is typically worse on movement and relieved by rest, with bony abnormalities sometimes being present; these include Heberden and Bouchard nodes (see *Fig. 10.2*)

E ≫ Bouchard nodes affect the PIP joints; and Heberden nodes affect the DIP joints (B comes before H in the alphabet).

10

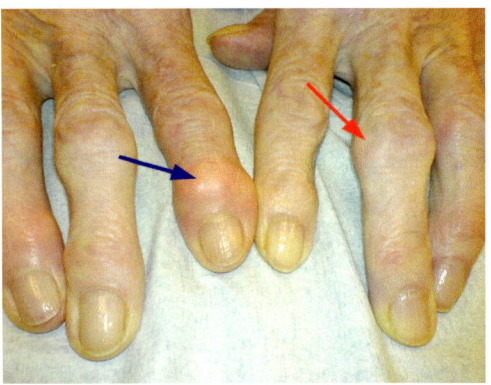

Fig. 10.2 *Heberden (blue arrow) and Bouchard (red arrow) nodes.*

Investigations

Stepwise plan:

1 **Assess the condition clinically**
- Check for activity-related joint pain, stiffness, BMI and physically examine the affected joint

2 **Arrange plain X-rays of the affected joint, looking for characteristic features of OA (see *Fig. 10.3*)**
- Bony osteophytes
- Joint space narrowing
- Cystic changes
- Subchondral sclerosis

3 **Diagnose osteoarthritis clinically without investigations if a person (NICE 2014, CG177)**
- Is 45 or over **and**
- Has activity-related joint pain **and**
- Has either no morning joint-related stiffness **or** morning stiffness that lasts no longer than 30 minutes

4 **Recommendations also include apt examination of a hot or swollen joint**
- Prompting consideration of an alternative diagnosis

P ≫ Blood tests are generally normal in OA. Measuring other parameters may be helpful in order to distinguish OA from another cause, such as rheumatoid arthritis. Joint aspiration may be helpful in particularly swollen joints. It is helpful to check baseline urea and creatinine before attempting to prescribe NSAIDs.

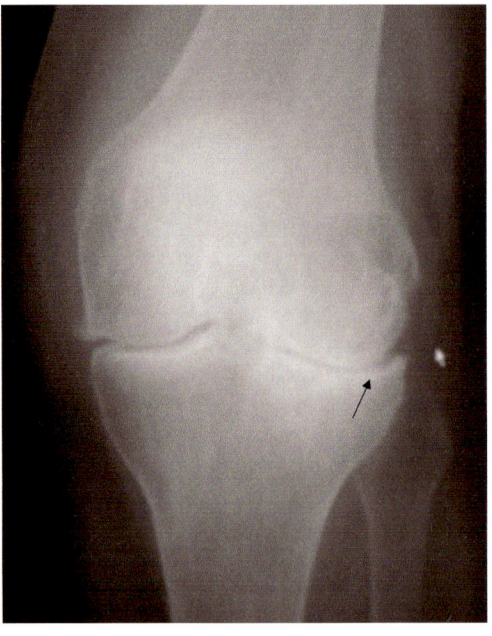

Fig. 10.3 *Left knee X-ray of a patient with knee OA, characterised by the loss of joint space (arrow), osteophytes and subchondral sclerosis.*

Management
Assess the patient holistically, taking into account psychosocial factors and potential necessary adjustments to the home or workplace. Take into account relevant comorbidities and agree on a treatment plan with the patient. Ensure that the patient is kept up to date and is adequately advised about the condition.

Stepwise management of osteoarthritis (NICE 2014, CG177)

1 **Carry out conservative management**
- Encourage the patient (if obese) to lose weight, engage in resistance training and improve general aerobic fitness
- The use of appropriate footwear should also be encouraged
- Acupuncture is **not recommended** in the management of OA

2 **Carry out medical management**
- **First line:** paracetamol and topical NSAIDs are recommended first-line treatments (note that topical NSAIDs are recommended for knee or hand OA only)

- **Second line:** oral NSAID/COX-2 inhibitor, co-prescribed with a PPI; note relevant side effect profiles
- **Third line:** intra-articular corticosteroid injections may be used as an adjunct in moderate or severe pain

3   Consider surgical management
- Consider surgical joint replacement (arthroplasty) if refractory to medical management

> **W** ≫ Topical **capsaicin** cream (derived from chilli) may be tried as an adjunct at this stage. Capsaicin is thought to inhibit transmission of substance P in sensory neurons when applied to achieve local stimulation.

> **P** ≫ Glucosamine, a normal component of articular cartilage, may sometimes be helpful in addressing symptoms, but its evidence and cost-effectiveness is limited, and it is not recommended by NICE.

10.2 Rheumatoid arthritis

Definition: rheumatoid arthritis (RA) refers to a chronic autoimmune inflammatory polyarthropathy that is generally symmetrical and causes deformity and restriction in function.

Epidemiology:
- Women are twice as likely to be affected as men
- Affects 1–2% of the population

Aetiology/pathophysiology:
- The exact pathogenesis is unknown, but HLA DRB1 has been associated with the development of the disease
- Smoking and infections have also been cited as potential risk factors
- Joint inflammation occurs secondary to infiltration of the synovium by white cells, and cytokine and matrix metalloproteinase proliferation are thought to contribute to overall joint destruction

Clinical features:
Arthritis
- RA typically presents as a symmetrical deforming polyarthritis that affects the MCP and PIP joints of the hands and feet

- Patients experience pain, swelling and tenderness, and various deformities may be observed on examination – these include ulnar deviation, subluxation of the MCPJs, swan-neck, boutonnière and Z-thumb deformities (see *Figs 10.4* and *10.5*)
- Patients are also likely to present with morning stiffness that lasts over an hour, and firm, tender rheumatoid nodules on the distal extremities
- RA affecting the cervical spine is also an important consideration and may lead to atlanto-axial subluxation. Patients with a history of RA should be assessed thoroughly, particularly if they are to undergo an operation

Systemic features
- RA may have other systemic complications, including:
  - Eyes – dry eyes (keratoconjunctivitis sicca), scleritis and Sjögren syndrome
  - Skin – rashes, vasculitides, rheumatoid nodules and ulcers
  - Cardiorespiratory symptoms – pericardial and pleural effusions, with associated pulmonary nodules or fibrosis

10

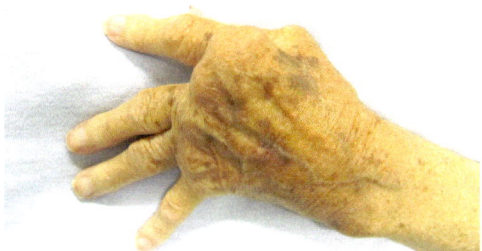

Fig. 10.4 *Left hand of a patient with severe RA. Note the ulnar deviation and subluxation of the MCPJs.*

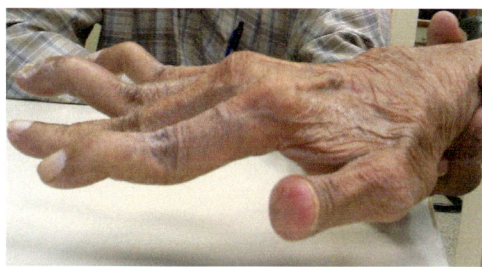

Fig. 10.5 *Extensive swan-neck and Z-thumb deformities.*

P ≫ Caplan syndrome: RA with pneumoconiosis and occupational dust exposure

Felty syndrome: RA with splenomegaly and neutropenia

An important point to bear in mind is that the arthritis in RA is rarely abrupt in onset. In the majority of patients it tends to get progressively worse from week to week, and from month to month.

– Neurological symptoms – peripheral neuropathies or entrapment, e.g. carpal tunnel syndrome

Investigations

The diagnosis of RA is largely clinical, with further investigation helping to rule out other conditions. The American College of Rheumatology/EULAR provides a criteria set for definitive diagnosis.

Stepwise plan:

1 **Assess the condition clinically, diagnosing at least four of the seven criteria:**
- Morning stiffness longer than an hour
- Arthritis affecting three or more joints
- Arthritis affecting the hands
- Symmetrical deforming pattern of disease
- Rheumatoid factor (RF) positive
- Presence of rheumatoid nodules
- Evidence of radiographic changes

2 **Arrange blood tests**
- Particularly **FBC**, **RF** and **anti-cyclic citrullinated** (CCP) antibodies and relevant radiographs (see *Fig. 10.6*)

E ≫ RF and anti-CCP antibodies are present in up to 70% of patients with RA. They are also associated with a poorer prognosis. Anti-CCP antibodies have a 95–98% specificity in the evaluation of rheumatoid arthritis.

3 **Apply the American College of Rheumatology/EULAR criteria**
- A score ≥6 criteria is required for definitive diagnosis

4 **Assess disease activity using appropriate scoring system**
- e.g. DAS 28

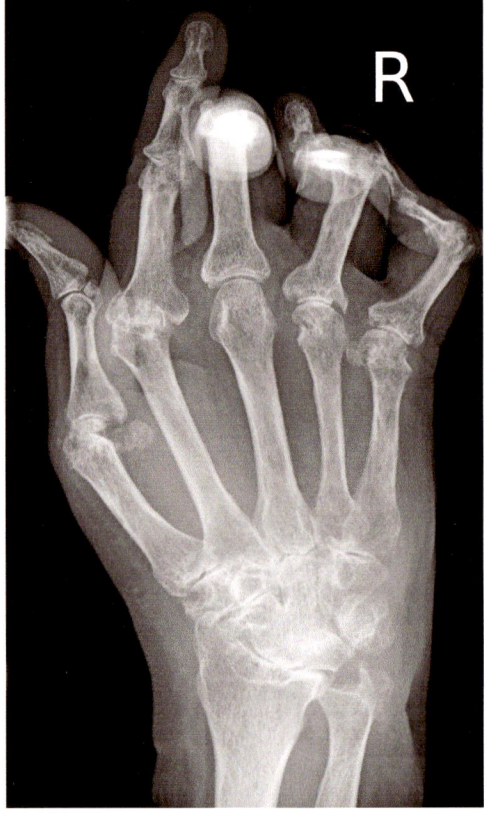

Fig. 10.6 *Right hand X-ray of a patient with severe RA. Note the diffuse loss of joint space, bony erosions and joint effusions.*

Management

Patients with RA should be managed by a multi-disciplinary team and be offered PT and OT assessment. NICE also recommends appropriate footwear and regular hand exercise for patients.

Stepwise management of rheumatoid arthritis (NICE 2015, CG79)

1 **Administer DMARDs and glucocorticoids**
- **First line:** early administration of disease-modifying anti-rheumatic drugs (DMARDs), plus short-term glucocorticoids, should be offered as soon as possible, ideally within 3 months of persistent symptoms
- **Offer a combination of DMARDs (methotrexate and at least one other DMARD) and glucocorticoids**
- DMARDs include:
  - **Methotrexate** – side effects include hepatotoxicity, pulmonary fibrosis and myelosuppression

- **Sulfasalazine** – side effects include hepatotoxicity and a lowered sperm count
- **Hydroxychloroquine** – side effects include retinopathy
- **Other agents** – less commonly used agents include gold, leflunomide and penicillamine

W >> Glucocorticoids in the initial context of disease are helpful in symptom control, as DMARDs may take a longer time to take effect.

2 Consider the use of biological agents
- Such as infliximab, adalimumab or etanercept.

E >> Biological agents may cause reactivation of tuberculosis and hepatitis B. They also carry with them an increased risk of infection.

3 Consider the use of other biologics, e.g. rituximab
- Rituximab is an anti-CD20 antibody used in RA cases that are unresponsive to biological agents

P >> Other agents that can be utilised at this stage include abatacept (which interferes with antigen presentation to T cells) or a newer agent, tofacitinib, which acts as a JAK pathway inhibitor, as opposed to other protein-based biologics. Tofacitinib carries with it an increased risk of dyslipidaemia and intestinal perforation.

4 Consider surgical management
- Surgery is indicated in the presence of debilitating deformity or loss of function, and early surgical referral is recommended if symptoms do not respond to medical therapy

10.3 Septic arthritis

Definition: septic arthritis refers to an infection that affects one or more (native or prosthetic) joints in the body.

Epidemiology:
- The incidence of the condition is greatly increased in patients with comorbid joint disease or prosthetic joints in particular
- The knee is the joint that is most commonly affected

Aetiology/pathophysiology:
- The most common infective organism is **Staphylococcus or Streptococcus**, but gonococcal arthritis should also be considered, particularly in young, sexually active individuals
- Patients with diabetes, joint surgery or immunocompromised individuals are at greater risk of developing the condition
- Inoculation with infective organisms occurs due to local or haematogenous spread

Clinical features:
- Patients with septic arthritis typically present as systemically unwell with a single, hot, swollen and painful joint (see *Fig. 10.7*)
- The knee is the most commonly affected joint in most cases
- An effusion around the area of swelling may also be present, and a decreased range of motion

P >> The disease may present slightly differently in children, with some children who are systemically unwell simply refusing to move the joint in question. Remember to maintain a high index of suspicion in patients with a prosthetic joint, particularly if they are systemically unwell.

10

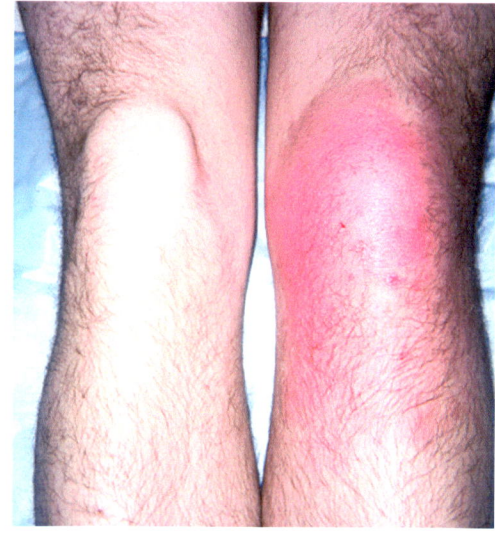

Fig. 10.7 *Septic arthritis of the left knee.*

Investigations

Stepwise plan:

1 If septic arthritis is suspected
- Arrange joint aspiration of synovial fluid for Gram stain, microscopy and culture, looking for an elevated white cell count

2 Arrange blood tests, including FBC, U&Es, ESR and CRP

> **E** ≫ Blood cultures should be taken before antibiotic therapy is instituted.

3 An MRI may be useful if underlying osteomyelitis is suspected

Management

Stepwise management of septic arthritis

1 Administer antibiotic therapy
- Start empirical antibiotic therapy before the results of blood cultures have been obtained

- Antibiotics are given IV for 2–3 weeks before being switched to oral preparations in the subsequent month
- An example of initial empirical therapy is IV vancomycin and cefotaxime

2 Drain purulent fluid

3 Assess response to treatment
- If the patient fails to respond to therapy, aspirate the joint again and reconsider the diagnosis; Lyme disease may also be considered
- Repeated aspiration may be helpful
- Surgical drainage may be attempted if patient remains unresponsive

4 Physiotherapy and splinting
- These may be offered as well, to promote wellbeing and recovery.

10.4 Crystal-induced arthritis

10.4.1 Gout

Definition: gout refers to a clinical state in which hyperuricaemia and monosodium urate crystal deposition in joints causes pain, inflammation and potential joint destruction.

Epidemiology:
- Affects significantly more men than women
- Pre-menopausal women are rarely affected
- More common in Asian populations

Aetiology/pathophysiology:

> **E** ≫ An important aetiological factor in the development of gout is diuretic therapy, particularly **thiazide** diuretics.

- Multiple aetiological factors are thought to be involved in the development or worsening of gout; these include:
  - Genetic susceptibility
  - Overproduction or under-excretion (more common) of uric acid
  - Being male
  - Consumption of red meat, seafood and alcohol
  - Associations with diabetes, heart disease and metabolic syndrome

> **W** ≫ Elevated urate levels in the body predispose an individual to the formation of monosodium urate crystals. Gout is more likely to occur in the first metatarsophalangeal joint and joints with concomitant osteoarthritis. Crystals provoke an inflammatory response by way of phagocytic interaction, causing chemokine stimulation, leukocytic infiltration and subsequent inflammation.

Clinical features:
- Gout typically presents with an acutely inflamed, hot, swollen joint that reaches peak pain intensity within 6–12 hours of the initial presentation, but this may also be suggestive of other crystal arthropathies
- The joint most likely to be affected (particularly in first presentations) is the first metatarsophalangeal (MTP) joint, also known as **podagra**, but it may affect other joints such as the knee
- Gouty **tophi** may also be present – masses of soft tissue swelling (e.g. at the pinna of the ear) that accrue as a result of urate crystal deposition (see *Fig. 10.8*)

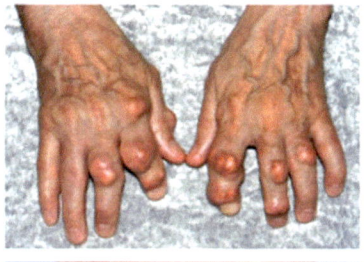
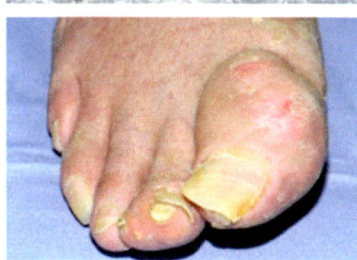
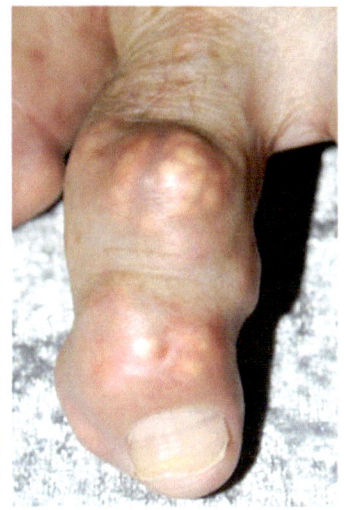

Fig. 10.8 *Gout affecting the hands and feet with its characteristic tophi.*

P ≫ **Lesch–Nyhan** syndrome, an inherited disorder that is characterised by the deficiency of hypoxanthine-guanine phosphoribosyltransferase (HGPRT), is associated with the build-up of urate in the body as a result of the aforementioned enzymatic deficiency. Patients present with severe gout early in life, learning disabilities and behaviours relating to self-mutilation.

Investigations

Stepwise plan:

1   **Gout can be diagnosed clinically**
- Especially if an acute monoarthritis affecting the first MTP joint is the initial presentation, but requires demonstration of monosodium urate crystals to be confirmed

2   **Arrange for synovial fluid aspiration (gold standard)**
- Monosodium urate crystals with **negatively** birefringent needle-shaped crystals when exposed to polarised light

3   **Blood tests may demonstrate an elevated serum urate level**

4   **Joint X-rays may demonstrate periarticular punched-out erosions**

Management

Patients with gout should be advised to maintain an optimal weight and restrict the amount of red meat and seafood they consume. Patients should also be advised not to binge-drink and to ensure they restrict their alcohol intake.

Stepwise management of gout (NICE, CKS 2015)

1   **Prescribe NSAIDs**
- NSAIDs are the **first-line treatment**, if they are not contraindicated (e.g. peptic ulcer disease or heart failure)

2   **Colchicine is recommended as an effective alternative to NSAID therapy**
- But patients should be warned about its gastro-intestinal side effects, particularly diarrhoea

3   **Consider steroids**
- Oral steroids may be used if NSAIDs and colchicine are contraindicated (e.g. in renal disease), or may be prescribed as an intra-articular injection

4   **Provide prophylaxis**
- Appropriate preventive measures should be taken
- Follow up the person 4–6 weeks after an acute attack of gout has resolved, and:
  - Check their serum uric acid level
  - Measure their blood pressure and take blood for fasting glucose, renal function and lipid profile
  - Identify and manage underlying conditions such as hypertension, diabetes or renal impairment, and assess the person's overall cardiovascular risk
  - Provide advice on risk factors such as obesity, diet, excessive alcohol consumption, and lack of exercise
  - Consider prophylactic medication if a person is having two or more attacks of gout in a year

10

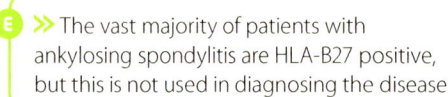 Allopurinol is the drug of choice in gout prophylaxis but should never be administered in the acute setting. The patient should be started on a low dose and titrated up to maintain serum urate levels below 300 micromol/L. Patients should be advised to continue taking allopurinol and not stop the drug during an acute attack. Another agent, febuxostat, is recommended by NICE if patients are allopurinol-intolerant.

10.4.2 Calcium pyrophosphate deposition (CPPD) disease (including pseudogout)

Calcium pyrophosphate deposition (CPPD) disease refers to a group of conditions that involve arthropathy caused by deposition of crystals. CPPD disease has several forms, including asymptomatic cartilage crystal deposition (chondrocalcinosis), acute crystal arthropathy (pseudogout), and a chronic inflammatory condition that may also present with underlying osteoarthritis.

Patients are typically older, and the condition has equal gender preponderance, unlike gout. Patients with diabetes, dehydration and hyperparathyroidism are also more at risk of the condition. The definitive investigation is joint aspiration, in which **rhomboid-shaped, positively birefringent crystals** may be observed. The management of an acute attack is similar to that for gout, with intra-articular steroids being the preferred treatment. If these are unsuitable, treat with NSAIDs (use carefully in older individuals), or colchicine may be offered instead.

10.5 Seronegative arthropathies

10.5.1 Ankylosing spondylitis

Definition: ankylosing spondylitis is a seronegative spondyloarthropathy, primarily affecting the axial skeleton, and the sacroiliac joints with potential systemic manifestations.

Epidemiology:
- Tends to affect more men than women
- Associated with early presentations, young people between 20 and 30

Aetiology/pathophysiology:

 The vast majority of patients with ankylosing spondylitis are HLA-B27 positive, but this is not used in diagnosing the disease.

- Despite clear associations with HLA-B27, the exact mechanism of the development of ankylosing spondylitis and its underlying aetiology and pathophysiology remain unclear.

Clinical features:
- Patients with ankylosing spondylitis typically present before the age of 30
- Characteristic features of the disease include:
  - Morning joint or back stiffness
  - Back or buttock pain that improves with activity or exercise
  - Back or joint pain at night which prompts waking

- Systemic features may or may not be present, e.g. fever, anterior uveitis (seen in 25%), episcleritis, heart block, valvular abnormalities
- Patients may also eventually develop thoracic kyphosis and hyperextension of the neck, leading to a 'question mark' posture
- A positive Schober test is also associated with the disease

Investigations

Stepwise plan:

1 **The diagnosis is usually suspected clinically, but NICE recommends that the modified New York criteria be used**
- Clinical criteria:
  - Lower back pain for more than 3 months, improved by exercise and not relieved by rest
  - Limitation of lumbar spine motion in both the sagittal and frontal planes
  - Limitation of chest expansion relative to normal values for age and sex
- Radiological criteria
  - Sacroiliitis on X-ray (see *Fig. 10.9* and *Fig. 10.10*)

>> Note that the classic 'bamboo spine' seen on X-ray in patients with the disease is a late and fairly uncommon feature.

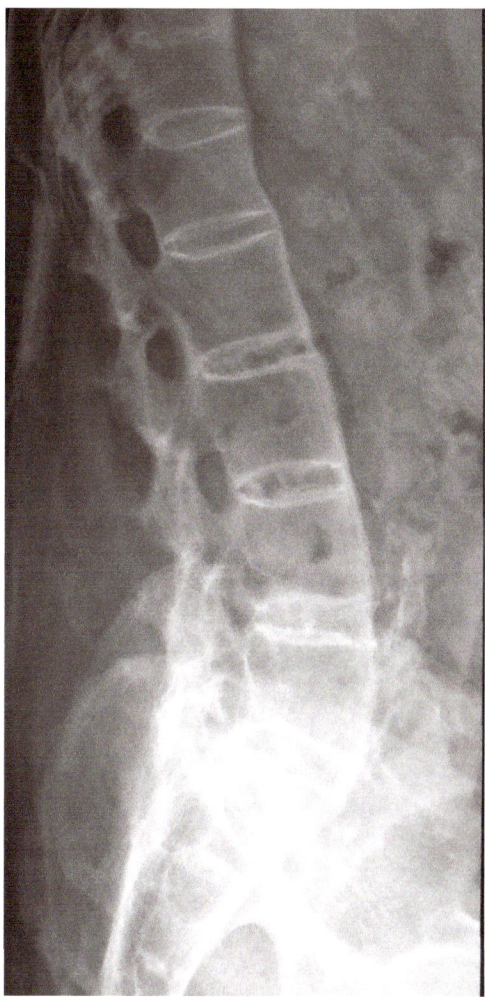

Fig. 10.9 *Lateral lumbar spine X-ray showing evidence of vertebral body squaring (bamboo spine) and syndesmophytic changes.*

> **P** » Blood tests are generally unhelpful in diagnosing ankylosing spondylitis.

2 Based on the modified New York criteria:
- **Diagnose definite ankylosing spondylitis** if the radiological criterion is present, plus at least one clinical criterion
- **Probable ankylosing spondylitis** if three clinical criteria are present alone, **or** if the radiological criterion is present but no clinical criteria are present

Management
There is generally no cure available for ankylosing spondylitis. Treatment goals include pain relief

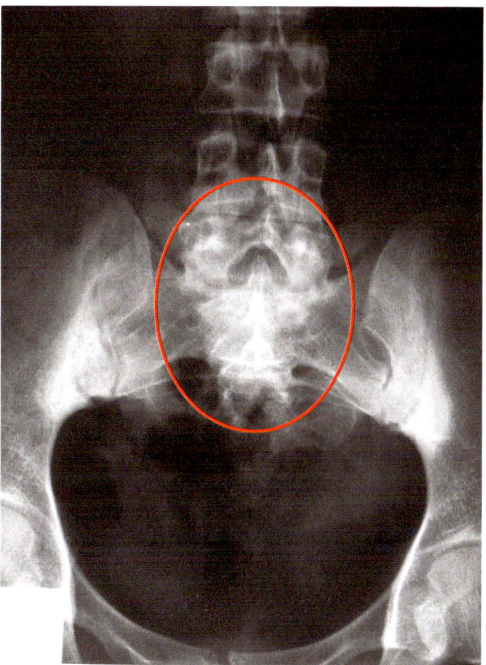

Fig. 10.10 *Lumbar spine X-ray showing evidence of sacroiliitis consistent with ankylosing spondylitis.*

and reducing functional limitation. Referral to a rheumatologist is recommended.

> **Stepwise management of ankylosing spondylitis (NICE 2017, NG65)**

1 Carry out conservative management
- Encourage the patient to undertake regular exercise and to attend structured physiotherapy

2 NSAID medications are used first line to control symptoms
- These should be co-prescribed with PPI cover for patients with an increased risk of gastrointestinal side effects

3 Prescribe steroids and pain relief
- Local corticosteroid injections may be of value, and a trial of other analgesics (including simple analgesia) may help if NSAID therapy is contraindicated or not well tolerated

4 Consider using biological agents
- NICE recommends **adalimumab, certolizumab pegol, etanercept, golimumab and infliximab** – if the diagnosis of ankylosing spondylitis has been

10

confirmed by the modified New York criteria, symptoms have persisted for at least 12 weeks and have not improved with NSAID therapy and no contraindications are present

5 Consider surgery
- In some cases, surgery may be needed to manage deformities or repair fractures that occur as a result of the condition
- Surgery may also be offered if the spinal deformity is significantly affecting the patient's quality of life

6 Provide follow-up care
- Patients with this condition should be monitored for cardiovascular disease and should be offered bisphosphonates according to specialist recommendation to prevent osteoporosis
- Osteoporosis screening should be conducted every 2 years

10.5.2 Reactive arthritis (includes Reiter syndrome)

Definition: reactive arthritis is a seronegative spondyloarthritis, also associated with HLA-B27, that describes arthritic pain, inflammation and extra-articular features that predominate after a preceding gastrointestinal or genitourinary infection.

Epidemiology:
- Most commonly affects adults

Aetiology/pathophysiology:

P ≫ Reactive arthritis that occurs post-infection is most commonly caused by *Campylobacter*, *Salmonella* or *Shigella* spp. if a gastrointestinal disease is suspected, and by *Chlamydia* spp. if a genitourinary cause is suspected.

- *Chlamydia trachomatis*, in particular, can trigger reactive arthritis, and may provoke undifferentiated arthritis
- Chlamydial proteins have been discovered in synovial fluid, indicating that these organisms have invaded the area
- The exact pathogenesis of the condition, and how it relates to genetic and HLA susceptibility, is incompletely understood

Clinical features:

E ≫ The classic features of Reiter syndrome (a subset of reactive arthritis) are: **arthritis** related to an infection, **conjunctivitis** and **non-gonococcal urethritis**. They may be helpfully remembered as 'a patient who can't see, can't pee and can't climb a tree'.

W ≫ The term Reiter syndrome has fallen out of favour in recent times, as Hans Reiter, the doctor who described the condition, performed numerous unethical experiments on concentration camp prisoners and was a member of the Nazi party.

- The arthritis typically develops 2 or more weeks post-infection, and patients may be systemically unwell
- Other dermatological features include erythema nodosum, nail changes, keratoderma blenorrhagica (yellow-brown waxy rash on the soles of the feet; see *Fig. 10.11*); circinate balanitis (formation of annular dermatitis on the glans penis) may also accompany the presentation

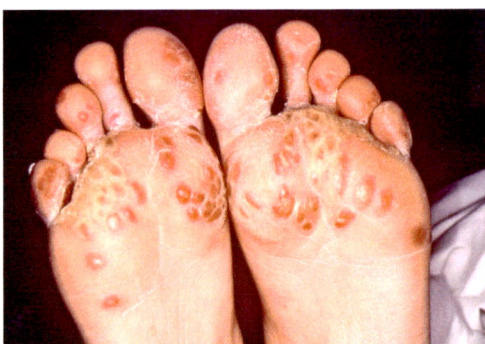

Fig. 10.11 *Keratoderma blenorrhagica.*

Investigations

Stepwise plan:

1 Arrange joint aspiration and synovial fluid analysis
- This will usually be negative for crystal deposition and help rule out other causes, but will generally have a higher white cell count

2 Obtain blood tests

- These will demonstrate a markedly elevated ESR and CRP, with RF and antibody tests usually proving negative in the majority of cases

3 Carry out cultures and PCR

- Urine chlamydia PCR and stool cultures may be helpful in identifying the organism in question, particularly if symptoms are dealt with early

4 Obtain plain radiographs of affected joints

- These may be useful in demonstrating any other abnormalities

Stepwise management of reactive arthritis

1 Prescribe NSAIDs

- NSAIDs are the first-line therapy when managing reactive arthritis

2 Prescribe corticosteroids

- Intra-articular steroids may be used if NSAID therapy is contraindicated, or as adjunct therapy in the acute setting
- Systemic steroids may be used if there is extensive polyarthritis

3 Prescribe antibiotics and DMARDs

- Antibiotics may treat the causative organism, but their long-term use in altering the course of arthritis is unsubstantiated
- Likewise, DMARD therapy may prove helpful in some patients, but only sulfasalazine has been shown to be effective in these instances

10.5.3 Psoriatic arthritis

Psoriatic arthritis occurs in approximately 10–20% of patients with psoriasis. Joint involvement often develops after cutaneous manifestations but may predate skin disease in 20% of cases. There are five patterns of joint involvement, most of which follow a relapsing-remitting course. *Table 10.1* describes these patterns and their clinical features.

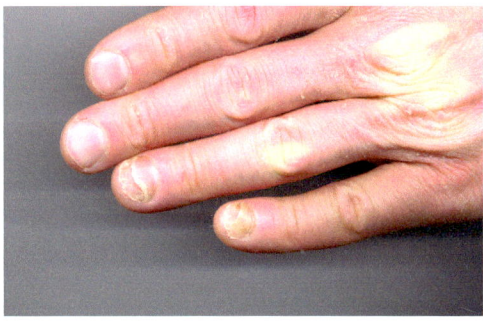

Fig. 10.12 *Onycholysis and some nail pitting, characteristic of a patient with psoriasis. Also note the psoriatic skin changes over the back of the hand.*

The management of psoriatic arthritis is similar to that of RA. NSAIDs are used for symptom control in the first instance. Intra-articular steroids may be used to relieve synovitis. DMARDs and anti-TNF therapy may be considered in refractory disease. The treatment of psoriasis is discussed in *Chapter 11*.

10.5.4 Enteropathic arthritis

Enteropathic arthritis is an inflammatory seronegative arthropathy that occurs in around 10–20% of patients with inflammatory bowel disease (IBD). It primarily affects the large joints with an asymmetrical pattern. The arthritis often develops during exacerbations of the bowel disease. Management mainly involves treatment of the underlying IBD. However, DMARDs and anti-TNF therapy may be required.

10

Table 10.1 *Patterns of psoriatic arthritis*

Asymmetrical oligoarthritis (40%)	• Presents insidiously, most often involving the hands and feet • Combination of synovitis and periarticular changes
Symmetrical polyarthritis (20%)	• More common in females • Similar to RA but nodules and extra-articular features are absent
Distal IPJ arthritis (~15%)	• More common in males • Isolated DIPJ involvement with concurrent nail dystrophy (see *Fig. 10.12*)
Arthritis mutilans (~5%)	• Erosive arthritis, often involving the digits, characterised by cartilage and bone destruction
Psoriatic spondylitis	• Similar presentation to ankylosing spondylitis

10.6 Connective tissue diseases

10.6.1 Systemic lupus erythematosus (SLE)

Definition: systemic lupus erythematosus (SLE) is a multisystem autoimmune inflammatory disorder.

Epidemiology:
- Affects up to 9 times more women than men
- More commonly seen in Asian and Afro-Caribbean populations

Aetiology/pathophysiology:
- The aetiology and pathophysiology of the disease are incompletely understood, but are thought to involve a combination of genetic, autoimmune and environmental factors (including drugs)
- One postulated pathway for disease is impairment in the body's ability to remove apoptotic waste products and immune complexes

> **P** ≫ SLE may be caused by some medications. This form, drug-induced lupus, presents with fewer features and less commonly affects the renal system. More commonly, it tends to present with skin and pulmonary symptoms. These patients are typically anti-dsDNA-negative, **but anti-histone antibody**-positive.

> **E** ≫ Common medications associated with drug-induced lupus are hydralazine, isoniazid and procainamide (HIP).

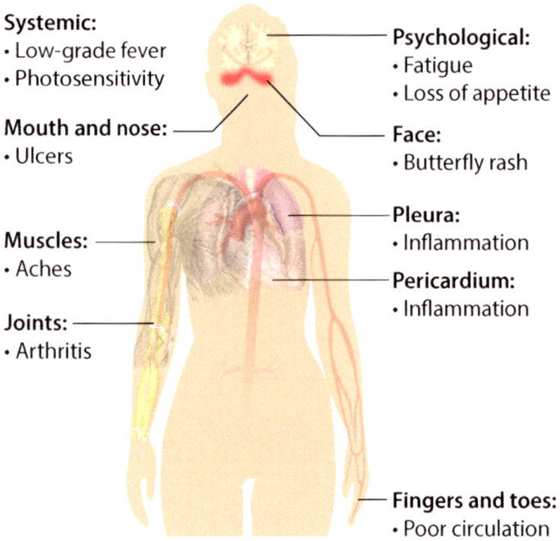

Clinical features:
- SLE may present with a wide variety of symptoms, and patients typically present with a relapsing-remitting history; patients most often have fatigue, fever, skin changes and arthralgia
- It may be helpful to classify other symptoms by system (see *Fig. 10.13*):
  - Skin – photosensitive, characteristic butterfly rash (see *Fig. 10.14*), mouth ulcers, discoid lupus (scaly, pruritic rash precipitated by sunlight that may cause alopecia)
  - Musculoskeletal – arthralgia
  - Pulmonary – pleurisy, fibrosing alveolitis
  - Cardiovascular – endocarditis, pericarditis

> **P** ≫ SLE causes LSE (Libman–Sacks endocarditis).

  - Neurological – seizures, psychosis
  - Thrombotic – antiphospholipid syndrome
  - Renal – glomerulonephritis, proteinuria
  - Increased risk of malignancy, particularly non-Hodgkin lymphoma

Systemic:
• Low-grade fever
• Photosensitivity

Mouth and nose:
• Ulcers

Muscles:
• Aches

Joints:
• Arthritis

Psychological:
• Fatigue
• Loss of appetite

Face:
• Butterfly rash

Pleura:
• Inflammation

Pericardium:
• Inflammation

Fingers and toes:
• Poor circulation

Fig. 10.13 *Common symptoms of SLE.*

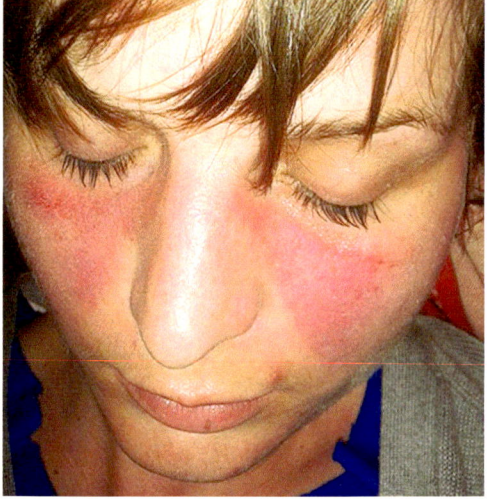

Fig. 10.14 *Malar (butterfly) rash.*

10

Investigations

Stepwise plan:

1. **The first step is to consider the American College of Rheumatology criteria**
   - If a patient has 4 out of 11 criteria, a diagnosis of SLE is likely

E ≫ The American College of Rheumatology has 11 criteria, which can be helpfully remembered with the mnemonic 'BUDAPEST AIR':

Butterfly (malar) rash
Ulcers
Discoid lupus
Arthralgia
Pleurisy/pericarditis
Exposure to sunlight (photosensitivity)
Seizures
Thrombocytopenia or other haematological issues
Positive **A**nti-nuclear antibody (ANA) titre
Immunological: anti-DNA antibody **or** anti-Smith **or** antiphospholipid antibodies
Renal disease (glomerulonephritis/proteinuria)

2. **Carry out other screening investigations**
   - These include FBC, U&Es, ESR, auto-antibody testing (ANA, anti-Smith anti-dsDNA in particular is very specific) and complement levels

P ≫ Patients with SLE often have reduced C3 and C4 and an elevated ESR.

Management

The treatment of SLE primarily involves symptomatic control and prevention of long-term sequelae. Patients should remain educated about their condition, be encouraged to stop smoking and avoid sunlight.

Stepwise management of systemic lupus erythematosus

1. **Prescribe medication**
   - NSAIDs, **hydroxychloroquine** (first-line), glucocorticoids (particularly useful for acute flares, but also thought to increase mortality as a result of infection)

2. **Protect the skin**
   - Avoid sunlight, wear sunscreen, topical steroids and oral care

3. **Consider biologics**
   - Biologics such as belimumab may be used in patients unresponsive to standard therapy

4. **In cases of lupus nephritis**
   - Prescribe cyclophosphamide (in very severe disease) or mycophenolate first line or tacrolimus and corticosteroids second line

10.6.2 Sjögren syndrome

Definition: Sjögren syndrome is a clinical condition that manifests with systemic symptoms, dryness and decreased secretions, particularly of the lacrimal and salivary glands, as a result of autoimmune lymphocytic infiltration.

Epidemiology:
- Female to male ratio 9:1

Aetiology/pathophysiology:
- Sjögren syndrome may be primary if it develops *de novo*, or secondary if it develops concomitantly with other autoimmune conditions (e.g. lupus, RA)
- The exact aetiology of the condition is unknown at this time, but is thought to involve a combination of genetic, autoimmune and viral (EBV) factors

Clinical features:
- The most common presenting complaints are dry eyes (keratoconjunctivitis sicca) and a dry mouth, but these may be attributed to a variety of causes
- A thorough history and examination should also assess if there are other autoimmune diseases or symptoms associated with Sjögren syndrome, including:
  - Parotid swelling
  - Vaginal dryness
  - Arthralgia, fatigue and myalgia
  - Vasculitis

Investigations

Stepwise plan:

1. **Attempt to confirm clinical criteria**
   - Look specifically for dry eyes, dry mouth and other features that may point to a diagnosis

2. **Perform the Schirmer test**
   - This involves using filter paper placed at the conjunctival eye sac for 5 minutes
   - If <5mm of tears stain the paper, it constitutes a positive test

10

3 Carry out auto-antibody testing
- Several auto-antibodies may be positive in investigating Sjögren syndrome (e.g. RF), but only two are clinically helpful in making the diagnosis – these are Anti-Ro and Anti-La antibodies

4 If the diagnosis is still uncertain, additional tests may be undertaken
- These include sialometry (testing salivary flow) and parotid gland biopsy

Management

No specific therapies exist for the treatment of this disease so it's best to provide symptomatic treatment – with artificial tears and drinking plenty of water. Arthralgia may be treated with NSAIDs, and other systemic complications may be dealt with symptomatically.

10.6.3 Systemic sclerosis (includes CREST syndrome)

Definition: systemic sclerosis (scleroderma) is a multi-system autoimmune disorder characterised by hardening and fibrosis of skin, blood vessels and viscera, resulting in abnormal structure or function. The term scleroderma comes from the Greek words *sclera* meaning 'hard', and *derma* meaning 'skin'. The disease is classified into two main types based largely on the extent of skin involvement:
- Limited cutaneous systemic sclerosis (also known as CREST syndrome – **C**alcinosis, **R**aynaud syndrome, (o)**E**sophageal dysmotility, **S**clerodactyly and **T**elangiectasia)
- Diffuse systemic sclerosis

> **P** ≫ **Raynaud phenomenon** may refer to **Raynaud disease** or **Raynaud syndrome**.
>
> **Raynaud phenomenon** classically produces symptoms of numbness, tingling and discoloration to the distal digits of the fingers and toes, thought to be due to vasospasm and triggered by emotional stress or the cold.
>
> **Raynaud disease** refers to the idiopathic form of the condition, while **Raynaud syndrome** refers to symptoms associated with an underlying connective tissue disease such as limited scleroderma.
>
> Management involves stopping smoking, reducing cold and stress exposure and using calcium channel blockers such as nifedipine if symptoms persist.

Epidemiology:
- Limited scleroderma is more common (affecting 70% of patients), while diffuse scleroderma affects 30%
- Women are usually affected up to 4 or 5 times more than men

Aetiology/pathophysiology:
- The exact pathophysiology and aetiology are unknown, but the condition is thought to arise as a result of interplay between genetic and autoimmune factors

Clinical features:
- Limited scleroderma:
  - Skin tightening typically affects the **face and distal extremities**
  - **Calcinosis, sclerodactyly** (see *Fig. 10.15*) and **telangiectasia** may also be present
  - Raynaud syndrome may be a presenting feature (see *Fig. 10.16*)
  - Associated with anti-centromere auto-antibodies
  - Indolent disease course, and progresses slowly
- Diffuse scleroderma:
  - More rapid progression
  - Fibrosis of internal organs such as lung, kidney, GI tract and heart, leading to pulmonary symptoms, arrhythmias, dysphagia and hypertensive crises
  - Associated with anti-Scl-70 auto-antibodies

> **E** ≫ Pulmonary hypertension is seen in 10–15% of patients with scleroderma and is an important contributor to early mortality.

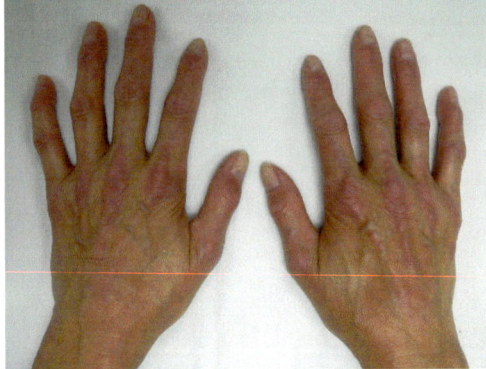

Fig. 10.15 *Calcinosis and sclerodactyly seen in the hands of a patient with scleroderma.*

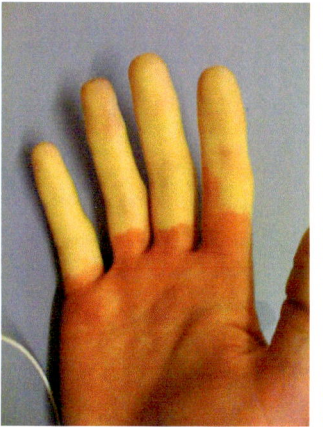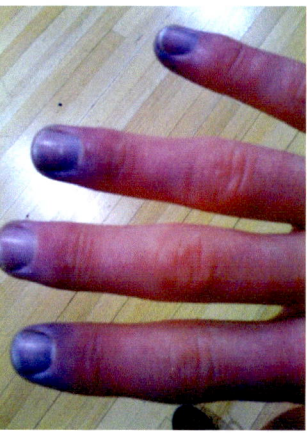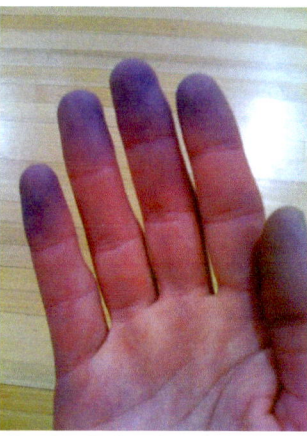

Fig. 10.16 *A series of photographs showing the progression of Raynaud phenomenon.*

Investigations

Note that patients may initially report suffering from Raynaud syndrome, or any number of associated conditions such as GORD, shortness of breath, dysphagia or weight loss. A careful, thorough history and examination should be conducted.

> **Stepwise plan:**

1 **Obtain initial blood tests**
   - Including FBC, U&Es, ESR and CRP

2 **Arrange auto-antibody testing:**
   - Anti-nuclear antibody (90%)
   - Anti-centromere antibody (limited scleroderma)
   - Anti Scl-70 or anti topoisomerase I (diffuse scleroderma)
   - Anti-RNA polymerase III (associated with an increased risk of renal crises)

3 **Arrange regular monitoring of systemic complications, using appropriate tests**
   - e.g. barium studies, ECG, CXR, PFTs, echocardiograms and monitoring renal function

Management

There is no specific therapy for the disease. The extent of organ involvement should be ascertained, and management should be centred on symptomatic control and prevention of complications.

> **Stepwise management of systemic sclerosis**

1 **Provide regular physiotherapy**
   - To strengthen muscles and joints, occupational therapy to help assist in activities of daily living

2 **Prescribe skin and immunosuppressive treatments**
   - Emollients for skin, and the use of immunosuppressives (such as cyclophosphamide or cyclosporin) have been shown to reduce skin and pulmonary fibrosis

3 **Provide treatment of GORD**
   - Conservatively with lifestyle changes and PPI

4 **Aim for early identification of pulmonary hypertension and treatment**
   - With endothelin receptor antagonists (such as bosentan) and phosphodiesterase-5 inhibitors (such as tadalafil)

> **E** ≫ Patients, particularly with diffuse scleroderma, may experience severe renal disease which may precipitate scleroderma renal crises. These may present with a sudden onset of hypertension, acute kidney injury and proteinuria, and may also present with headaches and fatigue. Patients at risk may be tested with anti-RNA polymerase III antibodies and should be treated with ACE inhibitors or dialysis if necessary.

10.6.4 Polymyositis

Polymyositis refers to a condition characterised by autoimmune-mediated muscle inflammation. Patients typically present with **symmetrical proximal muscle weakness** and sparing of the distal extremities. They may also experience dysphagia as a result of pharyngeal muscle weakening and will **generally have no rash**.

Initial investigations may demonstrate a markedly elevated creatine kinase (CK) and **anti-Jo-1** antibodies. Confirmatory testing involves electromyography and muscle biopsy.

> **E** » Both polymyositis and dermatomyositis may have systemic features, such as fever, arrhythmias and arthritis.

10.6.5 Dermatomyositis

Dermatomyositis presents with similar proximal muscle weakness associated with systemic features, but these patients often have dermatological complaints as an initial presenting feature. These are classically a heliotrope rash (peri-orbital purple rash; see *Fig. 10.17*) and Gottron papules on the knuckles, elbows and knees (see *Fig. 10.18*).

Patients may also be investigated initially with blood tests, which may demonstrate an elevated CK, anti-Mi-2 and ANA and may undergo confirmatory testing with electromyography and muscle biopsy.

> **E** » Anti-Mi-2 antibodies are highly specific for dermatomyositis but are only seen in about a quarter of patients.

> **P** » Both polymyositis and dermatomyositis can be associated with an underlying malignancy, and this should be investigated thoroughly. Treatment involves avoiding sun exposure and using sunblock (in dermatomyositis) and **steroids** first line, and immunosuppressive therapy with azathioprine or cyclophosphamide if unresponsive.

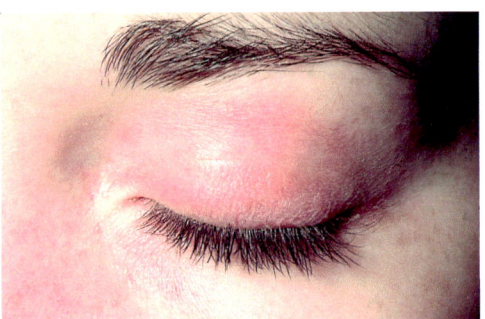

Fig. 10.17 *Heliotropic rash (confluent macular erythema).*

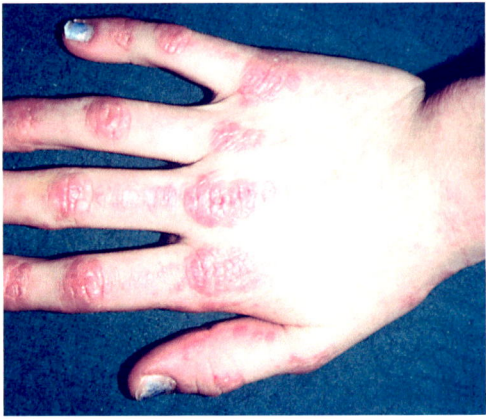

Fig. 10.18 *Gottron papules.*

10.7 Vasculitides

10.7.1 Giant cell (temporal) arteritis (GCA)

Definition: giant cell (temporal) arteritis refers to an autoimmune-mediated granulomatous vasculitis affecting medium and large arteries.

Epidemiology:
• Women are 2 to 4 times more likely to have the condition than men
• Patients are typically above the age of 50

Aetiology/pathophysiology:

> **E** » There is thought to be some degree of overlap in the disease processes of GCA and polymyalgia rheumatica.

W >> The inflammatory process is immuno-logically mediated, with infiltration of T-cells and macrophages eventually leading to granuloma formation. This disrupts the layer between the tunica intima and the media of the artery, whilst leucocyte proliferation and angiogenesis continue to take place. These processes narrow the vessel lumen, resulting in ischaemia and producing symptoms such as headaches or blindness, depending on which arteries are affected.

E >> It is essential not to delay treatment while waiting for confirmation of the temporal artery biopsy. If GCA is suspected, proceed immediately to treatment. In addition, the temporal artery biopsy can be negative in up to half of affected individuals, probably because the sampled area has remained unaffected by disease. Always prescribe steroids, particularly if visual symptoms predominate.

Clinical features:

- Patients typically present with **acute** onset of:
  - Headache
  - Visual disturbances
  - Jaw claudication
  - Scalp tenderness, often described as pain while combing hair
- Up to 30–50% of patients may also present with symptoms of polymyalgia rheumatica (see *Section 10.7.2*)
- Systemic upset may also be a much less common presentation

P >> Thoracic aortic aneurysms may still affect patients in the later course of the disease, even after successful management of GCA in the acute setting.

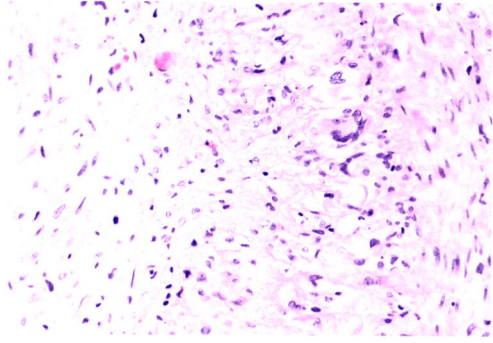

Fig. 10.19 *H&E stain of a temporal artery biopsy. Note the extensive leucocytic infiltration and oedematous changes.*

Investigations

Stepwise plan:

1 **Consider the American College of Rheumatology Criteria for GCA:**
- Age ≥50
- New onset of headache
- Temporal artery tenderness or pulsation
- Elevated ESR (≥50mm/hour)
- Abnormal artery biopsy, demonstrating granulomatous inflammation

2 **If 3 out of 5 of the criteria are met, the diagnosis of GCA can be made**

3 **Investigate the patient initially with blood tests, FBC, U&Es, LFTs, ESR and CRP**
- LFTs may be abnormal
- Some patients have a normochromic normocytic anaemia
- ESR is usually markedly elevated

4 **Refer patient for a temporal artery biopsy (see Fig. 10.19)**

Stepwise management of giant cell (temporal) arteritis (NICE CKS 2014)

1 **Prescribe oral prednisolone as first-line treatment**
- Visual symptoms: 60mg and same-day referral to an ophthalmologist
- No visual symptoms: 40–60mg daily
- Dose of prednisolone should be slowly tapered down over months to years

P >> Assess response to prednisolone over 48 hours. Patients with GCA typically respond quickly. If not, reconsider the diagnosis.

2 **Aspirin and PPI**
- Start aspirin 75mg and arrange PPI cover

10.7.2 Polymyalgia rheumatica

Definition: polymyalgia rheumatica (PMR) refers to a condition characterised by pain and stiffness of the neck, shoulder and pelvic girdles.

10

Epidemiology:
- Typically affects older people, more than 50 years of age
- Women are three times more likely to be affected than men

Aetiology/pathophysiology:

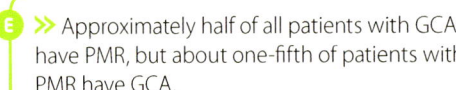
E ≫ Approximately half of all patients with GCA have PMR, but about one-fifth of patients with PMR have GCA.

- The aetiology and pathophysiology of the disease are unclear

Clinical features:
- Patients with PMR are likely to have pain and stiffness of the neck, shoulder and pelvic girdles that is worse in the morning
- They may describe being unable to get out of bed, and may also experience systemic symptoms, e.g. tenosynovitis and carpal tunnel syndrome

Investigations

Stepwise plan:

   1 Investigate the patient initially with blood tests, FBC, U&Es, LFTs, ESR, CRP and a CK
- ESR and CRP are likely to be elevated
- CK will be **normal**

Management
The goal of treatment is to alleviate symptoms and return the patients to a normal, baseline level of ESR and CRP.

Stepwise management of polymyalgia rheumatica

   1 Prescribe corticosteroids
- Patients generally respond dramatically
- Dose is tapered until treatment goals are achieved

   2 Prescribe NSAIDs
- May be used for symptomatic relief as necessary

10.7.3 Takayasu arteritis

Definition: Takayasu arteritis refers to an autoimmune-mediated vasculitis of large vessels that results in symptoms of arterio-occlusive disease and systemic features.

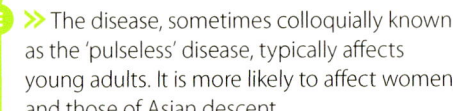
E ≫ The disease, sometimes colloquially known as the 'pulseless' disease, typically affects young adults. It is more likely to affect women, and those of Asian descent.

Clinical features:
- Patients classically present with non-specific symptoms such as fever and arthralgia
- These may eventually progress to occlusive symptoms such as limb claudication, cerebrovascular events such as a stroke or TIA, syncope, shortness of breath or heart failure

Investigations
On examination, a BP difference of >10mmHg may be observed in both arms, along with the inability to elicit a peripheral pulse. Blood tests may show an **elevated ESR**.

Management
The diagnosis is made on angiography (either invasive, CT or MR) and treatment involves **corticosteroids**. Patients who are unresponsive to steroids may benefit from immunosuppressive therapy such as azathioprine or methotrexate. Patients who remain unresponsive may be offered biologics such as rituximab.

10.7.4 Polyarteritis nodosa

Definition: polyarteritis nodosa (PAN) is a vasculitis that affects small or medium blood vessels. The exact aetiology is unknown, and the diagnosis can be difficult to make. The disease has been known to be associated with hepatitis B.

Clinical features:
- Patients may present with non-specific myalgia, fever and headaches
- The disease process is not predictable, in that various organ systems may be affected

Investigations
The American College of Rheumatology criteria may be helpful in ascertaining the diagnosis, citing features such as weight loss, livedo reticularis (purplish lattice-like skin discoloration), myalgia, kidney dysfunction, neuropathy and 'rosary-like' microaneurysms.

Management
The disease is not reliably related to ANCA titres but has an association with HBsAg. Patients should be offered corticosteroids first line, with other immunosuppressive medications being used if treatment remains ineffective.

10.7.5 Churg-Strauss syndrome

Churg–Strauss syndrome refers to a small to medium vessel vasculitis and has an association with asthma.

The American College of Rheumatology identifies six criteria:
- Asthma
- Sinusitis
- Peripheral blood eosinophilia >10%
- Pulmonary infiltrates
- Histological demonstration of vasculitis
- Polyneuropathy (or mononeuritis multiplex)

Any four of these confer a very high likelihood of the diagnosis. Just over one-third of patients are p-ANCA positive. Steroid therapy is usually effective, but immunosuppressive medications may be used in refractory cases.

> **E** » It may sometimes be difficult to remember the various types of vasculitis present. It is helpful to think of what vessel is affected first. As a rule of thumb, common associations (particularly in examinations) include:
> - Large vessel vasculitis – think of:
>   – Temporal pain? Jaw claudication? Visual problems? (GCA)
>   – Asian patient? Loss of peripheral pulses? (Takayasu arteritis)
> - Medium to small vessel vasculitis – think of:
>   – Young male? Smoker? Claudication? (Buerger disease)
>   – Non-specific symptoms? Renal disease? HBsAg? (PAN)
>   – Vasculitis? Asthma? (Churg–Strauss)

10.7.6 Henoch-Schönlein purpura

Definition: Henoch–Schönlein purpura is an IgA-mediated vasculitis of the small vessels.

Epidemiology:
- The vast majority of cases occur in children, teenagers or young adults
- More common in Asian and Caucasian populations
- Males are more affected

Aetiology/pathophysiology:
- The exact aetiology and pathophysiology are incompletely understood, but there are thought to be some similarities with IgA nephropathy

Clinical features:
- The disease most commonly occurs post-infection
- It's generally a URTI, causing a tetrad of:
  – Purpuric rash (usually over buttocks and extensor surfaces of upper and lower limbs; see *Fig. 10.20*)
  – Abdominal pain
  – Glomerulonephritis
  – Polyarthritis

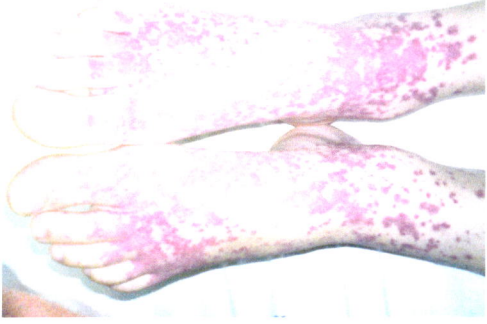

Fig. 10.20 *Henoch–Schönlein purpura over the feet.*

Investigations
The diagnosis of Henoch–Schönlein purpura is a clinical one, and no investigations are warranted.

Management
The condition (without severe renal impairment) is generally self-limiting and carries a good prognosis. Supportive therapy and symptomatic management are encouraged.

10.7.7 Buerger disease (thromboangiitis obliterans)

Definition: Buerger disease refers to inflammation of small to medium blood vessels of the distal extremities. The condition is most likely to affect male smokers and is associated with low socioeconomic status.

Aetiology/pathophysiology:
- Patients typically develop thrombosis, ischaemia and superficial thrombophlebitis that may present with limb claudication, ulceration and gangrene in severe cases
- The aetiology is thought to be multifactorial, but smoking has been implicated as a major risk factor

Management
The diagnosis is made on Doppler ultrasound and angiography, which demonstrates a classic **corkscrew**

10

appearance of the vasculature. Smoking cessation is an essential part of treatment, and while it does not stem progression, it reduces the severity of the condition. Medical therapies include prostacyclin analogues such as iloprost, which may be used initially. This should be followed by angioplasty and surgical amputation in cases where gangrene is present.

10.7.8 Behçet syndrome

Definition: Behçet syndrome is a multi-system disorder thought to arise from autoimmune-mediated vasculitis. Patients classically present with a triad of symptoms (with oral and genital ulcers, along with anterior uveitis) but often also describe a wide variety of systemic symptoms. They are usually of Middle Eastern or Mediterranean descent.

Management
The diagnosis is made on clinical grounds. Some patients have positive antiphospholipid antibodies;

and a **positive pathergy test** (needle-pricking produces papule formation) is seen in up to two-thirds of patients. Patients may benefit from topical corticosteroids for oral and genital ulceration, and systemic immunosuppressive therapy in more severe forms of the disease.

10.7.9 Relapsing polychondritis

Relapsing polychondritis is a rare multi-system disorder causing inflammation of connective tissues, particularly those that contain a large amount of proteoglycans. The presentation of the disease may vary, but the McAdams criteria indicate that chondritis of the ear, nasal and laryngotracheal cartilage with ocular inflammation and polyarthritis may be helpful in arriving at a diagnosis. Management of the condition is multi-disciplinary.

10.8 Other rheumatological conditions

10.8.1 Ehlers–Danlos syndrome

Ehlers–Danlos syndrome is an inherited autosomal dominant condition that involves joint hypermobility (see *Fig. 10.21*), increased elasticity of the skin (see *Fig. 10.22*) and fragility of connective tissue and blood vessels. Clues to the diagnosis may also be observed in the form of easy bruising and flexibility and the diagnosis is largely clinical. Patients with the condition have a higher risk of dissection or aortic rupture. These patients should be managed in a multi-disciplinary team with specialist input.

10.8.2 Marfan syndrome

Marfan syndrome is an inherited condition caused primarily by a mutation in the fibrillin-1 gene on chromosome 15. Patients with the condition may be asymptomatic, but do have 'classic features':
- Tall stature – ratio of arm span to height is >1.05 (see *Fig. 10.23*)
- Eyes – lens dislocation (ectopia lentis), myopia
- Mouth – high arched palate
- Chest – pectus excavatum, high risk of pneumothoraces, aortic rupture or dissection, valvular heart disease
- Joints – arachnodactyly (abnormally long, thin fingers) and arthralgia

10

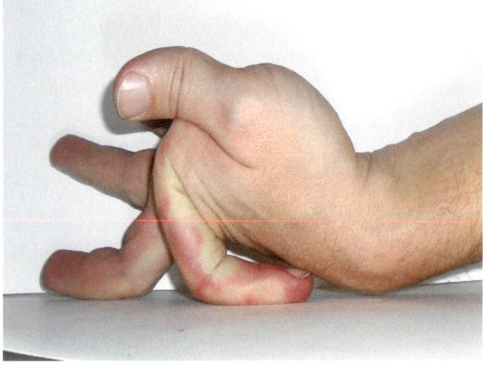

Fig. 10.21 *Finger hyperextension.*

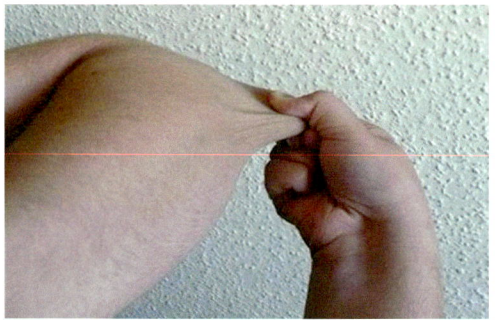

Fig. 10.22 *Skin hyperelasticity.*

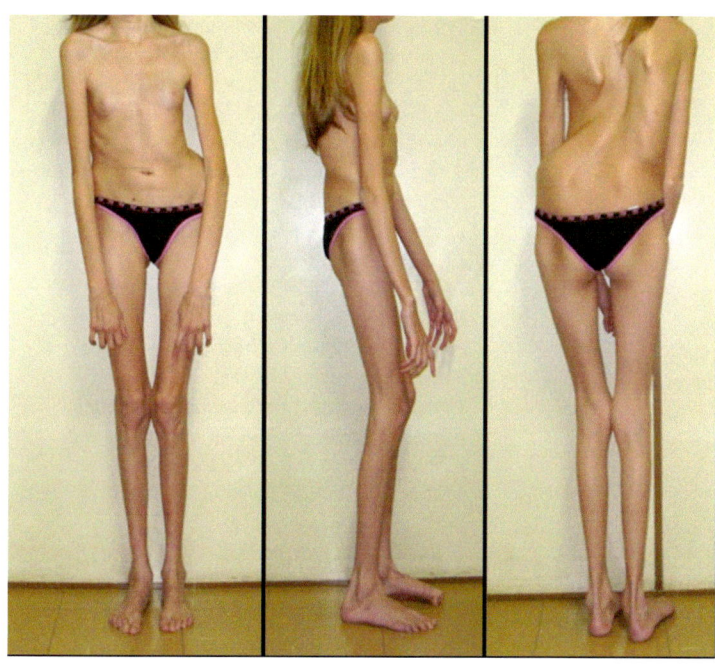

Fig. 10.23 *Marfanoid stature.*

Patients should be regularly followed up with ECGs and echocardiograms as well as spinal MRIs if necessary. ACE inhibitor therapy has been shown to be effective in patients with Marfan syndrome, but they have a reduced life expectancy, and mortality is often linked to cardiovascular sequelae or aortic rupture or dissection.

10.8.3 Carpal tunnel syndrome

Definition: carpal tunnel syndrome refers to symptoms and signs associated with compression of the median nerve within the carpal tunnel.

Aetiology/pathophysiology:
- Carpal tunnel syndrome develops from increased pressure or compression of the median nerve
- Patients who use their hands more often, have acromegaly or diabetes, or conditions that cause local pressure on the carpal tunnel, e.g. a gouty tophus or a ganglion, are more likely to develop the condition

> **P** ➤ Carpal tunnel syndrome is also more commonly seen in pregnant patients.

Clinical features:
- Patients with carpal tunnel syndrome often present with tingling and numbness of the thumb, index, middle and half of the ring finger and wasting of the **thenar** eminence

- Patients are also likely to describe having to shake their wrists to ease the sensation

> **E** ➤ A positive Tinel test (tapping on the median nerve at the wrist, producing tingling) or Phalen test (wrist flexion causes numbness and tingling) also help point towards the diagnosis.

Investigations
The diagnosis is usually made clinically, but electroneurography is the gold standard investigation if further confirmatory testing is required.

> **Stepwise management of carpal tunnel syndrome**

1 Adopt a 'watch and wait' strategy to see if symptoms resolve
- Alternatively, arrange for wrist splinting and advise patients to limit wrist activity in the meantime

2 Local corticosteroid injections have good efficacy
- These may be helpful in managing symptoms

3 Patients with more severe symptoms may be offered surgical decompression
- Although outcomes are good, patients may develop complications (e.g. chronic hand pain) as a result of surgical intervention

10

10.8.4 Fibromyalgia

Fibromyalgia is a chronic pain syndrome of unknown aetiology. Patients (who are almost always likely to be premenopausal women) typically experience widespread muscle aches and pains, fatigue, insomnia and depression. The diagnosis is largely clinical.

The American College of Rheumatology has a schematic diagram of 18 points (most on the axial skeleton), where 11 points would help point towards a diagnosis of fibromyalgia (see *Fig. 10.24*). Management of the condition should be multi-disciplinary, with patients being encouraged to exercise regularly and seek help if psychosocial symptoms predominate.

10.8.5 Osteogenesis imperfecta

Osteogenesis imperfecta (colloquially known as 'brittle bone disease') is an inherited condition that involves improper bone formation and poor bone health secondary to impaired formation of type I collagen. There are several variations of the disease:

- **Type I:** mild, the most common classic presentation with thin skin, **blue sclerae** (see *Fig. 10.25*), an increased fracture risk and erosion and discoloration of teeth as a result of enamel breakdown. **Bowing of bones** may also be seen on X-ray (see *Fig. 10.26*). **Cardiac valve abnormalities** and **aortic root dilation** are common. The underlying problem is abnormal pro-collagen peptide production.
- **Type II:** fractures occur *in utero*, and severe bone deformities occur during the perinatal period. Patients rarely survive beyond the first year of life.
- **Type III:** patients with this subtype experience milder symptoms early in life, but the disease progresses to be severely deforming, causing fractures, joint laxity and scleral and tooth discoloration later on.
- **Type IV:** this form is similar to type I with a poor quality of collagen, but is differentiated from type I by the presence of white sclera.

Other types exist – V, VI and VII. The diagnosis is made clinically, and management involves multi-disciplinary input with regular physiotherapy, surgical management of fractures and the use of bisphosphonates.

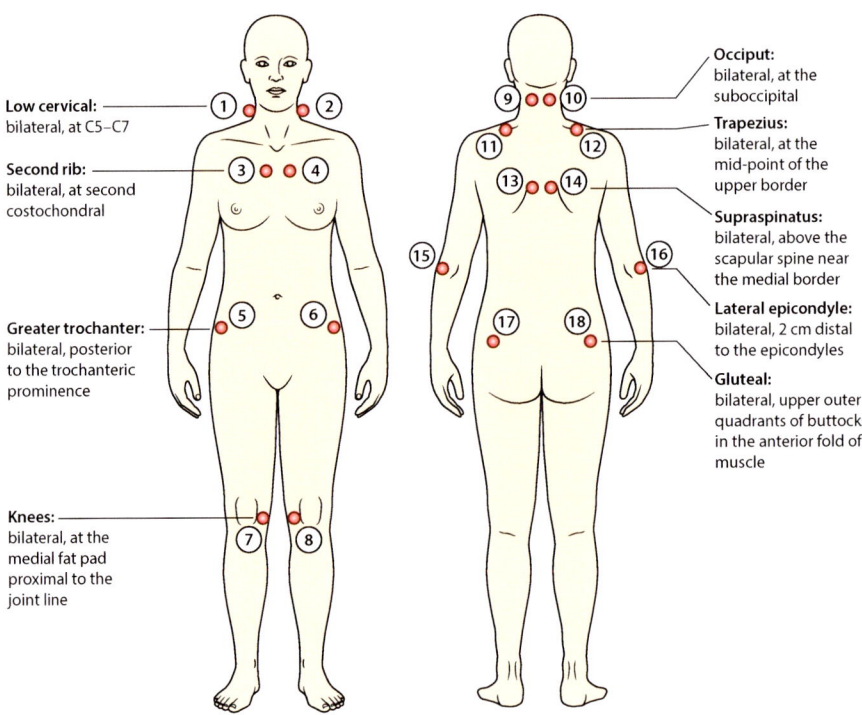

Low cervical: bilateral, at C5–C7

Second rib: bilateral, at second costochondral

Greater trochanter: bilateral, posterior to the trochanteric prominence

Knees: bilateral, at the medial fat pad proximal to the joint line

Occiput: bilateral, at the suboccipital

Trapezius: bilateral, at the mid-point of the upper border

Supraspinatus: bilateral, above the scapular spine near the medial border

Lateral epicondyle: bilateral, 2 cm distal to the epicondyles

Gluteal: bilateral, upper outer quadrants of buttocks in the anterior fold of muscle

Fig. 10.24 *Fibromyalgia tender points as per the American College of Rheumatology.*

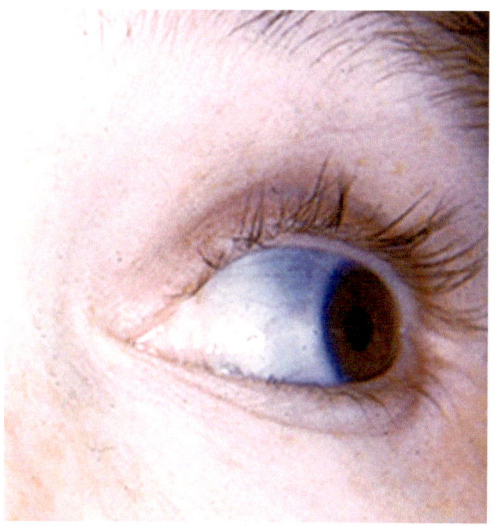

Fig. 10.25 *Characteristic blue sclera in a child with osteogenesis imperfecta.*

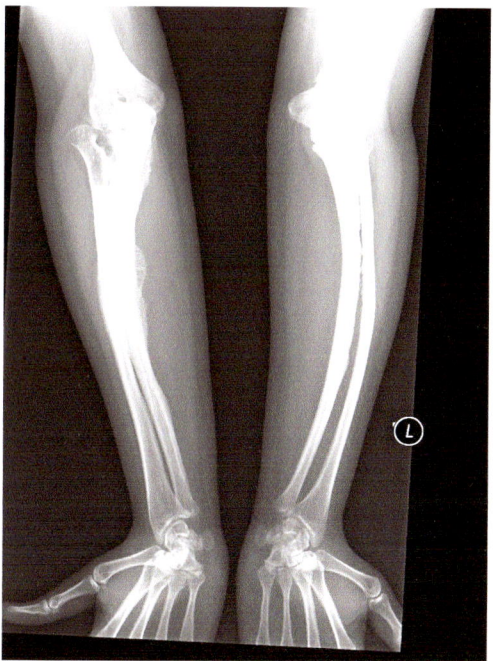

Fig. 10.26 *Bowing of the forearm bones and radial head dislocation.*

10.9 Immunology

10.9.1 Severe combined immunodeficiency (SCID)

SCID is characterised by the abnormal development of T and B cells. This condition is classified as a primary immunodeficiency and is the most severe form. This condition is also colloquially referred to as '**boy in a bubble syndrome**'. Most patients do not survive beyond the first year of life as a result of recurrent infection, unless they undergo bone marrow transplantation. However, patients are not diagnosed at birth because of the protection of circulating maternal antibodies.

10.9.2 DiGeorge syndrome

DiGeorge syndrome refers to a clinical condition caused by a gene deletion of chromosome 22q11.2.

Patients with DiGeorge syndrome also have cognitive impairment and are at increased risk of developing early Parkinson disease.

❻ » Patients with this disease may vary in presentation, but the much-used mnemonic '**CATCH-22**' is used to summarise key features:

Congenital heart disease (particularly tetralogy of Fallot)
Abnormal facies (hypertelorism – increased space between eyes or organs, hooded eyelids, large nose)
Thymic aplasia
Cleft palate
Hypoparathyroidism
22q11.2 gene deletion

10.9.3 Bruton agammaglobulinaemia

Bruton agammaglobulinaemia is an X-linked inherited disorder, characterised by absent production of B cells and immunoglobulins, leaving patients at risk for

10

recurrent infections. Treatment entails intravenous immunoglobulin for life, with antibiotic therapy as and when it is needed.

10.9.4 Hereditary angioedema

Hereditary angioedema is an autosomal dominant condition that causes recurrent episodic swelling of the face and limbs, as well as the GI tract, respiratory tract and genitals. It is associated with a deficiency of C1-INH, and in some forms accumulation of bradykinin. Patients should have C1-INH replacement therapy or fresh frozen plasma if specific therapy is not available.

10.9.5 IgA deficiency

Patients with IgA deficiency are susceptible to infections that affect the respiratory and GI tracts. This is the most common primary antibody deficiency and is characterised by absent serum IgA. Treatment with intravenous immunoglobulin is controversial, and antibiotic therapy is suggested to manage episodes of infection.

10.9.6 Chédiak-Higashi syndrome

Chédiak–Higashi syndrome is a rare, autosomal recessive disorder caused by a mutation in the lysosomal trafficking protein, causing impaired phagocytosis.

Patients have partial albinism (fair skin), photosensitivity, recurrent infections and peripheral neuropathy. No specific therapy exists, and treatment is centred on managing symptoms.

10.9.7 Common variable immunodeficiency (CVID)

CVID is the most common of the primary immunodeficiencies. It is characterised by low levels of immunoglobulin and antibodies. Patients with the condition produce normal levels of B cells, but these are unable to mature into plasma cells in the body. Treatment involves intravenous immunoglobulin and antibiotic therapy as needed.

10.9.8 Wiskott-Aldrich syndrome

Wiskott–Aldrich syndrome is a rare X-linked recessive disorder that is characterised by **recurrent infection**, bleeding secondary to **thrombocytopenia** and **eczema**. Patients with this condition are prone to the development of cancer (particularly leukaemia and lymphoma) and autoimmune disease. Patients may require regular platelet transfusions and intravenous immunoglobulins during severe infective episodes. The underlying mutation in the Wiskott–Aldrich syndrome protein (WASP), which is required for efficacious immune and platelet function.

Chapter 11
Dermatology

Senhong Lee, Adrian Mar and *Anastasios Stavrakoglou*

Basic principles

The skin is the largest organ of the human body. It plays an important role, not only in aesthetics, but also in immune defence, temperature regulation, vitamin D synthesis and the prevention of fluid loss. Severe loss of skin function may result in complications such as hypovolaemia, electrolyte imbalance, sepsis and even death. Dermatology is not about making a spot diagnosis but about looking beyond the surface.

Bridge to clinical medicine

Layers of the skin

- The skin is primarily made up of three layers – namely the epidermis, dermis and hypodermis (see *Fig. 11.1*)
- The epidermis is composed of stratified squamous epithelium, with layers of keratinocytes that are ectodermally derived
- The five layers of the epidermis, from outermost to innermost, are: stratum corneum, stratum lucidum, stratum granulosum, stratum spinosum and stratum basale
- Stratum lucidum is only seen in sites of thick skin (e.g. palms and soles)
- Keratinocytes differentiate as they move from the stratum basale to the stratum corneum; the terminally differentiated keratinocytes are flattened, dead, and will subsequently shed from the stratum corneum – this process takes around 4 weeks
- Melanocytes are interspersed amongst the basal keratinocytes. They produce melanin (skin pigments) that will be passed in packages (melanosomes) into the keratinocytes; this process results in skin pigmentation
- The dermis is composed of the papillary and reticular layers; the former is more superficial and contains a thinner arrangement of collagen fibres

- The epidermis is avascular and aneural, while the dermis is rich in blood vessels, lymphatics, nerves and sensory receptors
- The hypodermis (subcutaneous tissue) sits beneath the dermis

Types of hypersensitivity

There are four types of hypersensitivity reactions (ABCD – **A**naphylaxis, anti**B**ody, immune **C**omplex, **D**elayed). *Table 11.1* describes the types of reactions, their underlying immunology and examples of clinical conditions.

Table 11.1 *Types of hypersensitivity*

Type	Immunology	Conditions
I	IgE-mediated, immediate reaction	Anaphylaxis, allergic reaction
II	Antibody-mediated (IgM, IgG)	ANCA vasculitis, pemphigus vulgaris
III	Immune complex (antigen-antibody)-mediated	Serum sickness, polyarteritis nodosa (some cases)
IV	Cell-mediated (T cells), delayed reaction	Allergic contact dermatitis, tuberculosis

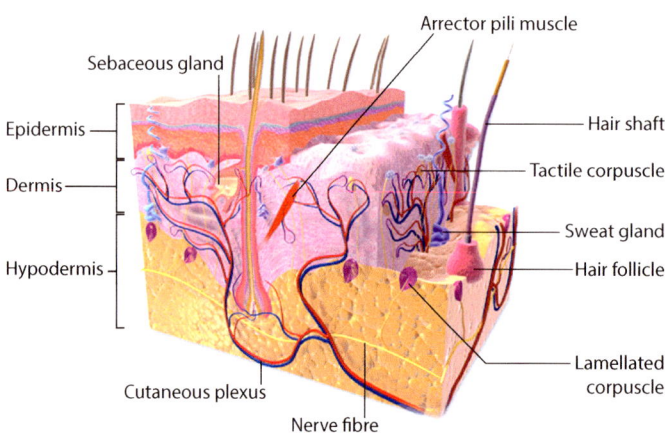

Fig. 11.1 *The anatomy of the skin.*

E ≫ Skin-prick testing detects type I hypersensitivity, while skin-patch testing detects type IV hypersensitivity.

Principles of topical therapy

- Emollients (moisturisers)
  - Emollient is the umbrella term for topical moisturising agents. There are various types of topical formulations, e.g. ointments, creams and lotions. Ointment is more oil-based, while cream and lotion are more water-based. Lotion is more watery than cream.
  - Oil-based products generally stay on the skin longer, are more effective (especially in eczema where they moisturise the affected skin, but also in general as skin occlusion enhances the penetration of the active ingredient) and sensitise the skin less (since oils do not require preservatives). However, they are associated with poorer compliance (as they are greasier and messier to use) and have more side effects from over-occlusion, e.g. acne and folliculitis.
- The potency of topical corticosteroids can be divided into four classes (according to the UK classification):
  - Class I (very potent), e.g. clobetasol propionate 0.05%
  - Class II (potent), e.g. betamethasone dipropionate 0.05%
  - Class III (moderate), e.g. betamethasone valerate 0.025%
  - Class IV (mild), e.g. hydrocortisone 0.1–2.5%

E ≫ Side effects of topical steroids include skin atrophy, telangiectasia, striae, acne, perioral dermatitis, glaucoma/cataracts (if used peri-orbitally), hypertrichosis, tachyphylaxis and Cushing syndrome.

- The thinner the skin, the greater the absorption of topical steroid. Therefore, mild and moderate potency topical steroids are generally used for the face, flexures and genitals. Potent and very potent topical steroids are usually avoided in these areas.
- The greatest danger of systemic absorption is in babies, whose skin surface area to body weight ratio is much greater than that of an adult.

Terminology

In dermatology, an accurate description facilitates efficient communication and helps in making a diagnosis.
- Flat, non-palpable lesions
  - Macule <0.5cm; patch >0.5cm
- Elevated lesions due to solid masses
  - Papule <0.5cm; plaque >0.5cm and flat-topped; nodule >0.5cm and dome-shaped
  - Wheal: pale area of dermal oedema
- Elevated lesions due to fluid-filled cavity
  - Vesicle <0.5cm; bulla >0.5cm
- Elevated lesions due to pus-filled cavity
  - Pustule <0.5cm; abscess >0.5cm
- Loss of skin
  - Atrophy: thinning of the epidermis or dermis
  - Erosion: partial epidermal loss; ulcer: complete epidermal loss
  - Fissure: a linear crack
- Vascular changes
  - Telangiectasia: visible superficial blood vessels (blanches)
  - Purpura: non-blanching extravasation of blood into the skin (usually around 2mm)
    - Petechiae: pinpoint areas of purpura; ecchymoses: purpura >2mm
- Surface changes
  - Scale: white flaking (implies epidermal pathology)
  - Crust: dried blood or serum
  - Lichenification: bark-like epidermal thickening (implies scratching)

11

11.1 Allergic contact dermatitis (ACD)

Definition: ACD is a type IV hypersensitivity reaction to contact allergens.

Epidemiology:
- The prevalence of ACD is suggested to be between 7% and 13% of the general population
- In the majority of these cases the contact allergy is to nickel in jewellery

Aetiology/pathophysiology:
- ACD is a delayed T-cell-mediated reaction
- The inflammatory response in ACD **requires a sensitisation phase**, which classically occurs within 5–16 days after first exposure
- Common allergens include cosmetics, metals (e.g. **nickel, cobalt and chromate**), topical medications, rubber additives, epoxy resin adhesives and plants (e.g. chrysanthemum)

Clinical features:

- ACD usually presents with a **pruritic** erythematous scaly rash (see *Fig. 11.2a*)
- It usually develops with contact, after a **delay** of many hours to several days
- The location of the rash is useful to identify the cause (e.g. cosmetics and eyelids, jewellery and finger/wrist/neck/ears)

Investigations

- ACD is diagnosed with **skin patch testing** (see *Fig. 11.2b*)

> **W** >> Why isn't latex allergy diagnosed with skin-patch testing? Latex allergy causes contact urticaria (type I hypersensitivity), in which symptoms typically present within minutes of contact. Skin-prick testing is used to diagnose this condition instead.

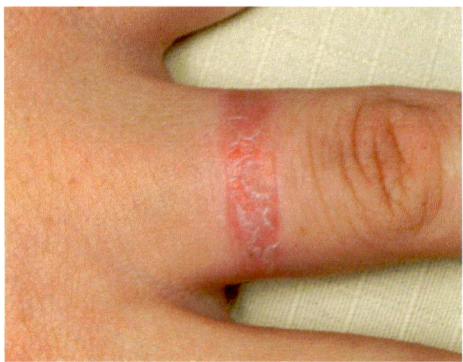

a)

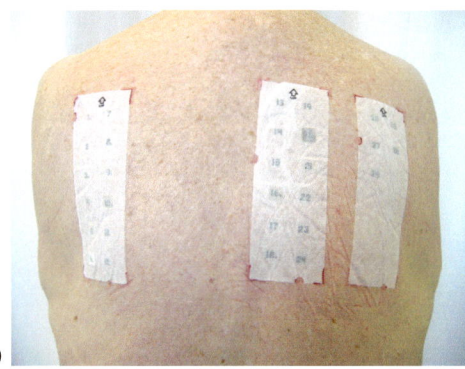

b)

Fig. 11.2 *(a) Well-demarcated erythematous scaly rash caused by ACD to nickel (found in jewellery) (b) Patch tests applied to the back.*

Management

> **Stepwise management of allergic contact dermatitis (NICE, CKS 2013)**

1 **Identify and avoid any stimulus**
- Encourage frequent application of emollients, emollient soap substitutes and protective clothing

2 **For acute contact dermatitis, treat patient with liberal use of emollients and topical corticosteroids (potency depends on location)**
- Consider short-term systemic steroids in severe cases

3 **Identify and treat any secondary infection**
- Perform a skin swab if indicated

4 **In cases with persisting symptoms, consider using a more potent topical steroid if initial response is poor**
- Also, reassess the patient's diagnosis, and consider ACD from topical meds

5 **Second-line treatments include phototherapy and immunosuppressants**
- e.g. cyclosporin, methotrexate

6 **Occupational contact dermatitis is notifiable to the Health and Safety Executive**
- Some patients may benefit from seeing a dermatologist specialising in occupational skin disease

11.1.1 Irritant contact dermatitis (ICD)

Definition: ICD is a non-immunologic localised skin reaction acquired through direct contact with irritants.

Epidemiology:
- Up to 80% of contact dermatitis is ICD

Aetiology/pathophysiology:
- ICD is caused by direct inflammatory pathways, without the need of prior sensitisation
- Common irritants include water, detergents, soaps, solvents, machining oils, reducing agents, acids, alkalis, soil and dust

Clinical features:
- ICD usually presents **within 48 hours** after exposure to an irritant. It could occur after an episode of exposure to a strong irritant (e.g. acids) or repeated exposure to weak irritants.

- ICD classically presents as an erythematous scaly rash affecting the site of exposure, e.g. hands (usually with involvement of the **webspace** and dorsum of the hands; see *Fig. 11.3*). The rash is usually **burning** and **stinging**.
- It is important to take an occupational history. Occupations at risk include hairdressers, healthcare workers and catering workers.

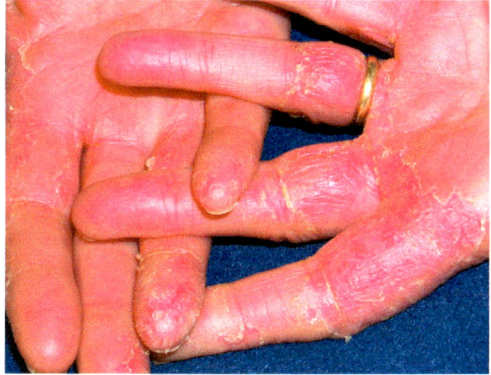

Fig. 11.3 *ICD involving the fingers (note the **webspace** involvement).*

Investigations
- The diagnosis of the condition is usually made clinically
- Skin-patch testing could be performed if ACD is suspected

Management (NICE CKS 2013)
The management of ICD is similar to that of ACD.

11.1.2 Atopic dermatitis

Definition: atopic dermatitis is a chronic relapsing inflammatory skin disease.

Epidemiology:
- Affects up to 20% of children and almost 3% of adults
- Around 80% of AD cases occur before 5 years of age
- No gender or ethnic predilection

Aetiology/pathophysiology:
- Likely multifactorial, involving: a genetic predisposition, impaired immunity, epidermal barrier dysfunction and environmental factors
- Has been perceived as a disease driven by **T helper 2 cells**
- Triggers include: soap and detergents, rough clothing or overheating, skin infection, animal dander (e.g. fur or hair), food (in patients with food allergy), dust mites, aeroallergens (e.g. pollens), stress and hormonal changes (e.g. premenstrual)

Clinical features:
- Typically presents as a **pruritic**, **poorly demarcated papulovesicular** rash associated with **xerosis** (dryness). The rash typically presents on the face, scalp and extensors in infants, whereas the flexural areas, hands and the face are more commonly involved in older patients.
- **Excoriation** (linear scratch marks) or **lichenification** may be seen (see *Fig. 11.4*).
- Follicular involvement is common in patients with darker skin.
- Secondary bacterial infection typically presents as **weeping**, **crusted** lesions. Pustules and surrounding cellulitis may be seen.
- Secondary viral infection (e.g. herpes simplex virus (HSV), varicella) may be seen. **Eczema herpeticum** is an extensive eruption of HSV infection, commonly seen in atopic dermatitis patients. It classically presents as painful monomorphic vesicles in clusters (see *Fig. 11.5*).
- Around 65% of children will outgrow the condition by the age of 7.

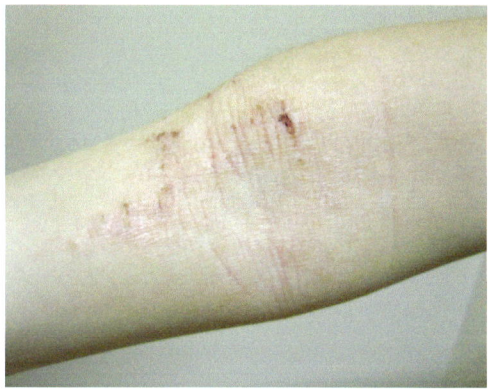

Fig. 11.4 *Poorly demarcated erythematous scaly rash with lichenification.*

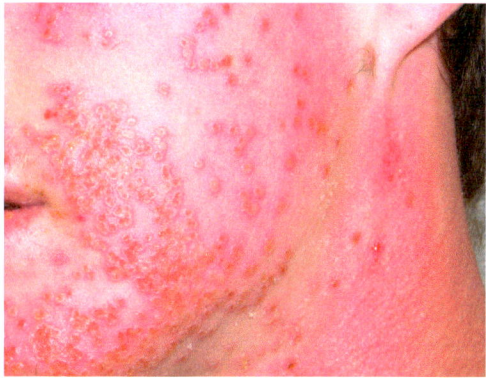

Fig. 11.5 *Monomorphic vesicles presenting in clusters, classic of eczema herpeticum.*

11

Investigations

Stepwise plan:

1 **The diagnosis of the condition is usually made clinically**

2 **Enquire about family and personal history of atopy, triggers, impact on quality of life, and sleep disturbance due to itch**

3 **Perform skin swabs if secondary infection is suspected**

4 **Most people do not need allergy testing**

Management

Stepwise management of atopic dermatitis (PCDS 2015)

1 **Education is important**
- Identify and avoid potential triggers (e.g. avoid irritating clothes, soaps or detergent)

2 **For long-term management, emollients are the mainstay of therapy**
- Use topical steroids of the lowest appropriate potency or topical calcineurin inhibitor (depending on the location) to inflamed skin
- Wet dressings and bandaging may be helpful

3 **For infrequent flare-ups, use a stronger topical steroid for the inflamed skin**
- Treat any secondary infection and consider a sedating antihistamine if sleep is disturbed

4 **For more frequent flare-ups, check treatment compliance**
- Perform skin and nasal swab (to detect *Staph. aureus* carriage), consider the possibility of allergic contact dermatitis and consider the use of steroid weekend regime (use steroids on two consecutive days of each week to the areas that tend to flare after the eczema is under control)

5 **For refractory disease, phototherapy or oral immunosuppressants (e.g. methotrexate and azathioprine) may be used**
- Eczema herpeticum requires urgent treatment with systemic acyclovir

11.1.3 Discoid eczema

Discoid ('disc-like') eczema, also known as nummular ('coin-like') eczema, is a type of eczema characterised by round or oval plaques. It typically affects younger to middle-aged patients. Its aetiology is likely multifactorial, involving environmental, allergic and emotional factors.

Discoid eczema typically presents as **pruritic round or oval** plaques located predominantly on the **limbs** (see *Fig. 11.6*). These lesions may have crusting and their borders fade gradually at the periphery. This type of eczema is usually diagnosed clinically.

The management of discoid eczema is similar to atopic dermatitis, as detailed above (PCDS 2014).

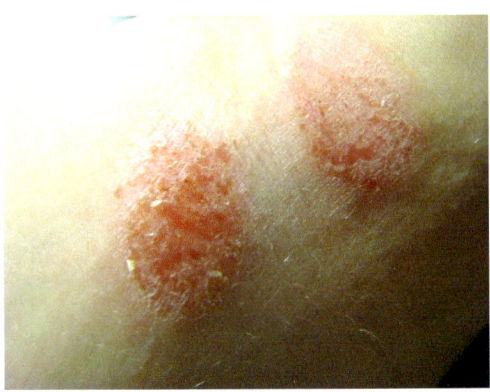

Fig. 11.6 *Coin-like plaques with some crusting, consistent with discoid eczema.*

11.1.4 Seborrhoeic dermatitis

Definition: seborrhoeic dermatitis is a chronic, relapsing inflammatory skin disorder with a predilection for regions that are rich in sebaceous glands.

Epidemiology:
- Commonly seen in infants younger than 3 months and adults 30–60 years of age
- The estimated prevalence is 1–5%
- More common in patients with **HIV infection and Parkinson disease**
- More prevalent in **winter**

Aetiology:
- Though the mechanism is unclear, SD is thought to be associated with yeasts of the genus *Malassezia*, which are lipophilic

Clinical features:
- Usually presents as scaly erythematous patches/plaques associated with mild **dandruff** or dense, adherent scale
- Commonly affects the **seborrhoeic region**, such as the scalp, nasolabial folds (see *Fig. 11.7*), eyebrows, behind the ears and chest
- In infants, seborrhoeic dermatitis may appear on the scalp as '**cradle cap**', presenting as large, greasy, yellow-brown scales/crusts (see *Fig. 11.8*)
- Infantile disease usually clears within a few weeks, while it displays a chronic relapsing trend in adults

11

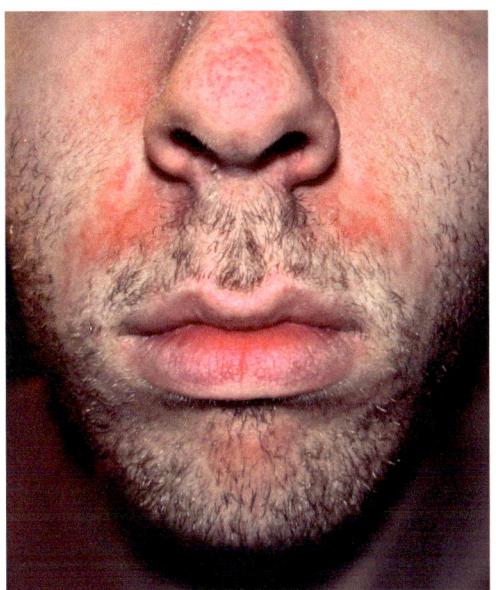

Fig. 11.7 *Seborrhoeic dermatitis involving the nasolabial folds and beard.*

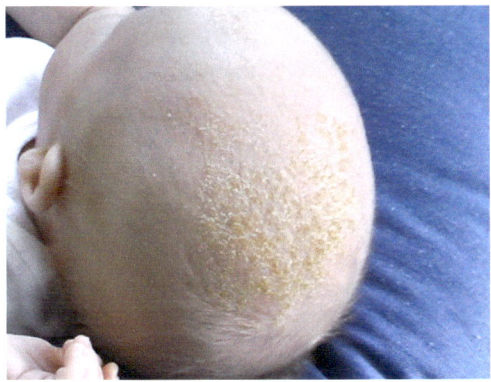

Fig. 11.8 *Seborrhoeic dermatitis involving cradle cap in infants.*

Investigations (NICE CKS 2013)

Stepwise plan:

1 **The diagnosis of the condition is usually made clinically**

2 **Skin scraping may be indicated to exclude tinea infection in the event of diagnostic uncertainty**

Management

Stepwise management of seborrhoeic dermatitis (NICE CKS 2013)

1 **In infants**
- Advise the parents to wash the scalp regularly with baby shampoo and brush the scalp gently with a soft brush
- Adherent scales/crusts can be soaked with baby oil, petroleum jelly or olive oil
- Topical imidazole is the next-line treatment

2 **For adults involving the scalp and beard**
- The first-line treatment is ketoconazole 2% shampoo, selenium sulphide shampoo or an anti-dandruff shampoo (containing coal tar or salicylic acid)
- A potent topical steroid application can be added for severe itching

3 **For adults involving the face and body**
- Topical imidazole is the first-line treatment, followed by mild topical steroids

4 **Patients with widespread disease**
- May require investigations for underlying immunosuppression based on clinical judgment

11.1.5 Venous eczema

Definition: also known as gravitational, varicose or stasis eczema, venous eczema is a form of eczema that is associated with chronic venous insufficiency (CVI).

Epidemiology:
- It is estimated that 20% of people over the age of 70 have venous eczema

Aetiology/pathophysiology:
- The exact mechanism is unknown; it is suggested that in patients with CVI, venous hypertension results in blood constituents leaking into the surrounding tissues
- This subsequently results in activation of inflammatory cells and fibroblasts
- Risk factors for CVI include obesity, physical inactivity, hypertension, diabetes, older age and PHx of DVT

Clinical features:
- Erythematous, scaly rash involving the **gaiter regions** (see *Fig. 11.9*)

11

P ≫ Other skin changes associated with CVI include varicose veins, oedema, skin pigmentation (from haemosiderin deposition), lipodermatosclerosis (indurated reddish-brown plaques from inflammation of the dermis and subcutis), atrophie blanche (star-shaped, white atrophic scars) and venous ulcers.

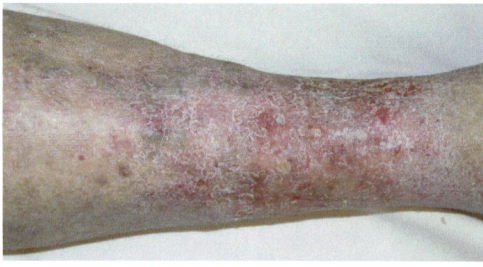

Fig. 11.9 *Erythematous scaly rash involving the gaiter region.*

Investigations

Stepwise plan:

1 **The diagnosis of the condition is usually made clinically**
- Perform a peripheral cardiovascular examination
- It is especially crucial to palpate for pedal pulses to assess arterial insufficiency

2 **Identify any associated CVI skin changes (as detailed above)**

3 **Perform an ankle-brachial index to exclude arterial insufficiency before recommending the use of compression stockings**

4 **Venous duplex ultrasound confirms the diagnosis of venous insufficiency and helps with planning for surgical interventions**
- It is also helpful when the clinical presentation is unclear or atypical

5 **Perform swabs if secondary bacterial infection is suspected**

Management

Stepwise management of venous eczema (PCDS 2012 and NICE CKS 2014)

1 **General advice should be given**
- e.g. elevate the legs

2 **Advise regular application of emollients and use topical steroids for acute flares**
- If topical steroids are needed on a regular basis, consider other topical immunomodulatory agents (e.g. tacrolimus)

3 **If symptoms persist**
- Consider using a topical steroid under occlusion and the possibility of an allergic contact dermatitis

4 **Recommend the use of compression stockings**
- To address underlying venous conditions after ruling out arterial insufficiency

5 **Treat secondary bacterial infection with antibiotics**

11.1.6 Pompholyx

Definition: pompholyx, also known as dyshidrotic eczema, is a vesiculobullous disease that affects the palmoplantar skin. It commonly affects people aged 20 to 40.

Aetiology:
- Pompholyx is associated with **tinea pedis**, atopic dermatitis, contact dermatitis, adverse drug eruption and hyperhidrosis
- It may be aggravated by hot weather, irritants, smoking or stress

Clinical features:
- Pompholyx typically presents as intensely pruritic **tapioca-like**, deep-seated vesicles that usually affect the palms and sides of fingers (see *Figs 11.10* and *11.11*)
- The vesicles may coalesce and form a bulla
- It typically peels off after a few weeks
- Secondary bacterial infection is not uncommon

Investigations
- Pompholyx is usually diagnosed clinically
- Perform swabs if secondary bacterial infection is suspected
- Investigations to exclude precipitants such as tinea pedis and contact allergies may be performed based on clinical suspicion

Management
Potent or very potent topical steroids are the cornerstone of treatment. These are commonly used in combination with a short course of oral steroids. Liberal application of ointment-based emollients is also essential. Identify and reverse any aggravating factors.

11

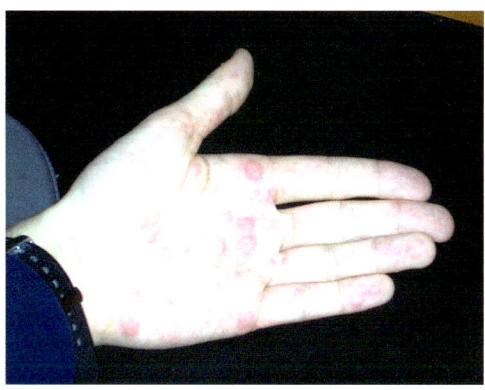

Fig. 11.10 *Pompholyx involving the palm.*

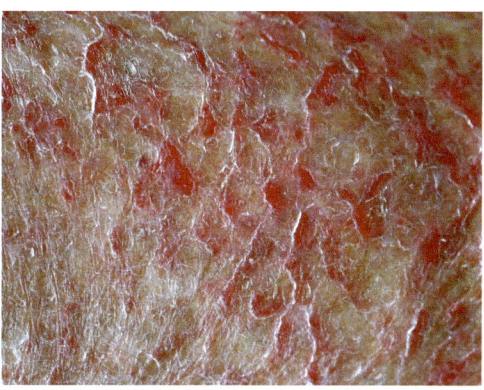

Fig. 11.12 *'**Crazy paving**'-like rash, classically seen in asteatotic eczema.*

Clinical features:

- It typically presents as an erythematous, scaly rash that exhibits a '**crazy paving**' pattern, characterised by interconnected superficial fissures (see *Fig. 11.12*)
- It commonly affects the shin, though it can be generalised
- Lesions are commonly pruritic or painful

Management (PCDS 2012)

Asteatotic eczema is usually diagnosed clinically. Liberal application of ointment-based emollients is the mainstay of treatment. It is also important to identify and avoid triggers that may exacerbate the skin condition – for example, skin degreasing by soap, excess washing, hot baths, and vigorous scrubbing and towelling. Topical steroid treatment is reserved for patients with a significant inflammatory component.

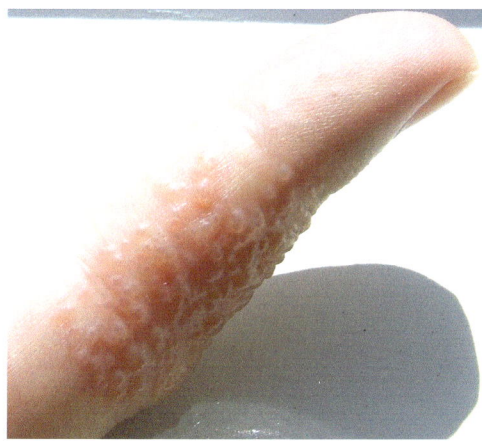

Fig. 11.11 *Classic tapioca-like vesicles seen in pompholyx.*

11.1.7 Asteatotic eczema

Definition: asteatotic eczema is a form of eczema that is associated with xerosis (abnormally dry skin). It commonly affects the elderly population during winter.

11.2 Papulosquamous disorders

11.2.1 Psoriasis

Definition: psoriasis is a common, immune-mediated genetic disorder manifesting in the skin or joints or both.

Epidemiology:

- Psoriasis affects 1–3% of the world's population
- Psoriasis affects both genders equally

Aetiology/pathophysiology:

- The **epithelial hyperproliferation** and dermal changes in psoriasis are probably mediated by macrophages, dendritic cells, **T cells** and various other immune cells, cytokines and chemokines
- Stress is often an exacerbating factor and psoriasis can typically occur at sites of skin **trauma (Koebner phenomenon – lesions occur at skin injury site)**, including sunburn

11

- **Streptococcal URTI** is often found to be the trigger for guttate psoriasis and smoking is known to be associated with palmoplantar pustulosis
- Less commonly, **drugs** (beta blockers, lithium, NSAIDs, antimalarials) and HIV infection could trigger psoriasis

Subtypes and clinical features

- Chronic plaque psoriasis (CPP; around 90% of cases) – characterised by **well-demarcated**, **erythematous plaques** covered by **silvery white scales** commonly found over the **extensor surfaces**, scalp, retroauricular, perianal and periumbilical regions (see *Fig. 11.13*) – lesions are usually asymptomatic
- Inverse/flexural psoriasis – a variant that affects the flexural or intertriginous regions; lesions are usually less scaly due to friction and moisture at these sites
- Guttate psoriasis – scaly, **raindrop**-shaped plaques on the trunk, commonly occurring following a **streptococcal URTI** (see *Fig. 11.14*)
- Pustular psoriasis – characterised by white coalescing pustules; it can be localised (palm and soles, fingers, toes) or generalised
- Erythrodermic psoriasis – when psoriasis affects more than 90% of body surface area; it is potentially life-threatening
- Nail psoriasis – associated nail changes include thickening of the nail plate, pitting, ridging, onycholysis, subungual hyperkeratosis (accumulated scale beneath the nail) and oil spots (yellow discoloration; see *Fig. 11.15*)

Assessment

- It is important to examine the patient's full body (including the scalp, nails, retroauricular, periumbilical and perianal regions)
- The Psoriasis Area and Severity Index (PASI) score is used to quantify disease severity
- Dermatology Life Quality Index (DLQI) questionnaire could be done to assess the impact of psoriasis on the patient

- Patient should be assessed for psoriatic arthritis
- Consider assessing for hypertension and other cardiovascular risk factors, diabetes and complications of obesity, as patients with psoriasis often have metabolic syndrome

Investigations (PCDS 2015)

- The diagnosis of the condition is usually made clinically

Management

Treatment focuses on CPP.

> **Stepwise management of psoriasis (PCDS 2015)**
>
> 1 **Provide general lifestyle advice, e.g. avoiding triggers**
>
> 2 **Encourage the application of emollients**
> - To soothe the skin and reduce the amount of scale
>
> 3 **A combined potent topical steroid and calcipotriol (vitamin D analogue) is the usual first-line option**
> - Other topical treatments include tar preparation, tazarotene and dithranol
> - Topical salicylic acid is used for thinning thick plaques
>
> 4 **Second-line options include phototherapy (e.g. narrow band UVB), cyclosporin, methotrexate and acitretin**

> **E** » Important side effects of cyclosporin include hypertension and renal toxicity. Methotrexate may cause hepatotoxicity and bone marrow suppression. Acitretin is teratogenic and should be avoided in women of child-bearing age.

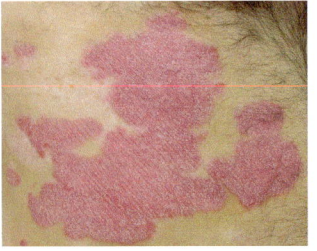

Fig. 11.13 CPP.

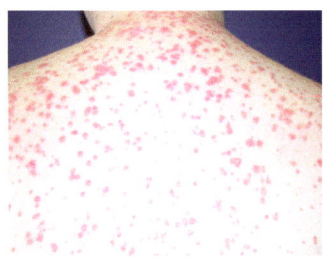

Fig. 11.14 Guttate psoriasis.

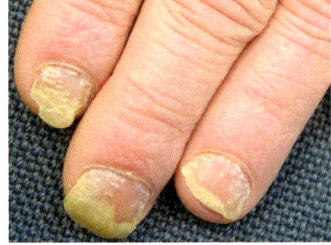

Fig. 11.15 Nail psoriasis.

5   **Biologics (e.g. etanercept, infliximab, adalimumab, ustekinumab and secukinumab) are very effective third-line treatment options**
- Consider the use of topical calcineurin inhibitor if there are concerns with the use of topical steroids
- Guttate psoriasis tends to respond well to phototherapy
- Nail psoriasis is difficult to treat
- Generalised pustular psoriasis and erythrodermic psoriasis require urgent referral to dermatology

11.2.2 Pityriasis rosea

Definition: pityriasis rosea is a self-limiting skin condition characterised by erythematous oval scaly eruption predominantly affecting the trunk.

Epidemiology:
- Mainly affects young adults (10–35 years old)
- More common in females

Aetiology:
- The exact aetiology is uncertain
- A viral aetiology has been proposed due to its seasonal variation and clinical features
- Human herpes viruses (HHV) 6 and 7 have been detected in the skin lesions

Clinical features:
- Usually begins as a **herald patch** – a salmon-coloured patch/plaque with peripheral **collarette scaling** (free edge of scale extends internally; see *Fig. 11.16*)
- Within days to three weeks, multiple smaller lesions of similar appearance develop over the trunk and proximal limbs symmetrically, giving rise to a **Christmas tree pattern** (lesions following the Langer lines; see *Fig. 11.17*)

> **P** ≫ Langer lines show the direction of the lowest naturally occurring skin tension. Incision following the Langer lines results in better wound healing.

- Some patients may have mild prodromic, flu-like symptoms
- Pruritus may be present

Investigations
- The diagnosis of the condition is usually made clinically
- Skin biopsy, HIV and syphilis testing could be considered in selected patients

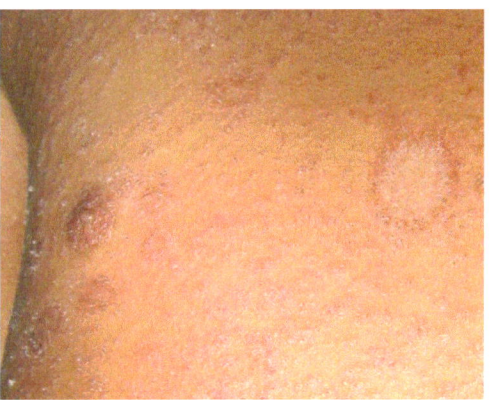

Fig. 11.16 *Herald patch with collarette of scale.*

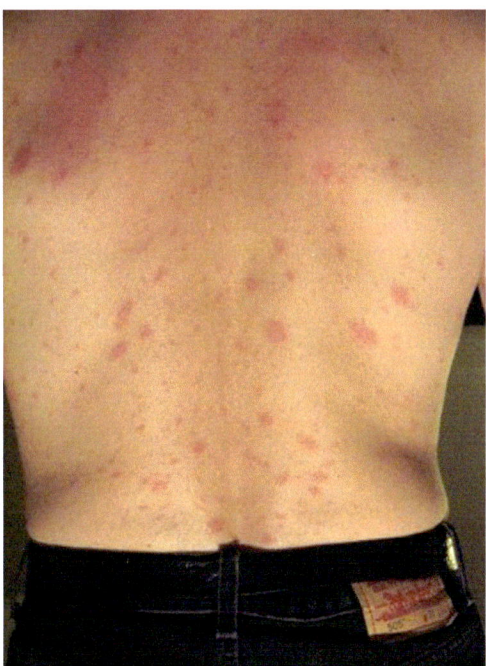

Fig. 11.17 *Christmas tree pattern rash.*

11

Management

> **Stepwise management of pityriasis rosea (NICE, CKS 2010)**
>
> 1   **Reassure the patient that the rash usually settles without treatment, within 2–3 months**
>
> 2   **Provide symptomatic treatment for itch**
> - Prescribe mild to moderate potency topical steroids or sedating oral antihistamine
>
> 3   **Refer to a dermatologist if the diagnosis is uncertain or the patient has extensive disease or uncontrollable itch**
> - Phototherapy is effective but simply shortens the course of the disease by a few weeks

11.2.3 Lichen planus (LP)

Definition: lichen planus is a chronic inflammatory disease that involves the skin, scalp, mucous membranes and nails.

Epidemiology:
- The estimated prevalence is 0.9–1.2% of the general population; it has a predilection for African Americans

Aetiology/pathophysiology:
- Considered to be a T-cell-mediated skin disease, expressing altered self-antigens on basal keratinocytes
- Associated with **hepatitis C virus** and certain **drugs** (e.g. antihypertensives, antibiotics, gold and penicillamine)

Clinical features:

> **E** ≫ Cutaneous lesions are described by 6 Ps – **p**ruritic, **p**lanar (flat-topped), **p**urple, **p**olygonal (many-sided), **p**apules or **p**laques.

- Classically presents as pruritic, flat-topped, papules and plaques (see *Fig. 11.18*), covered by **Wickham striae** (white reticular lines; see *Fig. 11.19*), involving the extremities (e.g. **ventral wrists**, forearms, ankles, legs), oral cavity and genitalia
- LP displays **Koebner phenomenon**
- **Nail changes**, such as longitudinal ridging, scarring and splitting, are commonly observed
- Scalp involvement may result in scarring alopecia

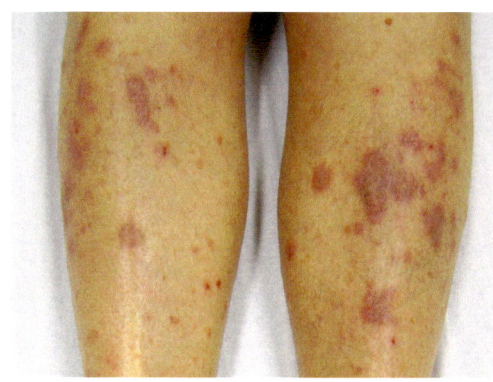

Fig. 11.18 *Multiple violaceous papules and plaques of lichen planus.*

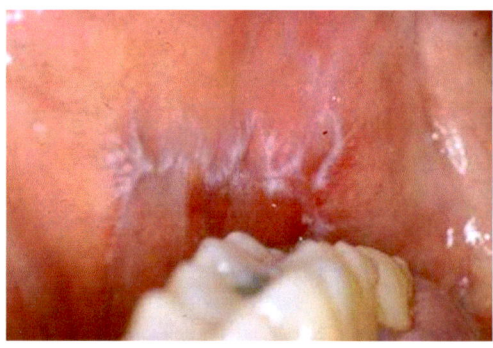

Fig. 11.19 *White lacy appearance of Wickham striae.*

Investigations
- The diagnosis of the condition is usually made clinically
- Skin biopsy may be performed if the diagnosis is uncertain
- LP will exhibit lichenoid changes on histopathology

Management

> **Stepwise management of lichen planus (PCDS 2015)**
>
> 1   **The mainstay of treatment is potent/very potent topical steroids**
> - Offer sedating antihistamine at night if sleep is affected
>
> 2   **The next line of treatment is intralesional or systemic steroids**
>
> 3   **Steroids are followed by phototherapy, hydroxychloroquine, cyclosporin and acitretin**
>
> 4   **Oral symptoms can be treated with a steroid inhaler**

11.3 Urticaria

Definition: urticaria is a transient eruption of dermal oedema.

Classification:

- Acute urticaria – short-lived bouts of urticaria
- Spontaneous urticaria (formerly chronic idiopathic urticaria) – chronic urticaria that lasts for over 6 weeks
- Physical urticaria – urticaria induced by physical stimuli (e.g. cold, heat, pressure, solar, exercise)
- Contact urticaria – urticaria that follows skin contact with certain biological or chemical agents, e.g. latex and foods (e.g. fruits)
- Urticarial vasculitis – defined as vasculitis on skin biopsy

Epidemiology:

- The estimated lifetime incidence of acute urticaria is 1 in 6 people (compared to 1 in 1000 people for spontaneous urticaria)

Aetiology/pathophysiology:

- Urticaria may be idiopathic, immune mediated (IgE, autoimmune or immune complex mediated) or non-immune mediated.
- Urticaria can be triggered by food (e.g. nuts, milk, eggs), stings/bites, drugs (e.g. antibiotics, opioids, NSAIDs, ACEi), physical stimuli or contact with chemical agents (e.g. latex)

Clinical features:

- Urticaria typically presents as **transient** (usually resolves within 24 hours), **non-scaly, smooth** plaques with surrounding erythema (see *Fig. 11.20*)
- Annular lesions result from central clearing
- Urticaria may be associated with **angioedema (oedema involving the deeper dermis, subcutis and submucosa) and anaphylaxis**

> **E** >> Urticarial vasculitis should be considered if the lesions: (1) stay longer than 24 hours, (2) are painful and (3) leave residual bruises.

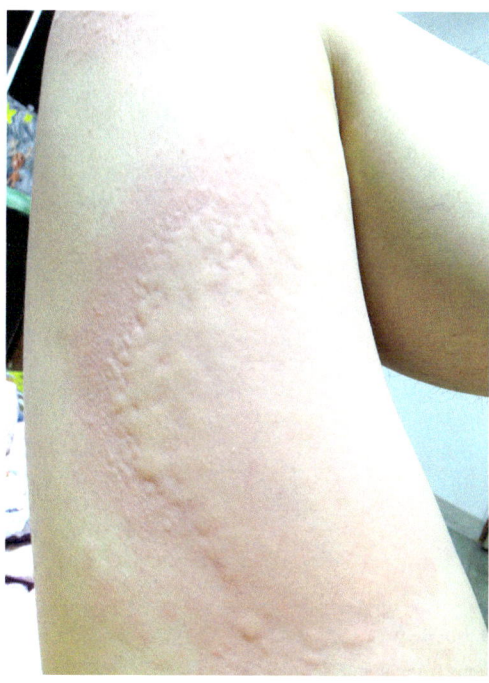

Fig. 11.20 *Non-scaly, smooth plaques with surrounding erythema.*

Investigations

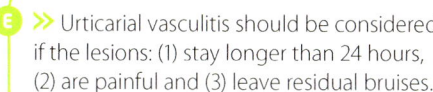

Stepwise plan:

1. **Urticaria is usually diagnosed based on history and clinical appearance**

2. **Skin-prick testing and RAST tests are reserved for patients with a history that suggests an IgE-mediated reaction to allergens**

3. **For spontaneous urticaria not responding to treatment, perform FBC, ESR, TFT and LFT to help identify an underlying cause**
   - e.g. autoimmune thyroiditis, bowel helminth infection and lupus

4. **Patients with possible urticarial vasculitis will require a skin biopsy and vasculitic screen (including complements)**

Management

Stepwise management of urticaria (BAD 2007 and PCDS 2012)

1. **Identify and avoid any triggers**
   - Non-specific triggers (e.g. stress, alcohol and NSAIDs/ACEi/opioids) should also be minimised

2. **Non-sedating antihistamine is the first-line therapy**
   - For resistant cases, double the standard licensed dose of the first antihistamine (off-label, but widely practised), or add on another H2 antihistamine/sedating antihistamine/anti-leukotrienes

11

3 A short course of oral corticosteroids could be given in severe acute urticaria
- Patients with anaphylaxis should be managed with intramuscular epinephrine

4 Immunosuppressants (e.g. cyclosporin) are needed for some patients with spontaneous urticaria or urticarial vasculitis

5 Patients with food allergies or anaphylactic reactions would benefit from referral to an immunologist

11.4 Acne, rosacea and related disorders

11.4.1 Acne vulgaris

Definition: acne vulgaris is a chronic inflammatory dermatosis characterised by comedones and inflammatory lesions.

Epidemiology:
- Most prevalent among adolescents and young adults
- An estimated 80% of people between the age of 11 and 30 have acne outbreaks at some point

Pathogenesis
The four main pathogenic features are:
1. Follicular hyperkeratinisation
2. *Propionibacterium acnes* colonisation
3. Increased sebum production
4. Complex inflammatory process involving both innate and acquired immunity

Aetiology:
- Factors that can cause/trigger acne include: hormonal factors (e.g. PCOS), stress, diet (associated with high glycaemic index diet, though link not strong), cosmetics and drugs (corticosteroids, anabolic steroids, lithium and cyclosporin)

Clinical features:
- May present as non-inflammatory lesions; these may be **comedones** or **whiteheads** (skin-coloured papules) and **blackheads** (black plugs caused by oxidised whiteheads) or inflammatory lesions (**papules, pustules and nodules**) involving the face, chest and back (see *Fig. 11.21*)
- There may be associated **seborrhoea** (greasy skin)
- Complications include scarring (atrophic or hypertrophic) and post-inflammatory hyperpigmentation
- Polycystic ovary syndrome (PCOS) or hyperandrogenism should be suspected in women with irregular periods, androgenic alopecia (male pattern hair loss) and hirsutism (increased hair growth in androgen-dependent areas)

Investigations (NICE, CKS 2014)
- The diagnosis of the condition is usually made clinically
- In women with suspected hyperandrogenism, consider the following investigations: total and free testosterone, LH/FSH ratio, serum DHEA, 17-hydroxyprogesterone, prolactin and 24-hour urinary-free cortisol

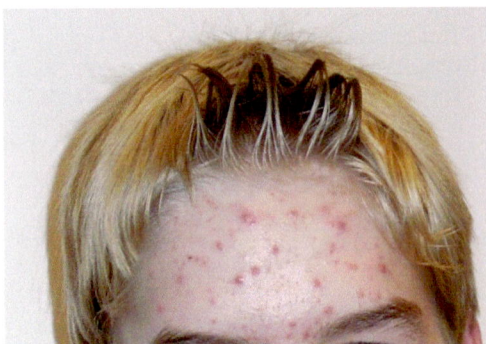

Fig. 11.21 *Papulopustular and comedonal lesions of acne vulgaris.*

Management

Stepwise management of acne vulgaris (PCDS 2016)

1 General advice includes using gentle cleanser and avoiding scrubbing, picking or excessive washing/use of make-up

2 For comedonal acne
- Topical retinoids are the first-line treatment, followed by topical azelaic acid

3 For mild inflammatory lesions
- Use a combination of two of the following: topical antibiotics (e.g. clindamycin or erythromycin), topical retinoids and topical benzoyl peroxide

11

4 For moderate inflammatory lesions
- Add an oral antibiotic (e.g. tetracycline, erythromycin) to the topical therapy
- Consider the use of anti-androgens (e.g. cyproterone acetate, spironolactone) in females without contraindication

5 Patients with severe, scarring or treatment-resistant acne, or severe psychological symptoms
- May benefit from dermatology review for other/additional treatments (e.g. oral isotretinoin)

E ≫ The side effects of oral isotretinoin include dry skin/mucous membrane, **teratogenicity**, photosensitivity, vision changes, mood changes, deranged LFT, elevated triglyceride and cholesterol levels, benign intracranial hypertension and acne flare.

11.4.2 Rosacea

Definition: rosacea is a chronic relapsing dermatosis that usually affects the face.

Epidemiology:
- Typically, first presents in patients between the ages of 30 and 50 years
- It has a predilection for patients with fair skin

Aetiology/pathophysiology:
- The exact pathogenesis of rosacea is unknown
- Aggravated by sunlight, caffeine, alcohol, spicy food, exercise, topical steroids and drugs that cause vasodilatation

Clinical features:
- Characterised by recurrent episodes of **facial flushing**, persistent erythema, **telangiectasia** and **papulopustular** lesions affecting the **central face** with sparing of the periocular skin (see *Fig. 11.22*)
- **Comedones are not present, unlike in acne vulgaris**
- Rosacea may also present as thickened, enlarged skin with irregular nodular surface (phymatous rosacea); when the nose is affected, it is called **rhinophyma**
- Patients may present with ocular symptoms, such as gritty eyes, conjunctivitis, blepharitis, episcleritis, chalazion and keratitis

The diagnosis of the condition is usually made clinically.

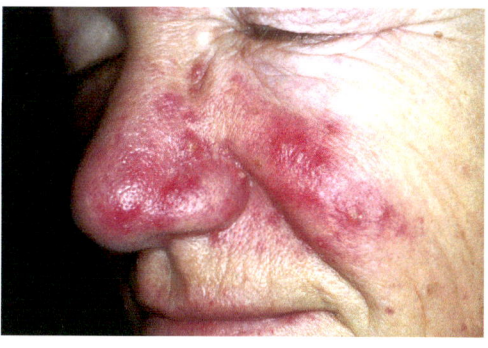

Fig. 11.22 *Papulopustular lesions on a background of erythema and telangiectasia; note the absence of comedones.*

Management

Stepwise management of rosacea (PCDS 2014)

1 Identify and avoid any aggravating factors

2 The first-line therapy for papulopustular lesions is topical metronidazole, or topical azelaic acid, followed by oral antibiotics (tetracycline, erythromycin)
- If symptoms are severe, consider other treatments such as low-dose isotretinoin

3 Non-selective beta blocker or clonidine may be used for flushing, while topical brimonidine and laser therapy could be used for erythrotelangiectatic symptoms

4 Rhinophyma responds well to CO_2 laser ablation

5 For ocular symptoms, encourage lid hygiene and artificial tears
- Oral tetracycline or erythromycin can also be used
- Patients with severe ocular symptoms require ophthalmology review to rule out keratitis

11.4.3 Perioral dermatitis (PD)

Definition: perioral dermatitis is an acneiform eruption involving the perioral area. It is termed periorificial dermatitis, if the lesions affect the perinasal or periorbital area.

Epidemiology:
- This condition is often found among women between the ages of 16 and 45, with no significant gender or racial predilection

11

Aetiology/pathophysiology:
- The exact pathogenesis of PD is unknown, but it is commonly preceded by **topical corticosteroid** use on the face

Clinical features:
- The condition is characterised by **monomorphic** papules and pustules involving primarily the perioral area with **relative sparing of the vermillion border** (see *Fig. 11.23*)
- Associated erythema and scaling are common
- The diagnosis of PD is usually made clinically

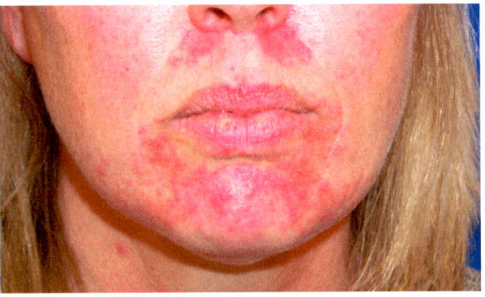

Fig. 11.23 *Monomorphic pustules over the perioral area with relative sparing of the vermillion border.*

Management

Stepwise management of perioral dermatitis (PCDS 2014)

1. **Identify and discontinue any topical steroids being used on the face or any facial creams that may be causing symptoms**
2. **Patients should be advised that their condition may initially worsen after stopping the topical steroids**
3. **Use topical antibiotics (e.g. clindamycin, erythromycin or metronidazole) for patients with mild perioral dermatitis**
4. **Oral antibiotics (e.g. tetracycline or erythromycin) should be reserved for patients with more severe perioral dermatitis**

11.5 Skin cancers

11.5.1 Basal cell carcinoma (BCC)

Definition: BCC is a slow-growing, locally invasive epidermal skin tumour arising from the basal cell.

Epidemiology:
- BCC accounts for around 80% of all skin cancer
- The estimated lifetime risk for BCC amongst Caucasians is dependent on UV exposure but may be up to 39% in some populations

Aetiology:
- Important risk factors for BCC include UV exposure, skin types I and II, increasing age, being male, smoking and immunosuppression

E ≫ There are six skin phototypes: type I burns easily and never tans (classically with red hair, blue eyes and freckles); type II burns easily and tans poorly; type III burns and tans moderately; type IV burns minimally and tans easily; type V rarely burns and tans easily; type VI never burns and always tans. Skin phototypes I–III are at increased risk of photo-ageing and skin cancers.

P ≫ Multiple BCCs presenting at a young age are a feature of basal cell naevus (Gorlin) syndrome, an autosomal dominant condition.

Subtypes
- Low-risk subtypes – nodular (nBCC), superficial (sBCC)
- High-risk subtypes – morpheic/sclerosing, basosquamous (histologically differentiated)

Clinical features:
- NBCC usually presents as a **pearly (shiny) nodule** with **telangiectasia** on the **head and neck region**; it tends to ulcerate with time and result in a **rolled edge** (see *Fig. 11.24*)
- SBCC usually presents as a slow-growing erythematous patch or plaque (see *Fig. 11.25*) that is usually found on the **trunk**
- Morpheic BCC is characterised by a shiny, scar-like plaque with ill-defined border
- BCC rarely metastasises

11

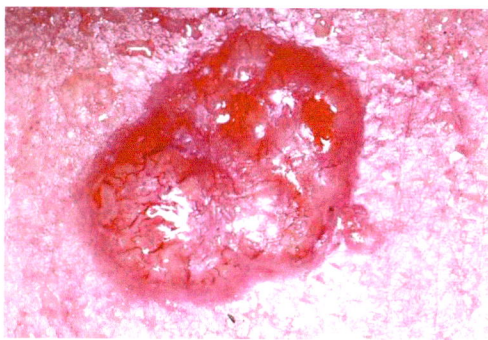

Fig. 11.24 *Nodular BCC – pearly nodule with telangiectasia and early signs of ulceration.*

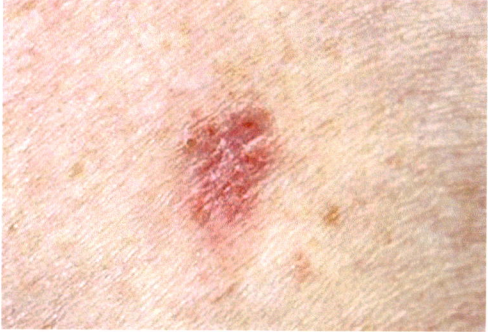

Fig. 11.25 *Erythematous scaly plaque of superficial BCC.*

Investigations (BAD 2008)
- The diagnosis of the condition is usually made clinically
- Biopsy is indicated when clinical doubt exists or when the histological subtype may influence treatment and prognosis

Management

> **Stepwise management of basal cell carcinoma (BAD 2008)**

1 **The aim of treatment is to eradicate the tumour, while preserving the function and cosmesis of the treatment site**

2 **Surgical excision with histological assessment of the margin is widely used to treat most BCCs**
- The target excision margin depends on the subtype (e.g. 3mm for nBCC)

3 **Destructive surgical and non-surgical techniques are reserved for low-risk BCCs**
- Destructive surgical techniques include curettage and cautery, cryosurgery

- Destructive non-surgical techniques include topical imiquimod (more for sBCC) and photodynamic therapy (PDT)

4 **Radiotherapy is a good treatment for primary and recurrent BCC**

5 **Mohs micrographic surgery is recommended for high-risk facial BCCs**

> **E** ≫ This technique combines staged resection with frozen section evaluation of the complete epidermal and deep surgical margins. It achieves the lowest recurrence rate of all treatment modalities and maximises tissue preservation.

11.5.2 Squamous cell carcinoma (SCC)

Definition: SCC is cutaneous carcinoma arising from the keratinocytes of the epidermis or its appendages.

Epidemiology:
- SCC is the second most common skin cancer
- The estimated incidence of SCC is 30/100,000 in the general population
- The incidence is higher in men

Aetiology/pathophysiology:
- SCC may arise *de novo* or from precursors (e.g. actinic keratosis (AK; *Fig. 11.26*) and SCC *in situ* – Bowen disease (BD; *Fig. 11.27*))
- Depending on the depth of epidermal dysplasia, AK (partial epidermal), BD (full epidermal) and SCC (invades beyond the epidermis/basement membrane) are considered a spectrum
- Risk factors for developing SCC include: skin phototype, **chronic UV radiation** (natural or artificial), co-carcinogens (e.g. smoking for lower lip SCC, HPV for genital or anal SCC), immunosuppression, chronic inflammation or chronic wound, genetic skin conditions (e.g. xeroderma pigmentosum, albinism) and arsenic poisoning

Clinical features:
- SCC usually presents as an **indurated** keratinising or crusted plaque or nodule at sun-exposed sites (e.g. dorsal hands and forearms, face)
- The lesion is typically symptomatic (e.g. pain, discomfort, bleeding, ulcerating, sensory changes)
- SCCs have different morphologies – well-differentiated (less aggressive; *Fig. 11.28*), and

11

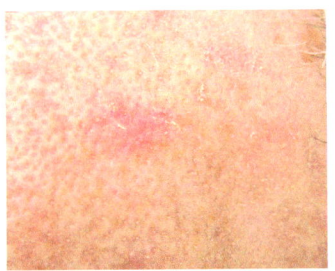

Fig. 11.26 Actinic keratosis – poorly defined erythematous scaly patch.

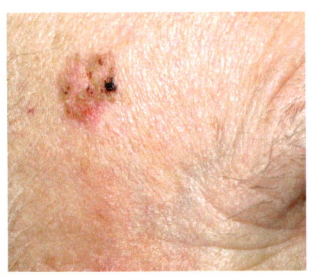

Fig. 11.27 Bowen disease – well-defined erythematous plaque.

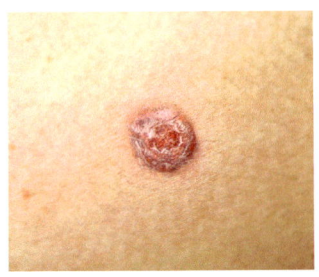

Fig. 11.28 Well-differentiated SCC – indurated nodule with ulceration.

moderately to poorly differentiated (more aggressive); the former is usually **scaly and grows slowly**, while the latter is often **non-scaly** and may appear like **granulation tissue**
- AK tends to present as multiple asymptomatic, erythematous scaly patches/plaques, while BD often presents as asymptomatic, well-defined erythematous, scaly (finer scale) patches/plaques

Investigations (BAD 2009)
- The diagnosis is usually established histologically
- Histology would also provide information on risk stratification

Management

> **Stepwise management of squamous cell carcinoma (BAD 2009)**
>
> 1 **SCCs should be classified into low risk or high risk, based on clinico-histological features (refer to BAD guidelines for details)**
>
> 2 **The cornerstone of treatment is surgical excision**
> - The recommended margin is 4mm for low-risk tumours, and 6mm for high-risk tumours
> - Wider margins may be needed if concerned
>
> 3 **Mohs surgery is reserved for patients with high-risk tumours needing wide margins or histological margin control**
>
> 4 **Radiotherapy is used for non-resectable tumours**
>
> 5 **Curettage and cautery, and cryotherapy could be considered in small, well-defined, low-risk tumours**
>
> 6 **Patient should be advised on sun protection**
>
> 7 **AK and BD can be managed with cryotherapy, topical chemotherapy (e.g. 5-fluorouracil (FU), imiquimod), or PDT**
> - If indicated, AK could just be observed

11.5.3 Melanoma

Definition: melanoma is a malignant tumour arising from melanocytes.

Epidemiology:
- In the UK, the lifetime risk of developing melanoma is 1 in 61 for men, and 1 in 60 for women
- The median age of diagnosis is 61 years old

Aetiology:
- Risk factors include solarium use, UV radiation exposure (especially intense, intermittent sun exposure), having multiple pigmented naevi, skin phototype I to III, family history and past history of melanoma, and having a giant congenital melanocytic naevus

Classification
- Predominantly radial growing – superficial spreading melanoma (SSM), acral lentiginous melanoma (ALM), lentigo maligna melanoma (LMM) or lentigo maligna if it is *in situ*
  - Follows the ABCDE rule: A – Asymmetry, B – Irregular border, C – Multi-coloured (variegated), D – Diameter >0.6cm, E – Evolution
  - Has potential to progress into vertical growth phase, which carries higher metastatic risks
- Predominantly vertical growing – nodular melanoma (NM)
  - May not exhibit ABCDE features and follows the EFG rule: E – Elevation, F – Firm, G – Growing
  - Prognosis is poorer as vertical growth phase starts earlier

11

Subtypes and clinical features:

- Remember the **ABCD** and **EFG rules**
- **Symptoms** (e.g. bleeding, ulceration, pain, itch, oozing and crusting) may be suggestive of a malignant lesion
- Some melanomas may be **amelanotic** (i.e. pink in colour)
- Beware of the **ugly duckling sign** – a lesion that stands out from others
- SSM is the most common subtype. It usually begins as a hyperpigmented patch/plaque growing radially (see *Fig. 11.29*)
- LMM is the second most common subtype; it most frequently occurs on the **faces** of **sun-damaged** elderly people
- ALM occurs on the palms, soles or nails (see *Fig. 11.30*); the extension of pigment onto the nail fold (the **Hutchinson sign**) raises suspicions of subungual melanoma – it is not associated with sun exposure and is more common in Afro-Caribbean and Asian people
- NM typically presents as a hyperpigmented/blue-black/amelanotic firm papule, nodule or plaque (see *Fig. 11.31*)

Investigations (BAD 2010)

Stepwise plan:

1 **Excisional biopsy with a 2mm margin is the gold standard investigation**
   - If this is not possible (e.g. face or acral region), incisional or punch biopsy is occasionally acceptable
   - Shave biopsy is not recommended as it may lead to incorrect diagnosis due to sampling error and inaccurate pathological staging

2 **Various prognostic factors are included in the pathology report**
   - Breslow thickness (BT), Clark level, lymphatic/vascular invasion, presence of ulceration, mitotic count and perineural infiltration

E ▶▶ BT refers to the vertical thickness of the melanoma in millimetres, while the Clark level refers to the level of melanoma invasion into the anatomical layers of skin. BT is more accurate in predicting prognosis and represents the T part of the TNM staging.

3 **The 2009 American Joint Committee on Cancer (AJCC) TNM classification is widely used. A simplified breakdown:**
   - Stage IV: when there is organ metastasis
   - Stage III: when there is lymph node involvement (Stage IIIA is when there is 1–3 nodal micrometastases but without ulceration)
   - Stage II: when BT >2mm or BT 1.01–2mm with ulceration
   - Stage I: when BT <1mm or BT 1.01–2mm without ulceration

4 **Consider sentinel lymph node biopsy**
   - This is highly sensitive and specific for diagnosing subclinical regional lymph node involvement
   - It should be introduced to patients as a staging procedure but they should understand that it has no proven therapeutic value

5 **Patients with stage I, II and IIIA melanoma**
   - Should not be routinely staged by imaging or other methods due to the low true positive rate and high false positive rate

6 **Patients with stage IIIB or IIIC melanoma**
   - Should have a CT head, chest, abdomen and pelvis done

7 **Patients with stage IV melanoma**
   - May benefit from PET or CT scan based on clinical need
   - LDH should also be measured

11

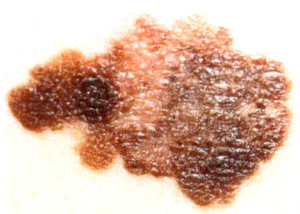

Fig. 11.29 *Melanoma – pigmented plaque displaying asymmetry, irregular border and colour variegation.*

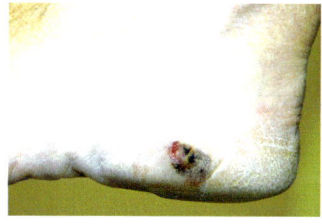

Fig. 11.30 *Acral lentiginous melanoma (ALM) on the foot.*

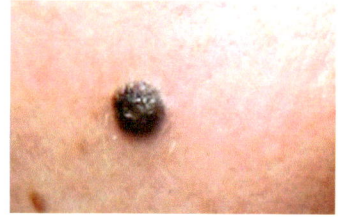

Fig. 11.31 *Nodular melanoma – hyperpigmented firm nodule.*

Management

Stepwise management of melanoma (BAD 2010)

1 **Surgical excision is the gold standard treatment. The recommended surgical margin is:**
- 5mm for *in situ* melanoma
- 1cm for Breslow thickness <1mm
- 1–2cm for BT 1.01–2mm
- 2–3cm for BT 2.1–4mm
- 3cm for BT >4mm

2 **Patients with confirmed positive lymph node metastasis should be reviewed for radical lymph node dissection**

3 **Chemotherapy and radiotherapy are reserved for selected patients**

4 **Patients with invasive melanomas should be reviewed regularly depending on their stage group**

5 **Patients should be advised on sun protection**

11.6 Dermatology in internal medicine

11.6.1 Pyoderma gangrenosum (PG)

Definition: pyoderma gangrenosum is a neutrophilic dermatosis characterised by cutaneous ulceration.

Epidemiology:
- The incidence is 3–10 per million per year
- Most commonly affects the middle-aged population without gender predilection

Aetiology:
- Around 50% of cases have an underlying systemic disease
- The three main groups are:
  - Gastrointestinal diseases (e.g. **IBD**, chronic active hepatitis)
  - Haematological malignancies (esp. **AML**)
  - Rheumatological diseases (e.g. **RA, SLE**)

Clinical features:
- Characterised by **rapidly enlarging, painful ulcers** with **granulomatous bases** and **undermined, violaceous edges**, typically found in the lower limbs (see *Fig. 11.32*)
- PG initially presents as a papule or pustule, commonly at the site of a minor injury (**pathergy**)

W >> How is pathergy different from the Koebner phenomenon? Although both terms describe the phenomenon of cutaneous lesions developing at the injury site, pathergy refers to an exaggerated skin reaction to trauma, characterised by the formation of papules or pustules, classically displayed by neutrophilic dermatoses.

- Ulcers typically heal with **cribriform** (sieve-like) scarring
- Other variants include pustular, bullous and vegetative PG

Investigations (PCDS 2015)
- Carry out **diagnosis of exclusion**
- Skin biopsies should be sent for histopathology and culture to exclude other conditions (e.g. malignancy and infection) – histopathology typically displays neutrophilic infiltrates, although this finding is non-specific and not always present
- Initial blood tests should include FBC, inflammatory markers, routine biochemistry, rheumatoid factor, plasma protein electrophoresis and cryoglobulins

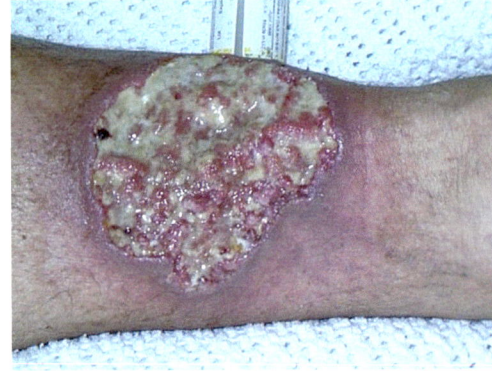

Fig. 11.32 *Classic pyoderma gangrenosum lesion that displays a granulomatous base and a violaceous edge.*

Management

Stepwise management of pyoderma gangrenosum (PCDS 2015)

1 **Provide appropriate wound care and pain relief**

2 **Topical therapy (e.g. steroids or tacrolimus) is essential in all cases**

3 **Systemic therapy is required in all but localised superficial cases**
- The mainstay of treatment is systemic corticosteroid ± cyclosporin
- Other adjuncts or alternatives include dapsone, minocycline, colchicine, sulfasalazine, azathioprine, methotrexate, cyclophosphamide, mycophenolate, biologics and IVIg

4 **Surgery (e.g. skin grafting) is reserved for selected cases**

11.6.2 Erythema nodosum (EN)

Definition: erythema nodosum is the most common type of panniculitis (inflammation of the subcutaneous tissue). It is considered a reactive process to various stimuli.

Epidemiology:
- Typically affects females in their teens and 20s
- The annual incidence of EN is 1–5/100,000 population

Aetiology/pathophysiology:
- Thought to be a delayed hypersensitivity reaction, though the exact mechanism remains elusive
- One-third of cases are idiopathic; common causes include infection (streptococci, tuberculosis, URTI, yersiniosis), drugs (penicillin, sulphonamides), autoimmune diseases (inflammatory bowel disease, sarcoidosis, rheumatoid arthritis, Behçet disease), hormonal changes (pregnancy, oral contraceptive pills) and malignancy (Hodgkin lymphoma)

Clinical features:
- Presents as an acute onset of **tender**, erythematous plaques and nodules that typically affect the lower limb bilaterally (especially the **shins;** see *Fig. 11.33*)
- Patients may have prodromal constitutional symptoms, e.g. low-grade fever, malaise and arthralgias

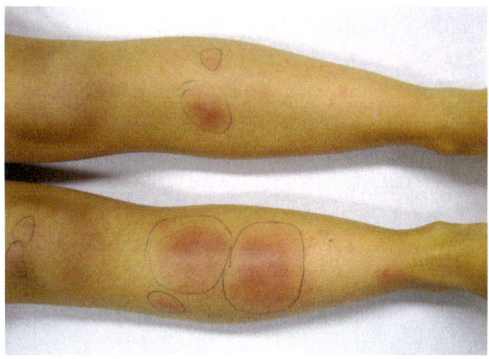

Fig. 11.33 *Erythematous plaques affecting the shins, typical of erythema nodosum.*

Investigations (PCDS 2014)

Stepwise plan:

1 **This condition is usually diagnosed clinically**

2 **Carry out initial evaluation**
- This should include FBC, inflammatory marker, serum ACE levels, ASOT, throat swab and CXR
- Other investigations can be ordered, based on suspected aetiology

3 **Elliptical biopsy can be performed in the event of diagnostic uncertainty**
- The classic histopathological picture is septal panniculitis without vasculitis

Management

Stepwise management of erythema nodosum (PCDS 2014)

1 **Identify and treat any underlying aetiology**

2 **Conservative management is the cornerstone of EN treatment as it tends to resolve spontaneously**
- This includes bed rest, compression bandages, elevation and NSAIDs

3 **Consider next-line therapy**
- Such as corticosteroids (systemic or intralesional), oral tetracycline, potassium iodide or colchicine

4 **Consider third-line therapy**
- Such as dapsone, hydroxychloroquine, anti-TNF biologics, thalidomide and methotrexate

11

11.6.3 Erythema multiforme (EM)

Definition: EM is an immune-mediated mucocutaneous condition that is commonly caused by herpes simplex virus (HSV). EM major refers to EM with mucosal involvement, whilst EM minor only involves the skin.

Epidemiology:
- The incidence of EM is postulated to be between 0.01% and 1%
- It commonly affects young adults, with a slight female predilection

Aetiology:
- Infection represents around 90% of triggered EM
- The most common infectious agent is **HSV**, followed by **Mycoplasma pneumoniae**
- **Drug**-induced EM is seen in <10% of cases – common culprits are NSAIDs, sulphonamides, anti-epileptics and antibiotics

Clinical features:
- EM classically presents as **acrally (typically the hands)** distributed **targetoid** lesions with **three zones** – a dusky central disc, surrounded by a pale oedematous ring, followed by an erythematous outermost ring; some lesions may only have two zones (see *Fig. 11.34*)
- Prodromal symptoms are usually mild or absent
- The lesions may coalesce into polycyclic configurations and they typically resolve within 1–2 weeks
- It may be accompanied by oropharyngeal, genital, ocular or upper respiratory mucosal erosions

Investigations (PCDS 2015)
- This condition is usually diagnosed clinically
- A biopsy may be performed to rule out other conditions

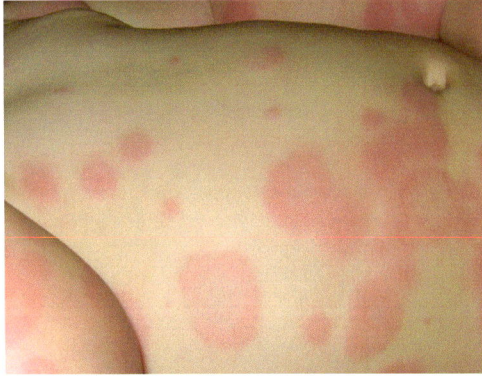

Fig. 11.34 Multiple targetoid lesions on the torso.

Management

> **Stepwise management of erythema multiforme**

1 **Identify and remove any inciting aetiology**
- Discontinue any offending medication
- Consider appropriate antibiotic for symptomatic *Mycoplasma pneumoniae* infection
- Antiviral therapy after the appearance of HSV-induced EM does not alter its clinical course

2 **The treatment of mucosal involvement depends on its severity and location**
- For mild disease, consider using high-potency topical steroids, oral antiseptic washes or oral anaesthetic solutions
- Systemic steroid is reserved for severe mucosal involvement
- Ophthalmology referral is essential for patients with ocular involvement

3 **The first-line therapy for HSV-associated or idiopathic recurrent EM (>6 episodes of EM per year) is continuous antiviral therapy for 6 months**
- Consider immunosuppressants for treatment-resistant recurrent EM

11.6.4 Granuloma annulare

Definition: granuloma annulare is a common cutaneous disorder classically presenting as smooth annular plaques without epidermal changes.

Epidemiology:
- Localised disease commonly occurs in patients under 30 years of age
- It has a 2:1 female to male predominance and no racial predilection

Aetiology:
- Its aetiology is unknown; however, due to its histological features, a delayed type hypersensitivity reaction is favoured
- Generalised, disseminated or atypical disease may in some cases be associated with diabetes mellitus (DM), thyroid disease, dyslipidaemia, malignancy, infections (e.g. HIV infection, hepatitis B) and drugs (e.g. infliximab)

Clinical features:
- Localised disease typically presents as a **smooth, annular plaque**, commonly involving the **dorsal hands and feet** (see *Fig. 11.35*); the plaques are usually **asymptomatic**
- Other subtypes include generalised disease (widespread annular plaques or disseminated

smooth papules), subcutaneous disease (presents as firm subcutaneous nodules, usually found in children) and perforating disease (presents as umbilicated papules)

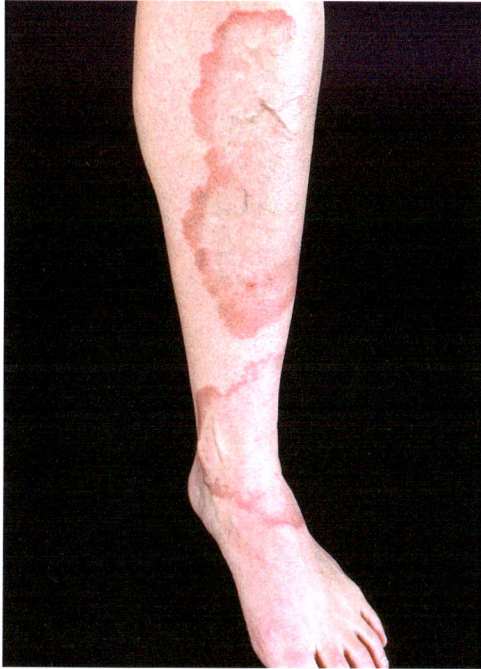

Fig. 11.35 *Multiple annular plaques of granuloma annulare.*

Investigations (PCDS 2015)

Stepwise plan:

1 **This condition is usually diagnosed clinically**

2 **A skin biopsy may be indicated if the diagnosis is uncertain**

3 **Carry out histology**
- This classically reveals dermal palisading granulomas with a central degeneration of collagen, in the presence of mucin

4 **In the appropriate clinical context, further investigations may be performed**
- To evaluate for any underlying DM, thyroid disease, dyslipidaemia and malignancy

Management
- For localised disease, lesions may sometimes resolve spontaneously
- Potent/very potent topical steroids or intralesional steroids are the common first-line therapy

- Other options include cryotherapy, topical tacrolimus, oral isotretinoin, phototherapy, photodynamic therapy and laser
- Topical therapy is usually insufficient to achieve clearance for generalised disease – treatments include hydroxychloroquine, fumaric esters, isotretinoin, phototherapy and biologic agents

11.6.5 Vitiligo

Definition: vitiligo is an acquired depigmenting disorder.

Epidemiology:
- Vitiligo is the most common depigmenting disorder, with an estimated global prevalence of 0.5–1%
- Its incidence is similar in all racial types but it is more visible in darker-skinned populations
- It affects both genders equally
- The majority of patients present before the age of 30

Pathophysiology:
- The autoimmune melanocyte destruction theory is the leading pathophysiological hypothesis – this is based on its association with other autoimmune disorders, such as **thyroiditis**, pernicious anaemia, Addison disease, alopecia areata and diabetes mellitus

Clinical features:
- Vitiligo typically presents as **depigmented**, non-scaly macules or patches with **well-demarcated borders** (see *Fig. 11.36*)
- The lesions are usually distributed symmetrically over the entire body (non-segmental vitiligo), though some may present in a unilateral and segmental distribution (segmental vitiligo)
- Vitiligo may display the Koebner phenomenon

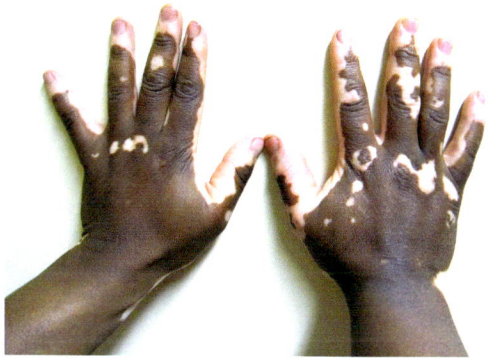

Fig. 11.36 *Multiple well-demarcated depigmented macules and patches affecting the acral region of a dark-skinned individual.*

11

Investigations (BAD 2008)

Stepwise plan:

1 **This condition is usually diagnosed clinically**

2 **A skin biopsy may be performed if the diagnosis is uncertain**
- Histological exam typically reveals an absence of melanocyte
- Lymphocytic infiltration may be seen in actively spreading lesions

3 **Thyroid function test should be considered**
- Due to the association between autoimmune thyroid disease and vitiligo

Management

Stepwise management of vitiligo

1 **Give patients advice on camouflage products and sun protection**

2 **The first-line therapy is topical steroid or topical calcineurin inhibitor**
- Depending on the site of involvement

3 **Phototherapy is an effective treatment**
- This should be considered in adult patients and all paediatric patients (of sufficient age to stand alone in the cabinet)

4 **Consider surgical treatments (e.g. tissue grafts and cellular grafts)**
- These are reserved for patients with non-active vitiligo for at least 12 months without the Koebner phenomenon

5 **Consider depigmentation treatment**
- This is reserved for patients with extensive or disfiguring vitiligo that is unresponsive to topical therapies and phototherapy

6 **The use of systemic agents is rarely indicated**
- Except for rapidly progressing vitiligo

11.7 Drug eruptions

11.7.1 Stevens-Johnson syndrome (SJS)/toxic epidermal necrolysis (TEN)

Definition: SJS and TEN are considered to occupy two ends of a spectrum of severe epidermolytic adverse cutaneous drug reactions. SJS is used when <10% of body surface area (BSA) is involved, while TEN affects >30% of the BSA. SJS/TEN overlap involves 10–30% of BSA.

Epidemiology:
- SJS and TEN affects approximately 1–2 cases/ million annually
- Its incidence is higher in the HIV-positive population

Aetiology/pathophysiology:
- Although the pathogenesis of SJS/TEN is not fully understood, CD8 T cells, cytolytic molecules FasL and granulysin have been found to play key roles

- SJS/TEN are commonly caused by drugs; common culprits are **allopurinol**, **sulphonamides**, **antibiotics**, **anticonvulsants**, **oxicam-type NSAIDs**
- Infections are occasionally reported as the sole cause

Clinical features:
- The onset of the disease is usually within the first 2 months when the culprit drug is commenced
- SJS/TEN classically presents as **painful**, **dusky erythema** with blisters and erosions (*Fig. 11.37*) that rapidly progress into confluent erythema with **sheet-like epidermal detachment** – the **Nikolsky sign** is positive (epidermis detached by mechanical pressure; *Fig. 11.38*)
- The rash is usually preceded by prodromal symptoms, such as fever, malaise, myalgia and arthralgia
- Mucosal involvement (e.g. the eyes, lips/mouth, oesophagus, upper respiratory tract and genitalia) is common

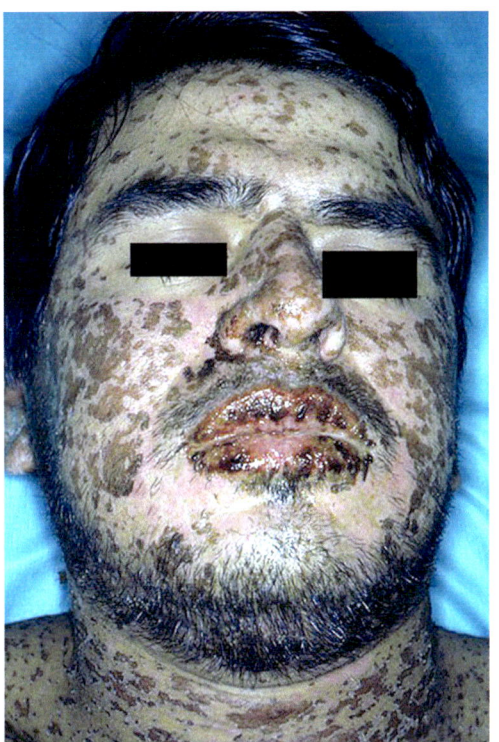

Fig. 11.37 *Dusky erythematous skin detachment associated with mucosal erosions.*

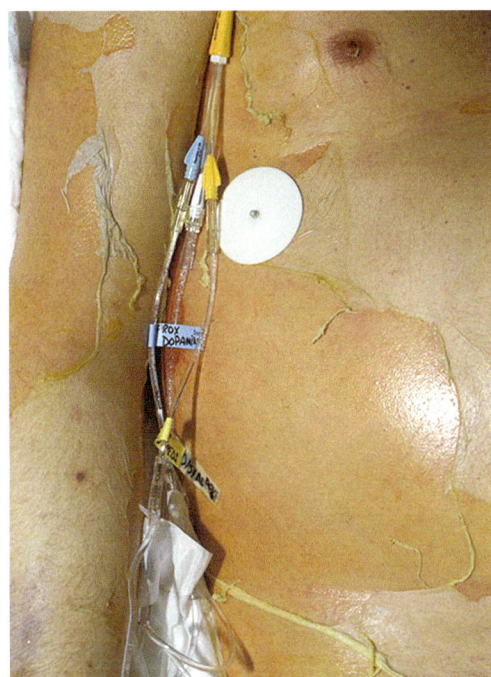

Fig. 11.38 *Sheet-like epidermal detachment seen in TEN.*

Investigations

Stepwise plan:

1 **Skin biopsy is required**
- To confirm the diagnosis of SJS/TEN and rule out other differentials
- Histology reveals widespread necrotic epidermis involving all layers

2 **Direct immunofluorescence (DIF) should be additionally performed**
- To rule out autoimmune blistering diseases
- DIF should be negative in SJS/TEN

3 **Blood tests (e.g. FBC, U&Es and LFT) are essential**
- To identify complications and assess prognosis

Management

Stepwise management of SJS/TEN

1 **Prompt withdrawal of the culprit drug is essential**

2 **Supportive care (e.g. fluids, electrolyte and wound management) is best delivered in an intensive care or burns unit**

3 **The early use of IVIg is recommended for TEN**
- Granulocyte-cell stimulating factor is administered to all patients with TEN in certain hospitals
- However, the concomitant use of systemic corticosteroids and immunosuppressants (e.g. cyclosporin) in SJS/TEN remains controversial

4 **The treatment of sequelae (cutaneous and mucosal involvement) is usually interdisciplinary**
- Early ophthalmology review is mandatory to identify and manage any eye involvement

Prognosis
- The mortality rate of SJS is 1–5% and the mortality rate for TEN is 25–35%

11

11.8 Autoimmune bullous disorders

11.8.1 Pemphigus vulgaris

Definition: pemphigus vulgaris is an epidermal immunobullous disease.

Epidemiology:
- Incidence ranges from 0.76 to 5 new cases/million/year
- The mean age of onset is 50–60 years
- This condition is more common in Ashkenazi Jews

Aetiology/pathophysiology:
- In pemphigus vulgaris, **IgG** auto-antibodies target mainly **desmoglein (DSG) 3**, but also DSG1, which are desmosomes of the keratinocytes
- This causes acantholysis (cell-cell detachment) in the epidermis, resulting in blister formation
- Usually occurs insidiously but can be triggered by drugs (e.g. thiol drugs and phenol drugs), viral infection, diet and stress

Clinical features:
- Characterised by **painful erosions** involving the mucosa, e.g. the **oropharyngeal mucosa**, genitalia and conjunctiva
- Cutaneous manifestation – **flaccid blisters** that easily rupture, leaving large **painful erosion** (see *Fig. 11.39*), usually involving the **trunk**, intertriginous areas and scalp
- The **Nikolsky sign** is positive in pemphigus vulgaris

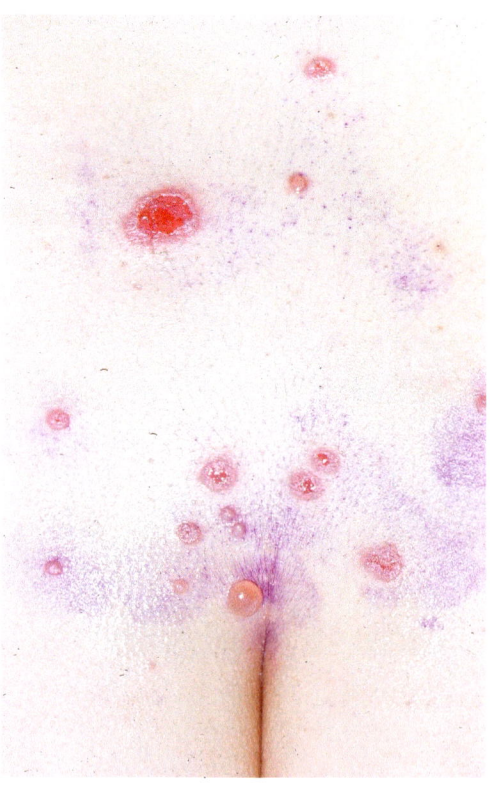

Fig. 11.39 *Flaccid blisters and erosions.*

Investigations (PCDS 2015)

Stepwise plan:

1 **Indirect immunofluorescence (IDIF) can be ordered**
- To detect anti-DSG3

2 **Arrange skin biopsies of the active lesion and the perilesional area**
- These are required for histology and **direct immunofluorescence** (DIF), respectively
- Histology typically reveals suprabasal clefts and blisters, with **acantholytic cells**
- DIF typically reveals a '**fishnet**' appearance with **IgG** ± C3 deposits in the epidermis (see *Fig. 11.40*)

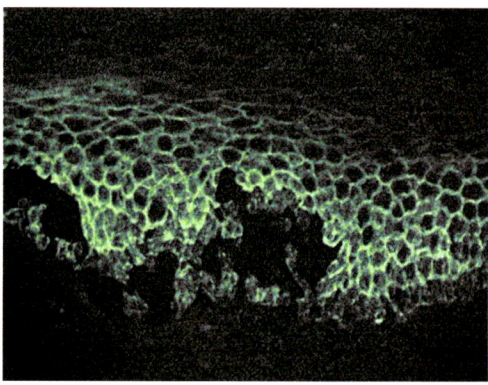

Fig. 11.40 *DIF revealing a '**fishnet**' appearance with IgG deposits in the epidermis.*

11

Management

Stepwise management of pemphigus vulgaris (PCDS 2015)

1 **General measures include wound care, emollients and antiseptic regimes**
   - To reduce risk of secondary infections

2 **Potent/very potent topical steroids are essential for wound healing**

3 **The preferred first-line treatment is systemic steroids (1mg/kg), with or without steroid-sparing agents**

4 **Common first-line steroid-sparing agents include azathioprine, mycophenolate mofetil and cyclophosphamide**
   - Newer second-line interventions include rituximab and IVIg

5 **Treatment goal is to induce and maintain remission, with a view to eventually tapering off treatment completely**

11.8.2 Bullous pemphigoid

Definition: bullous pemphigoid is an autoimmune sub-epidermal blistering disease.

Epidemiology:
- Classically affects the **elderly**
- Mean age of onset is 80 years old
- Incidence of 43 per million per year in the UK

Aetiology/pathophysiology:
- Auto-antibodies of mainly IgG-type attack adhesive components (**hemidesmosomes**) of the basement membrane zone (BMZ) resulting in subepidermal blistering
- The two main auto-antigens are BP230 and BP180
- This disease is associated with neurological diseases (e.g. dementia, Parkinson disease) and certain drugs (e.g. furosemide, spironolactone and neuroleptics)

Clinical features:
- Characterised by pruritic **tense blisters** that usually break after several days, leaving erosions and crusted lesions (see *Fig. 11.41*)
- Typically affects the trunk and flexural aspects of the extremities
- Although uncommon, the mucosal membrane may be involved

Investigations (BAD 2012)

Stepwise plan:

1 **Arrange skin biopsies of the active lesion and the perilesional area**
   - These are required for histology and **direct immunofluorescence** (DIF), respectively
   - Histology typically reveals sub-epidermal blisters with eosinophilic infiltrates
   - The **linear deposition** of **IgG ± C3** along the BMZ on DIF is characteristic of bullous pemphigoid (see *Fig. 11.42*)

2 **To differentiate bullous pemphigoid from epidermolysis bullosa acquisita, a DIF on salt-split skin may be performed**
   - The addition of normal saline cleaves the skin through the lamina lucida
   - Antigens are detected at the roof of the split skin, instead of the dermal aspect

3 **Indirect immunofluorescence could be performed on serum or blister fluids**

4 **ELISA test (to detect BP180 and BP230 antibodies) is a useful additional diagnostic tool but is not widely available in the UK**

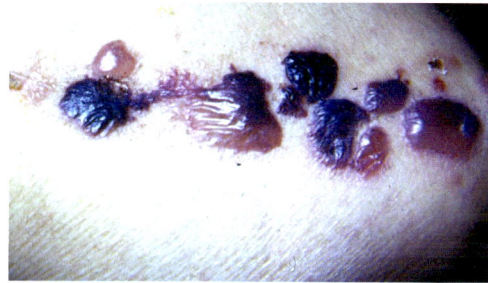

Fig. 11.41 *Multiple blood-filled tense bullae.*

11

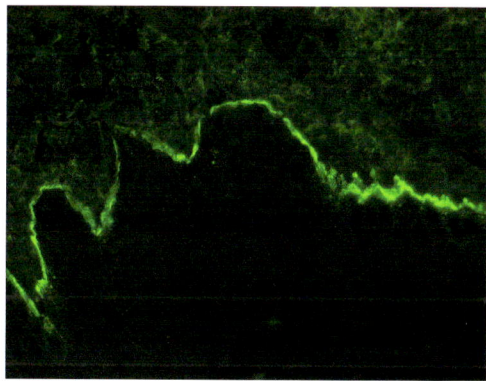

Fig. 11.42 *Linear deposition of IgG along the BMZ on DIF.*

Management

1 General measures include wound care, emollients and antiseptic regimes
- To reduce risk of secondary infections

2 For localised or mild disease
- Treat the patient with a very potent topical steroid
- Systemic steroids or anti-inflammatory antibiotics (e.g. doxycycline, erythromycin) could also be used

3 For moderate to severe disease
- Use systemic corticosteroids in combination with very potent topical steroids as the first-line therapy
- Anti-inflammatory antibiotics could also be used

4 For diseases not responding to existing treatment
- Consider adding immunosuppressive drugs, such as azathioprine, methotrexate or dapsone
- IVIg, mycophenolate mofetil, cyclophosphamide and plasmapheresis are reserved for refractory cases

11.8.3 Dermatitis herpetiformis (DH)

Definition: DH is an immunobullous condition associated with coeliac disease. DH typically affects Caucasians in their fourth and fifth decades. DH is considered the specific cutaneous manifestation of coeliac disease (CD). Both diseases share the same HLA haplotypes (DQ2 and DQ8) and patients with DH show typical CD alterations in the small bowel biopsy.

Clinical features:
- DH classically presents as a **symmetrical papulovesicular** rash that commonly involves the **extensors, shoulder and buttocks** (see *Fig. 11.43* and *Fig. 11.44*)
- The rash is **extremely pruritic**
- Therefore, the vesicles are often immediately excoriated, resulting in erosions, crusted papules or pigmentary changes
- Only a minority of patients will present with symptoms of CD, e.g. abdominal discomfort and bloating, diarrhoea or weight loss

Investigations (PCDS 2015)
- IgA, **anti-tissue transglutaminase (tTG) antibody**, FBC (folate deficiency) and iron studies (iron deficiency) should be performed in the investigation of DH

- Skin biopsies of the active lesion and the perilesional area are required for histology and **direct immunofluorescence** (DIF), respectively
- Histology typically reveals sub-epidermal blisters with neutrophilic infiltrates
- The finding of **granular IgA deposits** along the dermal-epidermal junction on DIF is characteristic of DH
- Positive results for anti-tTG and DIF are diagnostic of DH

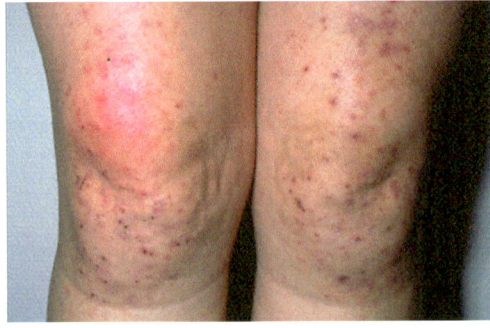

Fig. 11.43 *DH involving the knee.*

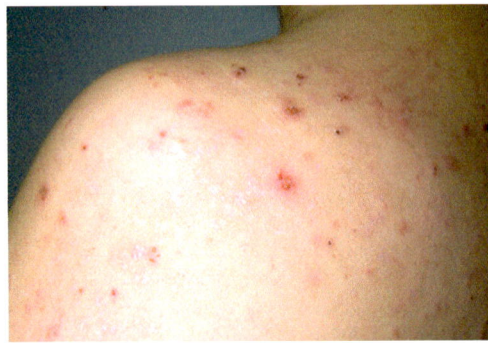

Fig. 11.44 *DH involving the shoulder.*

Management

1 Moderately potent topical steroids can be used for symptomatic relief in DH
- Oral dapsone is the first-line pharmacological treatment for DH
- Sulfapyridine can be used for patients who cannot tolerate dapsone

2 Other less effective treatments include colchicine, prednisolone, cyclosporin and azathioprine

3 **Refer the patient to a gastroenterologist for potential further work-up and management of CD**

4 **Patients should be referred to a dietitian for advice on a gluten-free diet**
- Adherence to a gluten-free diet is essential to lower the risk of intestinal lymphoma

11.9 Skin infections

11.9.1 Bacterial infections

11.9.1.1 Impetigo

Definition: impetigo is a superficial bacterial infection of the skin.

Epidemiology:
- Impetigo predominantly affects children
- In the UK, it has an annual incidence of around 2.8% in children up to 4 years of age

Aetiology:
- Non-bullous impetigo is commonly caused by *Staphylococcus aureus* (*Staph. aureus*) and *Streptococcus pyogenes* (*Strep. pyogenes*)
- Bullous impetigo is caused only by *Staph. aureus*

> 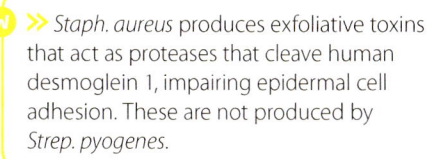 *Staph. aureus* produces exfoliative toxins that act as proteases that cleave human desmoglein 1, impairing epidermal cell adhesion. These are not produced by *Strep. pyogenes*.

- It is highly contagious and is usually spread via close contact
- Risk factors include pre-existing eczema, skin trauma, hot and humid climate, poor hygiene, crowding, day care settings and diabetes mellitus

Clinical features:
- Non-bullous impetigo is characterised by maculopapular lesions that transit rapidly into painful erosions covered by honey-coloured crust, commonly found over the face and extremities (see *Fig. 11.45*)
- Bullous impetigo is characterised by **flaccid bullae** over the trunk, axilla, extremities and intertriginous areas (see *Fig. 11.46*)
- As it ruptures, it oozes yellow fluid and leaves a **collarette of scales** around the erosions

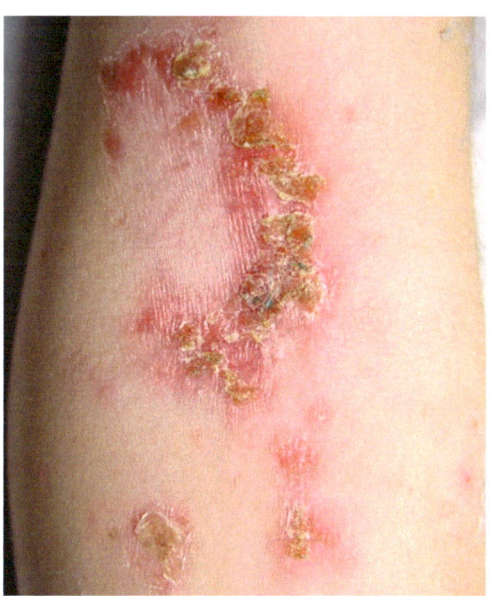

Fig. 11.45 *Classic honey-coloured crust of non-bullous impetigo.*

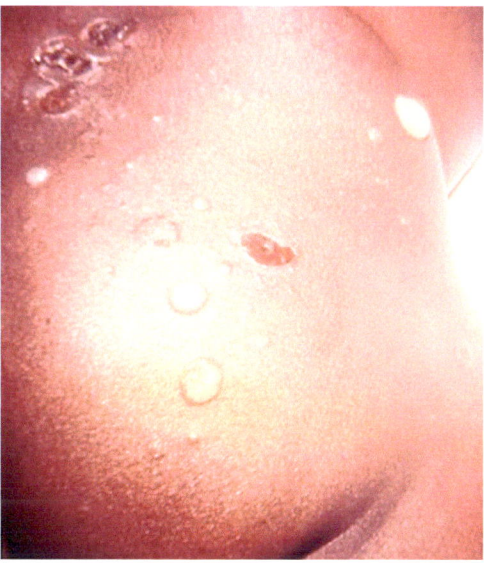

Fig. 11.46 *Flaccid bullae and characteristic collarette of scales in bullous impetigo.*

11

Investigations
- The diagnosis of the condition is usually made clinically
- Skin swab is not necessary **unless** the rash is extensive or severe, recurrent, suspected as being a community outbreak or suspected to be caused by MRSA

Management

> **Stepwise management of impetigo (NICE CKS 2015)**

1 Educate the patient
- Patient should stay away from school or work until the lesions are dry and scabbed over, or 48 hours after antibiotic treatment
- Patient should also avoid sharing personal items such as towels and flannels during that period

2 Prescribe appropriate medication
- Use topical fusidic acid for localised non-bullous impetigo, and oral antibiotics (flucloxacillin or clarithromycin/erythromycin) for extensive non-bullous impetigo or bullous impetigo

3 If lesions do not improve after 7 days of treatment
- Review the diagnosis, check treatment compliance, take a swab and revise antibiotics
- Consider topical retapamulin if topical fusidic acid was used
- If not, consider oral antibiotics
- Prolonged duration of antibiotics may be required

4 For patients with recurrent impetigo
- Consider nasal swabs to detect staphylococcal carriage

11.9.1.2 Cellulitis

Definition: cellulitis is an acute bacterial infection of the dermis and subcutis.

Epidemiology:
- The incidence of cellulitis ranges from 0.2 to 24.6 per 1000 person-years in different populations

Aetiology:
- The most common implicated organisms are *Strep. pyogenes* and *Staph. aureus*
- Risk factors include **trauma**, insect bites, ulcers, tinea pedis, venous insufficiency, lymphoedema, diabetes and obesity

Clinical features:
- Cellulitis is characterised by spreading erythema (with poorly demarcated margin) associated with pain, oedema and warmth (see *Fig. 11.47*)
- It is commonly found on the extremities (**unilaterally**) and face
- Patient may report constitutional features, e.g. fever and malaise
- Blisters, ulcers, lymphangitis or lymphadenopathy may be present

> **P** » Erysipelas is a bacterial infection involving the superficial dermis. The rash is well demarcated and commonly involves the face.
>
> Acute complications of cellulitis include necrotising fasciitis, myositis, subcutaneous abscess, septicaemia; its chronic complications are lymphoedema, recurrence and chronic ulcer.

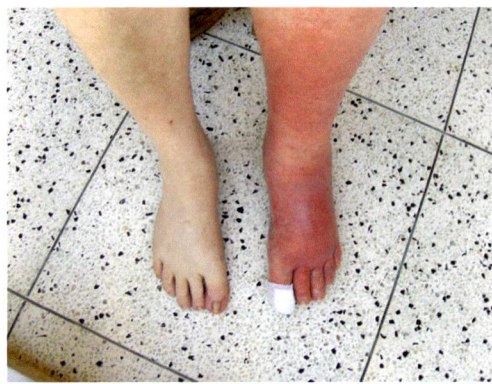

Fig. 11.47 *Cellulitis showing poorly demarcated erythema and oedema.*

Investigations and management
- **The Eron classification** of cellulitis is a useful guide for management (see *Table 11.2*)
- Identify and manage any underlying risk factors
- Consider ASOT or skin biopsy if the diagnosis is uncertain
- Prophylaxis for recurrent cellulitis (two or more episodes at the same site) is penicillin V or erythromycin for up to 2 years

11.9.2 Viral infections

Viral warts

Definition: viral warts are benign papillomas that are caused by the human papilloma virus (HPV).

Table 11.2 Eron classification

Eron classification	Investigation	Management
I – no signs of systemic toxicity and comorbidities	Clinical diagnosis	Managed with oral flucloxacillin/clarithromycin (if patient has penicillin allergy) as an outpatient
II – may be systemically well or unwell, but with a comorbidity (e.g. venous insufficiency)	As per Eron I + FBC, CRP, U&Es, culture any ulceration or blister fluid	Patient suitable for short-term hospitalisation (up to 48 hours) and IV antibiotics (flucloxacillin first line). Discharge on outpatient parenteral antibiotic therapy, if this service is available
III – significant systemic toxicity or unstable comorbidities	As per Eron II + blood culture	Immediate hospital admission and IV antibiotics (flucloxacillin first line)
IV – sepsis or necrotising fasciitis	As per Eron II + blood culture	Immediate hospital admission and IV antibiotics (benzylpenicillin + ciprofloxacin + clindamycin). Surgery may be indicated

Epidemiology:
- Prevalence in the general population is estimated to be 7–12%
- The infection is common in childhood

Aetiology:
- HPV can spread via direct contact or via the environment
- Risk factors include immunosuppression and activities that promote inoculation such as nail biting and walking barefoot

Subtypes
- Verruca vulgaris (common warts) – manifests as hyperkeratotic papules, often on the hands (see *Fig. 11.48*)
- Plantar warts – thick hyperkeratotic plaques beneath pressure points on the sole
- Gives rise to a 'mosaic' pattern in which plantar warts are grouped into clusters

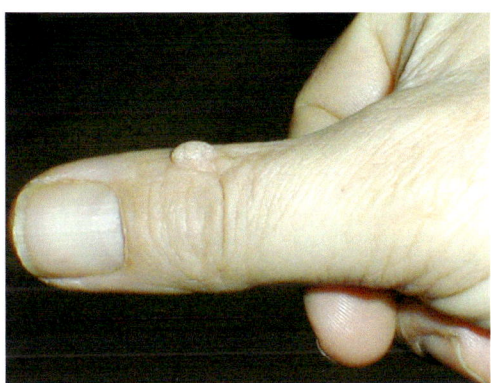

Fig. 11.48 Verruca vulgaris involving the thumb.

- Planar warts – flat-topped papules, commonly on the face
- Condyloma acuminata (anogenital warts) – cauliflower-like plaques over the anogenital region

Clinical features (for cutaneous viral warts):
- Can persist for years and are generally asymptomatic
- The presence of **thrombosed capillaries**, especially after paring, is characteristic of viral warts
- Spontaneous clearance within 1–2 years is common in children; this process is much slower in adults

Investigations
- The diagnosis of the condition is usually made clinically
- Histopathology may sometimes be required to distinguish viral warts from other keratotic skin diseases

Management

> **Stepwise management of cutaneous viral warts (PCDS 2012)**

1 **Educate the patient on lowering the risk of transmission**
- e.g. avoid sharing personal items, cover the wart with waterproof dressing when swimming, and avoid scratching or biting nails

2 **For patients with asymptomatic warts in non-cosmetically sensitive areas**
- Consider no treatment

11

3 If treatment is required
- Salicylic acid with regular paring and occlusion is the recommended first-line therapy
- This should be followed by cryotherapy, in combination with salicylic acid or duct tape (in children who can't tolerate pain well)

4 Consider third-line treatment
- This includes topical imiquimod, intralesional bleomycin, diphencyprone, curettage and cautery

5 Patients with anogenital warts
- Should be referred to a local genitourinary medicine service

11.9.3 Fungal infections

Dermatophytosis

Definition: dermatophytosis is a superficial fungal infection of keratinised tissues caused by dermatophytes.

Epidemiology:
- It is estimated that superficial fungal infections affect around 20–25% of the world population

Aetiology/pathophysiology:
- Dermatophytes are a specific group of fungi known as ringworms or tineas, comprising the following genera: *Microsporum*, *Trichophyton* and *Epidermophyton*

- Transmission is usually via direct contact with infected humans or animals, or indirectly via contaminated fomites, depending on whether the dermatophyte is anthropophilic (human host), zoophilic (animal host) or geophilic (lives in the soil)

Clinical features:
- Tinea typically presents as an asymmetrical, erythematous scaly plaque
- The rash is usually **annular (central clearing)** with an **advancing scaly edge** (see *Fig. 11.49*)
- Subtypes of dermatophyte present at different sites (see *Table 11.3*)

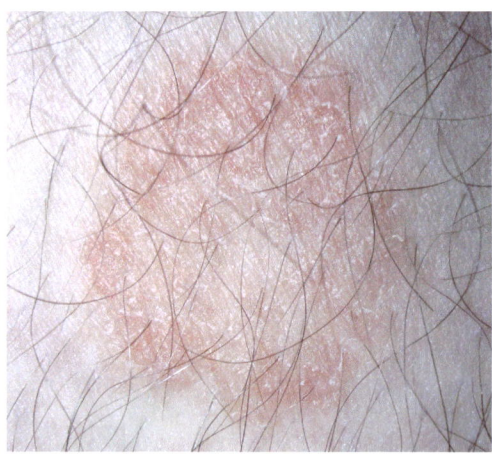

Fig. 11.49 *Advancing scaly edge with central clearing, typical of tinea.*

Table 11.3 *Subtypes of dermatophyte*

Site	Terminology	Clinical features
Face	Tinea faciei	
Beard/moustache area	Tinea barbae	• Presents as aggregated pustules, exudation or crusting
Hair	Tinea capitis	• Usually accompanied with scaling; involved areas may have broken hair stubs • Kerion is a highly inflamed tinea capitis, presenting as boggy masses and pustules
Body	Tinea corporis	
Groin	Tinea cruris	• Bilateral involvement is common • Satellite lesions not present as opposed to candidiasis
Hand	Tinea manuum	
Feet	Tinea pedis	• Athlete's foot • Interdigital involvement is common – skin becomes macerated and malodorous
Nail	Tinea unguium	• Also known as onychomycosis • Nails usually thicken and become yellow
Steroid-induced	Tinea incognito	• Initially patient feels better (due to reduced itch) but it progresses to become more pustular with less scale

11

Investigations
- The diagnosis of the condition is usually made clinically
- Skin scraping or nail clipping for microscopy and culture may be useful in the event of diagnostic uncertainty

> **Stepwise management of dermatophytosis (PCDS 2014/2015)**

1   Identify and correct risk factors

2   For tinea capitis
- Ketoconazole shampoo, in combination with oral terbinafine (due to risk of scarring alopecia)
- Prolonged treatment with oral terbinafine for kerion

3   For onychomycosis
- Oral terbinafine or itraconazole usually as first-line therapy, due to poor penetration with topical treatment

4   For tinea barbae
- Usually treated with oral terbinafine

5   For tinea corporis/cruris/manuum/pedis/faciei
- Topical terbinafine or imidazole as first-line treatment, followed by oral terbinafine

Pityriasis versicolor

Definition: pityriasis versicolor is a superficial fungal infection of the skin.

Aetiology:
- It is caused by yeasts of the genus *Malassezia*, which are lipophilic
- They are normal skin flora but can cause disease when converted to their pathogenic hyphal form

Epidemiology:
- Most commonly seen in teenagers and young adults, as they have increased sebum production
- Prevalence is significantly higher in tropical countries (up to 50%) than in the UK (around 1%)
- It is more common in summer than in winter

Clinical features:
- Commonly presents as well-demarcated thin plaques with fine scaling, involving the torso and occasionally the face (see *Fig. 11.50*)
- These plaques can be hyperpigmented, hypopigmented or erythematous and occasionally become confluent and widespread
- The fine scale on the rash can be accentuated with skin stretching

- Post-inflammatory pigmentary changes may persist for months despite eradication of infection

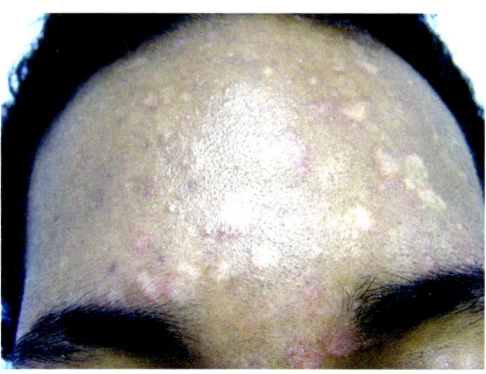

Fig. 11.50 *Well-demarcated hypopigmented plaques with evidence of active inflammation.*

Investigations
- The diagnosis of the condition is usually made clinically
- Microscopy confirmation is helpful when the diagnosis is uncertain
- Spores and hyphae resembling **'spaghetti and meatballs'** may be seen

> **Stepwise management of pityriasis versicolor (NICE CKS 2010)**

1   Educate the patient
- That this condition is not contagious and skin discoloration may persist for several weeks following successful eradication of the infection

2   Treat patient
- With either ketoconazole shampoo or selenium sulphide shampoo
- Imidazole antifungal cream can be applied if only small areas of skin are involved

3   Consider a second topical therapy
- Before considering oral antifungal drug, e.g. itraconazole or fluconazole

11.9.4 Parasitic infections

Scabies

Definition: scabies is a contagious skin infestation caused by the human parasite *Sarcoptes scabiei*.

Epidemiology:
- Approximately 300 million cases of scabies worldwide each year

11

- Individuals who are young, elderly, immuno-compromised or of a low socioeconomic status are more likely to develop scabies

Aetiology:

- Scabies is usually transmitted by direct skin-to-skin contact
- After being infested, patients develop a hypersensitivity reaction towards the mite or its byproducts, causing a generalised rash
- This reaction occurs more quickly during reinfestation

Clinical features:

- Classic presentation includes **linear burrows** (as the mites burrow into the epidermis; *Fig. 11.51*) and papular/papulovesicular rashes involving the **fingerwebs**, wrists, elbows, armpits, breasts and genital areas, as well as the feet and ankles (see *Fig. 11.52*)
- Patient commonly has generalised **intense pruritus** that is typically **worse at night**
- This rash usually develops within 2–6 weeks with initial infestation, and 1–3 days with reinfestation

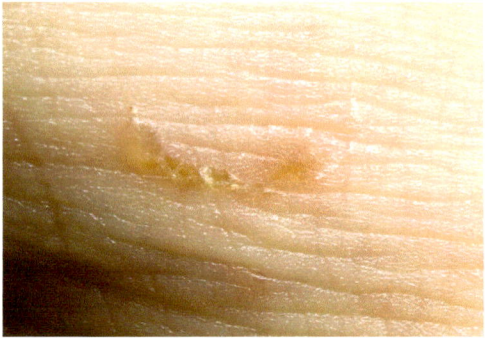

Fig. 11.51 *Linear burrows.*

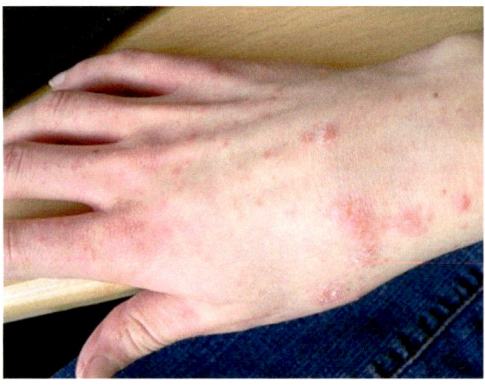

Fig. 11.52 *Papular rash involving the hand (note the fingerweb involvement).*

Investigations (NICE CKS)

- The diagnosis of the condition is usually made clinically
- If the diagnosis is uncertain, a burrow ink test can be carried out; taking skin scrapings of the burrows to identify any scabies mites, eggs or faeces is useful to confirm the diagnosis

Management

> **Stepwise management of scabies (NICE CKS 2011)**

1 **Treat the patient and all household members, close contacts and sexual contacts simultaneously with topical permethrin 5% cream**

- This should be applied twice, with applications 1 week apart, to eliminate the recently hatched eggs
- Use malathion 0.5% aqueous liquid if permethrin is contraindicated

2 **Machine wash (at 50°C or above) clothes, towels and bed linen on the day of application of first treatment**

3 **Patients should avoid close body contact with others until their close contacts have also been treated**

4 **Symptomatic treatments for itch include topical crotamiton and topical hydrocortisone 1%**

- Oral sedating antihistamine can be used at night if the itch interferes with sleep

5 **Treat secondary infection with an antibiotic**

6 **Oral ivermectin is commonly used in the context of an outbreak**

> **P** ≫ Norwegian (crusted) scabies is a severe form of scabies characterised by hyperinfestation with millions of mites, severe inflammation and hyperkeratotic reaction. It is associated with immunodeficiencies, e.g. HIV infection, haematological malignancies and autoimmune diseases. This condition is very contagious and requires more aggressive treatment.

11

Chapter 12
The emergency ladder

Hwan Juet Khaw

12.1 Acute coronary syndrome

Initial assessment

1. Obtain a quick history – **AMPLE** (**A**llergies, **M**edication, **P**MH, **L**ast ate/drank, **E**vents leading up to admission)
2. Consider cardiac risk factors

Airway

1. Ensure patient is maintaining own airway
2. **Sit patient up**
3. Obtain a set of observations
4. If acute coronary syndrome is suspected, and the patient's swallow is intact, administer:
   – **Aspirin** 300mg PO
   – **Antiplatelet agent**
     ○ **Clopidogrel** 300mg PO (some centres recommend 600mg if for PCI)
     ○ Newer agents include:
       • **Prasugrel** 60mg PO (if under 75 years of age and no history of CVA)
       • **Ticagrelor** 180mg PO

Breathing

1. Obtain SpO$_2$; **aim to keep sats 94–98%**
2. Give supplementary oxygen only if sats are below 90%

> **W** ≫ Some studies suggest that oxygen administration may prove harmful in acute coronary syndrome. However, this target has been set because there appears to be no clear benefit from administering oxygen, unless the patient is hypoxaemic or experiencing heart failure.

Circulation

1. Obtain **IV access**

2. Arrange for FBC, U&Es, blood glucose, lipid panel and **troponin**
3. Arrange for a 12-lead ECG and assess
4. Observe blood pressure; if SBP >90mmHg, offer **GTN** 2 puffs S/L for **pain relief**
5. Prescribe resuscitation fluids as necessary and:
   – **Morphine** 2.5mg–10mg IV
   – **Metoclopramide** 10mg IV
6. Ensure adequate control of blood glucose, aiming for a **level below 11mmol/L**

> **P** ≫ Some centres recommend the addition of metoprolol 5–10mg IV.

Disability & exposure

1. Contact Cardiology and consider admission to the Coronary Care Unit (CCU)
2. Assess type of presentation (i.e. STE-ACS or NSTE-ACS; see *Chapter 1*)
   – If STE-ACS, arrange immediate transfer for angiography and PCI, consider thrombolysis if patients are unable to receive PCI within 90–120 minutes of diagnosis
   – If NSTE-ACS, stratify risk using the GRACE score and manage accordingly (see *Chapter 1*)

> **E** ≫ Contraindications to thrombolysis:
> • Major trauma or surgery in the last 6 weeks
> • Previous stroke in the last 6 months
> • Hypertension >180/110
> • Coagulopathy or anticoagulant medication
> • Aortic dissection
> • Neurosurgery within the last year

12.2 Acute pulmonary oedema

Initial assessment

1. Obtain a quick history – **AMPLE** (**A**llergies, **M**edication, **P**MH, **L**ast ate/drank, **E**vents leading up to admission)
2. Consider fluid status; **stop** any current fluid prescription that may be contributing to fluid overload

Two major variants of acute pulmonary oedema:
- Cardiogenic: secondary to LV failure, infarction
- Non-cardiogenic: e.g. in ARDS, sepsis

> **E** ≫ A helpful mnemonic to remember the treatment for acute pulmonary oedema is '**LMNOP**' – **L**oop diuretic, **M**orphine, **N**itrates, **O**xygen, **P**osition (sit patient up).

Airway

1. Ensure patient is maintaining own airway
2. Sit patient up
3. Obtain a set of observations

Breathing

1. Obtain SpO$_2$
2. Give supplementary high flow oxygen 15L/min via a non-rebreather mask in the absence of respiratory disease
3. Arrange **CXR, looking for features of pulmonary oedema**

Circulation

1. Assess if patients are in cardiogenic shock
2. Obtain intravenous access

3. Arrange for FBC, U&Es, blood glucose, lipid panel, **troponin** and **B-type natriuretic peptide**
4. Arrange for a 12-lead ECG and assess
5. Observe blood pressure; if SBP >90mmHg, offer **GTN** 2 puffs S/L
6. Alternatively, if SBP >110mmHg, consider IV nitrates
7. Prescribe:
   - **Diamorphine** 2.5mg–5mg IV
   - **Furosemide** IV – 40mg, uptitrate as needed
   - **Thromboprophylaxis e.g. enoxaparin** 40mg SC

Disability & exposure

1. Continue to monitor patient clinically with observations, sats and urine output
2. If patients continue to decline, consider:
   - Increasing dose of furosemide to 80mg IV
   - NIV and CPAP

> **P** ≫ Do not arrange for nitrates or NIV if the patient has a SBP <90mmHg, as this may lower the BP further.

   - If refractory to NIV or CPAP, consider invasive ventilation
3. Once patient is stable, review medications, consider a low-salt diet and arrange CXR for assessment

12.3 Pericardial effusion/cardiac tamponade

Initial assessment

1. Obtain a quick history – **AMPLE** (**A**llergies, **M**edication, **P**MH, **L**ast ate/drank, **E**vents leading up to admission)
2. Consider aetiology of potential tamponade (Is this acute, e.g. trauma? Or is it chronic, e.g. malignancy?)

> **E** » Acute build-up of fluid or blood (up to as little as 100ml) may be sufficient to cause haemodynamic instability secondary to right atrial and ventricular compression. In practice, effusions rarely lead to tamponade.

Airway

1. Ensure patient is maintaining own airway
2. Sit patient up
3. Obtain a set of observations
4. Patients with cardiac tamponade may present with pulsus paradoxus

Breathing

1. Obtain SpO_2; aim to keep sats 94–98%
2. Give supplementary oxygen
3. Assess patient with a CXR

Circulation

1. Consider the **Beck triad:**
   - Hypotension
   - Elevated JVP
   - Muffled heart sounds
2. Obtain intravenous access
3. Arrange for FBC, U&Es, blood glucose, coagulation screen and troponin
4. Arrange for a 12-lead ECG and assess
5. Look for electrical alternans or low-voltage QRS complexes
6. Prescribe resuscitation fluids as necessary

Disability & exposure

1. Perform echocardiography, to assess cardiac function and to help with pericardiocentesis
2. Echocardiography-guided pericardiocentesis is the definitive therapy
3. Pericardiocentesis may be diagnostic, therapeutic, or both
4. Treat underlying cause
5. Emergency drainage below the xiphoid process should be attempted under echocardiographic guidance, so as not to perforate the right ventricle

12.4 Aortic dissection

Clinical features:
- Sudden onset, 'ripping/tearing' chest pain radiating through the back
- Hypotension, tachycardia
- Signs and symptoms of tamponade
- Absent pulse or increased BP differential in both arms

> **E** ≫ According to the Stanford classification, there are two types of aortic dissection:
> - Type A – involves the ascending aorta (surgical emergency)
> - Type B – does not involve the ascending aorta

Airway
1. Ensure patient is maintaining own airway
2. Provide airway support if necessary
3. Maintain airway
4. Obtain a set of observations

Breathing
1. Obtain SpO₂
2. Give supplementary high-flow oxygen 15L/min via a NRBM
3. Arrange an urgent CXR – typically shows a widened mediastinum

Circulation
1. Assess if patients are in shock
2. Obtain intravenous access
3. Provide careful fluid resuscitation with tight BP control

> **W** ≫ Strict BP control is important in the acute management of aortic dissection, and a systolic BP of 100–120mmHg should be the target. This is because high blood pressure can worsen the dissection and may eventually lead to rupture.

4. Arrange for FBC, U&Es, LFTs, blood glucose, coagulation screen, X-match, D-dimer (to exclude PE) and troponin
5. Arrange for a 12-lead ECG to exclude ACS
6. Note that ST-depression may be seen

> **P** ≫ The right coronary artery may be affected in Type A aortic dissections and may present as myocardial ischaemia or even infarction.

7. Prescribe:
   - Appropriate analgesia (**morphine** 2.5mg–10mg IV)
   - Consider antihypertensives
     - IV labetalol 50mg over 1 minute
     - GTN infusion 0.6–1.2mg/hour

Disability & exposure
1. Arrange for a CT aortogram when the patient is more stable
2. Type A dissections should be urgently referred for cardiothoracic surgery
3. Type B dissections are largely managed with medical therapy alone
4. Aortic dissection has a poor prognosis, with up to 20% of patients dying before they reach hospital

12.5 Ruptured abdominal aortic aneurysm

Clinical features:
- Abdominal pain radiating to the back, or frank back pain
- Hypotension, tachycardia, collapse (with or without recovery)
- Pulsatile abdominal mass
- Older patients who smoke are at greater risk

Airway
1. Ensure patient is maintaining own airway
2. Provide airway support if necessary
3. Maintain airway
4. Obtain a set of observations
5. **Immediate** vascular surgery referral

Breathing
1. Obtain SpO_2
2. Give supplementary high-flow oxygen 15L/min via a non-rebreather mask in the absence of respiratory disease

Circulation
1. Assess if patients are in shock

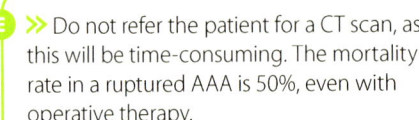 E >> Do not refer the patient for a CT scan, as this will be time-consuming. The mortality rate in a ruptured AAA is 50%, even with operative therapy.

2. Obtain intravenous access
3. Appropriate fluid resuscitation: **aim for 80mmHg systolic (i.e. permissive hypotension)**
4. Arrange for FBC, U&Es, LFTs, blood glucose, coagulation screen and troponin
5. Crossmatch 10 units of blood
6. Activate major haemorrhage protocol; retrieve O-negative blood if transfusion is required; transfuse 1 unit at a time
7. Arrange for a 12-lead ECG and assess
8. Prescribe:
    - **Morphine** 2.5–10mg IV
    - **Ceftriaxone** 1.5g and **metronidazole** 500mg IV prophylactically (based on local protocols)

Disability & exposure
1. Continue to monitor patient clinically with observations, sats and urine output
2. Consider rapid bedside ultrasound scan (FAST scan)

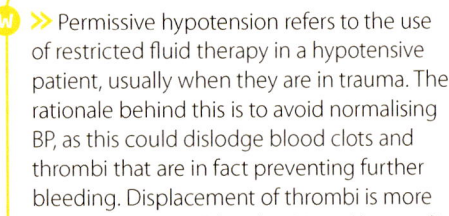 W >> Permissive hypotension refers to the use of restricted fluid therapy in a hypotensive patient, usually when they are in trauma. The rationale behind this is to avoid normalising BP, as this could dislodge blood clots and thrombi that are in fact preventing further bleeding. Displacement of thrombi is more likely to occur at BP levels >80mmHg systolic.

Administering fluid therapy also causes haemodilution, which may prevent adequate coagulation by the body. Evidence suggests that patients maintained at lower mean arterial pressures need less fluid and blood product replacement and also have lower mortality rates.

P >> The Hardman index delineates features that are indicative of a poor prognosis, and these are as follows:
- Age >76
- Loss of consciousness
- Hb <9g/dl
- Cr >180
- Signs of ischaemia on ECG.

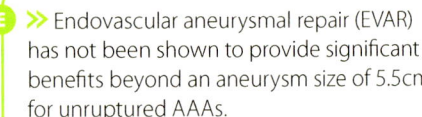 E >> Endovascular aneurysmal repair (EVAR) has not been shown to provide significant benefits beyond an aneurysm size of 5.5cm for unruptured AAAs.

12.6 Cardiac arrest

Initial assessment
1. Unconscious, unresponsive patient
2. Usually accompanied by respiratory arrest – apnoea or gasping
3. Pulseless

> **E** >> Initiate effective CPR without any delay. Put out an arrest call as per local protocol. Get as much help as you can.

Airway
1. Promptly check for a patent airway to ensure good delivery of oxygen

Breathing
1. Assess for breathing and check the pulse simultaneously; if no pulse or breathing is detected, start CPR immediately
2. The Resuscitation Council (UK) has recommended the following guidelines (see *Appendix 4*):
    - Compressions:
        o Compressions at the lower sternum to at least a depth of 5cm, at a rate of ≥100 compressions per minute
        o Allow sufficient recoil of the chest after each compression to promote filling of the heart and minimise interruptions in compressions
    - Ventilation:
        o Mouth-to-mouth or bag-mask ventilation is secondary in importance to compressions, as the primary aim is to ensure adequate circulation and oxygenation of tissues; hypoxia occurs later
        o Guidelines recommend performing ventilation only in the presence of other personnel, as disruption (however minimal)

to chest compressions in solo CPR markedly reduces the chances of survival
    o Two breaths are given after 30 chest compressions, aiming for 8–10 breaths per minute

Circulation
1. Assess cardiac rhythm and determine whether it is a shockable rhythm
    - Shockable – SVT, VT and VF
    - Non-shockable – asystole, pulseless electrical activity (PEA)

> **W** >> Asystole is deemed a non-shockable rhythm, as there is complete failure of the cardiac conduction system due to a major underlying cause (e.g. MI, hypoxia) disrupting its cellular environment. This prevents propagation of the conduction wave, despite any initial action potential generated by a shock.

2. Obtain intravenous access and administer IV adrenaline as appropriate:
    - 0.1mg/ml IV adrenaline should be given after the second shock and every 3–5 minutes subsequently

> **E** >> There are some reversible causes of a cardiac arrest, which are worth bearing in mind during any emergency. These can be remembered as 4 Hs and 4 Ts:
> - **4 Hs** – **H**ypokalaemia, **H**ypothermia, **H**ypoglycaemia, **H**ypoxia
> - **4 Ts** – **T**amponade (cardiac), **T**oxins, **T**ension pneumothorax, **T**hromboembolism

12.7 Bradycardia

Initial assessment

1. Obtain a quick history – **AMPLE** (**A**llergies, **M**edication, **P**MH, **L**ast ate/drank, **E**vents leading up to admission)
2. Cardiac history – previous known arrhythmias or drugs
3. Assess whether patient is symptomatic (i.e. dizziness, syncope)

Airway

1. Ensure patient is maintaining own airway

Breathing

1. Obtain SpO_2
2. Give supplementary oxygen to maintain SpO_2 >95%

Circulation

1. Measure heart rate and BP

 Differentiate bradycardia as follows:
- Asymptomatic >40bpm – treat conservatively
- Symptomatic <50bpm – provide urgent treatment

2. Obtain intravenous access
   - Give appropriate IV fluids to maintain haemodynamic stability
   - Send off baseline bloods, including U&Es, troponin
3. Arrange an urgent 12-lead ECG to assess underlying rhythm abnormalities
4. Prescribe appropriate medication

 Manage as follows:
- First line: consider IV atropine 0.5mg (max of 3g)
- Second line: isoprenaline infusion
- Urgent pacing (usually trans-venous) should be considered if patient is refractory to medical therapy

Disability & exposure

1. Ensure patient is transferred to a monitored bed
2. Arrange follow-up 24-hour Holter monitoring if no underlying cause/arrhythmias are found in the acute setting
3. Treat underlying cause
4. Consider permanent pacemaker insertion if indicated

P ⟫ Occasionally, bradycardia may be caused by beta blocker or calcium channel blocker overdose and is an important differential if no underlying cause is found or if the patient is unresponsive to medical therapy. The treatment for beta blocker overdose is glucagon. It is used because it exerts its chronotropic and inotropic effects via adenyl cyclase which bypasses beta-adrenergic receptors and calcium channels.

12.8 Narrow complex tachycardia

Common causes:
- Atrial fibrillation, atrial flutter
- AVNRT, AVRT

Initial assessment
1. Obtain a quick history – **AMPLE** (**A**llergies, **M**edication, **P**MH, **L**ast ate/drank, **E**vents leading up to admission)
2. Cardiac history – previous known arrhythmias or drugs
3. Assess whether patient is symptomatic (i.e. palpitations, dizziness, syncope)

Airway
1. Ensure patient is maintaining own airway

Breathing
1. Obtain SpO$_2$
2. Give supplementary oxygen to maintain SpO$_2$ >95%

Circulation
1. Measure heart rate and BP
   - Haemodynamically compromised – **urgent sedation and synchronised DC cardioversion**
   - Haemodynamically stable – medical management
2. Obtain intravenous access
   - Give appropriate IV fluids to maintain haemodynamic stability
   - Send off baseline bloods including U&Es, troponin, TFTs

P ≫ Fast AF (AF with a fast ventricular rate >100bpm), in patients with previously known AF, is usually triggered by an underlying cause (most commonly infection or dehydration) and should be treated. Rate control can normally be achieved using a beta blocker in the acute setting. However, patients not previously diagnosed with AF who present with acute AF, should be managed as described.

3. Arrange an urgent 12-lead ECG to assess underlying rhythm abnormalities
4. Use vagal manoeuvres in the first instance

W ≫ Vagal manoeuvres (e.g. carotid sinus massage and Valsalva manoeuvre) are used in tachycardias because they increase parasympathetic drive (vagal tone), inducing a temporary AV block and revealing the underlying atrial dysrhythmia.

5. Give IV adenosine if vagal manoeuvres were unsuccessful (in the setting of SVT)
   - Give as 6mg IV bolus, followed by a further 12mg bolus if not responding, and a third and final 12mg bolus after that
6. Consider anti-arrhythmic prophylaxis:
   - Digoxin IV 500mcg over 30 minutes
   - Amiodarone IV 300mg over 1 hour
   - Verapamil 5–10mg IV

E ≫ Adenosine is contraindicated in patients with co-existing asthma as it causes acute bronchoconstriction. Verapamil is used instead.

Disability & exposure
1. Ensure patient is transferred to a monitored bed
2. Arrange follow-up 24-hour Holter monitoring
3. Treat underlying cause
4. Consider prevention medication – beta blockers or verapamil

12

12.9 Broad complex tachycardia

Initial assessment
1. Obtain a quick history – **AMPLE** (**A**llergies, **M**edication, **P**MH, **L**ast ate/drank, **E**vents leading up to admission)
2. Cardiac history – previous known arrhythmias or drugs

Airway
1. Ensure patient is maintaining own airway

Breathing
1. Obtain SpO_2
2. Give supplementary oxygen to maintain SpO_2 >95%

Circulation
1. Measure heart rate and BP
   - Collapse and pulseless → **CPR!**
   - Haemodynamically compromised – **urgent sedation and synchronised DC cardioversion**
   - Haemodynamically stable – medical management

2. Obtain intravenous access
   - Give aggressive IV fluids to maintain haemodynamic stability
   - Send off bloods – U&Es (including K, Mg, Ca, PO_4) and troponin
   - Correct electrolyte disturbances as appropriate
3. Arrange an urgent 12-lead ECG to assess underlying rhythm abnormalities (note QTc interval) and consider:
   - Regular VT – amiodarone IV 300mg over 1 hour, followed by 900mg over 24 hours
   - Torsades de pointes – IV $MgSO_4$ 2g over 15–30 mins
4. Offer urgent synchronised cardioversion if unresponsive to medical therapy

Disability & exposure
1. Ensure patient is transferred to a monitored bed
2. Treat underlying cause
3. Seek Cardiology input
4. Consider ICD insertion if indicated

12.10 Acute asthma

Assessment of severe asthma (BTS 2014)

Moderate asthma:
- Increasing symptoms, PEFR >50–85% best or predicted
- No features of acute severe asthma

Acute severe asthma:
Any one of:
- PEFR 33–50% best or predicted
- RR >25, HR >100bpm
- Inability to complete sentences in one breath

Life-threatening asthma:
Any one of:
- PEFR <33% best or predicted
- SpO_2 <92%, PaO_2 <8kPa
- Normal $PaCO_2$
- Cyanosis; hypotension, poor respiratory effort, altered conscious level, arrhythmia
- Silent chest

Initial assessment
1. Obtain a quick history – **AMPLE** (**A**llergies, **M**edication, **P**MH, **L**ast ate/drank, **E**vents leading up to admission)
2. Obtain a PEFR (note that this may not always be possible); attempt every 15–30 minutes

Airway
1. Ensure patient is maintaining own airway
2. Sit patient up
3. Obtain a set of observations

Breathing
1. Obtain SpO_2; aim to keep sats 94–98%
2. Give supplementary oxygen; lack of pulse oximetry should not prevent the use of oxygen (BTS 2014)
3. Offer nebulised salbutamol (5mg) and repeat every 15–30 minutes
4. Add nebulised ipratropium bromide (0.5mg 4- to 6-hourly) to beta₂ agonist treatment for adults with acute severe or life-threatening asthma, or those with a poor initial response to beta₂ agonist therapy (BTS 2014)

Circulation
1. Obtain intravenous access
2. Monitor ECG
3. Obtain ABG

> **E** ≫ A normal or elevated $PaCO_2$ is a poor prognostic sign, indicating impending respiratory failure.

4. Steroids reduce mortality and should be given as early as possible in an acute attack – they may be given intravenously (hydrocortisone 200mg) or orally (prednisolone 40mg) if the patient is able to swallow

Disability & exposure
1. Consider giving a single dose of IV magnesium sulphate (1–2g, after discussion with specialist) in patients with poor response to therapy

> **E** ≫ Patients should be given oral prednisolone 40mg up to 5 days after the initial attack. This is especially important practically if the steroids were prescribed intravenously. Remember also to prescribe a short course of oral prednisolone.

> **P** ≫ Referral criteria for ITU:
> Refer any patient requiring ventilator support or with acute/life-threatening asthma in which there is altered mental status, acidaemia on ABG, hypercapnia or a deteriorating PEFR.

12

12.11 Acute exacerbation of COPD

Initial assessment

1. Obtain a quick history – **AMPLE** (**A**llergies, **M**edication, **P**MH, **L**ast ate/drank, **E**vents leading up to admission)
2. An exacerbation is defined as a sustained worsening of the patient's usual symptoms from their usual stable state, beyond normal day-to-day variations, and is acute in onset (NICE 2010)
3. *H. influenzae* and *S. pneumoniae* infections are commonly associated with acute exacerbations of COPD

Airway

1. Ensure patient is maintaining own airway
2. Sit patient up
3. Obtain a set of observations

Breathing

1. Obtain SpO_2; aim to keep sats 88–92%
2. Give supplementary oxygen, at 24%, via a Venturi mask
3. Obtain urgent ABG to allow assessment for escalation
4. Perform a CXR
5. Offer nebulised salbutamol (5mg) and repeat every 15–30 minutes
6. Add nebulised ipratropium bromide (0.5mg 4- to 6-hourly)

Circulation

1. Obtain intravenous access
2. Monitor ECG
3. Steroids should be given as early as possible in an acute attack; they may be given intravenously (hydrocortisone 200mg) or orally (prednisolone 40mg) if the patient is able to swallow – follow up with 40mg of prednisolone **for 7–14 days thereafter**
4. Antibiotic therapy should be offered (local guidelines may vary) to treat exacerbations of COPD

Disability & exposure

1. Physiotherapy should be offered to help with sputum clearance
2. Daily monitoring of FEV_1 should **not** be used, as variability in the measurement may be small post-exacerbation
3. Spirometry, however, should be monitored in all patients before discharge
4. Patients who have had an episode of respiratory failure should have satisfactory oximetry or ABG before discharge

---

P ≫ Non-invasive ventilation (NIV) should be considered, particularly if the pH is between 7.25 and 7.35. Invasive ventilation should be offered if pH falls below 7.25 or if response to NIV is poor.

Settings:
- Expiratory positive airway pressure (EPAP) = $5cm^2 H_2O$
- Inspiratory positive airway pressure (IPAP) = $15cm^2 H_2O$
- Back-up rate: 15 breaths per minute

E ≫ Hypoxaemic (Type I) respiratory failure is characterised by an arterial oxygen tension (PaO_2) of <8kPa (60mmHg) with normal or low arterial carbon dioxide tension ($PaCO_2$). Hypercapnic (Type II) respiratory failure is the presence of a $PaCO_2$ >6kPa (45mmHg) and PaO_2 <8kPa.

12.12 Pulmonary embolism

Initial assessment

1. Obtain a quick history – **AMPLE** (**A**llergies, **M**edication, **P**MH, **L**ast ate/drank, **E**vents leading up to admission)
2. Consider risk factors (e.g. pregnancy, immobility, post-surgery day 6–12; see *Chapter 2* for complete list)
3. Use Wells score to help assess probability of VTE

Airway

1. Ensure patient is maintaining own airway
2. Sit patient up
3. Obtain a set of observations

Breathing

1. Obtain SpO$_2$; aim to keep sats >95%
2. Give supplementary oxygen, 15L/min via a NRBM if there is no underlying respiratory disease
3. Perform a CXR
4. Urgent ABG – respiratory alkalosis, hypoxaemia

Circulation

1. Measure HR and BP

> **E** ≫ Thrombolysis should be considered if there is evidence of severe haemodynamic instability. Seek respiratory input and consider:
> • Alteplase 50mg IV bolus

2. Obtain intravenous access and bloods
   - Send off baseline bloods including a D-dimer and clotting
3. Monitor ECG – sinus tachycardia is the most common finding; there may occasionally be evidence of right heart strain (TWI and RBBB)
4. Offer appropriate analgesia – morphine IV 1–10mg titrated to pain and metoclopramide 10mg IV
5. Do not delay starting LMWH if there is high suspicion for a PE
   - Enoxaparin SC 1.5mg/kg/24 hours

Disability & exposure

1. TED stockings whilst in hospital
2. Perform CTPA to confirm diagnosis and consider Doppler US to look for peripheral DVTs
3. Commence concurrent warfarin, monitor INR and discontinue LMWH when INR therapeutic. Duration of long-term anticoagulation depends on whether there is an underlying cause for the PE:
   - Provoked – 3 months
   - Unprovoked – 6 months
   - Recurrent – lifelong

12

12.13 Anaphylaxis

Anaphylaxis is an acute and potentially life-threatening hypersensitivity reaction. It is often triggered by a substance (e.g. food, drugs), initially causing IgE-mediated mast cell release of histamine and other cytokines (Type 1 hypersensitivity). This is usually followed by eosinophilic accumulation, further exacerbating and sustaining the inflammatory response.

Clinical features:
- Sudden onset generalised urticaria, oedema, itching and sweating
- Wheeze (secondary to bronchospasm) and SOB (laryngeal oedema; potentially fatal if untreated)
- Palpitations, tachycardia and hypotension

Initial assessment
1. Obtain a quick history – **AMPLE** (**A**llergies, **M**edication, **P**MH, **L**ast ate/drank, **E**vents leading up to admission)

Airway
1. Secure a stable airway
2. Lay patient flat and elevate legs to improve airway
3. Look for airway obstruction and remove potential obstruction
4. Consider adjuncts (LMA or NP tube) to secure airway
5. **Contact Anaesthetics** for intubation in severe obstructive disease

Breathing
1. Obtain SpO$_2$
2. Give supplementary high-flow oxygen 15L/min via a NRBM
3. Offer nebulisers to alleviate wheeze: salbutamol 5mg nebs + ipratropium 0.5mg nebs

Circulation
1. Assess for signs of shock (hypotension, tachycardia)
2. Give **adrenaline 0.5mg IM** (0.5ml of 1:1000) without delay if anaphylaxis is suspected. This may be repeated after 5 minutes if required

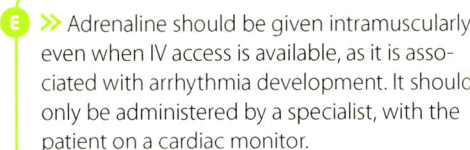
>> Adrenaline should be given intramuscularly, even when IV access is available, as it is associated with arrhythmia development. It should only be administered by a specialist, with the patient on a cardiac monitor.

3. Obtain intravenous access
4. Rapid fluid challenge (500ml of crystalloid solution STAT) to be administered
5. Patients may need more to maintain BP
6. Consider testing for serum mast-cell tryptase within 1–2 hours of symptom onset to support anaphylaxis diagnosis
7. Prescribe:
   - **Hydrocortisone IV 200mg**
   - **Chlorphenamine IV 10mg**
8. Arrange for a 12-lead ECG and assess

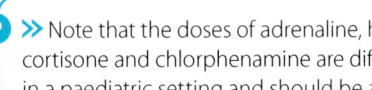
>> Note that the doses of adrenaline, hydrocortisone and chlorphenamine are different in a paediatric setting and should be age-adjusted.

Disability & exposure
1. Reassess A–E approach
2. Patients should be monitored for 6–12 hours post-event
3. Patient education and discharge with Epipen

12.14 Upper GI bleed

Initial assessment

1. Obtain a quick history – **AMPLE** (**A**llergies, **M**edication, **P**MH, **L**ast ate/drank, **E**vents leading up to admission)
2. Check for previous bleeds, liver status, known ulcers
3. Assess for signs of hypovolaemic shock – tachycardia, hypotension, low urine output (catheterise), cool peripheries
4. The two most common causes of UGI bleed are ulcer bleeds and variceal bleeds

Airway

1. Secure patient's airway
2. Place patient head down to minimise risk of aspiration
3. Suction may be required to clear blood/vomitus
4. Consider NP airway to facilitate suction

Breathing

1. Obtain SpO_2
2. Give supplementary high-flow O_2 15L/min

Circulation

1. Measure BP and heart pulse and monitor for signs of shock
2. Obtain IV access – ×2 wide-bore cannula (14G)
   - Aggressive fluid resuscitation 1L crystalloid solution STAT
3. Send off urgent bloods – FBCs (extent of anaemia and platelets), LFTs (pre-existing liver disease), U&Es (co-existing AKI, **urea rise**), clotting/ coagulation screen and ABG
4. **Cross-match blood at least 4 units RCC**
   - O –ve blood should be given if blood is needed before X-match available
   - NICE (CG141) recommends, for a patient who is actively bleeding:

   o With a platelet count $<50\times10^9$/L, offer platelet transfusion
   o With an APTT/PT >1.5 greater than normal, offer FFP
5. Other considerations if likely variceal bleed:
   - Prophylactic antibiotics (based on local protocols)
   - Terlipressin IV 1mg
6. Arrange for a 12-lead ECG and assess

> **E** ›› The use of IV PPI therapy pre-endoscopy is not recommended for patients with suspected non-variceal bleed. They can be offered this treatment after endoscopy.

Disability & exposure

1. Consider catheterisation for accurate fluid balance
2. Assess patients using Blatchford Bleeding score (pre-endoscopy) to assess urgency of UGIE
3. Urgent referral to Gastroenterology or Surgery for upper GI endoscopy

> **P** ›› The Glasgow Blatchford Bleeding score uses the following parameters:
> - Haemoglobin <12.9(m), <11.9(f)
> - Urea >6.5
> - Systolic blood pressure <109mmHg
> - Heart rate <100bpm
> - Presence of melaena
> - Presence of syncope
> - Hepatic disease
> - Cardiac failure.

12.15 Delirium tremens

Clinical features:

- Delirium tremens is an acute confusional and hyperadrenergic state often occurring 1–3 days after sudden alcohol withdrawal
- Varies slightly from acute alcohol withdrawal symptoms
- Presents with altered mental state, most commonly:
  - Hallucinations (auditory, visual)
  - Agitation
  - Confusion or delusions
- Often tremulous, tachycardic with nausea and vomiting
- Seizures (alcohol-related) may also occur

Airway

1. Ensure patient is maintaining own airway
2. Sit patient upright to reduce aspiration risk
3. Use suction to clear patent airway

Breathing

1. Measure SpO_2 and give supplementary O_2 to maintain sats >95%

Circulation

1. Measure BP and heart rate
2. Obtain intravenous access
   - IV fluids should be given to maintain a positive fluid balance, especially in drowsy patients
   - Give 2 pairs of IV Pabrinex I+II to prevent progression to Wernicke encephalopathy

- Sedation with benzodiazepines may be required; NICE (2010) recommends:
  - Oral lorazepam 2–4mg is the recommended first-line agent; multiple doses may be necessary
  - IV lorazepam, IM haloperidol 2mg or IM olanzapine 5–10mg may be used alternatively

> **E** » Care should be taken when giving multiple doses of sedation. Respiratory depression should be monitored and may require ventilation in ICU.

3. Send off bloods to assess for potential electrolyte disturbances (K, Mg, PO_4), glucose, LFTs and ABG (may show alcoholic ketoacidosis)
4. Arrange a 12-lead ECG – may show arrhythmias secondary to electrolyte disturbances

Disability & exposure

1. Measure blood glucose and correct any hypoglycaemia appropriately
2. Monitor for seizure activity
3. Continue IV Pabrinex TDS for up to 5 days
4. Monitor for withdrawal symptoms and treat as per CIWA
5. Consider ICU referral in very unwell patients, who could potentially require mechanical ventilation

12.16 Diabetic ketoacidosis (DKA)

Diagnostic criteria:
- Hyperglycaemia: plasma glucose >11.1mmol/L
- Ketosis: ketones ++ on urine dipstick
- Acidosis: pH <7.3 or HCO_3^- <18mmol/L

The principles of management of DKA (see *Chapter 4*) involve glycaemic control and correcting electrolyte as well as acid–base balance.

Airway
1. Ensure patient is maintaining own airway
2. Sit patient up
3. Obtain a set of observations

Breathing
1. Obtain SpO_2 and correct hypoxia with supplementary O_2
2. Watch for Kussmaul breathing, which may be present to compensate for metabolic acidosis

Circulation
1. Measure and monitor BP and heart rate; place patient on continuous monitoring
2. Obtain **at least two** IV access points (one for rehydration therapy and the other for insulin infusion)
   - Commence fluid therapy without delay, initially with 0.9% saline over 1 hour
   - An insulin infusion should be prepared at this stage (50 units of Actrapid in 50ml of 0.9% saline), infused at 6 units/hr; start infusion if serum K^+ levels >3.3mmol/L
   - Perform a bedside blood glucose and ketone test
3. Send off urgent bloods – FBC, U&Es including serum HCO_3 (establish baseline renal function and electrolyte status), ABG/VBG (assess extent of acidosis)

4. Arrange a 12-lead ECG – arrhythmias may be present due to hypokalaemia and severe acidosis

Disability & exposure
1. Measure temperature and initiate sepsis screen if patient is pyrexic

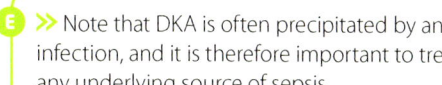
>> Note that DKA is often precipitated by an infection, and it is therefore important to treat any underlying source of sepsis.

2. Assess and monitor consciousness levels
3. Consider inserting a urinary catheter to monitor urine output
4. Give appropriate analgesia and anti-emetics if there is ongoing abdominal pain or vomiting
5. Perform hourly blood glucose, VBG and K^+ monitoring in the initial stages
6. Urgent referral to the Endocrinology/Diabetes registrar
7. Consider early HDU referral if there is:
   - Haemodynamic instability
   - Severe acidosis
   - Altered mental/conscious state
   - Severe respiratory distress
   - For ongoing management and resolution criteria of DKA, see *Chapter 4*

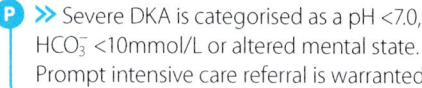
>> Severe DKA is categorised as a pH <7.0, HCO_3^- <10mmol/L or altered mental state. Prompt intensive care referral is warranted.

12

12.17 Hyperosmolar hyperglycaemic state (HHS)

Diagnostic criteria:
- Hyperglycaemia: plasma glucose >35mmol/L
- Hyperosmolality >320mmol/kg
- Hypovolaemia in the absence of acidosis or ketosis

The principles of managing HHS (much like DKA) involve rehydration, and correction of hyperglycaemia and electrolyte imbalance.

Airway
1. Ensure patient is maintaining own airway
2. Sit patient up
3. Obtain a set of observations

Breathing
1. Obtain SpO_2 and correct hypoxia with supplementary O_2
2. Early ICU admission may be warranted if there is severe respiratory distress or haemodynamic instability

Circulation
1. Measure and monitor BP and heart rate, and place patient on continuous monitoring
2. Send off a set of urgent bloods – FBC, U&Es, serum glucose, bicarbonate and an ABG ± blood cultures
3. Serum osmolality should be calculated using: [Serum osmolality = 2 (Na + K) + urea + glucose]
4. Perform bedside BM and ketones testing
5. Obtain **at least two** IV access points (one for rehydration therapy and the other for insulin infusion)

   – Commence fluid therapy without delay, initially with 1L of 0.9% saline over 1 hour
   – An insulin infusion should be prepared at this stage (50 units of Actrapid in 50ml of 0.9% saline), infused at 3 units per hour

> P >> An insulin infusion/replacement may not be necessary in some cases of HHS. Infusions should be commenced at a lower rate (compared to DKA), to prevent a sudden change in plasma osmolality.

   – Start infusion if serum K^+ levels >3.3mmol/L
6. Arrange a 12-lead ECG

Disability & exposure
1. Measure temperature and initiate sepsis screen if pyrexia is present
2. Consider inserting a urinary catheter to monitor urine output
3. Look for a precipitating cause – e.g. infection, MI, VTE, etc.
4. Arrange urgent referral to Endocrinology/Diabetes registrar
5. CVP monitoring and vasopressors may be considered in an ICU setting if haemodynamically unstable
6. For ongoing management and resolution criteria of HHS, see *Chapter 4*

12.18 Hypoglycaemia

Initial assessment

1. Obtain a quick history – **AMPLE** (**A**llergies, **M**edication, **P**MH, **L**ast ate/drank, **E**vents leading up to admission)
2. Ask about usual insulin/anti-glycaemic regimes
3. The two most common causes of hypoglycaemia are excess insulin and reduced sugar intake

E ≫ Diagnosis of hypoglycaemia is based on the Whipple triad:
  i.   Low BM
  ii. Hypoglycaemic symptoms
  iii. Resolution of symptoms post hypogly-caemia treatment

Airway

1. Secure patient's airway
2. Consider airway adjuncts (LMA, NP) if patient is unconscious and unable to maintain own airway
3. Obtain a set of observations

Breathing

1. Obtain SpO$_2$ and give supplementary high-flow O$_2$ 15L/min

Circulation

1. Measure capillary glucose (<3.0mmol/L)
2. Obtain intravenous access
   - Give 125ml of IV 20% dextrose or 250ml of IV 10% dextrose if patient is unconscious or unable to swallow
   - Alternatively, IM glucagon 1mg may be used
3. Monitor BP and heart rate

P ≫ Avoid using 50% dextrose, as it is highly viscous and irritant to the venous system, often causing thrombophlebitis. Its use has significantly decreased in recent years.

W ≫ Glucagon should not be used in patients with underlying chronic liver disease, as they have impaired hepatic gluconeogenesis. Glucagon may also provoke a rebound hypoglycaemia due to secondary insulin release.

Disability & exposure

- Offer oral 10–20g glucose (e.g. Glucotabs, or Glucogel) to stable and conscious patients who are able to swallow
- Check pupillary reflexes – may be affected in comatose patient secondary to cerebral oedema
- Repeat BM testing every 15–30 minutes to assess for response
- Consider ICU referral in patients with prolonged hypoglycaemic coma, requiring ventilatory or haemodynamic support
- Patient education is one of the most important interventions to prevent recurrence

12.19 Thyroid storm

Thyroid storm, or hyperthyroid crisis, is a potentially life-threatening condition caused by the overproduction of thyroxine. This is often precipitated by inter-current illness (e.g. infection, trauma or surgery) in a patient with underlying thyrotoxicosis.

Clinical features:
- Sudden onset, high fever (usually >40°C)
- Tachycardia and arrhythmias, occasionally resulting in hypotension and heart failure, may also be present
- Nausea, vomiting and acute abdominal pain
- Acute confusion and agitation

Initial assessment
1. Obtain a quick history – **AMPLE** (**A**llergies, **M**edication, **P**MH, **L**ast ate/drank, **E**vents leading up to admission), recent infection, surgery or trauma
2. Quickly assess thyroid status (medications, symptoms, previous episodes of thyroid storm)

Airway
1. Ensure patient is maintaining own airway
2. Use suction to prevent aspiration secondary to vomiting
3. NG tube may be used to reduce vomiting

Breathing
1. Obtain SpO$_2$ and maintain >95% with supplementary O$_2$
2. Perform ABG

Circulation
1. Measure BP and heart rate
2. Obtain intravenous access
   - Aggressive fluid resuscitation with crystalloid solution (usually 0.9% saline to replace gastric losses)
   - Send off bloods, including TFTs, U&Es, FBC, CRP and blood cultures, to look for an infective source
3. Arrange 12-lead ECG – often revealing AF or SVTs
   - First line: IV propranolol 5mg
   - Second line: diltiazem or digoxin (if beta blockers are contraindicated, e.g. asthma)

Disability & exposure
1. Measure temperature – usually significantly pyrexial
   - Give paracetamol and cooling with tepid sponging
   - Ice baths may be used in extreme cases
2. Consider chlorpromazine for severe agitation
3. Treat underlying cause
4. Seek endocrinology input

 ≫ 5. Anti-thyroid therapy:
- Oral carbimazole 5mg or propylthiouracil
- Lugol solution given 4 hours post-carbimazole
- IV hydrocortisone 200mg is recommended

12.20 Myxoedema coma

E ≫ The term myxoedema coma is a misnomer, as most patients present with neither oedema nor coma. However, these symptoms may be present in later/advanced stages of the condition.

Clinical features:

- Myxoedema coma represents a rare endocrine malignancy, sitting at the extreme end of the hyperthyroid spectrum; it is sometimes used synonymously with severe hypothyroidism
- Similar to thyroid storm, the condition is often triggered by an underlying infection or systemic illness
- The most common precipitate is sudden onset hypothermia and hypoglycaemia
- Altered mental state – low mood, confusion and sometimes coma
- Hypotensive and bradycardic (secondary to compensatory vasoconstriction)
- Hypoventilation and hypoxia

Initial assessment

1. Obtain a quick history – **AMPLE** (**A**llergies, **M**edication, **P**MH, **L**ast ate/drank, **E**vents leading up to admission)
2. Quickly assess thyroid status (medications, symptoms, previous episodes of myxoedema coma)

Airway

1. Ensure patient is maintaining own airway
2. Secure airway with manoeuvres and adjuncts in particular patients with reduced consciousness levels

Breathing

1. Obtain SpO_2 and maintain sats >95% with supplementary O_2

2. Monitor respiratory rate and do not delay ICU referral for ventilator support
3. Perform ABG and consider CXR to look for pleural effusions

Circulation

1. Measure BP and heart rate
2. Obtain intravenous access
   - Aggressive fluid resuscitation with crystalloid solution
   - Send off bloods, including TFTs, U&Es, FBC, CRP, cortisol and blood cultures, to look for an infective source

P ≫ Cortisol levels are obtained to rule out a diagnosis of adrenal insufficiency secondary to hypopituitarism.

3. Arrange 12-lead ECG – often revealing bradycardia and heart blocks ± prolonged QTc

Disability & exposure

1. Measure temperature – usually significantly hypothermic
   - Warming blankets and bear-huggers may be used
2. Monitor BMs and treat any hypoglycaemia
3. Check pupillary reflexes – may be affected in comatose patients
4. Treat any underlying triggers
5. Seek Endocrinology input
6. IV hydrocortisone 100mg should be given to all patients until adrenal insufficiency can be excluded
7. Thyroid replacement therapy
   - IV T_4 with initial loading dose of 100–500mcg, followed by a maintenance dose of 75–100mcg orally daily

12

12.21 Acute cerebrovascular event

Initial assessment

1. Prompt assessment and recognition of FAST symptoms, prior to arrival at hospital, improves outcomes
2. A 'stroke call/pathway', as per hospital protocol, should be initiated as soon as possible – allowing for early neurology/neurosurgical registrar involvement and rapid access to imaging
3. Ascertain the exact onset of symptoms, as this will determine further management, i.e. thrombolysis/stent retrieval

Airway

1. Ensure patient is maintaining own airway
2. Secure airway with manoeuvres and adjuncts, particularly in patients with reduced consciousness levels

> **P** ≫ Intubation should only be attempted if a patient is non-responsive, as it may cause severe hypertension, provoking further bleeding.

Breathing

1. Obtain SpO_2 and maintain SpO_2 >95% with supplementary oxygen

Circulation

1. Measure BP and HR, and ensure patient is haemodynamically stable

> **E** ≫ Patients presenting with an acute cerebrovascular event are often hypertensive. BP should not be reduced, as this pressure is crucial to maintain cerebral perfusion.

2. Obtain intravenous access
   - Gentle fluid resuscitation – do not overhydrate patient
3. Bedside blood glucose testing should be performed
   - Correct any hypoglycaemia or hyperglycaemia
4. Send off a set of baseline bloods – FBC (extent of bleed if any), U&Es, Coags studies (which will guide decision to thrombolyse), glucose, lipid studies
5. Arrange 12-lead ECG and place patient on continuous cardiac monitoring

Further management:

1. An **urgent neuroimaging (CT ± CTA/MRI)** should be performed without delay to exclude any primary haemorrhage
2. Once a haemorrhage stroke has been excluded, administer high-dose aspirin 300mg
3. Patients with suspected dysphagia should be made NBM until speech and language therapist review; consider NGT insertion if there is a high risk of aspiration
4. Prompt stroke registrar/consultant referral for consideration of thrombolysis
5. Refer to neurosurgical team for surgical management of a haemorrhagic stroke

> **E** ≫ Thrombolysis is contraindicated in patients who are hypertensive (BP >185/110).

12.22 Meningitis

Initial assessment
- Obtain a quick history – **AMPLE** (**A**llergies, **M**edication, **P**MH, **L**ast ate/drank, **E**vents leading up to admission)
- Meningitis should be suspected in patients presenting with a fever, headache, neck stiffness and photophobia

> **E** >> Rapid recognition and prompt treatment are essential as bacterial meningitis is fatal within hours.

Airway
1. Ensure patient is maintaining own airway
2. Secure airway with manoeuvres and adjuncts, particularly in patients with reduced consciousness levels

Breathing
1. Obtain SpO$_2$ and maintain SpO$_2$ >95% with supplementary oxygen

Circulation
1. Measure BP and heart rate and place patient on continuous cardiac monitoring
2. Obtain intravenous access
   - Aggressive fluid resuscitation with crystalloid solution
   - Send off bloods, including FBC, U&Es, coagulation studies, serum glucose levels, lactate, CRP, ABG and blood cultures, to look for an infective source

> **E** >> Empirical IV antibiotics (as per hospital protocol) should be commenced without delay, even prior to further imaging or lumbar puncture.

3. Arrange early ICU referral if patient is in septic shock, for consideration of vasopressors and CVP monitoring
4. Arrange 12-lead ECG

Disability & exposure
1. Perform a thorough head-to-toe examination, looking for evidence of rashes or neurological signs
2. Monitor consciousness levels (GCS)
3. Isolate patient, as per local hospital infection control guidelines
4. Consider urinary catheter insertion and monitor urine output
5. Arrange an urgent CT brain, once initial resuscitation has been completed
6. Perform an LP unless contraindicated (see below); for CSF analysis, see *Chapter 5*
7. Consult appropriate infectious disease/microbiology registrar for further management advice

> **P** >> Contraindications to LP:
> - Signs of raised ICP – reduced consciousness levels, focal neurology, mass lesion/evidence of coning on imaging
> - ↑Bleeding risk – thrombocytopenia, deranged coagulation studies
> - Haemodynamically unstable.

12.23 Status epilepticus

Status epilepticus is defined as continuous seizure activity or sequential seizures occurring back to back, without any recovery, lasting for more than 30 minutes.

Initial assessment

1. Obtain a quick history – **AMPLE** (**A**llergies, **M**edication, **P**MH, **L**ast ate/drank, **E**vents leading up to admission)
2. Take protective measures – protect head, and move into recovery position if appropriate

Airway

1. Ensure patient is maintaining own airway
2. Assess and secure stable airway
3. Adjuncts (NP, LMA) may be required
4. Suction may be used to clear secretions to reduce aspiration risk
5. Contact Anaesthetics/ICU if intubation required

Breathing

1. Obtain SpO$_2$ and give high-flow O$_2$ as appropriate
2. Perform ABG

Circulation

1. Measure observations – BP and HR

2. Obtain IV access
   – Send off bloods – FBC, U&Es, LFTs, glucose, Ca, Mg, PO$_4$, anti-epileptic drug levels ± toxic screen
3. Arrange for cardiac monitoring; 12-lead ECG may be difficult to perform, due to seizure activity
4. Prescribe:
   – First line: IV diazepam 2mg up to 10mg boluses over 5 minutes, repeat after 15 minutes up to a total of 20mg
     ○ lorazepam 4mg IV may be used alternatively
   – Second line: phenytoin 15mg/kg IV infusion at 50mg/min

Disability & exposure

1. Check blood glucose and correct for any evidence of hypoglycaemia
2. Monitor pupillary reflexes and GCS levels
3. Contact Anaesthetics/ICU early, in particular for patients with refractory seizures who may require general anaesthetic
4. Send urine for toxicology screen
5. Consider IV thiamine (Pabrinex) if likely alcohol-related

12.24 Spinal cord compression

Clinical features:

- Spinal cord compression is a neurosurgical emergency; it also represents one of the oncological emergencies
- Major trauma involving the spine
- Underlying malignancy either primary or secondary mets
- Acute disc prolapse
- Infection

Initial assessment

1. Obtain a quick history – **AMPLE** (**A**llergies, **M**edication, **P**MH, **L**ast ate/drank, **E**vents leading up to admission), (previously known spinal problems, underlying malignancy), recent infection or trauma

> **E** ≫ 2. Look out for signs of cauda equina syndrome
> - Back pain (most commonly lower back) ± radicular pain
> - Sensorimotor disturbances – paraesthesia, weakness
> - Urinary retention or faecal incontinence, reduced anal tone, saddle paraesthesia (late signs)

Airway

1. Ensure patient is maintaining own airway
2. Secure airway ± C-spine in the case of spinal trauma; a modified jaw thrust may be used in patients with C-spine injury requiring neck immobilisation

3. Suction should be used to clear secretions and eliminate obstruction
4. Consider early intubation in patients with acute respiratory failure or reduced GCS (<9)
5. Contact Anaesthetics urgently

Breathing

1. Obtain SpO_2 and give supplementary O_2
2. Monitor for respiratory depression
3. Perform ABG if indicated

Circulation

1. Measure BP and HR and look for signs of shock
2. Obtain IV access
   - Urgently correct any haemodynamic instability with rapid fluid challenges of crystalloid solutions
   - Send off baseline bloods
3. Arrange 12-lead ECG and cardiac monitoring
4. Prescribe appropriate analgesia – IV morphine titrated to pain

Disability & exposure

1. Measure temperature and ensure appropriate warming
2. Monitor BMs, GCS and pupillary reflexes
3. Perform full neurological examination when patient is stable
4. Arrange for an urgent spinal MRI
5. Consider IV dexamethasone 16mg bolus within 8 hours of diagnosis
6. Urgent referral to Neurosurgery
7. Consider radiotherapy

12

12.25 Neutropenic sepsis/septic shock

Clinical features:

- Neutropenic sepsis is an oncological emergency, occasionally seen in patients receiving chemotherapy or with an underlying haematological malignancy
- NICE (2012) defines the diagnosis of neutropenic sepsis as: neutrophil count $<0.5 \times 10^9$/L with **either** temperature $>38.0°C$ **or** other clinical signs of sepsis

Initial assessment

1. Obtain a quick history – **AMPLE** (**A**llergies, **M**edications, **P**MH (underlying malignancy, last chemotherapy cycle), **L**ast ate/drank, **E**vents leading up to admission), recent infection
2. Look for clinical signs of sepsis and initiate **Sepsis Six** bundle

> **E** ≫ The Sepsis Six bundle should be initiated within 1 hour of diagnosis. It can be remembered as 'give 3, take 3':
> Give: Take:
> - Oxygen   • Blood cultures
> - IV fluids   • Lactate, FBC
> - Antibiotics   • Urine output

> **W** ≫ The Sepsis Six bundle was first introduced in 2006 as an educational tool by the UK Sepsis Trust. This has led to significant improvements in mortality, and has also reduced the need for HDU beds as well as the length of hospital admissions.

Airway

1. Ensure patient is maintaining own airway

Breathing

1. Obtain SpO_2 and give supplementary high-flow O_2 at 15L/min

2. Give nebuliser (0.9% saline or salbutamol 5mg) if indicated
3. Perform ABG (allows early assessment for escalation, may also provide a quick lactate level)
4. Consider a CXR if chest source is suspected

Circulation

1. Measure and monitor BP and HR
2. Look for signs of septic shock
3. Obtain IV access – ideally two large-bore cannulas
   - Rapid fluid challenges with IV crystalloid solution
   - Send off bloods – FBC, U&Es, LFT, CRP, lactate and blood cultures
4. Initiate empirical antibiotic therapy for neutropenic sepsis – **IV piperacillin-tazobactam (Tazocin) 4.5g** if not contraindicated
5. NICE advises against the use of an aminoglycoside agent and/or the removal of central venous catheters in the initial management of neutropenic sepsis
6. Arrange a 12-lead ECG and consider cardiac monitoring

Disability & exposure

1. Measure and monitor temperature, BMs and GCS
   - Use appropriate cooling measures (i.e. paracetamol, fan, ice packs may be required in severe pyrexia)
2. Insert urinary catheter and carefully monitor fluid balance
3. Patient should be isolated to a side room and barrier-nursed
4. Obtain further cultures (e.g. throat, sputum, urine, skin) to look for potential source/s of sepsis
5. Seek HDU/ICU input if patient is not clinically improving with initial measures

12.26 Acute renal colic

 ≫ Indications for hospital admission:
- Severe symptoms unresponsive to treatment
- Solitary kidney or chronic kidney disease
- Previous renal transplant
- Fever

E ≫ The possibility of a dissecting AAA needs to be excluded in patients over the age of 60 presenting with signs and symptoms of renal colic.

Initial assessment
1. Obtain a quick history – **AMPLE** (**A**llergies, **M**edications, **P**MH (underlying renal disease), **L**ast ate/drank, **E**vents leading up to admission), pregnancy

Airway
1. Ensure patient is maintaining own airway

Breathing
1. Obtain a set of observations
2. Maintain SpO_2 >95%

Circulation
1. Measure BP and HR
2. Look for signs of shock
3. Obtain IV access
   - Send off baseline bloods – FBC, U&Es, Ca, urate, CRP
   - Encourage hydration orally but supplement with IV fluids if not able to tolerate oral intake
4. Prescribe analgesia:
   - NSAIDs – diclofenac 50mg oral or 100mg PR or 75mg IM
   - Opioids – morphine IV titrated to pain
5. Arrange a 12-lead ECG and assess

Disability & exposure
1. Measure temperature – take blood and urine cultures if pyrexial
2. Perform urinalysis and urine pregnancy testing – may show haematuria in acute renal colic
3. Arrange for an urgent non-contrast CT KUB
4. Consider antibiotics if high clinical suspicion for underlying pyelonephritis
5. Consider follow-up lithotripsy or seek Urology input in the event of abnormal CT findings

12.27 Hyperkalaemia

Definition (according to European Resuscitation Guidelines):

- Mild: 5.5–5.9mmol/L
- Moderate: 6.0–6.4mmol/L
- Severe: >6.5mmol/L

> **E** >> Common causes include:
> - Renal impairment: AKI, CKD, acidosis
> - Drugs – ACEi, spironolactone, NSAIDs
> - Excessive exogenous potassium replacement.

Initial assessment

1. Obtain a quick history – **AMPLE** (**A**llergies, **M**edications, **P**MH (presence of renal disease), **L**ast ate/drank, **E**vents leading up to admission)
2. Look for symptoms of tachycardia – chest pain, palpitations, muscle weakness

Airway

1. Ensure patient is maintaining own airway

Breathing

1. Obtain SpO$_2$ and give supplementary O$_2$ to maintain sats >95%
2. Perform ABG (allows early quantification of K$^+$ levels and the presence of acidosis may point to an underlying cause)

Circulation

1. Measure BP and HR – likely tachycardic
2. Obtain intravenous access
   - Send off bloods – formal U&Es, Mg^{2+}

3. Arrange a 12-lead ECG and cardiac monitoring (if possible)
   - Look out for typical ECG changes associated with hyperkalaemia (see *Chapter 8*)
   - Urgently prescribe **10ml of 10% calcium gluconate IV**, if there are ECG changes

> **W** >> Calcium gluconate will usually improve ECG changes within 1–3 minutes. Note that rapid administration may result in arrhythmias. Therefore, patients should be on a cardiac monitor/ECG when it is given. Calcium gluconate functions only as cardiac protection and does not treat the actual hyperkalaemia.

Disability & exposure

1. Measure BM and temperature
2. Review drug chart and stop all relevant offending medications
3. Prescribe:
   - 5–10 units of a short-acting insulin (usually Actrapid or Novorapid) in 50ml of 50% dextrose to shift K into cells; alternatively, 125ml of 20% dextrose can be used
   - Salbutamol 5mg nebs. Caution: this may produce a rebound hyperkalaemia 2–3 hours after administration
   - Calcium resonium 15g TDS for 4–5 days
4. Contact Renal Team/HDU in cases of refractory hyperkalaemia for consideration of sodium bicarbonate infusion or haemofiltration
5. Reassess and repeat U&Es after treatment

12.28 Burns

Classification of burns:

Superficial	Erythema and painful
Partial thickness	*Superficial* – dermis intact, presence of painful blisters *Deep* – some loss of dermis, very painful, no blisters
Full thickness	Complete loss of dermis Charred, waxy, greyish skin Often non-painful

E >> Use **Wallace rule** of 9s to calculate percentage of body surface area burnt:
- Head and neck – 9%
- Arms – 9% each
- Torso – 18% front, 18% back
- Legs – 18% each
- Groin, palm – 1%

Airway
1. Ensure patient is maintaining own airway
2. Perform a careful examination of the oral and nasal cavities, looking for any evidence of soot deposition, burnt nasal hairs or stridor, suggestive of respiratory burns
3. Consider airway adjuncts or manoeuvres
4. Intubation and ventilation may be required in severe cases

Breathing
1. Obtain SpO_2 and give high-flow (100%) oxygen
2. Perform an ABG, to look for carboxyhaemoglobin (COHb) levels if there is any evidence of carbon monoxide exposure

Circulation
1. Measure BP and HR and place on continuous cardiac monitoring
2. Obtain intravenous access – two wide-bore cannulas (14G)
   - Aggressive fluid resuscitation – crystalloid solution, ideally 2L during initial resuscitation
3. Send off a set of bloods – FBC, U&Es, Coags, G&S/X-match

P >> The use of colloid solutions remains controversial, with little evidence to support its use during initial burn management.

E >> Use **Parkland Formula** to guide fluid replacement:
- Patient's weight × %BSA × 4 = ml of crystalloid solution required in the first 24 hours.

Disability & exposure
1. Perform a thorough head-to-toe examination to assess %BSA burnt, using **Wallace rule**
2. Give appropriate analgesia as per hospital pain protocol
3. Consider urinary catheter insertion to monitor urine output – guide response to fluid replacement therapy
4. Administer tetanus immunisation
5. Consider commencing IV antibiotic therapy if wound appears infected
6. Urgent Plastics Registrar referral for dressings advice and consideration of surgical debridement
7. Admission to specialist burns unit if available

12

Appendix 1
The management of atrial fibrillation

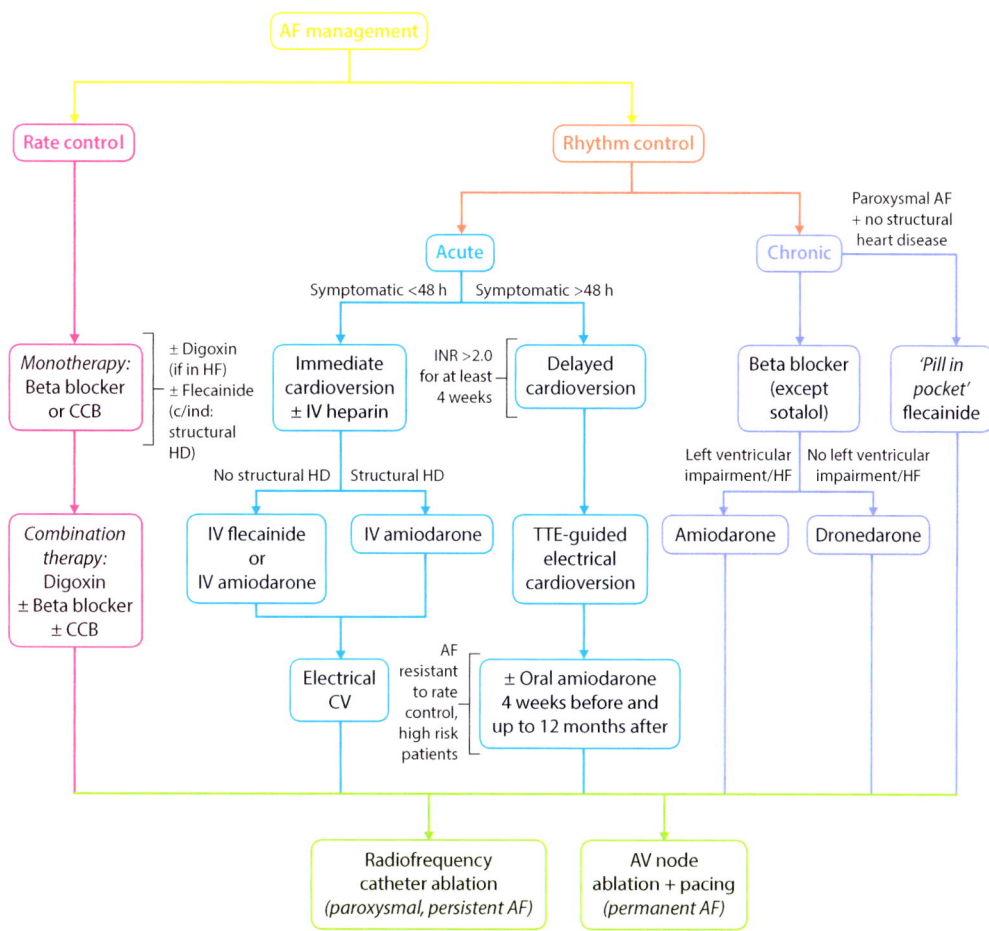

Based on NICE 2014, CG180.

Appendix 2

Clinical Institute Withdrawal Assessment for Alcohol, revised version (CIWA-Ar)

Patient:_____ **Date:**_____ **Time:**_____ (24 hour clock, midnight = 00:00)

Pulse or heart rate, taken for one minute:_____ **Blood pressure:**_____

NAUSEA AND VOMITING – Ask "Do you feel sick to your stomach? Have you vomited?" Observation.

0 no nausea and no vomiting

1 mild nausea with no vomiting

2

3

4 intermittent nausea with dry heaves

5

6

7 constant nausea, frequent dry heaves and vomiting

TACTILE DISTURBANCES – Ask "Have you any itching, pins and needles sensations, any burning, any numbness, or do you feel bugs crawling on or under your skin?" Observation.

0 none

1 very mild itching, pins and needles, burning or numbness

2 mild itching, pins and needles, burning or numbness

3 moderate itching, pins and needles, burning or numbness

4 moderately severe hallucinations

5 severe hallucinations

6 extremely severe hallucinations

7 continuous hallucinations

TREMOR – Arms extended and fingers spread apart. Observation.

0 no tremor

1 not visible, but can be felt fingertip to fingertip

2

3

4 moderate, with patient's arms extended

5

6

7 severe, even with arms not extended

AUDITORY DISTURBANCES – Ask "Are you more aware of sounds around you? Are they harsh? Do they frighten you? Are you hearing anything that is disturbing to you? Are you hearing things you know are not there?" Observation.

0 not present

1 very mild harshness or ability to frighten

2 mild harshness or ability to frighten

3 moderate harshness or ability to frighten

4 moderately severe hallucinations

5 severe hallucinations

6 extremely severe hallucinations

7 continuous hallucinations

PAROXYSMAL SWEATS – Observation.

0 no sweat visible

1 barely perceptible sweating, palms moist

2

3

4 beads of sweat obvious on forehead

5

6

7 drenching sweats

VISUAL DISTURBANCES – Ask "Does the light appear to be too bright? Is its color different? Does it hurt your eyes? Are you seeing anything that is disturbing to you? Are you seeing things you know are not there?" Observation.

0 not present

1 very mild sensitivity

2 mild sensitivity

3 moderate sensitivity

4 moderately severe hallucinations

5 severe hallucinations

6 extremely severe hallucinations

7 continuous hallucinations

ANXIETY – Ask "Do you feel nervous?" Observation.

0 no anxiety, at ease

1 mildly anxious

2

3

4 moderately anxious, or guarded, so anxiety is inferred

5

6

7 equivalent to acute panic states as seen in severe delirium or acute schizophrenic reactions

HEADACHE, FULLNESS IN HEAD – Ask "Does your head feel different? Does it feel like there is a band around your head?" Do not rate for dizziness or lightheadedness. Otherwise, rate severity.

0 not present

1 very mild

2 mild

3 moderate

4 moderately severe

5 severe

6 very severe

7 extremely severe

AGITATION – Observation.

0 normal activity

1 somewhat more than normal activity

2

3

4 moderately fidgety and restless

5

6

7 paces back and forth during most of the interview, or constantly thrashes about

ORIENTATION AND CLOUDING OF SENSORIUM – Ask "What day is this? Where are you? Who am I?"

0 oriented and can do serial additions

1 cannot do serial additions or is uncertain about date

2 disoriented for date by no more than 2 calendar days

3 disoriented for date by more than 2 calendar days

4 disoriented for place/or person

Total **CIWA-Ar** Score _____

Rater's Initials _____

Maximum Possible Score 67

The **CIWA-Ar** is *not* copyrighted and may be reproduced freely. This assessment for monitoring withdrawal symptoms requires approximately 5 minutes to administer. The maximum score is 67 (see instrument). Patients scoring less than 10 do not usually need additional medication for withdrawal.

Sullivan, J.T.; Sykora, K.; Schneiderman, J.; Naranjo, C.A.; and Sellers, E.M. Assessment of alcohol withdrawal: The revised Clinical Institute Withdrawal Assessment for Alcohol scale (**CIWA-Ar**). *British Journal of Addiction* 84:1353–1357, 1989.

Appendix 3
Warfarin reversal management

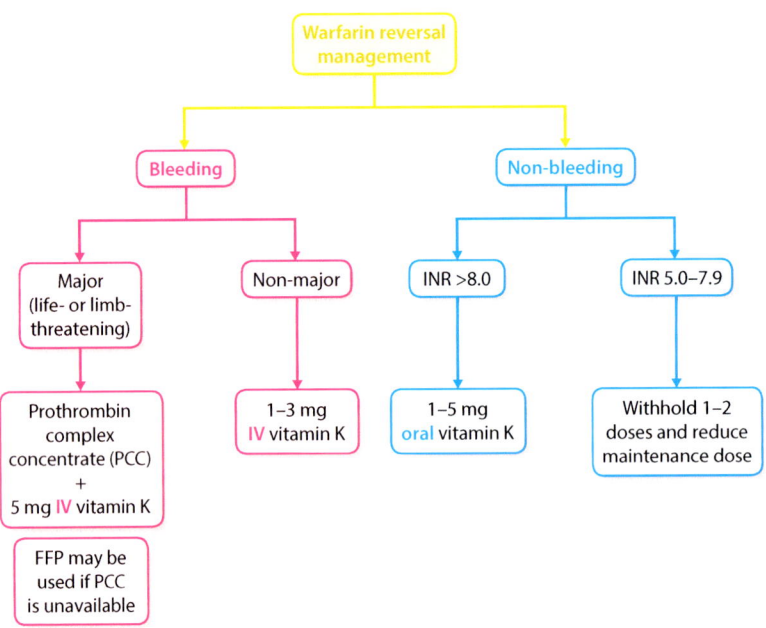

(*Adapted from Keeling* et al. *(2011) Guidelines on oral anticoagulation with warfarin – fourth edition.* British Journal of Haematology.)

Appendix 4
Adult Advanced Life Support (ALS) algorithm

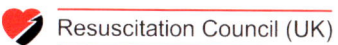 Resuscitation Council (UK) Adult Advanced Life Support

Unresponsive and not breathing normally

Call resuscitation team

CPR 30:2
Attach defibrillator/monitor
Minimise interruptions

Assess rhythm

Shockable (VF/Pulseless VT)

Return of spontaneous circulation

Non-shockable (PEA/Asystole)

1 Shock
Minimise interruptions

Immediate post cardiac arrest treatment
- Use ABCDE approach
- Aim for SpO₂ of 94-98%
- Aim for normal PaCO₂
- 12-lead ECG
- Treat precipitating cause
- Targeted temperature management

Immediately resume CPR for 2 min
Minimise interruptions

Immediately resume CPR for 2 min
Minimise interruptions

During CPR
- Ensure high quality chest compressions
- Minimise interruptions to compressions
- Give oxygen
- Use waveform capnography
- Continuous compressions when advanced airway in place
- Vascular access (intravenous or intraosseous)
- Give adrenaline every 3-5 min
- Give amiodarone after 3 shocks

Treat Reversible Causes
- Hypoxia
- Hypovolaemia
- Hypo-/hyperkalaemia/metabolic
- Hypothermia
- Thrombosis - coronary or pulmonary
- Tension pneumothorax
- Tamponade – cardiac
- Toxins

Consider
- Ultrasound imaging
- Mechanical chest compressions to facilitate transfer/treatment
- Coronary angiography and percutaneous coronary intervention
- Extracorporeal CPR

Reproduced with the kind permission of the Resuscitation Council (UK).

Appendix 5
Image sources

Diagrams not shown in this list were created by the authors.

Chapter 1

Fig. 1.1 *(adapted)*
Licensed under: Creative Commons Attribution 3.0 Unported
Additional attribution: Openstax College
Available at: http://cnx.org/content/col11496/1.6/

Fig. 1.2 *(adapted)*
Licensed under: Creative Commons Attribution 3.0 Unported
Additional attribution: Openstax College
Available at: http://cnx.org/content/col11496/1.6/

Fig. 1.3 *(adapted)*
Licensed under: Creative Commons Attribution-Share Alike 2.5 Generic license
Additional attribution: Wikimedia Commons
Available at: https://commons.wikimedia.org/wiki/File:Wiggers_Diagram.svg

Fig. 1.4 *(adapted)*
Licensed under: Creative Commons Attribution 3.0 Unported
Additional attribution: Openstax College
Available at: http://cnx.org/content/col11496/1.6/

Fig. 1.13
Licensed under: Creative Commons Attribution-Share Alike 3.0 Unported
Additional attribution: CardioNetworks
Available at: http://en.ecgpedia.org/wiki/File:De-12leadpericarditis.png

Fig. 1.14
Licensed under: Public Domain
Available at: https://commons.wikimedia.org/wiki/File:Splinter_hemorrhage.jpg

Fig. 1.15
Licensed under: Creative Commons Attribution-Share Alike 4.0 International
Additional attribution: Roberto J. Galindo
Available at: https://commons.wikimedia.org/wiki/File%3AOsler_Nodules_Hand.jpg

Fig. 1.16
Licensed under: Creative Commons Attribution 2.0 Generic

Available at: https://www.flickr.com/photos/58146070@N07/8621673540/in/photostream/

Fig. 1.17
Licensed under: Creative Commons Attribution 2.0 Generic
Additional attributions: Daisuke Koya, Kazuyuki Shibuya, Ryuichi Kikkawa and Masakazu Haneda
Available at: https://bmcnephrol.biomedcentral.com/articles/10.1186/1471-2369-5-18

The following ECGs are reproduced under the Creative Commons Attribution-ShareAlike 4.0 International License; reproduced with permission from Life in the Fast Lane (https://lifeinthefastlane.com): Figs 1.18–1.27, 1.29–1.37

Chapter 2

Fig. 2.1 *(adapted)*
Licensed under Creative Commons Attribution 4.0
Additional attribution: OpenStax
Available at: https://cnx.org/contents/FPtK1zmh@8.108:udJfuR_E@5/The-Lungs

Fig. 2.2 *(adapted)*
Licensed under Creative Commons Attribution-Share Alike 3.0 Unported
Additional attribution: Vihsadas
Available at: https://commons.wikimedia.org/wiki/File:Lungvolumes.svg

Fig. 2.4
Licensed under Creative Commons Attribution-Share Alike 3.0 Unported
Additional attribution: James Heilman, MD
Available at: https://commons.wikimedia.org/wiki/File:BullaCXR.PNG

Fig. 2.5
Licensed under Public Domain

Fig. 2.6
Licensed under Creative Commons Attribution-Share Alike 3.0 Unported
Additional attribution: Hellerhoff
Available at: https://commons.wikimedia.org/wiki/File:Massive_Bronchiektasen_-_CT_LF_axial_001.jpg

Fig. 2.7
Licensed under Creative Commons Attribution-Share Alike
3.0 Unported
Additional attribution: Drriad
Available at: https://commons.wikimedia.org/wiki/
File:Pulmon_fibrosis.PNG

Fig. 2.8
Licensed under Creative Commons Attribution-Share Alike
3.0 Unported
Additional attribution: James Heilman, MD
Available at: https://commons.wikimedia.org/wiki/
File:ENlegs.JPG

Fig. 2.9
Licensed under Creative Commons Attribution-Share Alike
3.0 Unported
Additional attribution: Jonathan Trobe, MD
Available at: https://commons.wikimedia.org/wiki/
File:Anterior-uveitis.jpg

Fig. 2.10
Licensed under Creative Commons Attribution-Share Alike
4.0 International
Additional attribution: James Heilman, MD
Available at: https://commons.wikimedia.org/wiki/File:Hilar_
Adenopathy_from_Sarcoidosis.jpg

Fig. 2.11
Public Domain

Fig. 2.12
Licensed under Creative Commons Attribution-Share Alike
2.0 Generic
Additional attribution: Yale Rosen
Available at: https://commons.wikimedia.org/wiki/
File:Nodular_sarcoidosis_Case_228_(7310281902).jpg

Fig. 2.13
Licensed under Creative Commons Attribution-Share Alike
3.0 Unported
Additional attribution: Hellerhoff
Available at: https://commons.wikimedia.org/wiki/
File:Sarkoidose_der_Lunge_Stadium_4_nach_Scadding.jpg

Fig. 2.14
Licensed under Creative Commons Attribution-Share Alike
3.0 Unported
Additional attribution: Samir
Available at: https://commons.wikimedia.org/wiki/
File:ARDS_X-Ray.jpg

Fig. 2.15
Licensed under Creative Commons Attribution 2.0 Generic
Additional attribution: Yale Rosen
Available at: https://www.flickr.com/photos/pulmonary_
pathology/15350007817/in/photolist-poqNxc-6wrsAp-
zEsAD-NqZ3x1-WwVo73-5ujjb2-dbvnAK-coTkF-WAvexH-
3KyXNn-WwVHjw-cnXNof-UPWpNw-6wrs3H-oFLmUg-
pW4Zwj-VjfwhY-s7mRht-6wrtbn-6wrro4-4GfQiy-cstW2u-
a2FZzy-csu1wh-ej1Vdd-6vRUui-M62Xyo-co6Gih-6wvAUo-
akEmFa-a96cbK-c3u5zo-4NuLB5-aetUKU-WoNUG8-c6Y6TE-
cnXNuE-WoNM7i-5BvxsB-aUktfa-nvZd6k-5XB3U9-5a97tA-
4NuLy3-WAvgCV-dLzUAJ-eXfaW5-pECkVD-LGZmF-cHGsxQ

Fig. 2.16
Licensed under Creative Commons Attribution-Share Alike
3.0 Unported
Additional attribution: James Heilman, MD
Available at: https://commons.wikimedia.org/wiki/
File:MesotheliomaCXR.png

Fig. 2.17
Licensed under Creative Commons Attribution-Share Alike
3.0 Unported
Additional attribution: Hellerhoff
Available at: https://commons.wikimedia.org/wiki/File:03-01-
Infiltrat_Ausgang.png

Fig. 2.18
Licensed under Creative Commons Attribution-Share Alike
2.0 Generic
Additional attribution: Yale Rosen (Flickr user)
Available at: https://www.flickr.com/photos/pulmonary_
pathology/7471756830

Fig. 2.19
Licensed under Creative Commons Attributions 2.0 Generic
Additional attribution: Yale Rosen
Available at: https://www.flickr.com/photos/
pulmonary_pathology/5390379081/in/photolist-abyXxu-
a1N1mK-b1AeTr-b1AeMz-a1QSKA-9dk73B-9dkgPx-
9dodmY-9dodiS-9dk7Kr-ajkU98-6DnxTk-8PWems-6DrFWf-
9dkhBT-9dk6Un-9dodpW-9doePf-9dodp3-9dk7M4-9dk8FV-
9dk8br-4BqE15-7CsizC-4Bmnge-5oiRLb-mSPdPs-5ZzwRh-
7CotHa-9fuc1N-fmBhMo-9dk8JH-9Md9zE-9dnKVr

Fig. 2.20
Public Domain

Fig. 2.21
Licensed under Creative Commons Attribution-Share Alike
2.5 Generic
Additional attribution: PhilippN
Available at: https://commons.wikimedia.org/wiki/File:Left-
sided_Pleural_Effusion.jpg

Fig. 2.22
Licensed under Creative Commons Attribution-Share Alike
3.0 Unported
Additional attribution: Karthik Easvur
Available at: https://commons.wikimedia.org/wiki/
File:Pneumothorax_gif_1.gif

Fig. 2.23
Licensed under Creative Commons Attribution-Share Alike
3.0 Unported
Additional attribution: James Heilman, MD
Available at: https://commons.wikimedia.org/wiki/
File:Tpneumopneumomed.png

Fig. 2.25
Licensed under Creative Commons Attribution-Share Alike
3.0 Unported
Additional attribution: James Heilman, MD
Available at: https://commons.wikimedia.org/wiki/
File:LungCACXR.PNG

Fig. 2.26
Licensed under Creative Commons Attribution-Share Alike
3.0 Unported
Additional attribution: Lange123
Available at: https://commons.wikimedia.org/wiki/
File:Thorax_CT_peripheres_Brronchialcarcinom_li_OF.jpg

Fig. 2.27
Licensed under Creative Commons Attribution- Share Alike
4.0 International
Additional attribution: LifeintheFastLane
Available at: https://lifeinthefastlane.com/wp-content/
uploads/2011/12/Massive-PE2.jpg

Fig. 2.28
Licensed under Creative Commons Attributions-Share Alike
4.0 International
Additional attribution: Rvahudson
Available at: https://commons.wikimedia.org/wiki/
File:CTA_Chest_With_Massive_Pulmonary_Embolism_and_
Complete_Occlusion.jpg

Fig. 2.29
Licensed under Creative Commons Attribution 2.5 Generic
Additional attribution: Westgate EJ, FitzGerald GA
Available at: https://commons.wikimedia.org/wiki/
File:Pulmonary_embolism_scintigraphy_PLoS.png

Chapter 3

Fig. 3.1 (adapted)
Licensed under Creative Commons Attribution License 3.0
Additional attribution: Openstax
Available at: http://cnx.org/contents/14fb4ad7-39a1-4eee-
ab6e-3ef2482e3e22@7.16:158/The-Stomach

Fig. 3.2 (adapted)
Licensed under Creative Commons Attribution License 3.0
Additional attribution: Openstax
Available at: http://cnx.org/contents/14fb4ad7-39a1-4eee-
ab6e-3ef2482e3e22@7.16:159/The-Small-and-Large-
Intestines

Fig. 3.3 (adapted)
Licensed under Creative Commons Attribution License 3.0
Additional attribution: Openstax
Available at: http://cnx.org/contents/14fb4ad7-39a1-
4eee-ab6e-3ef2482e3e22@7.16:160/Accessory-Organs-in-
Digestion-

Fig. 3.5 (adapted)
Licensed under Creative Commons Attribution License 3.0
Additional attribution: Openstax
Available at http://cnx.org/contents/14fb4ad7-39a1-4eee-
ab6e-3ef2482e3e22@7.16:160/Accessory-Organs-in-
Digestion-

Fig. 3.7
Licensed under Creative Commons Attribution-Share Alike
3.0 Unported
Additional attribution: Hellerhoff
Available at: https://commons.wikimedia.org/wiki/
File:Achalasie_Stadium_1_mit_typischem_Tropfen.jpg

Fig. 3.8
Licensed under Creativekfc Commons Attribution-Share
Alike 3.0 Unported
Additional attribution: Bernd Brägelmann
Available at: https://commons.wikimedia.org/wiki/
File:ZenkerSchraeg.gif

Fig. 3.9
Licensed under Creative Commons Public Domain
Additional attribution: Samir
Available at: https://commons.wikimedia.org/wiki/
File:Barretts_esophagus.jpg

Fig. 3.13
Licensed under Creative Commons CC0 1.0 Universal Public
Domain Dedication
Additional attribution: Klinikum Dritter Orden, München,
Abteilung Innere Medizin
Available at: https://commons.wikimedia.org/wiki/
File:Pseudomembranoese_Colitis_Endo1.jpg

Fig. 3.14
Licensed under Creative Commons Attribution-Share Alike
3.0 Unported
Additional attribution: BallenaBlanca
Available at: https://commons.wikimedia.org/wiki/
File:Dermatitis_Herpetiforme_1.jpg

Fig. 3.15
Licensed under Creative Commons Attribution-Share Alike
3.0 Unported
Additional attribution: Nephron
Available at: https://commons.wikimedia.org/wiki/
File:Celiac_disease_-_high_mag.jpg

Fig. 3.16
Licensed under Creative Commons Attribution-Share Alike
4.0 International
Additional attribution: Hellerhoff
Available at: https://commons.wikimedia.org/wiki/File:Toxic_
Megacolon_in_Ulcerative_Colitis.jpg

Fig. 3.17
Licensed under Creative Commons Attribution-Share Alike
3.0 Unported
Additional attribution: Hellerhoff
Available at: https://commons.wikimedia.org/wiki/
File:Colitis_ulcerosa_-_Haustrenverlust_-_Fahrradschlauch.
jpg

Fig. 3.18
Licensed under Creative Commons Attribution-Share Alike
3.0 Unported
Additional attribution: Hellerhoff
Available at: https://commons.wikimedia.org/wiki/
File:Morbus_Crohn_MR-Sellink_T2FS_cor.jpg

Fig. 3.19
Licensed under Creative Commons Attribution-Share Alike
3.0 Unported
Additional attribution: Samir
Available at: https://commons.wikimedia.org/wiki/File:CD_
colitis.jpg

Fig. 3.20
Licensed under Creative Commons Attribution-Share Alike
3.0 Unported
Additional attribution: CoRus13
Available at: https://upload.wikimedia.org/wikipedia/
commons/7/7b/Lymphocytic_colitis%2C_high_mag.jpg

Fig. 3.21
Licensed under Creative Commons Attribution 2.0 Generic
Additional attribution: Ed Uthman
Available at: https://commons.wikimedia.org/wiki/
File:Collagenous_Colitis_(6263982703).jpg

Fig. 3.22
Licensed under Creative Commons Attribution-Share Alike
3.0 Unported
Additional attribution: Biswarup Ganguly
Available at: https://commons.wikimedia.org/wiki/
File:Erythema_nodosum_-_Kolkata_2012-01-03_7753.JPG

Fig. 3.23
Licensed under Public Domain
Additional attribution: Crohnie
Available at: https://commons.wikimedia.org/wiki/
File:Crohnie_Pyoderma_gangrenosum.jpg

Fig. 3.24
Licensed under Creative Commons Attribution-Share Alike
3.0 Unported
Additional attribution: Jonathan Trobe, M.D.
Available at: https://commons.wikimedia.org/wiki/
File:Anterior-uveitis.jpg

Fig. 3.25
Licensed under Creative Commons Attribution-Share Alike
4.0 International
Additional attribution: Imrankabirhossain
Available at: https://commons.wikimedia.org/wiki/
File:Episcleritis.jpg

Fig. 3.26
Licensed under Creative Commons Attribution-Share Alike
3.0 Unported
Additional attribution: Samir
Available at: https://commons.wikimedia.org/wiki/
File:Ulcerative_colitis.jpg

Fig. 3.27
Licensed under Creative Commons Attribution-Share Alike
3.0 Unported
Additional attribution: Samir
Available at: https://commons.wikimedia.org/wiki/File:CD_
colitis_2.jpg

Fig. 3.28
Licensed under Creative Commons Attribution-Share Alike
3.0 Unported
Available at: https://commons.wikimedia.org/wiki/
File:Ulcerative_colitis_(1)_active.jpg

Fig. 3.29
Licensed under Creative Commons Attribution-Share Alike
3.0 Unported
Additional attribution: Nephron

Available at: https://commons.wikimedia.org/wiki/
File:Crohn%27s_disease_-_colon_-_very_high_mag.jpg

Fig. 3.30
Licensed under Creative Commons Attribution License 3.0
Additional attribution: James Heilman, MD
Available at: https://commons.wikimedia.org/wiki/
File:Ischemicbowel.PNG

Fig. 3.31
Licensed under Creative Commons Attribution-Share Alike
3.0 Unported
Additional attribution: Nephron
Available at: https://commons.wikimedia.org/wiki/
File:Lymphocytic_colitis_-_high_mag.jpg

Fig. 3.32
Licensed under Creative Commons Attribution 2.0 Generic
Additional attribution: Ed Uthman
Available at: https://commons.wikimedia.org/wiki/
File:Collagenous_Colitis_(6263982645).jpg

Fig. 3.33
Licensed under Creative Commons Attribution 2.5 Generic
Available at: https://commons.wikimedia.org/wiki/
File:Endomucosal_resection_1.jpg

Fig. 3.34
Licensed under Creative Commons Attribution 2.5 Generic
Available at: https://commons.wikimedia.org/wiki/
File:Polyp-2.jpeg

Fig. 3.35
Licensed under Creative Commons Attribution-Share Alike
3.0 Unported
Additional attribution: Samir
Available at: https://commons.wikimedia.org/wiki/
File:Familial_adenomatous_polyposis_as_seen_on_
sigmoidoscopy.jpg

Fig. 3.36
Licensed under Creative Commons Attribution License 3.0
Additional attribution: Abdullah Sarhan
Available at: https://commons.wikimedia.org/wiki/File:Peutz-
Jeghers-Syndrom.JPG

Fig. 3.37
Licensed under Creative Commons Attribution-Share Alike
3.0 Unported
Available at: https://commons.wikimedia.org/wiki/
File:AscendensKarzinomBiopsie.PNG

Fig. 3.38
Licensed under Creative Commons Attribution-Share Alike
4.0 International
Additional attribution: James Heilman, MD
Available at: https://commons.wikimedia.org/wiki/
File:ColonCaWithMetsMark.png

Fig. 3.39
Licensed under Creative Commons Attribution-Share Alike
3.0 Unported
Additional attribution: Nephron
Available at: https://commons.wikimedia.org/wiki/
File:Cirrhosis_high_mag.jpg

Chapter 4

Available at: https://cnx.org/contents/
FPtK1zmh@8.108:kaX2y2XZ@4/The-Adrenal-Glands

Fig. 4.23 *(adapted)*
Licensed under Public Domain

Fig. 4.24
Licensed under Public Domain

Fig. 4.25 *(adapted)*
Licensed under Creative Commons Attribution-Share Alike
4.0 International
Additional attribution: OpenStax
Available at: https://cnx.org/contents/
FPtK1zmh@8.108:6sIw0Wr4@5/Development-of-
the-Male-and-Fe

Fig. 4.26
Licensed under Creative Commons Attribution 2.0 Generic
Additional attribution: Johannes Nielsen
Available at: https://commons.wikimedia.org/wiki/File:Neck_
of_girl_with_Turner_Syndrome_(before_and_after).jpg

Chapter 5

Fig. 5.1 *(adapted)*
Licensed under Creative Commons Attribution-Share Alike
4.0 International
Additional attribution: OpenStax
Available at: https://cnx.org/contents/
FPtK1zmh@8.108:mYoZvS9p@5/Nervous-Tissue

Fig. 5.2 *(adapted)*
Licensed under Creative Commons Attribution-Share Alike
4.0 International
Additional attribution: OpenStax
Available at: https://cnx.org/contents/
FPtK1zmh@8.108:QBrzNCkw@5/The-Action-Potential

Fig. 5.3 *(adapted)*
Licensed under Creative Commons Attribution-Share Alike
4.0 International
Additional attribution: OpenStax
Available at: https://cnx.org/contents/FPtK1zmh
@8.108:mYoZvS9p@5/Nervous-Tissue

Fig. 5.4 *(adapted)*
Licensed under Creative Commons Attribution-Share Alike
4.0 International
Additional attribution: OpenStax
Available at: https://cnx.org/contents/FPtK1zmh
@8.108:DcB5rjNc@3/Circulation-and-the-Central-Ne

Fig. 5.5 *(adapted)*
Licensed under Creative Commons Attribution-Share Alike
4.0 International
Additional attribution: OpenStax
Available at: https://cnx.org/contents/
FPtK1zmh@8.108:94Iv8wHH@5/The-Central-Nervous-System

Fig. 5.6 *(adapted)*
Licensed under Creative Commons Attribution-Share Alike
3.0 Unported

Additional attributions: Polarlys and Mikael Häggström
Available at: https://commons.wikimedia.org/wiki/
File:Spinal_cord_tracts_-_English.svg

Fig. 5.7 *(adapted)*
Licensed under Creative Commons Attribution-Share Alike
4.0 International
Additional attribution: OpenStax
Available at: https://cnx.org/contents/
FPtK1zmh@8.108:DcB5rjNc@3/Circulation-and-
the-Central-Ne

Fig. 5.8 *(adapted)*
Licensed under Creative Commons Attribution-Share Alike
4.0 International
Additional attribution: OpenStax
Available at: https://cnx.org/contents/
FPtK1zmh@8.108:5QEuK48_@7/The-Peripheral-Nervous-
System

Fig. 5.9 *(adapted)*
Licensed under Public Domain

Fig. 5.10 *(adapted)*
Licensed under Creative Commons Attribution-Share Alike
4.0 International
Additional attribution: Miquel Perello Nieto
Available at: https://commons.wikimedia.org/wiki/
File:Human_visual_pathway.svg

Fig. 5.11
Licensed under Creative Commons Attribution-Share Alike
3.0 Unported
Additional attribution: James Heilman, MD
Available at: https://commons.wikimedia.org/wiki/
File:Bellspalsy.JPG

Fig. 5.12
Licensed under Creative Commons Attribution-Share Alike
3.0 Unported
Additional attribution: Dr Laughlin Dawes
Available at: https://commons.wikimedia.org/wiki/File:Hsv_
encephalitis.jpg

Fig. 5.13
Licensed under Creative Commons Attribution-Share Alike
3.0 Unported
Additional attribution: Hellerhoff
Available at: https://commons.wikimedia.org/wiki/File:Brain_
abscess_-_MRI_T1_KM_axial.jpg

Fig. 5.14
Licensed under Creative Commons Attribution-Share Alike
3.0 Unported
Additional attribution: James Heilman, MD
Available at: https://commons.wikimedia.org/wiki/
File:StrokeMCA.png

Fig. 5.15
Licensed under Creative Commons Attribution-Share Alike
3.0 Unported
Additional attribution: James Heilman, MD
Available at: https://commons.wikimedia.org/wiki/
File:Subarach.png

Fig. 5.16
Licensed under Creative Commons Attribution-Share Alike 3.0 Unported
Additional attribution: Lucein Monflis
Available at: https://commons.wikimedia.org/wiki/File:Ct-scan_of_the_brain_with_an_subdural_hematoma.jpg

Fig. 5.17
Licensed under Creative Commons Attribution-Share Alike 3.0 Unported
Additional attribution: Jpogi
Available at: https://commons.wikimedia.org/wiki/File:Traumatic_acute_epidual_hematoma.jpg

Fig. 5.18
Licensed under Public Domain

Fig. 5.19
Licensed under Creative Commons Attribution-Share Alike 3.0 Unported
Additional attribution: James Heilman, MD
Available at: https://commons.wikimedia.org/wiki/File:Menigioma.PNG

Fig. 5.20 (adapted)
Licensed under Public Domain

Fig. 5.21 (adapted)
Licensed under Creative Commons Attribution-Share Alike 3.0 Unported
Additional attribution: Tvil
Available at: https://commons.wikimedia.org/wiki/File:ThreeNeuronArc.png

Fig. 5.22
Licensed under Creative Commons Attribution-Share Alike 3.0
Additional attribution: Niels Olson
Available at: https://en.wikipedia.org/wiki/File:Cord-en.png

Fig. 5.23 (adapted)
Licensed under Creative Commons Attribution-Share Alike 3.0
Additional attribution: Niels Olson
Available at: https://en.wikipedia.org/wiki/File:Cord-en.png

Fig. 5.24
Licensed under Creative Commons Attribution-Share Alike 3.0 Unported
Additional attribution: Benefros
Available at: https://commons.wikimedia.org/wiki/File:Charcot-marie-tooth_foot.jpg

Fig. 5.25
Licensed under Creative Commons Attributions-Share Alike 2.0 Generic
Additional attribution: Sheffield, Herman Bernard
Available at: https://commons.wikimedia.org/wiki/File:Modern_diagnosis_and_treatment_of_diseases_of_childern;_a_treatise_on_the_medical_and_surgical_diseases_of_infancy_anf_childhood_(1911)_(14801659623).jpg

Fig. 5.26
Licensed under Creative Commons Attribution 1.0 Generic
Additional attributions: Herbert L. Fred, MD, Hendrik A. van Dijk
Available at: https://commons.wikimedia.org/wiki/File:Myotonic_dystrophy_patient.JPG

Fig. 5.27
Licensed under Creative Commons Attribution-Share Alike 4.0 International
Available at: https://commons.wikimedia.org/wiki/File:Cutaneous_neurofibroma_(MedMedicine).jpg

Fig. 5.28
Licensed under Creative Commons Attribution-Share Alike 3.0 Unported
Additional attribution: Accrochoc
Available at: https://commons.wikimedia.org/wiki/File:NF-1-Tache_cafe-au-lait.jpg

Fig. 5.29
Licensed under Public Domain

Fig. 5.30
Licensed under Creative Commons Attribution 2.0 Generic
Additional attributions: M. Sand, D. Sand, C. Thrandorf, V. Paech, P. Altmeyer, F.G. Bechara
Available at: https://commons.wikimedia.org/wiki/File:Adenoma_sebaceum_01.jpg

Fig. 5.31
Licensed under Creative Commons Attribution 2.0 Generic
Additional attributions: Herbert L. Fred, MD, Hendrik A. van Dijk
Available at: https://commons.wikimedia.org/wiki/File:Whitemacules.jpg

Fig. 5.32
Licensed under Public Domain

Chapter 6

Fig. 6.1 (adapted)
Licensed under Creative Commons Attribution 4.0
Additional attribution: OpenStax
Available at: https://cnx.org/contents/FPtK1zmh@8.108:IUrEdFyf@7/An-Overview-of-Blood

Fig. 6.2 (adapted)
Licensed under Creative Commons Attribution 4.0
Additional attribution: OpenStax
Available at: https://cnx.org/contents/FPtK1zmh@8.108:AZ9CODIR@5/Production-of-the-Formed-Eleme

Fig. 6.3 (adapted)
Licensed under Creative Commons Attribution License 4.0
Additional attribution: OpenStax
Available at: https://cnx.org/contents/FPtK1zmh@8.108:QFNYp9m0@6/Hemostasis

Fig. 6.4
Licensed under Creative Commons Attribution 2.0 Generic

Chapter 7

Fig. 7.1 *(adapted)*
Licensed under Creative Commons Attributions-Share Alike 4.0 International
Additional attribution: OpenStax
Available at: https://cnx.org/contents/
FPtK1zmh@8.108:XJvfBd1g@4/Microscopic-Anatomy-of-the-Kid

Fig. 7.2 *(adapted)*
Licensed under Creative Commons Attributions-Share Alike 4.0 International
Additional attribution: OpenStax
Available at: https://cnx.org/contents/
FPtK1zmh@8.108:CATSMth@5/Tubular-Reabsorption

Fig. 7.3 *(adapted)*
Licensed under Creative Commons Attributions-Share Alike 4.0 International
Additional attribution: OpenStax
Available at: https://cnx.org/contents/
FPtK1zmh@8.108:XJvfBd1g@4/Microscopic-Anatomy-of-the-Kid

Fig. 7.4
Licensed under Creative Commons Attributions-Share Alike 3.0 Unported
Additional attribution: James Heilman, MD
Available at: https://commons.wikimedia.org/wiki/
File:RhabdoUrine.JPG

Fig. 7.5
Licensed under Creative Commons Attributions-Share Alike 3.0 Unported
Additional attribution: Nephron
Available at: https://commons.wikimedia.org/wiki/
File:Membranous_nephropathy_-_pas_-_very_high_mag.jpg

Fig. 7.6
Licensed under Creative Commons Attributions-Share Alike 3.0 Unported
Additional attribution: Nephron
Available at: https://commons.wikimedia.org/wiki/
File:Membranous_nephropathy_-_cropped_-_mpas_-_very_high_mag.jpg

Fig. 7.7
Licensed under Creative Commons Attribution 2.0 Generic
Additional attributions: Lazarus Karamadoukis, Linmarie Ludeman and Anthony J Williams
Available at: https://commons.wikimedia.org/wiki/
File:Henoch-Sch%C3%B6nlein_nephritis_IgA_immunostaining.jpg

Fig. 7.8
Licensed under Creative Commons Attributions-Share Alike 3.0 Unported
Additional attribution: Nephron
Available at: https://commons.wikimedia.org/wiki/File:Post-infectious_glomerulonephritis_-_very_high_mag.jpg

Fig. 7.9
Licensed under Creative Commons Attributions-Share Alike 3.0 Unported
Additional attribution: Nephron
Available at: https://commons.wikimedia.org/wiki/
File:Crescentic_glomerulonephritis_-_very_high_mag.jpg

Fig. 7.10
Licensed under Creative Commons Attribution 2.0 Generic
Additional attributions: Zeina A.R., Vladimir W., and Barmeir E.
Available at: https://commons.wikimedia.org/wiki/
File:Renal_artery_angiography_in_a_patient_with_fibromuscular_dysplasia_(1).jpg

Fig. 7.11
Licensed under Creative Commons Attributions-Share Alike 3.0 Unported
Additional attribution: Steven Fruitsmaak
Available at: https://commons.wikimedia.org/wiki/
File:CT_scan_autosomal_dominant_polycystic_kidney_disease.jpg

Fig. 7.12
Licensed under Creative Commons
Additional attribution: James Heilman, MD
Available at: https://commons.wikimedia.org/wiki/
File:3mmstone.png

Chapter 8

Fig. 8.5
Licensed under Creative Commons Attribution-Share Alike 4.0 International
Additional attribution: Life in the Fast Lane
Available at: https://lifeinthefastlane.com/wp-content/
uploads/2011/02/ECG-Potassium-9.2.jpg

Fig. 8.6
Licensed under Creative Commons Attribution-Share Alike 4.0 International
Additional attribution: Life in the Fast Lane
Available at: https://lifeinthefastlane.com/wp-content/
uploads/2011/02/U-waves-in-hypokalaemia.jpg

Fig. 8.8
Licensed under Creative Commons Attribution 2.0 Generic
Additional attribution: Dr Caroline LeBreton, CHU Raymond Poincaré, Garches, France
Available at: https://commons.wikimedia.org/wiki/
File:Morbus_Fabry_DXA_01.jpg

Fig. 8.9
Licensed under Creative Commons Attribution-Share Alike 3.0 Unported
Additional attributions: Chen GL, Yang DH, Wu JY, Kuo CW, Hsu WH
Available at: https://commons.wikimedia.org/wiki/
File:Urine_of_patient_with_porphyria.png

Fig. 8.10
Licensed under Creative Commons Attribution-Share Alike 3.0 Unported

Additional attribution: Chern
Available at: https://en.wikipedia.org/wiki/File:Prfr1.jpg

Chapter 9

Fig. 9.1 *(adapted)*
Licensed under Creative Commons Attribution 4.0 license
Additional attribution: OpenStax
Available at: http://cnx.org/contents/GFy_h8cu@10.54:nnx1QFeU@11/Structure-of-Prokaryotes

Fig. 9.2
Licensed under Public Domain
Additional attribution: Centers for Disease Control and Prevention's Public Health Image Library
Available at: https://commons.wikimedia.org/wiki/File:Borrelia_burgdorferi_(CDC-PHIL_-6631)_lores.jpg

Fig. 9.5
Licensed under Public Domain
Additional attribution: Centers for Disease Control and Prevention's Public Health Image Library
Available at: https://commons.wikimedia.org/wiki/File:Secondary_Syphilis_on_palms_CDC_6809_lores.rsh.jpg

Fig. 9.6
Licensed under Creative Commons Attribution-Share Alike 3.0 Unported license
Additional attribution: SOA-AIDS Amsterdam
Available at: https://commons.wikimedia.org/wiki/File:SOA-epididymites.jpg

Fig. 9.7
Licensed under Public Domain
Additional attribution: Centers for Disease Control and Prevention's Public Health Image Library (PHIL)
Available at: https://commons.wikimedia.org/wiki/File:Chancroid_lesion_haemophilus_ducreyi_PHIL_3728_lores.jpg

Fig. 9.8
Licensed under Public Domain
Available at: https://commons.wikimedia.org/wiki/File:Donovanosis.JPG

Fig. 9.9
Licensed under Creative Commons Attribution-Share Alike 3.0 Unported license
Additional attribution: SOA-AIDS Amsterdam
Available at: https://commons.wikimedia.org/wiki/File:SOA-Chlamydia-trachomatis-female.jpg

Fig. 9.10
Licensed under Creative Commons Attribution-Share Alike 4.0 International license
Additional attribution: Øyvind Holmstad
Available at: https://commons.wikimedia.org/wiki/File:Vannkopper_chickenpox.JPG

Fig. 9.11
Licensed under Creative Commons Attribution-Share Alike 3.0 Unported license
Additional attribution: Fisle

Available at: https://commons.wikimedia.org/wiki/File:Herpes_zoster_chest.png

Fig. 9.12
Licensed under Creative Commons Attribution-Share Alike 3.0 Unported license
Additional attribution: Michael Gaither
Available at: https://commons.wikimedia.org/wiki/File:Leukoplakia02-04-06.jpg

Fig. 9.13
Licensed under Public Domain
Additional attribution: Centers for Disease Control and Prevention's Public Health Image Library (PHIL)
Available at: https://commons.wikimedia.org/wiki/File:Kaposi%E2%80%99s_sarcoma_intraoral_AIDS_072_lores.jpg

Fig. 9.14
Licensed under Creative Commons Attribution-Share Alike 2.5 Generic license
Available at: https://commons.wikimedia.org/wiki/File:Scharlach.JPG

Fig. 9.15
Licensed under Creative Commons Attribution-Share Alike 3.0 Unported
Available at: https://commons.wikimedia.org/wiki/File:Ostermyelitis_Tibia.jpg

Fig. 9.16
Licensed under Public Domain
Additional attribution: Dr F.C. Turner
Available at: https://commons.wikimedia.org/wiki/File:G.vaginalis.jpg

Fig. 9.17
Licensed under Public Domain
Additional attribution: Pierre Arents
Available at: https://commons.wikimedia.org/wiki/File:Leprosy.jpg

Fig. 9.18
Licensed under Public Domain
Additional attribution: US Department of Health and Human Services
Available at: https://commons.wikimedia.org/wiki/File:Leprosy_thigh_demarcated_cutaneous_lesions.jpg

Fig. 9.19
Licensed under Public Domain
Additional attribution: Centers for Disease Control and Prevention's Public Health Image Library (PHIL)
Available at: https://commons.wikimedia.org/wiki/File:PHIL_tetanus.jpg

Fig. 9.20
Licensed under Public Domain
Additional attribution: Tim Vickers
Available at: https://commons.wikimedia.org/wiki/File:Plasmodium.jpg

Chapter 10

Fig. 10.1 *(adapted)*
Licensed under Creative Commons Attribution 4.0 License
Additional attribution: Openstax
Available at: https://cnx.org/contents/
FPtK1zmh@8.25:bFtYymxt@4/Synovial-Joints

Fig. 10.2
Licensed under Creative Commons Attribution-Share Alike
3.0 Unported license
Additional attribution: Drahreg01
Available at: https://commons.wikimedia.org/wiki/
File:Heberden-Arthrose.JPG

Fig. 10.3
Licensed under Creative Commons Attribution-Share Alike
3.0 Unported license
Additional attribution: James Heilman, MD
Available at: https://commons.wikimedia.org/wiki/
File:Osteoarthritis_left_knee.jpg

Fig. 10.4
Licensed under Creative Commons Attribution-Share Alike
3.0 Unported license
Additional attribution: James Heilman, MD
Available at: https://commons.wikimedia.org/wiki/
File:Rheumatoid_Arthritis.JPG

Fig. 10.5
Licensed under Creative Commons Attribution-Share Alike
3.0 Unported license
Available at: https://commons.wikimedia.org/wiki/
File:Swan_neck_deformity_in_a_65_year_old_Rheumatoid_
Arthritis_patient-_2014-05-27_01-49.jpg

Fig. 10.6
Licensed under Creative Commons Attribution-Share Alike
3.0 Unported license
Additional attribution: Bernd Brägelmann Braegel Mit
freundlicher Genehmigung von Dr. Martin Steinhoff
Available at: https://commons.wikimedia.org/wiki/
File:RheumatoideArthritisAP.jpg

Fig. 10.7
Licensed under Creative Commons Attribution-Share Alike
4.0 International
Available at: https://www.omicsonline.org/india/septic-
arthritis-peer-reviewed-pdf-ppt-articles/

Fig. 10.8
Licensed under Creative Commons Attribution 2.0
Generic license
Additional attribution: Arthritis Research UK Primary Care
Centre, Primary Care Sciences, Keele University, Keele, UK
Available at: https://commons.wikimedia.org/wiki/
File:Tophaceous_gout.jpg

Fig. 10.9
Licensed under Public Domain
Available at: https://commons.wikimedia.org/wiki/
File:Ankylosing_spondylitis_lumbar_spine.jpg

Fig. 10.10
Licensed under Public Domain
Available at: https://commons.wikimedia.org/wiki/
File:Rad_1300095.JPG

Fig. 10.11
Licensed under Public Domain
Available at: https://commons.wikimedia.org/wiki/File:Feet-
Reiters_syndrome.jpg

Fig. 10.12
Licensed under Creative Commons Attribution-Share Alike
3.0 Unported license
Additional attribution: CopperKettle
Available at: https://commons.wikimedia.org/wiki/
File:Onycholysis_left_hand_34yo_male_ring_and_little_
fingers_non-fungal.jpg

Fig. 10.13 *(adapted)*
Licensed under Public Domain
Available at: https://commons.wikimedia.org/wiki/
File:Symptoms_of_SLE.svg

Fig. 10.14
Licensed under Creative Commons Attribution-Share Alike
4.0 International license
Available at: https://commons.wikimedia.org/wiki/
File:Lupusfoto.jpg

Fig. 10.15
Licensed under Creative Commons Attribution-Share Alike
4.0 International license
Additional attribution: James Heilman
Available at: https://commons.wikimedia.org/wiki/
File:CREST1.JPG

Fig. 10.16
Licensed under Creative Commons Attribution-Share Alike
3.0 Unported license
Additional attribution: Tcal at English Wikipedia
Available at: https://commons.wikimedia.org/wiki/
File:Raynaud_phenomenon.jpg

Fig. 10.17
Licensed under Creative Commons Attribution-Share Alike
3.0 Unported license
Additional attribution: Elizabeth M. Dugan, Adam M. Huber,
Frederick W. Miller, Lisa G. Rider
Available at: https://commons.wikimedia.org/wiki/
File:Dermatomyositis9.jpg

Fig. 10.18
Licensed under Creative Commons Attribution-Share Alike
3.0 Unported license
Additional attribution: Elizabeth M. Dugan, Adam M. Huber,
Frederick W. Miller, Lisa G. Rider
Available at: https://commons.wikimedia.org/wiki/
File:Dermatomyositis.jpg

Fig. 10.19
Licensed under Creative Commons Attribution-Share Alike
3.0 Unported license
Additional attribution: Nephron
Available at: https://commons.wikimedia.org/wiki/
File:Giant_cell_arteritis_--_high_mag.jpg

Chapter 11

Figs. 11.14 and 11.15
Image reproduced with permission from DermNet
New Zealand (www.dermnetnz.org)

Fig. 11.16
Licensed under Creative Commons Attribution-Share Alike
3.0 Unported
Additional attribution: Grook Da Oger
Available at: https://commons.wikimedia.org/wiki/
File:Pityriasis_ros%C3%A9_de_Gibert_-_peau_noire_-
_d%C3%A9tails.jpg

Fig. 11.17
Licensed under Public Domain

Fig. 11.18
Licensed under Creative Commons Attribution-Share Alike
3.0 Unported
Additional attribution: James Heilman, MD
Available at: https://commons.wikimedia.org/wiki/
File:Lichen_Planus_(2).JPG

Fig. 11.19
Licensed under Creative Commons Attribution-Share Alike
3.0 Unported
Additional attributions: James, Candice, Mai
Available at: https://commons.wikimedia.org/wiki/
File:Lichen_planusWickham%27s.jpg

Fig. 11.20
Licensed under Creative Commons Attribution-Share Alike
3.0 Unported
Additional attribution: John
Available at: https://commons.wikimedia.org/w/index.
php?curid=32178972

Fig. 11.21
Licensed under Public Domain

Fig. 11.22
Licensed under Creative Commons Attributions 2.0 Generic
Additional attributions: M. Sand, D. Sand, C. Thrandorf,
V. Paech, P. Altmeyer, F. G. Bechara
Available at: https://commons.wikimedia.org/w/index.
php?curid=15606564

Fig. 11.23
Image reproduced with permission from DermNet
New Zealand (www.dermnetnz.org)

Figs. 11.24 and 11.25
Licensed under Public Domain

Fig. 11.26
Licensed under Creative Commons Attribution-Share Alike
4.0 International
Additional attribution: Future FamDoc
Available at: https://commons.wikimedia.org/w/index.
php?curid=36814600

Fig. 11.27
Licensed under Creative Commons Attribution 3.0 Germany
Additional attribution: Klaus D. Peter, Gummersbach,
Germany

Available at: https://commons.wikimedia.org/w/index.
php?curid=6265931

Fig. 11.28
Licensed under Creative Commons Attribution-Share Alike
4.0 International
Additional attribution: BruceBlaus
Available at: https://commons.wikimedia.org/w/index.
php?curid=44924607

Fig. 11.29
Licensed under Public Domain

Fig. 11.30
Licensed under Creative Commons Attribution-Share Alike
3.0 Unported
Additional attribution: Will Blake
Available at: https://commons.wikimedia.org/w/index.
php?curid=1598913

Fig. 11.31
Licensed under Creative Commons Attribution-Share Alike
3.0 Unported
Additional attribution: 0x6adb015
Available at: https://commons.wikimedia.org/w/index.
php?curid=10738017

Fig. 11.32
Licensed under Public Domain

Fig. 11.33
Licensed under Creative Commons Attribution-Share Alike
3.0 Unported
Additional attribution: James Heilman, MD
Available at: https://commons.wikimedia.org/w/index.
php?curid=11520780

Fig. 11.34
Licensed under Creative Commons Attribution-Share Alike
3.0 Unported
Additional attribution: Grook Da Oger
Available at: https://commons.wikimedia.org/wiki/
File:Erythema_Multiforme_EM_01.jpg

Fig. 11.35
Licensed under Creative Commons Attribution-Share Alike
2.0 Generic
Additional attribution: Kreuter *et al.*
Available at: https://commons.wikimedia.org/wiki/
File:Generalized_granuloma_annulare.JPEG

Fig. 11.36
Licensed under Creative Commons Attribution-Share Alike
3.0 Unported
Additional attribution: James Heilman, MD
Available at: https://commons.wikimedia.org/wiki/
File:Vitiligo2.JPG

Fig. 11.37
Licensed under Creative Commons Attribution-Share Alike
3.0 Unported
Additional attribution: Dr Thomas Habif
Available at: https://commons.wikimedia.org/w/index.
php?curid=9699327

References

Chapter 1

Adler *et al.* (2015) 2015 ESC Guidelines for the diagnosis and management of pericardial disease. *Eur Heart J*, **36**:2921.

Expert Panel on Detection, Evaluation, and Treatment of High Blood Cholesterol in Adults (2001) Executive Summary of the Third Report of the National Cholesterol Education Program (NCEP). *J Am Med Assoc*, **285**:2486.

Habib *et al.* (2015) 2015 ESC Guidelines on prevention, diagnosis and treatment of infective endocarditis. *Eur Heart J*, **36**:3075.

NICE (2008, updated 2013) PH10: *Stop smoking services.*

NICE (2010) CG108: *Chronic heart failure in adults: management.*

NICE (2011) CG126: *Management of stable angina.*

NICE (2011) CG127: *Hypertension in adults: diagnosis and management.*

NICE (2014) CG180: *Atrial fibrillation: management.*

NICE (2014) CG181: *Cardiovascular disease: risk assessment and reduction, including lipid modification.*

NICE (2014) TA88: *Dual-chamber pacemakers for symptomatic bradycardia due to sick sinus syndrome and/or atrioventricular block.*

Nishimura *et al.* (2014) 2014 AHA/ACC Guideline for the management of patients with valvular heart disease. *Circulation*, **129**:e521.

Thygesen *et al.* (2012) Third universal definition of myocardial infarction. *Circulation*, **126**:2020.

Chapter 2

British Thoracic Society (2010) Guideline for non-CF bronchiectasis. *Thorax*, **65**: Suppl 1.

British Thoracic Society (2010) Pleural disease guideline. *Thorax*, **65**: Suppl 2.

NICE (2010) CG101: *Chronic obstructive pulmonary disease in over 16s: diagnosis and management.*

NICE (2011) CG121: *Lung cancer: diagnosis and management.*

NICE (2012) CG144: *Venous thromboembolic diseases: diagnosis, management and thrombophilia testing.*

NICE (2013) CG136: *Idiopathic pulmonary fibrosis in adults: diagnosis and management.*

NICE (2014) CG191: *Pneumonia in adults: diagnosis and management.*

NICE (2016) NG33: *Tuberculosis.*

NICE (2017) NG12: *Suspected cancer: recognition and referral.*

SIGN (2016) 153: *BTS/SIGN British guideline on the management of asthma.*

Wells *et al.* (2000) Derivation of a simple clinical model to categorize patients probability of pulmonary embolism: increasing the models utility with the SimpliRED D-dimer. *Thromb Haemost.* **83(3)**:416–20.

Chapter 3

NICE (2010) CG106: *Barrett's oesophagus: ablative therapy.*

NICE (2010) TA208: *Trastuzumab for the treatment of HER2-positive metastatic gastric cancer.*

NICE (2012) CG152: *Crohn's disease: management.*

NICE (2013) CG166: *Ulcerative colitis: management.*

NICE (2013) DG11: *Faecal calprotectin diagnostic tests for inflammatory diseases of the bowel.*

NICE (2014) CG61: *Irritable bowel syndrome in adults: diagnosis and management.*

NICE (2014) CG118: *Colorectal cancer prevention: colonoscopic surveillance in adults with ulcerative colitis, Crohn's disease or adenomas.*

NICE (2014) CG131: *Colorectal cancer: diagnosis and management.*

NICE (2014) CG184: *Gastro-oesophageal reflux disease and dyspepsia in adults: investigation and management.*

NICE (2014) CG188: *Gallstone disease: diagnosis and management.*

NICE (2014) NG49: *Non-alcoholic fatty liver disease (NAFLD): assessment and management.*

NICE (2015) Do Not Do: *Alpha-1 antitrypsin replacement therapy is not recommended for patients with alpha-1 antitrypsin deficiency.*

NICE (2015) NG20: *Coeliac disease: recognition, assessment and management.*

NICE (2015) TA337: *Rifaximin for preventing episodes of overt hepatic encephalopathy.*

NICE (2015) TA476: *Paclitaxel as albumin-bound nanoparticles with gemcitabine for untreated metastatic pancreatic cancer.*

NICE (2016) CG141: *Acute upper gastrointestinal bleeding in over 16s: management.*

World Gastroenterology Organisation (2014) *Dysphagia Global Guidelines.*

Chapter 4

NICE (2007) TA117: *Cinacalcet for the treatment of secondary hyperparathyroidism in patients with end-stage renal disease on maintenance dialysis therapy.*

NICE (2011) CKS: *Hypothyroidism.*

NICE (2015) NG17: *Type 1 diabetes in adults: diagnosis and management.*

NICE (2015) NG18: *Diabetes (type 1 and type 2) in children and young people: diagnosis and management.*

NICE (2015) NG28: *Type 2 diabetes in adults: management.*

World Health Organization (2006) *Definition and diagnosis of diabetes mellitus and intermediate hyperglycaemia.*

Chapter 5

European Society of Cardiology (2009) Guidelines on diagnosis and management of syncope. *Eur Heart J,* **30**:2631.

International Headache Society (2013) *International Classification of Headache Disorders*, 3rd edition [www.ichd-3.org – accessed 6 June 2018]

International League Against Epilepsy (2014). Definition of epilepsy.

NICE (2008) CG68: *Stroke and transient ischaemic attack in over 16s: diagnosis and initial management.*

NICE (2010) CG102: *Meningitis (bacterial) and meningococcal septicaemia in under 16s: recognition, diagnosis and management.*

NICE (2010) CG103: *Delirium: prevention, diagnosis and management.*

NICE (2011) CKS: *Labyrinthitis.*

NICE (2012) CG150: *Headaches in over 12s: diagnosis and management.*

NICE (2012) CKS: *Bell's palsy.*

NICE (2012) CKS: *Ménière's disease.*

NICE (2013) CKS: *Benign paroxysmal positional vertigo (BPPV).*

NICE (2014) CG186: *Multiple sclerosis in adults: management.*

NICE (2015) CKS: *Epilepsy.*

NICE (2016) NG59: *Low back pain and sciatica in over 16s: assessment and management.*

NICE (2017) NG71: *Parkinson's disease in adults.*

NINCDS-ADRDA (1984). *Clinical diagnosis of Alzheimer's disease. Neurology,* **34**:939.

SIGN (2015) 143: *Diagnosis and management of epilepsy in adults.*

Chapter 6

British Society of Haematology (2011) Guidelines on oral anticoagulation with warfarin – 4th edition. *Br J Haemotol,* **154**:311.

NICE (2009) CG81: *Advanced breast cancer: diagnosis and treatment.*

NICE (2011) CG80: *Early and locally advanced breast cancer: diagnosis and treatment.*

NICE (2011) CG122: *Ovarian cancer: recognition and initial management.*

NICE (2014) CG175: *Prostate cancer: diagnosis and management.*

NICE (2016) NG35: *Myeloma: diagnosis and management.*

NICE (2016) NG52: *Non-Hodgkin's lymphoma: diagnosis and management*.

World Health Organization (2015) *The global prevalence of anaemia in 2011*.

Chapter 7

European Urology Association (2015) *EAU Guidelines on urolithiasis*.

NICE (2013) CG169: *Acute kidney injury: prevention, detection and management*.

NICE (2014) CG182: *Chronic kidney disease in adults: assessment and management*.

NICE (2015) CKS: *Urinary tract infection* (UTI).

Chapter 8

BNF (2017) Emergency treatment of poisoning. *British National Formulary 74*.

European Resuscitation Council (2015) *Resuscitation guidelines*. [www.resus.org.uk – accessed 6 June 2018]

NICE (2004) CG16: *Self-harm in over 8s: short-term management and prevention of recurrence*.

NICE (2017) CG174: *Intravenous fluid therapy in adults in hospital*.

World Health Organization (2008) *WHO Criteria for diagnosis of osteoporosis*.

Chapter 9

British HIV Association (2015) *BHIVA Guidelines for the Treatment of HIV-1-positive Adults with Antiretroviral Therapy 2015* (2016 interim update) [www.bhiva.org/hiv-1-treatment-guidelines – accessed 21 August 2018]

NICE (2014) CKS: *Bacterial vaginosis*.

NICE (2014) CKS: *Lyme disease*.

Chapter 10

NICE (2014) CG177: *Osteoarthritis: care and management*.

NICE (2015) CG79: *Rheumatoid arthritis in adults: management*.

NICE (2015) CKS: *Gout*.

NICE (2015) NG65: *Spondyloarthritis in over 16s: diagnosis and management*.

Chapter 11

British Association of Dermatologists (2007) Guidelines for evaluation and management of urticaria in adults and children. *Br J Dermatol*, **157**:1116.

British Association of Dermatologists (2008) Guidelines for the management of basal cell carcinoma. *Br J Dermatol*, **159**:35.

British Association of Dermatologists (2008) Guidelines for the diagnosis and management of vitiligo. *Br J Dermatol*, **159**:1051.

British Association of Dermatologists (2009) *Multi-professional guidelines for the management of the patient with squamous cell carcinoma*.

British Association of Dermatologists (2010) Revised UK guidelines for the management of cutaneous melanoma 2010. *Br J Dermatol*, **163**:238.

British Association of Dermatologists (2012) Guidelines for the management of bullous pemphigoid 2012. *Br J Dermatol*, **167**:1200.

NICE (2010) CKS: *Pityriasis rosea*.

NICE (2010) CKS: *Pityriasis versicolor*.

NICE (2011) CKS: *Scabies*.

NICE (2012) CKS: *Rosacea*.

NICE (2013) CKS: *Dermatitis – contact*.

NICE (2013) CKS: *Seborrhoeic dermatitis*.

NICE (2014) CKS: *Acne vulgaris*.

NICE (2014) CKS: *Psoriasis*.

NICE (2014) CKS: *Venous eczema and lipodermatosclerosis*.

NICE (2015) CKS: *Eczema – atopic dermatitis*.

NICE (2015) CKS: *Impetigo*.

Primary Care Dermatology Society (2012) *Asteatotic eczema*. [www.pcds.org.uk – accessed 6 June 2018]

Primary Care Dermatology Society (2012) *Eczema: gravitational*. [www.pcds.org.uk – accessed 6 June 2018]

Primary Care Dermatology Society (2014) *Basal cell carcinoma – an overview*. [www.pcds.org.uk – accessed 6 June 2018]

Primary Care Dermatology Society (2014) *Eczema: contact allergic dermatitis*. [www.pcds.org.uk – accessed 6 June 2018]

Primary Care Dermatology Society (2014) *Eczema: discoid*. [www.pcds.org.uk – accessed 6 June 2018]

Primary Care Dermatology Society (2014) *Erythema nodosum*. [www.pcds.org.uk – accessed 6 June 2018]

Primary Care Dermatology Society (2014) *Hand (and foot) eczema*. [www.pcds.org.uk – accessed 6 June 2018]

Primary Care Dermatology Society (2014) *Nodular BCC*. [www.pcds.org.uk – accessed 6 June 2018]

Primary Care Dermatology Society (2014) *Perioral dermatitis*. [www.pcds.org.uk – accessed 6 June 2018]

Primary Care Dermatology Society (2014) *Rosacea*. [www.pcds.org.uk – accessed 6 June 2018]

Primary Care Dermatology Society (2014) *Squamous cell carcinoma*. [www.pcds.org.uk – accessed 6 June 2018]

Primary Care Dermatology Society (2014) *Tinea capitis (scalp)*. [www.pcds.org.uk – accessed 6 June 2018]

Primary Care Dermatology Society (2014) *Tinea faciei (face) and barbae (beard)*. [www.pcds.org.uk – accessed 6 June 2018]

Primary Care Dermatology Society (2014) *Urticaria: acute*. [www.pcds.org.uk – accessed 6 June 2018]

Primary Care Dermatology Society (2015) *Dermatitis herpetiformis*. [www.pcds.org.uk – accessed 6 June 2018]

Primary Care Dermatology Society (2015) *Eczema: atopic dermatitis*. [www.pcds.org.uk – accessed 6 June 2018]

Primary Care Dermatology Society (2015) *Erythema multiforme*. [www.pcds.org.uk – accessed 6 June 2018]

Primary Care Dermatology Society (2015) *Granuloma annulare*. [www.pcds.org.uk – accessed 6 June 2018]

Primary Care Dermatology Society (2015) *Lichen planus*. [www.pcds.org.uk – accessed 6 June 2018]

Primary Care Dermatology Society (2015) *Pemphigus vulgaris*. [www.pcds.org.uk – accessed 6 June 2018]

Primary Care Dermatology Society (2015) *Psoriasis*. [www.pcds.org.uk – accessed 6 June 2018]

Primary Care Dermatology Society (2015) *Pyoderma gangrenosum*. [www.pcds.org.uk – accessed 6 June 2018]

Primary Care Dermatology Society (2015) *Tinea corporis (body), cruis (groin) and incognito (steroid exacerbated)*. [www.pcds.org.uk – accessed 6 June 2018]

Primary Care Dermatology Society (2015) *Tinea manuum (hands), pedis (feet), and unguium (nails)*. [www.pcds.org.uk – accessed 6 June 2018]

Primary Care Dermatology Society (2015) *Warts*. [www.pcds.org.uk – accessed 6 June 2018]

Primary Care Dermatology Society (2016) *Acne vulgaris*. [www.pcds.org.uk – accessed 6 June 2018]

Primary Care Dermatology Society (2016) *Urticaria: spontaneous*. [www.pcds.org.uk – accessed 6 June 2018]

Chapter 12

Resuscitation Council UK (2015) *Adult advanced life support algorithm*. [www.resus.org.uk – accessed 6 June 2018]

Index

Bold indicates main entries

Related titles

Remember, you can order any Scion books at 35% discount from: www.scionpublishing.com/medicalstudents

Simply add the books to your basket and enter the promotional code **miam35** when prompted.

Whilst there, don't forget to sign up for our medical student newsletter to hear first about new books, special offers, giveaways, etc.

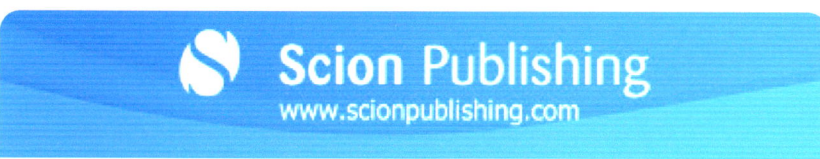

Welcome to the latest medical student newsletter
Scroll down for free samples.....

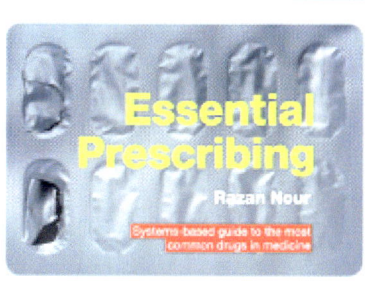

Just Published!

Essential Prescribing
Razan Nour
Apr 2018
Spiral bound – ISBN 9781911510000
Price: £19.99

View sample chapter here

Free Samples this month

Click to access free sample chapters

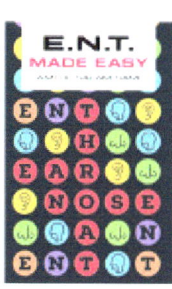
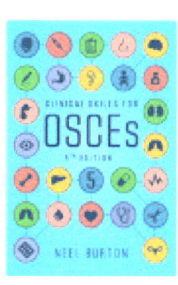
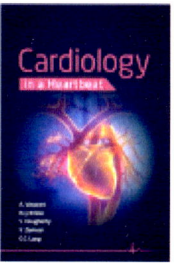
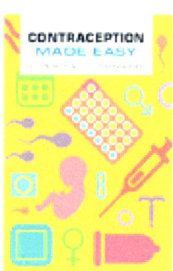

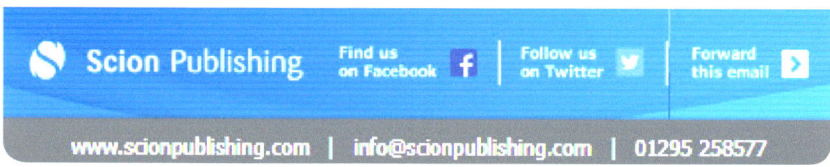

www.scionpublishing.com | info@scionpublishing.com | 01295 258577

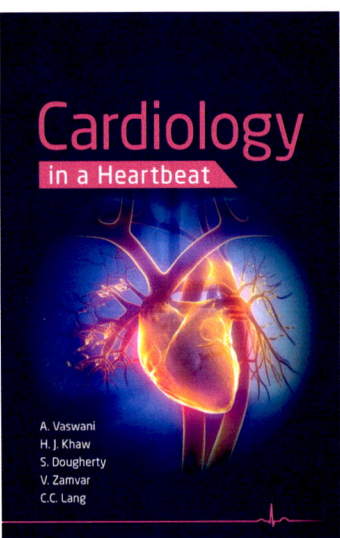

Use your QR reade
to access more
information and
sample material.

Cardiology in a Heartbeat

Amar Vaswani, Hwan Juet Khaw, Dr Scott Dougherty, Mr Vipin Zamvar and Professor Chim Lang

Paperback, 320pp, ISBN 9781907904783, Price: £25.99

Compiled by a team of students and practising doctors and consultants from the University of Edinburgh Medical School, *Cardiology in a Heartbeat* provides practical advice to enable the reader to get to grips with the subject quickly and easily. This unique author team brings the reader the best of both worlds: the student authors focus on what students need to know whilst the contributions from senior medics ensure the book is accurate and covers the subject completely.

The attractive full-colour layout and short, consistent chapters mean the book is easy to navigate through; this is especially useful when the reader wants to quickly brush up on a particular topic or find an answer to a specific question.

Reviews:

'A fantastic and up to date cardiology guide for undergraduate medical students and foundation doctors.' ★★★★★

'An excellent guide to cardiology. Full of concise up-to-date information, in a very practical and easy to read format.
I would definitely recommend it to anyone undergoing a cardiology rotation.' ★★★★★

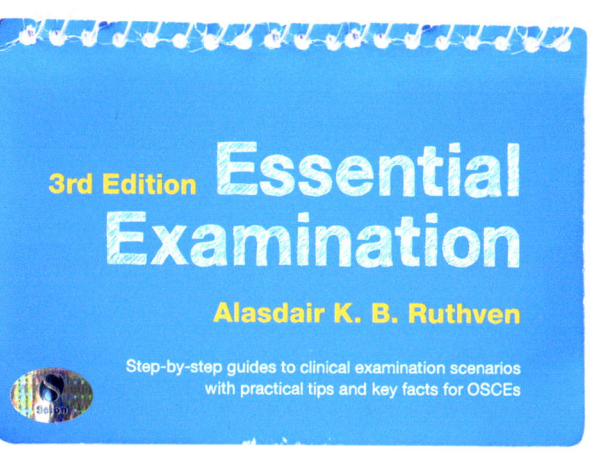

Use your QR reader to access more information and sample material.

Essential Examination, third edition

Alasdair K.B. Ruthven

Spiral bound, 154pp, ISBN 9781907904103, Price: £19.99

** Number 1 Bestseller on Amazon! **

If you are learning how to examine patients, or preparing for an OSCE, then you need *Essential Examination!*

Essential Examination is one of the bestselling texts for medical students in the UK. Students love its concise format, with easy access to the core information.

The success of the book lies in its unique format and approach:

Clear, step-by-step guides to each examination, including useful things to say to the patient (or an examiner), detailed descriptions of special tests, etc.

In a separate column is a collection of key information: potential findings, differential diagnoses of clinical signs and practical tips.

On the following pages there are facts relating to that particular examination and, in many sections, there are also tips on how to present your findings succinctly – a skill which is crucial to master for exam success.

Reviews:

'I rarely write a rave review but this one is warranted. This textbook is AMAZING' ★★★★★

'This book is by far the best purchase I have made at medical school' ★★★★★

'I love the fact that this book is really condensed – has everything that you need to know about each examination in a couple of pages.' ★★★★★

'The best and only book you need for undergraduate OSCE revision' ★★★★★

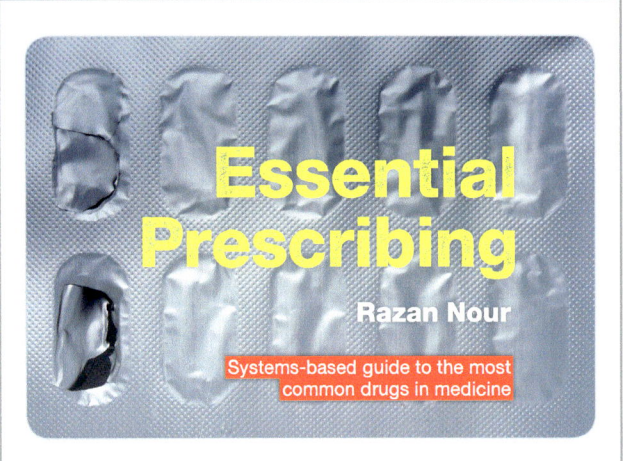

Use your QR reader to access more information and sample material.

Essential Prescribing

Razan Nour

Spiral bound, 186pp, ISBN 9781911510000, Price: £19.99

Essential Prescribing is a brand new text aimed at providing medical students with an easy-to-follow overview of the drugs they are most likely to encounter at medical school and as they start their medical careers. The book benefits from the same landscape format and approach as Scion's bestselling *Essential Examination*.

Each class of drug is detailed using a common tabular format, based on the following sections:

Examples, Mode of Action, Routes of Delivery, Indications, Cautions and contraindications, Interactions, Monitoring, Side-effects, Patient counselling.

This consistent approach helps the reader quickly find the pertinent information for the common drugs and situations they are likely to come across, so they can become confident of prescribing the correct drugs for the patient in appropriate doses.

Review:

'This book is a wealth of information! Well written in a simple concise way, easy to follow guidelines for prescribing medications, oxygen, intravenous fluids ... and is divided by the system involved and has a section specifically for patient counselling which makes this book unique.' ★★★★★

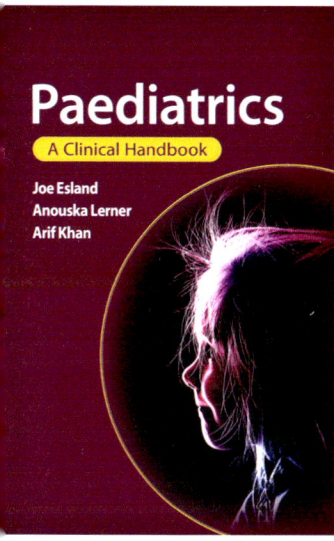

Paediatrics: A Clinical Handbook

Joe Esland, Anouska Lerner and Arif Khan

Paperback, 288pp, ISBN 9781907904851, Price: £21.99

Paediatrics: A Clinical Handbook provides all the essential information required for a successful paediatrics rotation. Written by two recently qualified junior doctors and a consultant paediatrician, the book offers an exam-centred, reader-friendly style backed up with concise clinical guidance.

Building on the success of the other 'Clinical Handbook' titles (*Rheumatology* and *Psychiatry*), *Paediatrics: A Clinical Handbook* provides student-friendly coverage of the material with many key features (such as mnemonics and OSCE tips) to help the reader get to grips with the subject.

Paediatrics: A Clinical Handbook is ideal for medical students and junior doctors; like the other books in the series it will have a secondary market amongst medics who want a quick refresher of the subject.

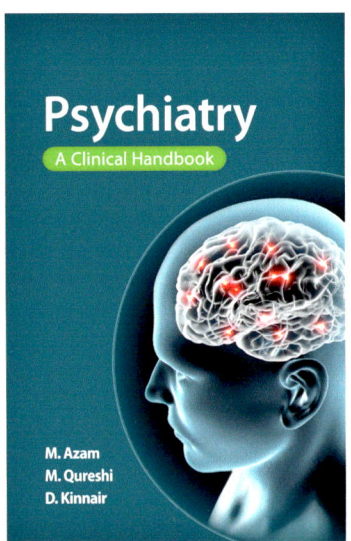

Use your QR reader to access more information and sample material.

Psychiatry: A Clinical Handbook

Mohsin Azam, Mohammed Qureshi and Daniel Kinnair

Paperback, 282pp, ISBN 9781907904813, Price: £23.99

Psychiatry: A Clinical Handbook provides all the essential information required for a successful psychiatry rotation. Written by two recently qualified junior doctors and a consultant psychiatrist, the book offers an exam-centred, reader-friendly style backed up with concise clinical guidance.

The book covers diagnosis and management based upon the ICD-10 Classification and the latest NICE guidelines. For every psychiatric condition:

- the diagnostic pathway is provided with suggested phrasing for sensitive questions
- the relevant clinical features to look out for in the mental state examination are listed
- a concise definition and basic pathophysiology/aetiology is outlined.

Self-assessment questions are provided at the end of each chapter. A chapter is dedicated to OSCE scenarios to aid practising with colleagues in preparation for exams. SBA questions with detailed answers written by a Consultant Psychiatrist are also provided.

Reviews:

'One of the best psychiatry books I have ever read. It is organised in a neat, concise manner with tables, colours, mnemonics, OSCE tips to name but a few.' ★★★★★

'Great book for undergraduate psychiatry. Lots of useful mnemonics and colour coded to aid commit facts to memory.' ★★★★★

'Finally a psychiatry book great for quick referencing, with a design made for the modern reader.' ★★★★★

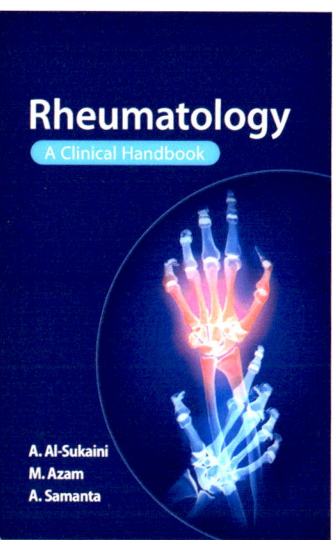

Rheumatology: A Clinical Handbook

Ahmad Al-Sukaini, Mohsin Azam and Ash Samanta

Paperback, 168pp, ISBN 9781907904264, Price: £19.99

Rheumatology: A Clinical Handbook is an essential resource for medical students who need an introduction, understanding and overview of the subject. Most competing texts either burden medical students with information they do not require, or cover rheumatology alongside orthopaedics and as a result compromise fundamentals of rheumatology. This book is different – it provides all the information students need during their rheumatology placement and signposts them to where they can find further information.

Reviews:

'For me this book ticks all of the boxes for being a fine modular text. I was completely lost when it came to rheumatology before I picked up this book.' ★★★★★

'Excellent layout. Clear, concise and informative condition summaries, plenty of images and self-assessment.
'Must-read for all Medical Students' ★★★★★

'Best rheumatology guide for medical students' ★★★★★

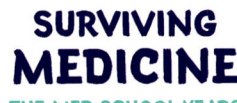

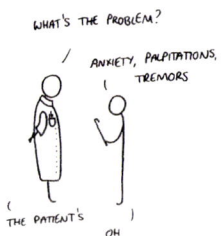

Surviving Medicine

Will Sloper

Paperback, 154pp, ISBN 9781911510253, Price: £14.99

Medicine is one of the most wonderfully ridiculous professions in the world and the cartoons in this book are light-hearted reflections on life as a medical student.

Most of the situations described in this book will crop up at some point as you progress through medical school and beyond. Consider them a rite of passage as you rack up the experience and confidence to look back and think, *I can't believe I was scared of that...!*

But more than that, the book offers advice on surviving ward rounds, coping with doubt and anxiety, preparing for exams, and lots more besides!

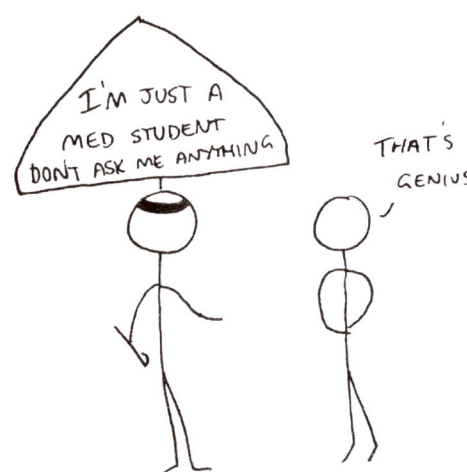